ROUTLEDGE INTERNATIONAL HANDBOOK OF NURSE EDUCATION

While vast numbers of nurses across the globe contribute in all areas of healthcare delivery from primary care to acute and long-term care in community settings, there are significant differences in how they are educated, as well as the precise nature of their practice. This comprehensive handbook provides a research-informed and international perspective on the critical issues in contemporary nurse education.

As an applied discipline, nursing is implemented differently depending on the social, political and cultural climate in any given context. These factors impact on education, as much as on practice, and are reflected in debates around the value of accredited programmes, and on-the-job training, apprenticeship, undergraduate and postgraduate pathways into nursing. Engaging with these debates amongst others, the authors collected here discuss how, through careful design and delivery of nursing curricula, nurses can be prepared to understand complex care processes, complex healthcare technologies, complex patient needs and responses to therapeutic interventions, and complex organizations. The book discusses historical perspectives on how nurses should be educated; contemporary issues facing educators; teaching and learning strategies; the politics of nurse education; education for advanced nursing practice; global approaches; and educating for the future.

Bringing together leading authorities from across the world to reflect on past, present and future approaches to nurse education and nursing pedagogy, this handbook provides a cutting-edge overview for all educators, researchers and policy-makers concerned with nurse education.

Sue Dyson is Professor of Nursing at the University of Derby, United Kingdom. Sue is a nurse and midwife by professional background. Her research focuses on volunteerism and volunteering, and is concerned with exploring links between student volunteering, critical thinking, compassion and critical pedagogy.

Margaret McAllister is Professor of Nursing at Central Queensland University, Australia. With a background in nursing, mental health nursing, education and cultural studies, Margaret teaches in the Master of Mental Health Nursing and has research expertise in Narrative Therapy and Narrative Research.

ROUTLEDGE INTERNATIONAL HANDBOOK OF NURSE EDUCATION

Edited by Sue Dyson and Margaret McAllister

Routledge
Taylor & Francis Group

LONDON AND NEW YORK

First published 2020
by Routledge
4 Park Square, Milton Park, Abingdon, Oxon OX14 4RN
605 Third Avenue, New York, NY 10017

First issued in paperback 2023

Routledge is an imprint of the Taylor & Francis Group, an informa business

British Library Cataloguing-in-Publication Data
A catalogue record for this book is available from the British Library

Library of Congress Cataloging-in-Publication Data
A catalog record has been requested for this book

ISBN: 978-1-03-257025-9 (pbk)
ISBN: 978-0-8153-5886-2 (hbk)
ISBN: 978-1-351-12167-5 (ebk)

DOI: 10.4324/9781351121675

Typeset in Bembo
by Swales & Willis, Exeter, Devon, UK

Publisher's Note
The publisher has gone to great lengths to ensure the quality of this reprint but points out that some imperfections in the original copies may be apparent.

CONTENTS

FIGURES

TABLES

BOXES

ACKNOWLEDGEMENTS

As authors, we are indebted to our respective universities, the University of Derby, UK, and Central Queensland University, Australia, for providing the encouragement and support to enable us to prepare this work.

Sue would like to say thank you to Simon: ever constant, always encouraging. To Emma von Pahlen (née McCartney) and Matt McCartney: my reason to be, and Nina and Toby von Pahlen and Henry McCartney: the little gifts that keep on giving. To colleagues in the Health and Social Care Research Centre: for your commitment and dedication to research for the benefit of others. To Margaret McAllister, my colleague and now good friend: without whom this book would not have made it to publication. To our intrepid authors: for committing precious time in the knowledge this book may be of some help to the global community of nurse educators. And last, but not least, to those very nurse educators who strive to find new ways to ensure nurses of the future have the knowledge and skills for all that lies ahead: thank you.

CONTRIBUTORS

Helen Allan is Professor of Nursing at Middlesex University. She qualified as a nurse in 1978 and went into nurse teaching after her time as a ward sister in Intensive Care at University College Hospital, where "a lot of the job was about teaching and making sure the students felt safe". Dr Allan registered as a nurse teacher in 1992 and has worked in education and research since then. Her research with Karen Evans, Pam Smith and Carin Magnusson while at the University of Surrey into learning environments of overseas nurses, student nurses and newly qualified nurses has been a major part of her research career since 2003. At Middlesex University, her work has focused on routes into nursing for overseas nurses and apprentices.

Keryn Bolte is an experienced registered nurse-midwife educator at the University of Melbourne, with extensive clinical experience in critical care, aeromedical retrieval and also rural health education. She is a passionate advocate for rural health workforce development. Keryn has worked across the clinical and academic sectors both in nursing and as an interprofessional practitioner.

Helga Bragadóttir is Professor and Chair Nursing Administration at the University of Iceland Faculty of Nursing and Landspítali University Hospital, Iceland. Dr Bragadóttir's area of research is work and the work environment of nurses and the safety and quality of care. In the past decade she has led studies on the work of nurses in acute care, missed nursing care and nursing teamwork. Her main teaching area is nursing administration and leadership in healthcare. Dr Bragadóttir has been active in international research and development projects as well as teaching, and with Dr Teddie Potter is a pioneer in Collaborative Online International Learning (COIL) in nursing. She has served on several committees, boards and working groups within nursing and healthcare nationally and internationally.

Katrina Campbell is a lecturer in nursing at the Australian Catholic University, Australia. With a clinical background in acute and crisis mental health nursing, Katrina teaches into the mental health courses within the undergraduate nursing and paramedic programs. Katrina is currently part-way through her PhD exploring clinical decision making surrounding the diagnosis of borderline personality disorder.

Shirley Ching, Kin Cheung and Yim-wah Mak are associate professors at the School of Nursing of the Hong Kong Polytechnic University. Dr Ching focuses her research on cancer and survivorship care, and mental health of nursing and healthcare students. Dr Cheung studies extensively on workforce health and wellness, musculoskeletal health and academic support to transfer students in university. Dr Mak conducts studies on smoking cessation, protecting children from health risk behaviours and promoting the well-being of nursing students and families with children by using acceptance and commitment therapy and other psycho-social interventions.

Rachelle Cole is a lecturer in nursing and simulation coordinator within the School of Nursing, Midwifery and Social Sciences at Central Queensland University, Australia. With a clinical background in critical care, chronic disease management and palliative nursing as well as health service management, Rachelle teaches into the nursing courses within the undergraduate nursing programme. Rachelle has a keen interest in bridging the theory-to-practice gap and, whilst new to academe, has already been actively involved in research projects in simulation and co-authoring nursing textbooks.

Wendy Couchman is Emeritus Professor of Social Work at London South Bank University and is also an artist. Research interests are the use of the arts in social work education and practice, particularly in services for older adults. She has applied art in qualitative research both as a method and as a means of communicating findings more widely. As an artist, she works with a range of media to evoke the flux and vulnerability of human experience, drawing on her professional background in health and social care.

Roger Dunston joined the Faculty of Arts and Social Sciences, University of Technology, Sydney, Australia in 2007. Roger is an associate professor located in the Faculty of Health where, in partnership with over nine Australian universities, he has led the development of a programme of interprofessional education and interprofessional and collaborative practice research and development studies that commenced in 2007. The development of the programme remains active through the work of the national research translation project: "Securing an interprofessional future for Australian health professional education and practice".

Sue Dyson is Professor of Nursing and Head of the Health and Social Care Research Centre at University of Derby. Dr Dyson's research focuses on volunteering and volunteerism, educational experiences of international nursing students, the educational experiences of young people with sickle cell disorder and pedagogic research to inform nursing and midwifery education. Sue has authored four books: *Fundamental Aspects of Transcultural Nursing, Fundamental Aspects of Research for Nurses, Research Skills for Nurses and Midwives* (with Dr Peter Norrie) and *Critical Pedagogy in Nursing: Transformational Approaches to Nurse Education in a Globalized World*. Sue is an associate editor for BMC Health Services Research.

Sandra Egege is currently an academic within the Centre for Learning and Teaching at Flinders University, Australia. She has a Diploma of Teaching, a Certificate IV in teaching of English to speakers of other languages (TESOL) and a PhD in philosophy. While she has delivered a range of academic workshops in teaching programmes across the university since 2003, her main area of speciality has been teaching critical thinking. In this capacity, she has developed a series of workshops on critical thinking for pre-entry students, commencing local and international students and higher degree research students. Her recent research interest is in how to teach critical thinking effectively. She is currently under contract with Macmillan to write a study skills book on critical thinking.

Karen Evans is Emeritus Professor at UCL Institute of Education, University College London, based in the Department of Education, Practice and Society. She is a leading researcher in the UK Economic and Social Research Council's Research Centre LLAKES, investigating Learning and Life Chances in Knowledge Economies and Societies. Her research interests focus on learning and working life, throughout the life course. She has directed major studies of learning and work in Britain and internationally. Her most recent co-authored book *How Non-permanent Workers Learn and Develop* was published by Routledge in 2019. Karen Evans is a Fellow of the Academy of Social Sciences.

Dawn Forman is a professor of academic leadership at the University of Derby, UK, and adjunct professor at both Auckland University of Technology, New Zealand and Curtin University, Australia. For the last 12 years Dawn has been a co-owner and director of Interactive Leadership and Management Development, a consultancy specialising in governor and executive coaching, leadership and interprofessional education and academic writing. Dawn has been privileged to work on a freelance basis with universities and health services internationally. Dawn is an active researcher and is widely published, including eight books and over 120 peer-reviewed articles.

Sue Fyfe is adjunct professor in the faculty of Health Sciences, Curtin University, Australia. She is an epidemiologist, anatomist, speech pathologist and teacher with educational research interests in interprofessional education, collaborative practice and innovative approaches to teaching and learning. She has held senior leadership and management roles at Curtin University as inaugural Dean of Teaching and Learning in the Faculty of Health Sciences, Head of School of Public Health and Professor of Medical Education. She has taught both anatomy and physiology to students in nursing and was instrumental in developing interprofessional units for all first-year degree courses in health sciences. She has published and presented widely on learning innovation and change.

Trish Hafford-Letchfield is Professor of Social Work, University of Strathclyde, Scotland. She is a qualified nurse and social worker. Her research interests concern the experiences of older people from marginalised communities using social care services and how to engage them in quality improvement. Her doctoral studies were in educational gerontology. She has specific interests in LGBTQI issues in social work and social care education. Trish has used the arts in pedagogy to facilitate co-production. Trish has published extensively in gerontology; sexuality; ethics and values in professional practice; arts-based pedagogy; and leadership and management.

Leeanne Heaton is a lecturer and Head of Course for undergraduate nursing at Central Queensland University. She has had a number of roles in leadership and academia over the last decade involved in undergraduate, postgraduate and offshore programmes relating to nursing, midwifery and paramedicine. Leeanne has a diverse range of experience working in healthcare as a registered nurse, registered midwife and paramedic. She has experience working in rural and remote parts of Australia as a flight nurse with the Royal Flying Doctor Service.

Kwadwo Ameyaw Korsah is a senior lecturer at the University of Ghana. He holds a PhD in nursing from De Montfort University, Leicester, in the United Kingdom. He is a nurse by profession and has practised for 22 years. He is an experienced nurse educator with a recordable teaching qualification. Dr Korsah has many years' experience teaching and supervising graduate and undergraduate students. He is well grounded in qualitative research methodologies and his publications include book chapters and articles in peer-reviewed journals. His research work focuses on chronicity of disease, diabetes care and coping.

Renee S. Kumpula is Assistant Professor and Director of Continuing Professional Development at University of Minnesota, USA. Renee earned an EdD at the University of St. Thomas, honors dissertation and a Masters at Bethel University. She teaches bachelor to doctoral programmes. Her career includes acute/end-of-life care, public health/community/ school nursing, educational consulting and leadership across settings. She contributes to university teams, curricular development, online programmes, accreditation and community partnerships. Her research includes end-of-life/spiritual care, adult learning/developmental theory, educational design, interprofessional education, continuing education/lifelong learning and programme evaluation. Her leadership includes STTI chapters and the Midwest Nursing Research Society. She presents research/scholarly work at regional/national conferences.

Marion Jones is Professor of Interprofessional Learning and Dean of University Graduate Research School at Auckland University of Technology, New Zealand. She is a member of the Executive Board of Interprofessional Global and a director of the National Centre for Interprofessional Education and Collaborative Practice in New Zealand. She is a visiting professor of interprofessional education at Derby University in the UK. She is a registered nurse and her PhD was in "The shaping of interprofessional team practice"; at present she is involved in co-editing a fourth book on interprofessional leadership, resilience and sustainability. Marion has a strong commitment to interprofessional practice, research supervision, nursing and health practice nationally and internationally.

Kate Leonard is a senior lecturer at Royal Holloway, University of London. She is a registered social worker with extensive experience as a supervisor and practitioner. Until recently she was the course director for the MA Practice Education at London South Bank University, an interprofessional course for nurses, midwives and social workers. She has published in the areas of: interprofessional learning; applying arts-based pedagogies; working with service users to provide creative learning opportunities; decision making in children and families social work. Her current research interests include the understanding and use of critical reflection in social work.

Sandra Lewenson is a professor of nursing at Pace University, College of Health Professions, Lienhard School of Nursing in New York. Her research explores public health nursing, education and diversity and inclusivity in nursing. Sandy is a fellow of the American Academy of Nursing and the recipient of the R. Louise McManus Award for Outstanding Leadership in Nursing from Teachers College, Columbia University. Her most recent book, with co-editors Annemarie McAllister and Kylie Smith, *Nursing History for Contemporary Role Development*, won the prestigious Mary Roberts Award from the American Association for the History of Nursing. She currently serves as the chair of the Barbara Bates Center for the Study of Nursing History at the University of Pennsylvania.

Mzwandile A. Mabhala is Professor of Public Health Epidemiology as the University of Chester, UK. Dr Mabhala is a Fellow and member of the Faculty of Public Health, Fellow of the Royal Society of Public Health, and Fellow of the Royal Society of Medicine. His research centres on socio-economic determinants of inequalities in health and social justice. Dr Mabhala's recent research work has focused on marginalised population groups and under-researched subjects, including homeless, substance users. His research on homelessness won the 2018 EducateNorth award. He is co-editor of *Health Improvement and Well-Being: Strategies* *for Action*, which was highly commended in the British Medical Association's Medical Book Awards 2015, and co-edited *Key Concepts in Public Health* (2009).

Carin Magnusson is health services researcher and university lecturer in the School of Health Sciences at the University of Surrey. Her research has mainly focused on health professional education and training, quality improvement, patient safety and human factors. Most of her research has involved carrying out ethnographic case studies in NHS Acute Care, collecting data using in-depth interviewing, participant observations, focus groups and documentary analysis.

Rachael Major is a senior lecturer at the Institute of Health and Social Care Studies in Guernsey where she is currently the Post-registration Lead and the Disability Lead. She has 18 years' experience in nurse education, supporting both students and registered nurses, with and without dyslexia, to achieve their academic ambitions. Rachael completed a Doctorate in Education exploring registered nurses' personal and professional experiences of dyslexia in lifelong learning in 2017 and has presented her research at international conferences and in journals.

Priya Martin is Advanced Clinical Educator – Interprofessional, Cunningham Centre, Darling Downs Health, Toowoomba, Queensland, Australia and Adjunct Research Fellow, Rural Clinical School, University of Queensland, Toowoomba, Queensland, Australia. Dr Martin is a health professional educator and a health services researcher. Although she trained as an occupational therapist, she has worked in interprofessional roles since 2013. In her current role, she works with post-registration health professionals, including nurses, doctors, dentists and allied health professionals, across the state of Queensland in Australia. In 2018, she completed a multi-award-winning PhD in Health Sciences. She is passionate about interprofessional education and collaborative practice in the post-registration period and undertakes research in this area. She is a member of the Centre for the Advancement of Interprofessional Education international liaison group, as well as a steering committee member for the Australasian Interprofessional Practice and Education Network.

Annemarie McAllister is the Dean at the Cochran School of Nursing/St John's Riverside Hospital in New York. She received a Master's degree in administrative studies and her EdD at the Executive Program for Nurses at Teachers College, Columbia University. Her research interests include the way nurses are educated in the United States and the advent of the associate degree model in nursing. She is the book review editor for *Nursing History Review* and serves on the advisory board of the Barbara Bates Center for the Study of the History of Nursing at the University of Pennsylvania School of Nursing. Her edited book, with co-authors Sandy Lewenson and Kylie Smith, entitled *Nursing History for Contemporary Role Development*, received the Mary Roberts Award from the American Association for the History of Nursing.

Margaret McAllister is Professor of Nursing in the School of Nursing, Midwifery and Social Sciences at Central Queensland University, in Noosa, Australia. She is also an adjunct professor at the University of Technology Sydney and an award-winning educator and is experienced in working across disciplines. Her research and teaching focus includes narratives of health and well-being, mental health promotion and transformative learning. She has co-authored several books: *Paradoxes in Nurses' Identity, Culture and Image*, *Empowerment Strategies for Nurses*, *The Clinical Helper*, *Stories in Mental Health*, *The Resilient Nurse* and *Solution Focused Nursing*.

Tracey McClean is Head of the Institute of Health and Social Care Studies, States of Guernsey. Dr McClean has had a long career within health, starting as a nursing auxiliary in 1984 before going on to train as a registered nurse at St Bartholomew's School of Nursing in London. Tracey returned to Guernsey in 1989 to take up post as a surgical nurse, moving into education in 1996. She has held a number of key positions, including pre-registration lead and post-qualifying lead. Tracey has undertaken a range of qualifications, including a postgraduate certificate in education and a Professional Doctorate in Health. Tracey is a reviewer for the *Nurse Education Today* journal.

Margaret McMillan is Emeritus Professor and Editor-in-Chief, *International Journal of Prob-lem-Based Learning*, and conjoint professor in the School of Nursing and Midwifery at the University of Newcastle, Australia. Dr McMillan has over 40 years' experience in health professional education in workforce initiatives. She has research, policy and capacity-building expertise gathered through working in clinical practice, higher education, health service governance, policy work and consultancy activity. She has researched and published articles on clinical education, health workforce education and training and reform; curriculum design and evaluation; change management and practice development. Margaret has been involved with health service governance for over 19 years, serving on Ministerial Committees. She continues to be actively involved in health service governance, and health service and workforce evaluation.

Simeon K. Mining is Professor of Immunology and Director of Research at Moi University, Kenya. He serves as Director of the Kenya National Innovation Agency, President and member of the Kenya Society of Immunology, Senior Advisor, Moi-Linkoping Universities-funded projects, Chairman of the Medical Education Committee, Planning Curriculum Implementation and International Linkages for Medical and Nursing programmes for student and staff exchange. Simeon has contributed to book chapters in *Leadership Development for Interprofessional Education and Collaborative Practice* and *Routledge International Handbook of Medical Education*. He is an external examiner at the universities of Nairobi and Makerere, Catholic University of Health and Allied Sciences, Bugando and Muhimbili University of Health and Allied Sciences for both nursing and medical students.

Steve Parker was until recently a teaching specialist in the College of Nursing and Health Sciences at Flinders University, Australia. Dr Parker is a registered nurse, has a Bachelor of Education (Secondary Education), and a PhD in nursing. His areas of teaching have been critical thinking, communication/interpersonal skills ethics, and the supervision of research for higher degree students. Dr Parker's research areas have included the theory–practice gap, assessment alignment and factors in the first year that influence student success. His PhD was in the field of professional autonomy. He taught for over 30 years in the higher education sector in Australia until his retirement in 2019. He enjoys exploring new technologies that support life, work and learning.

Teddie Potter is Clinical Professor and Coordinator of the Doctor of Nursing Practice in Health Innovation and Leadership; and Director of Inclusivity, Diversity and Equity at the University of Minnesota School of Nursing. Dr Potter has spoken nationally and internationally about partnership-based healthcare and the BASE of nursing. She co-authored with Riane Eisler the award-winning book, *Transforming Interprofessional Partnerships: A New Framework for Nursing and Partnership-Based Health Care*. In addition, she founded and is Executive Editor of the *Interdisciplinary Journal of Partnership Studies*. She has also partnered with Dr Helga Bragadóttir to bring Collaborative Online International Learning to the field of nursing. Dr Potter currently leads movements to address the health impacts of climate change and other issues impacting planetary health.

Kerry Reid-Searl has been involved in the Central Queensland University undergraduate nursing programme for the past 30 years and is a world leader in simulation education and design. She is currently the Deputy Dean of Simulation in the School of Nursing, Midwifery and Social Sciences. Kerry is also Adjunct Professor at Monash University. Her current simulation work is focused on patient safety and strategies for "the teacher in role". In particular, she works with silicone humanistic props and has designed a unique modality in simulation called Mask-Ed (KRS Simulation). Mask-Ed stands for masking the educator, whilst KRS represents knowledgeable, realistic and spontaneous simulation. The technique is now gaining a national and international reputation, as reflected in her extensive invitations to present her work in Australia, New Zealand, Japan, the USA and the UK.

Ruta Renigere is a guest lecturer at Riga Medical College of the University of Latvia and Riga Stradiņs University. Since 2009, she has developed and been implementing a study course on the Ecological Approach in Patient Care at Riga Medical College of the University of Latvia. Together with her co-authors, she has published a monograph *Nurse and Patient from an Ecological Perspective: Education and Patient Care* (2008). She has been a speaker at various international conferences (in Portugal, Italy, Turkey and the USA) promoting the ecological approach in education and healthcare. She has had 16 international publications.

David Robertshaw is a registered nurse and registered nurse teacher, Fellow of the Higher Education Academy and Fellow of the Royal Society for Public Health and holds a BA-(Hons) in Nursing and an MSc in Critical Care. He is currently Head of Pre-qualifying Healthcare at the University of Derby, UK, supporting the development of nursing associates, assistant practitioners and operating department practitioners. David designed, developed and delivered the University of Derby's first massive open online course on dementia between 2015 and 2017, and regularly uses technology-enhanced learning approaches to teaching in nursing. David is currently studying for a PhD.

Colleen Ryan is a lecturer in Nursing at Central Queensland University, Australia. With a background in nursing and health professionals education, Colleen works with industry partners in supporting nursing students' clinical learning, which is also the focus of her doctoral studies.

Gemma Sinead Ryan is Lecturer in Nursing and Co-qualification Director Nurse Degree Apprenticeship and Nurse Associate, in the Faculty of Wellbeing, Education and Language Studies, at the Open University in the UK. She has a diverse background as a qualified teacher with Qualified Teacher in Learning and Status/Qualified Teacher Status and as a registered adult nurse and nurse teacher. Her previous experience includes secondary, further and higher education (mathematics, biology, science, health and social care, research methods, independent study supervision); research management and leadership; private and NHS healthcare (community, residential care and acute settings). Gemma has extensive experience in development and delivery on online and distance education at a range of academic levels with research interests spanning e-professionalism, professional accountability, (critical) realist methodology, systematic review and education involving nurses and students from health and social care backgrounds.

Alison Steven is Professor of Health Professions Education at Northumbria University, Newcastle upon Tyne, UK. Dr Steven has over 20 years' experience in research and academic activity related to health professions education and professional practice, and has authored a range of publications spanning nursing, medicine and allied health professions. Her research has focused on educational initiatives, the development of professional knowledge and the implementation and embedding of new knowledge and practices. She led the five-country European Union-funded Sharing Learning from Practice for Patient safety (SLIPPs) project exploring students' practice-based learning experiences, and has been involved in a range of nationally and internationally funded projects with particular focus on student experience, patient safety, mentoring and professional well-being.

Teresa E. Stone is Editor-in-Chief, *Nursing and Health Sciences*, and visiting professor in a number of universities across Asia and in Australia. Dr Stone has received awards for both her teaching and her research. Research areas in which she has a particular interest are health beliefs, therapeutic intent, leadership and cross-cultural interpretation of well-being and mental health.

Michael Traynor is Professor of Nursing Policy at Middlesex University, London, UK, where he jointly leads the Centre for Critical Research in Nursing and Midwifery. Michael Traynor came to Middlesex University in 2004 after working at the London School of Hygiene and Tropical Medicine in the only policy research centre focusing on research in nursing and the allied health professions. Michael's research interests include a critical view of political and professional issues in nursing, professional identity, managerialism in healthcare, job satisfaction and methodological issues, including discourse analysis, post-structuralism and psychoanalytic approaches. Michael has recently been awarded a fellowship of the Royal College of Nursing.

Alistair Turvill lectures in child health and development on the Early Childhood Studies programme at the University of Derby, UK, and is currently undertaking a PhD investigating the impact of pain management programmes in collaboration with the Royal Derby Hospital. This has a focus on understanding the role and long-term impact of multidisciplinary teams on self-reported health-related quality of life in chronic pain patients. Other areas of research interest include the impact of technology and media on children and parents, and the use of technology in the process of pain evaluation and management for children and vulnerable adults.

Bill Whitehead is Deputy Dean of the College of Health and Social Care at the University of Derby, UK. Bill has a professional interest in clinical nurse education, preceptorship, research philosophy and nursing ethics. Prior to working in higher education Bill practised as a hospital-based nurse and educator from 1987 to 2005. He maintains a close involvement with the healthcare industry through local partnership working and national networks such as the Clinical Nurse Educator Network. He is Fellow of the Higher Education Academy and National General Secretary of the Clinical Nurse Educator Network.

Tagrid Yassine is Senior Program Manager at the Health Education and Training Institute, New South Wales Health, Australia. Tagrid has a background in organisational learning and adult education. She has worked with universities to develop and renew health curricula at undergraduate and postgraduate levels. Tagrid's more recent work has been in project management and research, specifically in the field of interprofessional education (IPE) and practice. Projects she has contributed to include an audit of IPE in Australian universities, as well as an initiative to implement a national IPE governance framework.

FOREWORD

There is no doubt that the world is increasingly complex, uncertain, ambiguous, ever-changing, and interconnected, and all predictions indicate that these challenges will expand as each day passes by. Knowledge is exploding at an unimaginable rate; technology is ubiquitous and evolving rapidly; the health-related, environmental, economic, and justice issues faced by individuals and societies are increasingly multifaceted and have no easy solutions; and there are more and more options in all arenas of life. Sitting squarely amid this complexity is nursing education and the demands placed upon it to prepare a workforce that will take a leadership role in primary, secondary, and tertiary health-promoting interventions; policy development; and improving the health and well-being of individuals and communities.

This *Handbook of Nurse Education* provides readers with an overview of the social, political, and economic forces that are challenging nurse educators worldwide to re-think where, when, and how we design and deliver nursing education. Included among these forces are the continually evolving role of the nurse, new discoveries related to health problems and approaches to managing them, new insights about how people learn and how best to facilitate the learning process, increasing demands from patients and learners to have more involvement in decisions related to their care or education, demands for evidence-based clinical and teaching practice, and patient and learner populations that are unique and exceptionally diverse. The expectation of nurse educators is to design and implement relevant curricula, as well as evidence-based teaching/learning strategies and assessment/evaluation methods that will best prepare graduates for a lifetime career in a healthcare environment we can hardly imagine today. Obviously, this is no small challenge.

The nurse educator of today needs to be armed with knowledge about generational differences, learning preferences, student disabilities, technology, and a variety of pedagogical approaches, as well as the personal, financial, and familial demands placed on learners. Additionally, the educator must know how to use this knowledge to construct curricula that are innovative, evidence-based, and flexible. Knowledge in these and many other areas also must be used to design courses and learning experiences that are engaging, build on and expand previous learning, and attend to the development of learners as knowledgeable, skilled nurses who can think critically, make sound clinical judgments, collaborate with colleagues from other disciplines to plan and provide care, function as leaders and change agents, bring a scholarly perspective to their practice, and have a commitment to caring, social justice, and excellence.

The chapters in this book attest to these challenges and offer thoughtful and innovative ways to help nurse educators meet them. Contributing authors provide a context for thinking about nursing education from a global perspective and help educators realize that, despite the uniqueness of people, cultures, and educational systems around the world, many in nursing education are facing similar challenges, constraints, and opportunities. In this era of collaboration, this understanding provides opportunities for multi-site and multi-cultural studies about nursing education and the most effective ways to facilitate and assess/evaluate learning, as well as united efforts to advance the profession.

This book also helps the reader understand the many contemporary issues that affect nursing education. How do we design curricula that are flexible enough to allow for discussions of emerging health problems, new discoveries in genetics, new models of healthcare delivery, and the ever-evolving treatments and technologies used to help patients/families manage their health? How do we design curricula and learning experiences to accommodate students who have disabilities, whose native language is not that of the schools in which they are enrolled, who learn in very different ways, who need more than the typical amount of time to complete a program or who can meet all program requirements in less than the typical amount of time, who are homeless or need to forgo meals in order to pay tuition, or who have extensive family responsibilities while enrolled in a nursing program?

Nurse educators also are challenged to think in new ways about the approaches we use to facilitate learning and to more fully appreciate the need to address development of students as whole persons, citizens, and contributing members of their communities, as well as care providers in many different settings. What we are coming to understand about learning suggests that students need to be more engaged, active, and self-directed; they need to learn how to work effectively on teams and deal with the conflicts that inevitably arise in such situations; they need to see themselves as leaders and scholars who will help shape a preferred future for nursing; and they need to be able to engage in honest, constructive self- and peer-evaluation in order to ensure that high-quality care is provided and the environments in which they live and work continually strive for excellence.

Finally, nurse educators need to be aware of how the role and expectations of the nurse are continually changing, and many contributing authors address these issues. From considerations of the type and nature of doctoral education for nurses, to the need for nurses to be involved politically, influence decisions that affect patient care and nursing practice, and be resilient readers, who are exposed to the world, and how we can and must continue to be the conscience, heart, and soul of patient care.

As you read this book, you are urged to keep an open mind, to look beyond your particular school or environment, and to engage in honest self-assessment about what *you* can do to continually advance nursing education and the profession of nursing. Our students and the patients/families/communities for whom they and we care deserve our sincere efforts to strive for excellence.

Theresa M. "Terry" Valiga, EdD, RN, CNE, ANEF, FAAN
Professor Emerita
Duke University School of Nursing
Durham, North Carolina, USA

SECTION 1

Global perspectives on nurse education

Foreword: Margaret McAllister

This section aims to provide a global view of nursing education by training a historical lens on the changes to nursing that took place in various countries. The series of chapters explores nursing education in England, Australia, the Bailiwick of Guernsey, Hong Kong, African countries including Botswana, Ghana and Nigeria and the United States. A chapter also explores the nature of working and studying across countries – a practice that offers the opportunity to create a truly global nursing profession and an approach to working globally that is sensitive to being participatory, rather than dominant.

Bill Whitehead provides an overview of the British nursing system of education concentrating on the periods between the mid to late 1800s through to the present day and explains how the clinical teaching role played a vital role in stimulating the advancement of nursing education. McAllister, Campbell and Ryan provide an overview of nursing education in Australia. Ching, Cheung and Mak provide an account of nursing in Hong Kong, detailing that country's movement from a model of apprenticeship to one of the most advanced systems of education for nursing in the world. Korsah traces developments in three African countries that were heavily influenced by colonial rule, and the health of these nations very much challenged by endemic tropical diseases. In these nations, political independence heralded possibilities for reform to nursing, which in turn triggered improvements to flow to primary, secondary and tertiary healthcare across Africa. The Channel Islands – though home to a small population – have a fascinating history that McClean elaborates. Sandra Lewenson and Annemarie McAllister summarise developments in the United States of America.

Teresa Stone and Margaret McMillan, drawing on their years of experience working in countries other than their home base in Australia, discuss opportunities to broaden horizons by working with nurses in foreign lands.

Potter and Bragadóttir provide a timely discussion of the COIL programme – a global curriculum development approach that is grounded in principles of collaboration and respect. In today's commodification of education, where education providers are seeking markets for their courses, it is vital that nursing scholars provide principles for ethical engagement and to guide the development of relevant, inspiring curriculum that is fit for purpose.

This important section tracing the history of nurse education globally reminds us how learning from history has many benefits – it helps one to notice change or continuity, struggle, achievements and ongoing needs for change in nursing. Historical awareness gives learners a wide vision of nursing, and in this way can illuminate thinking on what directions nursing could and should be headed towards in the future. This series of chapters shows that nurses across the world have been united in their determination to provide reliable, safe and technically skilled care to patients by establishing systems of education that provide relevant training, support and knowledge to students.

1

A HISTORY OF NURSE EDUCATION AND THE CLINICAL NURSE EDUCATOR

Bill Whitehead

Introduction

This chapter will provide a brief historical perspective of British nurse education from the 1860s to the present day. From a secular viewpoint this can be dated precisely to the time of the first Nightingale school at St. Thomas' Hospital in June 1860 (Seymer, 1957).

It is necessary to gain a historical context in order to understand contemporary nurse education in any depth. Historical knowledge also ensures that we learn from the successful policies of the past and avoid repeating mistakes. Much of the ethos and content of training courses was based on the principles emanating from the late nineteenth century (Bradshaw, 2001a). Consequently, it is necessary to look back to the origins of nurse training, because this is a model to which many nurses educating and practising in the early twenty-first century refer (Rideout, 2000). The chapter is organised around the historical events influencing nurse education over this one hundred and fifty-year period. An underlying theme is the three factors of recruitment, retention and skills modernisation which have continually driven the changing delivery of nurse education throughout. For example, one turning point was a paper written following a review of a major London teaching hospital at the end of the 1950s. In this research study, it was found that students were so pressured to provide care for the inpatients that between 30% and 50% left before they reached the end of their training (Menzies, 1960). This report, amongst other factors, led to the widespread adoption of the clinical teacher (CT) role in the years that followed. The account will continue up to the current day and will comment on the resonance of these historical initiatives with contemporary British Government and Nursing and Midwifery Council (NMC) policy (DH, 2016; NMC, 2017a).

Woven throughout the account will be the clinical nurse educator roles which have fulfilled the need for student nurses to receive clinical training and education in practice. This important aspect of the infrastructure of nurse education begins during World War One with the appointment and training of the first "sister tutors" at St. Thomas' Hospital (Martin, 1989). The majority of clinical education continued to be provided by ward sisters, but repeated attempts have been made to professionalise the role. The most well remembered of these was the CT role which was first trialled in Scotland in 1955 (McNaught, 1957) and continued until the changes brought about by the introduction of Project 2000 in the late 1980s and early 1990s (Morris, 1998). It will then examine the roles which followed the CT, such as the lecturer practitioner, practice teacher, practice education facilitator and clinical nurse educators. The chapter will end with the potential roles which will be engendered by the new NMC standards and framework for nurse education (NMC, 2017b).

History

When writing any historical account, it is both difficult and important to decide upon the starting point. Bradshaw convincingly argues, through research based on the core textbooks spanning one hundred years of nurse education, that much of the ethos and content of training courses was based on the principles emanating from the late nineteenth century (2001a). Consequently, it is necessary to look back to the origins of the apprenticeship nurse training model, because this is a model to which many nurses educating and practising in the early twenty-first century refer (Rideout, 2000). It is often seen as an ideal type for producing competent and caring nurses. It goes without saying that this is a debatable point. As an oppressed group, nurses struggle to see beyond the terms of reference of their suppression (Freire, 1972; Marcuse, 1964; Marx and Engels, 1845; Whitehead, 2010). Therefore, it is understandable that many nurses see apprenticeship training, with its accoutrements of servitude to the medical profession and self-sacrifice to the hospital administration, as a historical golden age. However, even politically aware and critical academic nurses have begun to question whether the direction of travel for nursing away from the hands-on, clinical, "knowledgeable doer", described by the United Kingdom Central Council for Nursing, Midwifery and Health Visiting (UKCC) in Project 2000 (1986), has gone too far in the direction of the "knowledgeable" from the "doer" (Drennan and Hyde, 2009).

Origins of the apprenticeship model

The beginning of apprenticeship nurse education appears to be a good starting point, whichever explanation is selected for this phenomenon. From a secular British viewpoint this can be dated precisely to the time of the first Nightingale school at St. Thomas' Hospital in June 1860 (Seymer, 1957). That is not to suggest that nursing began in 1860. There were nurses or people who cared for the sick going back into pre-history. Nurse historians such as Dock have attempted to trace its origins back beyond recorded history (Dock and Stewart, 1938).

In this account Dock and Stewart (1938) provides a creation mythology which is important to the sense of imagined community she was attempting to foster amongst the profession (Anderson, 1991; Samuel and Thompson, 1990). Starting with prehistoric proto-nurses, Dock charts an irregular progression from Stone Age carers through to the nineteenth-century Kaiserworth School for Protestant Deaconesses. The founders provided broad training including pharmacy, ethics and anatomy as well as cooking, cleaning and other practical skills related to the care of the sick. Kaiserworth was where Nightingale gained her inspiration for nurse training (Dock and Stewart, 1938). Nurses had been taught things prior to this and the hospitals which became the illness factories of the nineteenth century required skilled operatives to run them (Foucault, 2003). In addition, there were, of course, women who nursed the sick in warzones prior to and contemporaneously to Nightingale's time in Scutari. Some of these were remembered either in their own words, such as Mary Seacole

(Seacole, 1857), or through local campaigns of charitable giving for their retirement, such as Agnes Harkness (BBC, 2008). However, the identity of the nurse at the time was increasingly of the untrained nurse described in Dickens' 1844 novel *Martin Chuzzlewit* (Dickens, 1844) and illustrated in Dock's curve above as the "secular servant nurse". Nursing at the time was depicted as "a particularly repugnant form of domestic service for which little or no education or special training was necessary" (Kalisch and Kalisch, 1987: 14).

This concept of dangerously incompetent care in British hospitals was supported by Nightingale's experience in the Crimea. The Crimean War death rate had been in main part caused by disease exacerbated by poor care. This led to support for formal nurse training. Nightingale was the founder of this first real secular school of nursing at St. Thomas' Hospital in 1860. However, it must be considered likely that some such course of events would have taken place with or without her. The hospitals were becoming an area for treatment rather than a repository for the sick poor. In addition, women were at this stage beginning to be accepted into higher education (HE) and the professions. This was, in part, a response to the radical and liberal challenges to patriarchy by thinkers such as Wollstonecraft (1792) and Mill (1869). However, it was also an empirical phenomenon that was, arguably, happening independently of philosophical theorising. For example, the first woman to join the medical register in the UK was registered in 1868. She had gained her medical degree in the USA in 1849 and she formed the women's medical college in England in 1869 (LeClair *et al.*, 2007). Contemporaneously, as part of this movement of history, capable women were encouraged to become student or probationer nurses in this newly professionalised discipline.

Probationer nurses

The probationers had a set period of one year at the outset. There were weekly lectures but the main form of education took place on the wards with the matron in charge of the day-to-day education and discipline. According to Bradshaw (2001a), a strict timetable of supervision and certification was imposed on the probationers. The range and content of the nurses' duties and skills are a matter of historical dispute. Relying on official records it is tempting to point to the contents of primary source documents such as the 1860s St. Thomas' School application form which listed duties such as: "dressing of blisters"; "application of leeches"; "bandaging, making bandages and rollers, lining of splints" and "strict observation of the sick" (Dingwall *et al.*, 1988: 54–55).

However, Baly (2007) and Dingwall *et al.* (1988) convincingly cast doubt on this by citing evidence from late nineteenth-century probationers' contemporary diaries and reports. These indicate that tasks such as temperature, pulse and respiration taking and recording were done by medical students; and the nurse's involvement in wound dressing was mainly in preparing poultices. This disconnection between theory and practice is something which would continue to be an issue in nurse education throughout the next century to the present day. The point that Baly (2007) and Dingwall *et al.* (1988) were making was that this implied a lower status for the standard of education and actual work undertaken than for that laid out by the school authorities. It also meant that St. Thomas' saw "probationers as a cheap source of labour" (Dingwall *et al.*, 1988: 53) rather than teaching them valuable skills. The question that must be asked is: what makes the cleaning of patients and the provision of essential care less important than recording temperatures? This was precisely the point that Nightingale made over and over to her probationers and to the governing class at the time (1898, 1914). It remains an issue for nurses in the twenty-first century. In more recent years the Royal College of Nursing (RCN) debated the conference motion "are we too posh to wash?" with regard to expanding nursing careers and the retreat from the bed-side (Bore, 2004; O'Dowd, 2004) and the debate continues with the new standards for nurse education being introduced (Wade, 2018). Nevertheless, whether probationers were learning how to record observations or how to make beds, they were undergoing a certificated training course.

Certification or registration

At the end of the year the probationer became a hospital nurse and was entered on the hospital register as a certified nurse. This was prior to compulsory national registration and in later years when this was discussed, Nightingale was a staunch opponent of compulsory registration. "[S]he felt it would do great damage to the cause of nursing" (Abel-Smith, 1960: 65). "Seeking a nurse from a Register" she wrote "is very much like seeking a wife from a Register, as is done in some countries" (Nightingale, cited in Abel-Smith, 1960: 65 [original capitals retained]). Other nurses, such as Bedford Fenwick, and doctors, such as Acland, argued that nurses, similarly to medical practitioners, should be registered to ensure quality and consistency of training (Bradshaw, 2001a; Dingwall *et al.*, 1988). However, Nightingale was influential and well connected and partially due to her interventions national registration for nurses, and the regulation of minimum educational standards which comes with it, would have to wait until well into the twentieth century.

Nurses Registration Act

In 1904 and 1905 parliamentary select committees were convened to discuss the issue of com-pulsory nurse registration. Despite strong argument from the anti-registrationists they found in favour of registration. Nevertheless, state registration and the professional standing which came with it were not to be enacted until the 1919 Registration Act (Hart, 2004). Bradshaw sees the Act following directly from the intellectual arguments put forward at the committees (2001a). However, this delay of fourteen years cannot be dismissed easily. It would appear likely that the registration of nurses came when it did because of events in the wider political, social and economic context. This was immediately after the war and the extension of the electoral franchise to all working-class men and to all women over thirty. It was in a period of increased industrial militancy during a brief period of economic boom (Pribicevic, 1959; Rosenberg, 1987). The factors influencing other workers were also affecting nurses. Nurses, especially asylum workers, were beginning to unionise and take industrial action (COHSE, 1993; Hart, 2004). One of the issues at stake was that of the Voluntary Aid Detachment (VAD) nurses. These volunteer carers had little or no training and were recruited in large numbers during the war. Dingwall *et al.* go so far as to say that "VADs gave the nurses a common enemy against whom they could unite" (1988: 74). This was similar to the con-cerns of other trades during the war which had been required to accept unqualified workers into their fields of employment (Mann, 1967). Also, the issue of women's suffrage had an effect on the priorities of parliamentarians, as evidenced by the comments of an incumbent of the House of Lords in the year just prior to the Act. Earl Russell said:

> [t]he position is this, women now have the vote, they have to be considered more than they used to be. It is not so easy to say "I don't like this registration of nurses". Women are now likely to get what they insist on having … .
>
> *(Earl Russell, 1919)*

These combined forces were compelling and led to a radical change in the composition of British social life. This was the beginning of the rise of labour in both a political and industrial sense (Hobsbawm, 1978). The government responded with initiatives in social reform such as the creation of a Department of Health and with attempts to de-radicalise potentially organised labour. This encouraged the setting up of regulations to control professions. Nursing as one of the largest was on the front line for regulation. This initiative would organise nurses under what government saw as appropriate senior members of the profession. The more positive aspect of this for the profession was that it would give them "what they insist on having" by regulating their training and restricting the membership to those licensed to practise. The General Nursing Council (GNC) was formed as a result of the legislation. From shortly after its inception to near its end it required a set syllabus and state final examinations for all training courses. These requirements for registration, in continually evolving form, continued as the basis of the profession until 1977. The registration of nurses was an important step for nursing to be recognised as a legally defined occupational group. However, it did not lead to a radical change in the methods or content of training. Bradshaw argues, with strong historical evidence, that this continued the ethos of the Nightingale nurse education method. That is that nurses needed to be of high moral character and be practically skilled rather than theoretically knowledgeable (2001a).

Recruitment and retention

Other issues faced by nurses and their employers, such as recruitment, retention and the attainment of appropriate skills, also remained the same after registration and still concern these groups today. It would appear self-evident that the two factors of the Nightingale ethos and falling recruitment were linked. The continued oppressed position in which this put the profession would be raised continually in the reports of numerous attempts at understanding the problems facing the profession.

In the following fifty years there were many reports and studies, and all indicated that apprenticeship training was inadequate but that it should continue in a modified form. It will be useful to illustrate the transition from early registration to the beginning of university-based education by reference to these reports.

The Lancet Commission on Nursing

The first of these reports was the *Lancet* Commission on Nursing, set up in 1932 to "inquire into the reasons for the shortage of candidates for nursing" (Martin, 1989: 9). They concluded that part of the problem was poor working conditions, lack of trust, over-work and under-pay. This led to an attrition rate of approximately a third. A high drop-out rate on top of inadequate recruitment was creating acute shortages (*Lancet* Commission on Nursing, 1932). The report recommended that preliminary classroom training should become universal before students went out on to the wards. This was already the case in 60–70% of hospitals and subsequently became the norm. Therefore, they accepted the necessity of lectures by nurse teachers. The widely accepted practice in America by this stage was for learner nurses to be full-time students. Nevertheless, the Commission did not recommend that British trainee nurses become supernumerary students. This was because they felt that the practical skills were best maintained by hands-on direct nursing care (Martin, 1989).

The Athlone Report

The Athlone Report was published in 1939. Its terms of reference were the same as the *Lancet* Commission: recruitment, retention and skills. The RCN put forward evidence for a register of trained tutors and for student status for trainees. These were rejected, as again the committee considered that nurses required primarily practical training. Its recommendations roundly supported the conclusions of the previous report and also recommended government regulation of maximum working hours of a ninety-six-hour fortnight and minimum wages. However, these were rejected by the government because they did not feel it was appropriate for them to become involved in setting salaries for a profession (Ministry of Health, 1939).

The Wood Report

During World War Two VADs were again deployed, and along with many other trades, nurses were temporarily forced to work alongside untrained volunteers and hastily educated workers. In 1947 a working party on the recruitment and training of nurses reported. This was known as the Wood Report and was widely critical of the London-based GNC. It proposed giving the power to standardise and regulate training to regional committees appointed by the Ministry of Health (1947). The recommendations were partly brought into being by the Nurses Act of 1949. This also changed the composition of the GNC to include more nurse educators (Nursing Times, 1950). A further recommendation of the report was that there appeared to be little sign of actual ward-based teaching. The committee reported that there was a paucity of research evidence about the work of nurses, and partly as a consequence, research was commissioned which reported in 1953 (Goddard, 1953). This reiterated the view that there was little or no ward teaching occurring. It stated that most learning was from more senior students and advised that selected ward sisters be provided with a course of teacher training to become teaching sisters. These should be set apart to undertake bedside teaching on behalf of the managing sister. The logical conclusion was for specially trained and separately funded clinical tutors to be created. Clinical skills were theoretically prioritised throughout this period, as shown by the outcomes of these reports. However, it was now becoming evident that the acquisition of these skills was haphazard and often left to the efforts of the student and chance.

A case-study in the functioning of social systems as a defence against anxiety

It was hardly surprising that gaining the skills and knowledge required was haphazard under the existing circumstances. For example, the administration of a London teaching hospital was so concerned that the status quo was not an option that it commissioned a study into developing new methods of nursing organisation. The statistics published with this research alone illustrate the problem. Student nurses numbered five hundred and fifty out of a nursing workforce of seven hundred at the hospital. This left only one hundred and fifty matrons, sisters and staff nurses in total to train and supervise them. The students as a result were so pressured to provide the care for the seven hundred inpatients that between 30% and 50% left before they reached the end of their training (Menzies, 1960). Menzies (later to be known as Menzies-Lyth) took a psycho-social methodological approach to this study and concluded that the organisation was a pathological example of a social defence system against the otherwise unbearable anxiety in which the nurses and students were placed, due to their workplace position as essential carers. She took the final position that, unless the structural organisation systems such as task lists and decision avoidance were modified to less alienating and more empowering systems, the nursing social structure was heading towards crisis (Menzies, 1960). Clearly, education would be an important component of any changes required. The CT would be a central part of the educational reform introduced.

The origins of the clinical teacher

The GNC syllabus and final examination instructions were highly prescriptive to provide national conformity of education and achievement. This included the use of a nationally agreed "nurse's chart" which was designed to record when the probationer had achieved proficiency in a list of procedures (Bradshaw, 2000). Therefore, from the beginning of the GNC's reign there was supposed to be formal and regulated assessment of clinical skills by ward-based staff. The appropriate person to do this was seen as the most senior and experienced nurse at ward level. However, there were no regulations governing the ability of these clinical experts to teach or assess. That is not to say that there was no training of ward-based educators. The first sister tutors were appointed in 1914. In 1918, the first course for tutors was established at King's College (Martin, 1989). However, the main educator and assessor from the late nineteenth century on was the ward sister and the vast majority of these had no formal training in teaching or supporting students. This state of affairs continued through World War Two into the foundation of the National Health Service (NHS) in 1948. At this time the hospital-based nurse training schools became part of the NHS. Nurse education remained the responsibility of the hospital. However, following the Wood Report (1947) and the Nurses Act (1949, cited in Nursing Times, 1950) the funding for some of the educational costs was removed from the hospital budget and the regional committees set up by the Act were given powers to instigate experimental training courses. As a result of one of these attempts in Scotland in 1955, a by-product was the employment of the first CTs in the UK.

The CT can be seen as the first real fully committed role in the UK to teaching practical skills at the bedside. CTs were entirely employed by the school of nursing and directed towards teaching pre-registration students. Nevertheless, the correlation which nurses in the twenty-first century make between these roles and those of clinical nurse educators is a fair one in this primary purpose at least (Whitehead & Allibone, 2014). The CT was similar in function to the already existing clinical instructors used in the USA. Their remit was to teach clinical skills at the bedside and in the clinical simulation room of the school of nursing. The first of these spent four months in Canada, where the role was already in existence. There she underwent preparation for the work and later wrote up her experiences for a *Nursing Times* article (McNaught, 1957). The CTs were required for an experimental course at the Glasgow Royal Infirmary. The experimental course itself was not well reviewed, but the CT role was welcomed from the outset and came out of the formal evaluation well (Scottish Home and Health Department, 1963).

As a consequence of good initial feedback, new CT posts were created to assist with the teaching and assessment of students on traditional courses nationwide. The first in England were at Leicester Royal Infirmary but most hospitals' schools of nursing followed suit during the ensuing years. The RCN was the first to devise a course purely for the instruction of CTs. This began as a six-month course in 1959 and several others were created in the years following. The main differences between these courses and the full nurse tutor courses were that the CT courses were shorter and were based on the teaching of practical clinical skills rather than on the student's professional development. As a consequence of this and of academic prejudice against skills rather than theory teaching, these roles would be described as transitional roles for those wishing to see if teaching suited them. This would continue to be the attitude of many nurse academics (Rowan and Barber, 2000). Another consequence of the 1949 Nurses Act was the upgrading of what had been termed assistant nurses to state enrolled nurses (SENs) who had to meet a level of competence set by the GNC and were registered. Learners preparing for SEN status began to be called pupil nurses to differentiate them from the state registered nurse (SRN) students. Pupil nurses had to complete a two-year instead of a three-year course to register. Pupils had less time in the school of nursing but similar amounts on the wards to students. They were prepared in the practical aspects of nursing but less so in the theoretical (Iley, 2004).

A special six-month training course was created for teachers of pupil nurses and this was eventually merged with the CT course in 1968. There was a long period of dispute over the status and requirements of CTs. They were often used as lecturers in the school to the detriment of their position in the clinical area. It would not be until 1970, long after their presence had become the norm across the country, that they were finally given the status of a registered clinical nurse teacher by the GNC. This ensured that they had a minimum level of teacher training which was the City and Guilds Further Education Teaching Certificate.

In 1977 the required qualifications for CT registration were extended to include a diploma in nursing as well as their initial registration and teaching certificate. This state of affairs continued until the amalgamation of the registered nurse teacher (RNT) and CT roles in 1988 (Martin, 1989). This is in contrast with the current position of certified nurse educators (CNEs). The majority of CNE employers require little or no post-registration educational attainment and at best minimal teaching qualifications. The NMC introduced requirements for the registration of nurse educators in 2006 which appeared to reintroduce a skills teacher level in the guise of the practice teacher (PT) alongside the NMC "mentor" (NMC, 2006). However, there was no requirement for roles such as CNEs to be registered as PTs. The new NMC standards for education introduce a split in the roles supporting student nurse practice-based education. The "supervisor" role is to facilitate student learning and can be fulfilled by any registered professional. The "practice assessor" role has the purpose of providing high-quality objective assessment to ensure that students are practising at a level fit to join the register. This will require experience and education and would fit the CNE job description well. Nevertheless, CTs were in the workplace from the late 1950s.

The modernisation of nursing

During this period of the rise of the CT there were very great changes going on in nurse education, nursing and British life in general. During the 1960s the same social forces which led to Wilson's "white heat of technology" speech (Wilson, 1963) resulted in changes in the educational system at both school age and beyond. In nursing this allowed the GNC for the first time to stipulate minimum entry requirements of 2 "O" levels for entry to nurse training. Changes in the social status of women, the aspirations of the newly invented teenagers (Hamblett and Deverson, 1964) and the expansion of HE of all kinds changed the possible life choices of applicants who previously had more restricted options and made nursing with its strict hierarchy and long hours look less appealing. Consequently, continued poor recruitment and high attrition rates resulted in further investigations and reports on nursing and nurse education such as the Salmon Report (Ministry of Health, Scottish Home and Health Department, 1966).

The Salmon Report

This report into senior nurses and nurse administration marked a clear change from the past. It created a new set of nurse administrators which signed the death knell for the old dominance of the matron. It was not a report on nurse education as such but it had a definite effect. In Martin's research into the period, one of the nurse lecturers interviewed in the late 1970s said: "Salmon set all us tutors free" (Martin, 1989: 24). This was because one of the results of the report was that management of schools of nursing on a day-to-day basis was put into the hands of a nurse educator and recruitment of students was left entirely to the school. The major report which had the most influence on nurse education in the late twentieth century was about to be commissioned.

The Briggs Report

The move from hospital-based to university-based education in nursing is usually traced back to this report from the early 1970s. The Briggs Report (DHSS, 1972) was set up as one of the final acts of the outgoing Labour administration in 1970. The report of the Committee on Nursing was finally published in 1972. The committee did wide-ranging and in-depth research to examine its terms of reference. They presented their research findings as well as their interpretations and recommendations in the published report. In relation to the teaching of clinical skills on wards, which was supposed to be the centre of the curriculum, there were some worrying results, as can be seen in Table 1.1.

Table 1.1 shows that a majority of nurses saw the balance of working and learning on ward placements as too much working and not enough learning. This was one of numerous pieces of evidence presented to show that the existing system of education was not sustainable. The committee presented carefully costed plans to radically overhaul nurse education. The costings had to take into account the removal of the student nursing workforce because Briggs intended that student nurses should cease to be workers and become full-time students. This was initially shelved on publication as too costly but in the late 1970s was picked up again. Another aspect of the committee's recommendations was that the GNC and the other nine "separate bodies across the United Kingdom" should unite as the UKCC. Both the recommendations for nurse education and for the regulatory body were eventually adopted almost in full with the passing of the Nurses, Midwives and Health Visitors Act (1979).

Table 1.1 Balance between learning and working

Balance between learning and working in wards	All trainees and recent trainees†	Registered nurses	Enrolled nurses	Student nurses	Pupil nurses
Weighted base	3,027	714	566	1,142	388
Too much learning	–	–	–	1%	–
Too much working	56%	49%	46%	70%	48%
Balance right	42%	51%	47%	28%	52%
Don't know	2%	–	8%*	1%	–

* Columns may not sum to one hundred due to rounding.
† Recent trainees are staff who completed basic training less than five years ago (DHSS, 1972: 65).

End of the General Nursing Council national syllabus

This was the beginning of the end for the apprenticeship system of nurse education. Bradshaw argues that the end came when the Briggs recommendations were accepted in 1977, which led to the final publication of the GNC national syllabus in that year (2001a, 2001b). There can be no doubt that, with the benefit of hindsight, it is possible to trace back the eventual implementation of HE-based nurse education to this point. However, the form of nurse training which incorporated most of the time working as a salaried employee of the hospital continued until the mid-1990s. The CTs and hospital-based schools of nursing continued with them. Therefore, the experience of the students undergoing this training remained the same, whatever government or professional body policy was. Essentially, most student nurses remained apprentices until then. CTs were kept busy in both classroom teaching and assessing the four ward-based practical assessments which were introduced in 1969 by the GNC and were only rescinded with the advent of Project 2000 (Bradshaw, 2000). These assessments required demonstration of an acceptable level of proficiency in four separate skills. These clinical skills were the drug assessment; aseptic technique; total patient care; and management of a ward (Elliott *et al.*, 1973). Along with the final examination, these formed the mainstay of the assessment of nurses until the implementation of Project 2000.

Continuous assessment

With Project 2000 this series of four practical examinations was to be replaced by continuous assessment by ward-based mentors. These mentors would be existing ward nurses, either staff nurses or sisters. They would observe students throughout their placement and make a judgement as to whether they had achieved a list of competencies at every stage of their nurse education (UKCC, 1986).

Project 2000 was the final materialisation of the recommendations which Briggs made in 1972. As stated earlier, these were accepted in 1977. However, the process of implementation would take a further ten years to be accepted and it would not be until the mid-1990s that all student nurses were finally given full supernumerary student status. The next section will examine the road to supernumerary and bursary rather than salaried employee status, which radically changed the nature of nurse education. This would be especially the case for the practical skills aspect of the course.

Nurses, Midwives and Health Visitors Act

The 1979 Nurses, Midwives and Health Visitors Act went on to the statute books at the transition between the Labour and Conservative administrations of that year. In fact, the incoming Conservative Government attempted to stop its implementation, but backed down following an outcry from the profession (Martin, 1989). The Act included many aspects of the Briggs recommendations. There would be one single UK body to regulate nurses, midwives and health visitors. This took the place of ten geographical and professional bodies (Department of Health and Social Security, 1972). There would be a separation of responsibility for nurse education to four national boards. The government for the first time devolved the responsibility for regulation and education to the profession. This was in sharp contrast to the previous regime of the GNC, which had been both interdependent with medical staff and constantly interfered with by the Department of Health. The new self-regulatory bodies were brought into being by this Act in 1983.

All of this was again happening during a period of great social, political and economic change. The decision to implement the move to HE for nurse education and the move to professional self-regulation took place in the years after Prime Minister James Callaghan's Ruskin College speech and the Great Debate about the purpose of education which followed (1976). Nursing would be as affected as other professions by the forces which led to vocational courses being brought into line with transferable values. As a vocational training course, it would be part of the new wave of educational programmes which, two decades later would dominate the HE landscape. One of the biggest shocks of the age was that, after decades of almost full employment, mass unemployment was reaching highs of over three million out of work. In nursing this led to less pressure on recruitment, as nurse education became comparatively a more attractive option and qualified nurses had fewer career options to move out of the profession. The women's movement had won several victories, including the Equal Pay Act (1970) and the Sex Discrimination Act (1975). In addition to this legislative feminist success, the profession had become more active in industrial relations. This was especially marked in the pay disputes of 1974 (Hart, 2004). As a consequence, the history of unquestioned subservience of nurses to doctors and management was being challenged (Whitehead, 2010). It is no coincidence that during this period the leaders of the profession felt confident enough to implement the "nursing process" nationwide. This professionally empowering intervention was, however, done in a typically authoritarian manner by providing a nursing Kardex which ensured that the four stages of the process were completed by all hospital nurses. These stages were the steps developed in the mid-1970s of assessing, planning, implementing and evaluating patient care (Walker Seaback, 2000). This process marked nursing as a separate and autonomous profession because it implied that there were aspects of patient care to which the nurse was the primary assessor as well as deliverer of treatment (Habermann and Uys, 2005). With this background the profession could feel confident enough to call for and implement the changes in education and status for students and qualified staff that had been suggested by those who had been in favour of raised professional status for some time.

Project 2000

The result of these calls for professional education to match professional status was what would come to be known as Project 2000. This was initially a paper produced by the UKCC in 1986. It called for many of the reforms outlined in the Briggs Report and in some ways went further. It saw the future of nursing as residing outside of hospitals and claimed that by the year 2000 there would be few nurses working in general hospitals. Those who would be left working in institutions would be in highly specialised and technological fields such as intensive care units and coronary care units. This was extrapolated from the reduction in hospital beds which was taking place at the time and from moves that were taking place in mental health to reduce hospital admission to a minimum. The UKCC argued that, when asked, the majority of patients said that they would prefer to be cared for at home. Consequently, the health professions would have to provide care in the future which delivered this aspiration and thus move away from most nursing occurring in hospitals. This, they argued, required a very different type of nurse for the future. The training which had gone before, which relied on experience of a series of hospital wards, would not be appropriate for this new kind of nursing (United Kingdom Central Council for Nursing, Midwifery and Health Visiting, 1986).

The single-status nurse followed on from this. Briggs had suggested retaining the two status levels of nursing but changing the second-level nurse from SEN to certified nurse. These would have completed the same first eighteen months of their course with the registered nurses (RNs) but then stepped off (Department of Health and Social Security, 1972). The Project 2000 proposal was for one level of RN. In addition, for the first time there would be a requirement for achievement of an academic standard as well as a professional one for registration. The academic standard would be at diploma in HE level. Previously to this there had been no academic equivalence for the majority of nurses achieving registration. A minority of nursing students had been on degree programmes which usually achieved registration in four years rather than three. However, these were unusual. The requirement for diploma of HE level was in line with other government initiatives to give academic status to vocational courses. In addition, the UKCC argued that academic education would provide the sort of inquiring, evidence-based nurses that would be required for the new world of nursing that they envisaged (Davies, Beach and Beech, 2000).

A logical consequence of single status for initial registration was that nurse educators, who had for decades been divided into CTs and nurse tutors, should both be given the same status. The new nurse tutor would be a combination of both of the previous clinical and theoretical educators (Jolly, 1997). All tutors would be required to spend a proportion of their time in clinical practice as well as the classroom. The UKCC envisaged that this would help to close the theory-to-practice divide which at that time appeared to be widening.

The final proposal was that students and their teachers would be removed from the NHS and placed into a small number of HE institutions. This would ensure that education staff and students could not be used as clinical staff by the hospitals. It also, as Briggs had anticipated, would remove a mainstay of the nursing workforce at a stroke. The proposal was to replace these with a new type of carer called support workers (UKCC, 1988) and later re-branded by the Secretary of State (Kenneth Clarke) as health care assistants. These would be trained on the job with National Vocational Qualifications.

The end of the Nightingale ethos

The government of the day surprised most nurses and their representative bodies by accepting the proposals almost completely as they were requested. This was perhaps surprising at first as the proposals would be expensive and fall entirely on to the taxpayer. This was at the time of the ambulance dispute and the Poll Tax. Both of these disputes had involved nurses and other health workers in bitter confrontation with government (Kerr and Sachdev, 1992; Whitehead, 1997). This political and industrial activism was not the only newsworthy event at the time which would change the governmental and social perception of nurses.

The year after the Poll Tax campaign, serial murderer Beverly Allitt killed four children in her care. She had recently qualified as an SEN and her betrayal of trust would affect the way that all nurses were perceived by the general public (Batty, 2007). The case of Harold Shipman, which came to light in the late 1990s, had the same effect for the medical profession (*The Guardian*, 2019). A result of these extreme serial murder cases and concerns about the general competence level of nurses led to action being taken to reintroduce governmental control of the nursing profession in the shape of the NMC. The NMC was an event for the future at this time but other changes were occurring.

A return to apprenticeship

In recent years, learning while in paid work in modern apprenticeships has been reintroduced as a twenty-first-century UK Government policy. However, in the late 1980s and 1990s the direction of modernisation was supposed to be towards HE and the increased professional status this was intended to bring with it. The first Project 2000 courses were commenced in September 1989 (Bradshaw, 2001b). As previously asserted, these were, at that time, a minority of courses and many nurses continued to be educated under the apprenticeship system until the mid-1990s. Nevertheless, the gradual introduction of Project 2000 to all schools of nursing had been agreed and set on track. Therefore, the reality of the new type of preparation for registration was now foremost in the minds of nurse regulators and managers. This would lead to concerns about the ability of the new regimen to produce competent skilled nurses. As Project 2000 and continuous assessment were being introduced, CTs were being removed from practice and the UKCC proposals for the content of future pre-registration education did not specify the skills which should be acquired by nursing students. It could be argued that Project 2000 removed clinical examinations and specified clinical educators and as a consequence, in clinical education, it was moving back to a previous definition of apprenticeship rather than forward into HE; that is, the old kind of time-served apprenticeship without any full-time practice educators, just mentors trying to provide education support in addition to their primary clinical care role. This approach to learning was an expectation that, by spending enough time in the company of experts doing the job, expertise would be acquired by the apprentice. In theory this was not the case, as each student had a mentor who was allocated to solely monitor his or her progress. However, this mentor was primarily a care provider and often a very busy one. Consequently, many students were left to pick up what clinical skills learning they could, or not, without any specific guidance (Cahill, 1996).

Continuing professional development

The next stage to the implementation of the new order in nurse self-regulation would be the concept of compulsory post-registration education and practice, which would be introduced as a UKCC project in 1990 (Post-Registration Education and Practice Project: PREPP) (O'Bryne, 1990; UKCC, 1990). This was designed to ensure that, once nurses qualified, they would be expected and encouraged to continue studying to remain competent. In addition to maintaining educational proficiency they would be monitored to ensure that they were working sufficient hours in an appropriate role to remain on the register. This twin system of assessing the continuing ability of RNs again emphasised the apprenticeship concept of "time-served" as a measure of ability rather than regular examinations or some other objective method of academic assessment. However, this time it was during, rather than prior to, the RN's practice.

The proposals were finalised in 1994 and became known as PREP as it was no longer a project (UKCC, 1994; 1995). The project had also introduced the idea of preceptorship for the first time. Newly qualified nurses (NQNs) were perceived to be in need of a period when they could be supported by a more senior nurse following registration. The space of time was not specified but a period of four to six months was suggested. This was recommended as good practice rather than made compulsory by the NMC. Part of the reason for the introduction of preceptorship was concern that nurses were not sufficiently competent in clinical skills following registration. The theory was that, as they had previously been paid employees as students they would have learned the ropes. However, under Project 2000 this could not be guaranteed and therefore a period of adjustment after qualifying should be allowed for. This sounds like an admission that they were not entirely convinced that the move to continuous assessment would be effective in ensuring sufficient assessment. As such, the move to provide a period of supervision after qualifying would appear to be a sensible insurance policy.

However, the issue of staffing reduction following the withdrawal of cheap student labour had not gone away. There had never previously been a grade of staff required to support NQNs as they were expected to progress along a continuum seamlessly from being a senior student. Consequently, as no one else was available, existing staff nurses and ward sisters were expected to take on the role of preceptor in addition to their primary caring role and new responsibilities as continuous assessment mentors. As a result, a period of real preceptorship was an expensive luxury that significant numbers of NQNs did not receive. This brought back the necessity of ensuring that, when students qualified, they could "hit the ground running" as fully formed and able, qualified nurses. Preceptorship has now been generally accepted by employers, although still not required by the NMC (Whitehead *et al.*, 2016). Nevertheless, the practical reality for most NQNs in the 1990s was that they were in a position of accountability from the start. This would usually include having complete responsibility for a group of acutely ill patients for a shift at a time.

Concerns about competence

In the latter half of the 1990s Project 2000 had been fully implemented nationwide. All of the students qualifying had gained registration under this system and in some parts of the UK this had been the case for many years. Those nurses in positions of authority within the educational and regulatory establishment remained committed to the professionalisation agenda. All nurses now qualifying had diplomas in HE as a minimum requirement for registration and the logical next step was to convert nursing to a graduate profession. However, outside of these hallowed circles, the front-line carers, their managers and the patients in their trust were sceptical that this was the route of most benefit to them (Cowan *et al.*, 2007). This became highlighted in governmental circles most effectively when prominent politicians were able to observe, as hospital inpatients, at close quarters the nursing care delivered, both good and bad. One such was the former academic and active politician Lord Morris. As he said in the opening speech on a debate on nurses and the NHS:

> [t]he facts are not in dispute. We are facing the worst nurse shortage crisis in 25 years: the first ever shortfall in applications for nurse education places in England. In 1993/4 there were 18,100 applications for 12,000 places. In 1996/7 there were 15,400 applications for 16,100 places. Turnover among registered nurses was 21 per cent. in 1997, up from 12 per cent in 1992. Vacancies remain unfilled. One report in 1997 suggested that there was a shortage of more than 8,000 full-time posts across Britain. The Royal College of Nursing reports that the number of nurses aged over 55 will double over the next five years, with 25 per cent of registered nurses in the NHS eligible for retirement by the year 2000. (...)
>
> One thing comes through again and again about pre-registration training: practical clinical skills are not sufficiently achieved by the student. The clinical teacher role has gone and quite senior clinicians have to waste their time teaching new nurses how to do things on the wards. Perhaps an internship for the diplomates at the end of their course is necessary. After all, new nurses are in law accountable for their practice from day one.
>
> *(Morris, 1998: Column 1540).*

This neatly sums up the issues as Morris and many others saw them. There were not enough nurses to provide quality care; the ones that were left were likely to leave soon; attempts to increase the number of those in training to remedy this had not been met with sufficient applicants; CTs were no longer available, which put the burden of teaching clinical skills on to "clinicians"; and Project 2000 was not producing nurses with skills fit for purpose without a period of "internship". Clearly, something must be done, and simply expanding the number of places on Project 2000 courses would not be a remedy. Further research and reports such as that presented by Aston *et al.* (2000) for the English National Board (ENB) would highlight the need for nurse teachers to fulfil a practice education role.

Making a difference and fitness for practice

Two policy documents would provide a blueprint for the changes to nurse education. The first was the UKCC's *Fitness for Practice* (1999). This endorsed the concerns that nurses were qualifying without sufficient skills and put forward recommendations including a competency-based curriculum; the use of clinical skills laboratories; earlier exposure to clinical practice placements; a three-month final placement and the implementation of proper preceptorship. *Making a Difference* was the second influential document. Produced by the Department of Health (1999), it took on board many of the recommendations made in the UKCC paper and gave them governmental impetus. The document laid out plans to commence pilot sites at ten universities in September 2000 and added that practising clinical staff should be provided with teaching roles in conjunction with universities. This commitment to modern-day CTs appeared to be based on the existing, very limited provision of lecturer practitioners (Leigh *et al.*, 2002). However, this was not specifically stated and thus allowed universities and hospital trusts to experiment with new practice education roles. A particularly popular model would become the clinical nurse educator employed by hospital and community care providers.

Conclusion

Nurses from the mid nineteenth century to the present have been required to obtain an adequate level of skills to practise safely. Since the beginning nurses have attempted to ensure that their education and supervision would make this happen. For most of the history of nursing there have been problems recruiting and retaining enough nurses. Exacerbating and often defining these issues has been the socially oppressed position of the nursing profession. This has led to insufficient resources being allocated and constant interference from the medical profession and politicians.

Across the country many novel attempts to meet a need for support of practical skills achievement and to provide preceptorship for NQNs have been made in recent years. These new roles are constantly expanding and have formed a national network to avoid isolation and to gain a voice independent of HE and practice employers (Sprinks, 2015).

This history of the past one hundred and fifty years of nurse education indicates that many of the challenges currently facing nursing and nurse education, such as recruitment, retention and skills acquisition, are recurring themes which have generated repeated reports, investigations and sometimes even radical action. At time of writing nurse education is facing up to the latest set of changes intended to address these issues. It is unknown whether they will be successful or not. What can be certain is that they will not be the last set of policy changes. Health care technology and treatment improve apace and the demand for ever more complex and demanding nursing care will continue to expand.

References

Abel-Smith B (1960) *A History of the Nursing Profession*. London: Heinmann.

Anderson B (1991) *Imagined Communities*. London: Verso.

Aston L, Mallik M, Day D and Fraser D (2000) An Exploration into the Role of the Teacher/Lecturer in Practice: Findings from a Case Study in Adult Nursing, *Nurse Education Today, 20*(3): 178–188.

Baly M (2007) *Florence Nightingale and the Nursing Legacy*, 2nd edn. London: Wiley.

Batty D (2007) *Serial Killer Nurse Allitt must Serve 30 Years*, [online] Available from: <www.guardian.co.uk/uk/2007/dec/06/ukcrime.health> [Accessed 6 October 2008].

BBC (2008) *Agnes Harkness: Heroine of Matagorda, Making History, broadcast BBC Radio 4 3pm-3.30pm 30 September 2008* Available from: <www.bbc.co.uk/radio4/history/making_history/making_history_20080930.shtml> [Accessed 6 January 2019].

Bore J (2004) Are We Really Too Posh to Wash? *Nursing Standard, 18*(38): 28.

Bradshaw A (2000) Competence and British Nursing: A View from History, *Journal of Clinical Nursing, 9*(3): 321–329.

Bradshaw A (2001a) *The Nurse Apprentice, 1860-1977*. Aldershot: Ashgate.

Bradshaw A (2001b) *The Project 2000 Nurse: The Remaking of British General Nursing, 1978-2000*. London: Whurr.

Cahill HA (1996) A Qualitative Analysis of Student Nurses' Experiences of Mentorship, *Journal of Advanced Nursing, 24*(4): 791–799.

Callaghan J (1976) *Towards a National Debate, 18 October*, [online] Available from: <www.educationengland.org.uk/documents/speeches/1976ruskin.html> [Accessed 12 January 2019].

Confederation of Health Service Employees (1993) 12 Page History Special, *COHSE Journal*, June, 11–22.

Cowan DT, Norman I and Coopamah VP (2007) Competence in Nursing Practice: A Controversial Concept – A Focused Review of Literature, *Accident and Emergency Nursing, 15*(1): 20–26.

Davies C Beach A Beech A (2000) *Interpreting Professional Self-Regulation: A History of the United Kingdom Central Council for Nursing, Midwifery and Health Visiting*. London: Routledge.

Department of Health (1999) *Making a Difference: Strengthening the Nursing, Midwifery and Health Visiting Contribution to Health and Healthcare*. London: HMSO.

Department of Health (2016) *Nursing Degree Apprenticeship: Factsheet*, Available from: www.gov.uk/government/publications/nursing-degree-apprenticeships-factsheet [Accessed30 December 2017].

Department of Health and Social Security (1972) *Report of the Committee on Nursing. Cmnd. 5115.* London: HMSO.

Dickens C (1844) *Martin Chuzzlewit*, [Project Gutenberg EBook] Available from: <www.gutenberg.org/ebooks/968> [Accessed 12 January 2019].

Dingwall R, Rafferty AM and Webster C (1988) *An Introduction to the Social History of Nursing*. London: Routledge.

Dock L and Stewart I (1938) *A Short History of Nursing: From the Earliest Times to the Present Day*, 4th edn. London: Putnam's.

Drennan J and Hyde A (2009) The Fragmented Discourse of the 'Knowledgeable Doer': Nursing Academics' and Nurse Managers' Perspectives on a Master's Education for Nurses, *Advances in Health Sciences Education, 14*(2): 173–186.

Earl Russell (1919) *House of Lords Debates 27 May 1919*, col. 846 Available from: <https://hansard.parliament.uk/lords/1919-05-27/debates/fe6202b7-a8fa-4522-8f24-6cfc64aa1ae4/NursesRegistrationBillHl> [Accessed 12 January 2019].

Elliott J, Jones V and Spoor J (1973) Ward-Based Practical Examinations, *Nursing Times, 69*(23): 744–745.

Foucault M (2003) *The Birth of the Clinic: An Archaeology of Medical Perception*. London: Routledge.

Freire P (1972) *Pedagogy of the Oppressed*. Harmondsworth: Penguin.

Goddard HA (1953) *The Work of Nurses in General Hospital Wards. Report of a Job Analysis*. London: Nuffield Hospital Provincial Hospital Trusts.

Great Britain (1970) *Equal Pay Act 1970: Elizabeth II*, Available from <www.opsi.gov.uk/acts/acts1970/pdf/ukpga_19700041_en.pdf> [Accessed 19 January 2019].

Great Britain (1975) *Sex Discrimination Act 1975: Elizabeth II*, Available from: <www.opsi.gov.uk/acts/acts1975/pdf/ukpga_19750065_en.pdf> [Accessed 19 January 2019].

Great Britain (1979) *Nurses, Midwives and Health Visitors Act 1979: Elizabeth II*, Available from: <www.legislation.gov.uk/ukpga/1979/36/pdfs/ukpga_19790036_en.pdf> [Accessed 19 January 2019].

Habermann M and Uys L (eds.) (2005) *The Nursing Process: A global concept*. London: Churchill Livingstone.

Hamblett C and Deverson J (1964) *Generation X*. London: Gibbs.

Hart C (2004) *Nurses and Politics: The Impact of Power and Practice*. Houndmills: Palgrave.

Hobsbawm E (1978) The Forward March of Labour Halted? *Marxism Today*, September, 279–286, Available from: <www.amielandmelburn.org.uk/collections/mt/pdf/78_09_hobsbawm.pdf> [Accessed 19 January 2019].

Iley K (2004) Occupational Changes in Nursing: The Situation of Enrolled Nurses, *Journal of Advanced Nursing, 45*(4): 360–370.

Jolly U (1997) *The First Year Nurse Tutor: A qualitative study*. Dinton: Quay.

Kalisch PA and Kalisch BJ (1987) *The Changing Image of the Nurse*. Wokingham: Addison Wesley.

Kerr A and Sachdev S (1992) Third among Equals: An Analysis of the 1989 Ambulance Dispute, *British Journal of Industrial Relations, 30*(1): 127–143.

LeClair K, White J and Keeter S (2007) *Three 19th-century Women Doctors: Elizabeth Blackwell, Mary Walker and Sarah Loguen Fraser*. New York: Hofmann Press.

Leigh J, Monk J, Rutherford J, Windle J and Neville L (2002) What is the Future of the Lecturer Practitioner Role – a Decade on? *Nurse Education in Practice, 2*(3): 208–215.

Mann T (1967) *Memoirs*. London: MacGibbon and Kee Ltd.

Marcuse H (1964) *One Dimensional Man*. London: Sphere.

Martin L (1989) *Clinical Education in Perspective*. Harrow: Scutari.

Marx K, and Engels F (1845) The German Ideology [selections] in Wooton, D. (Ed.) (1996) *Modern Political Thought: Readings from Machiavelli to Nietzsche*. Cambridge: Hackett. 775.

McNaught E (1957) Clinical Instruction, *Nursing Times Occasional Paper, 54*: 53–58.

Menzies IEP (1960) A Case Study in the Functioning of Social Systems as a Defence against Anxiety: A Report on a Study of the Nursing Service of a General Hospital, *Human Relations, 13*(2): 95–121.

Mill JS (1869) The Subjection of Women in Wooton, D. (Ed.) (1996) *Modern Political Thought: Readings from Machiavelli to Nietzsche*. Cambridge: Hackett. 652.

Ministry of Health Board of Education (1939) *Inter-departmental Committee on Nursing Services (Athlone report)*. London: HMSO.

Ministry of Health, Department of Health for Scotland and Ministry of Labour and National Service (1947) *Report of the Working Party on the Recruitment and Training of Nurses (Wood report)*. London: HMSO.

Ministry of Health, Scottish Home and Health Department (1966) *Report of the Committee on Senior Nursing Staff (Salmon report)*. London: HMSO.

Morris B (1998) *Nurses in the NHS, Hansard House of Lords Debates 16 Jun 1998, HL 180616-26*. London: HMSO. Available from: <www.publications.parliament.uk/pa/ld199798/ldhansrd/vo980616/text/80616-26.htm> [Accessed 31 December 2017].

Nightingale F (1898) *Notes on Nursing: What It Is, and What It Is Not*, [Project Gutenberg EBook] Available from: <www.gutenberg.org/files/12439/12439-8.txt> [Accessed 12 January 2019].

Nightingale F (1914) *Florence Nightingale to her Nurses: A selection from Miss Nightingale's addresses to probationers and nurses of the Nightingale School at St. Thomas's Hospital*. London: MacMillan.

Nursing and Midwifery Council (2006) *Standards to Support Learning and Assessment in Practice*. London: NMC.

Nursing and Midwifery Council (2017a) *NMC Announces Radical Overhaul of Nursing Education*, Available from: <www.nmc.org.uk/news/press-releases/nmc-announces-radical-overhaul-of-nursing-education/> [Accessed 30 December 2017].

Nursing and Midwifery Council (2017b) *Programme of Change for Education*, Available from: <www.nmc.org.uk/education/programme-of-change-for-education> [Accessed 31 December 2017].

Nursing Times (1950) Nurses Act, 1949: Its educational scope and potentialities, *Nursing Times, 46*(27): 707–709.

O'Bryne K (1990) PREPP: Linking Study, Education and Practice, *Nursing Standard, 5*(7): 16–17.

O'Dowd A (2004) 'Too Posh to Wash' Motion Dismissed Convincingly, *Nursing Times, 100*(20): 5.

Pribicevic B (1959) *The Shop Stewards' Movement and Workers' Control: 1910 – 1922*. Oxford: Blackwell.

Rideout E (2000) *Transforming Nursing Education through Problem-Based Learning*. Sudbury: Jones and Bartlett.

Rosenberg C (1987) *1919: Britain on the Brink of Revolution*. London: Bookmarks.

Rowan P, Barber P (2000) Clinical Facilitators a New Way of Working, *Nursing Standard, 14*(52): 35–38.

Samuel R, Thompson P (eds.) (1990) *The Myths We Live By*. London: Routledge.

Scottish Home and Health Department (1963) *Experimental Nurse Training at Glasgow Royal Infirmary*. Edinburgh: HMSO.

Seacole M (1857) *The Wonderful Adventures of Mrs Seacole in Many Lands*. London: Blackwood's London Library.

Seymer LR (1957) *A General History of Nursing*. London: Faber and Faber.

Sprinks J (2015) Call for Support and Standardising of Clinical Nurse Educator's Role, *Nursing Standard*, *30*(3): 11.

The Guardian (2019) *Harold Shipman the Guardian*, [online] Available from: <www.guardian.co.uk/uk/shipman> [Accessed 19 January 2019].

The Lancet (1932) The Lancet Commission On Nursing, *The Lancet*, *219*(5663): 585–588, Available from: <https://doi.org/10.1016/S0140-6736(00)91039-0> [Accessed 12 January 2019].

United Kingdom Central Council for Nursing, Midwifery and Health Visiting (1986) *Project 2000: A New Preparation for Practice*. London: UKCC.

United Kingdom Central Council for Nursing, Midwifery and Health Visiting (1988) *Position Paper on the Development of the Support Worker Role*. London: UKCC.

United Kingdom Central Council for Nursing, Midwifery and Health Visiting (1990) *The Report of the Post-Registration Education and Practice Project*. London: UKCC.

United Kingdom Central Council for Nursing, Midwifery and Health Visiting (1994) *The Future of Professional Practice- The Council's Standards for Education and Practice Following Education*. London: UKCC.

United Kingdom Central Council for Nursing, Midwifery and Health Visiting (1995) PREP and You – Your Questions Answered, *Register*, *16*: 4–5.

United Kingdom Central Council for Nursing, Midwifery and Health Visiting (1999) *Fitness for practice: The UKCC Commission for Nursing and Midwifery Education*. London: UKCC.

Wade T (2018) Too Posh to Wash? *RCN Students*, Autumn/Winter 18/19: 10–11Available from: <www.rcn.org.uk/-/media/royal-college-of-nursing/documents/bulletins/2018/students-autumn-winter-2018.pdf> [Accessed 12 January 2019].

Walker Seaback W (2000) *Nursing process: Concepts and application*. Florence: Delmar.

Whitehead B (1997) The Goldfish and the Revolutionary Anti-Poll Tax Campaign: Derby Student Nurses Against the Poll Tax, [unpublished dissertation], Ruskin College Oxford.

Whitehead B (2010) Will Graduate Entry Free Nursing from the Shackles of Class and Gender Oppression? *Nursing Times*, *106*(21): 19–22.

Whitehead B and Allibone L (2014) *Britain's First National Network for Clinical Nurse Educators has been Launched*. Available from: <www.derby.ac.uk/cnenet> [Accessed 12 January 2019].

Whitehead B, Owen P, Henshaw L, Beddingham E and Simmons M (2016) Supporting Newly Qualified Nurse Transition: A Case Study in a UK Hospital, *Nurse Education Today*, *36*: 58–63.

Wilson H (1963) The White Heat of Technology in Hill P. (Ed.) (1996) *Great Political Speeches: Lloyd George, Hugh Gaitskell, Harold Wilson, Nye Bevan, Margaret Thatcher, Tony Benn, Winston Churchill, Neil Kinnock Audiobook*. London: Hodder & Stoughton Audio Books.

Wollstonecraft M (1792) *A Vindication of the Rights of Woman*, [Project Gutenberg EBook] Available from: <www.gutenberg.org/ebooks/3420> [Accessed 13 January 2019].

2

NURSING EDUCATION IN AUSTRALIA

Margaret McAllister, Katrina Campbell and Colleen Ryan

About Australia

In 2019, according to the United Nations estimates, the Australian population reached 25 million. While a vast land mass – the world's largest island, and the sixth largest country after Russia, Canada, China, Brazil and the USA – the continent of Australia has many parts that are sparsely populated because of its arid climate. Indeed, 35% of Australia receives so little rain it is effectively desert. As a result, most of the population lives along the coastline in urban areas, particularly the large cities such as Melbourne, Sydney, Brisbane and Perth.

The country of Australia has been inhabited for over 50,000 years. It became a British colony in 1788, and a Federation in 1901 – with the right to govern in its own right. At this time, Australia was referred to as the *Commonwealth of Australia*. The federation still consists of six states and two territories. Indigenous Australians, who comprise about 4% of the population, are the Aboriginal and Torres Strait Islander peoples who are descended from groups that existed in Australia and surrounding islands before this colonisation. At the time of European settlement, over 250 languages were spoken. Today, about half these languages remain, as a result of an explicit policy of cultural assimilation (Langton, 2018). This attempt to erase Aboriginal and Torres Strait Islander culture has resulted in much grief and loss for the original Australians and there continue to be social and health disparities that result in unacceptably high morbidity and early death that need to be resolved (Pascoe, 2018).

Nursing in Australia

It is estimated that there are over 360,000 registered nurses and midwives in Australia (Australian Institute of Health and Welfare, 2016). Of these, about 260,000 were registered as a registered nurse only, 60,000 were registered as an enrolled nurse (EN) only and 3,600 were registered as a midwife only. The Australian Health Practitioner Regulation Agency (AHPRA) is the regulatory body. Approximately 90% of registered nurses are female. Amongst midwifery, the figure is even higher, at 98%.

Because Australia was a British colony, the modern system of nursing closely parallels that British history, with some important differences. The first nurses to be employed in Australian hospitals were reformed convict women, when the Sydney Infirmary first opened in 1811. Just 50 years after colonisation, in 1839 five Irish Sisters of Charity arrived to provide nursing care to convicts in the female factory at Paramatta in Sydney (Bessant, 1999). Despite this, the standard and reach of care were not considered acceptable, prompting medical officers to request that more nurses be trained and the care extended (Yuginovich, 2000).

Twenty years later the New South Wales Governor, Henry Parkes, wrote to Florence Nightingale requesting her assistance to reform nursing and improve the standard of care provided to Australian patients. Nightingale sent a small group of newly trained nurses to institute the Nightingale training system throughout Australia. Lucy Osburn, who was among this group, was appointed as the first Lady Superintendent of the Sydney Infirmary and dispensary – what would later become known as Sydney Hospital (Godden & Helmstadter, 2009). Osburn and her colleagues were tasked with reforming the Sydney Infirmary over a period of 3 years, which included providing adequate training for nurses. Ms Osburn and her colleagues were appointed as matrons by Governor Parkes, with the idea for all nurses to be trained at the Sydney Infirmary and then move to country locations to then train prospective trainees for rural and remote locations (Yuginovich, 2000). Osburn is regarded as the founder of modern nursing in Australia (Godden, 2006).

The Nightingale training system comprised an approach for women to: learn nursing skills, raise the quality of care provided to patients and institute more order and discipline amongst nurses so that standards of care could be instituted. According to McDonald (2010), Nightingale never explicitly documented this method of training, but it consisted of:

- nursing skills development
- raising the status and comportment of nurses, including the maintenance of modest and practical uniforms
- a requirement that all nurses be trained in a civilian (not military) hospital, so that they would see a broad range of clinical issues and develop a strong set of skills
- apprentice-style learning, where students worked in the wards under the guidance of the ward sister
- classroom learning provided by medical doctors
- decent working conditions, including provision of a probationer's home, hot meals, adequate bathing and toileting facilities and a home-like atmosphere
- supervision from a trained nurse
- certificates of nursing completion, which were time-limited.

This system of learning was instituted at hospitals such as the Sydney Infirmary, the Alfred Hospital in Melbourne, the Brisbane Infirmary, Adelaide and Perth Colonial Hospitals and the Gladesville Hospital for the Insane (McDonald, 2010).

As Australia continued to develop and regional centres were established, district nurses were required. Thus, in 1885 district nursing, modelled on the English system, was established and by 1904, the Melbourne district nursing service was seeing nearly 1,000 patients and making 28,000 visits in 1 year (Bessant, 1999). With the increasing need for nursing services came an increased need for more rigorous training and education.

Accreditation, regulation and registration

As nursing developed within Australia, there was a recognition for the need to set minimum standards to ensure quality of hospital apprenticeship-type training and quality of nursing care. The first professional organisations were the Victorian Trained Nurses Association and the Australian Trained Nurses Association, which lobbied to introduce standardisation of nursing training within hospitals and were responsible for the introduction of a register for trained nurses (Lusk, Russell, Rodgers, & Wilson-Barnett, 2001).

Throughout the 20th century, each state had its own regulatory body for nursing registration until 2010 when the nationally focused Nursing and Midwifery Board of Australia (NMBA) was established. The NMBA implements policies and laws, such as professional standards and codes of practice which regulate nursing. AHPRA is the national organisation that all health professionals use to register themselves annually and to declare they meet the requirements for currency to practise.

Separate nursing specialisation certificates, which operated as licence to practise in specialty areas, were instituted. For example, in New South Wales, six specialty nursing certificates included General, Psychiatric, Geriatric, Mental retardation, Midwifery and Mothercraft. These specialty areas were adopted across each of the states and territories, although some offered other specialties (Lusk et al., 2001).

The Australian Nursing and Midwifery Accreditation Council (ANMAC), established in 1992, holds a crucial role in the accreditation of nursing and midwifery education programmes (Ralph, Birks, & Chapman, 2015). ANMAC oversees the accreditation of approximately 480 programmes of study within nursing that are offered across approximately 160 Australian educational institutions spanning the two tertiary education sectors – higher education and vocational training (Ralph et al., 2015).

Nursing education in Australia

State processes for training and accreditation continued until the 1960s. Around this time – with the world-wide influence of feminism and social justice movements – nursing within Australia was motivated by a renewed impetus to politicise and professionally develop, particularly in regard to access to tertiary education, which was considered the main way for nursing to emancipate.

In line with achieving equity in education, on a par with other health professions, nursing organisations lobbied hard for nurses in training to be able to access tertiary education. The arguments were to retain the hospital-based apprenticeship model, to transfer the education into colleges of advanced education (vocational training/diploma) or to completely transfer all training to university level (Lusk et al., 2001). Despite resistance and concern, in the 1980s Australia's education system for nursing shifted towards diploma-based training in tertiary institutions.

The national shift from hospital-based training to the higher education sector began in 1984 when the federal government announced its support to transfer nurse training from hospital-based to colleges of advanced education (Lusk et al., 2001). A later decision made by the Australian Education Council suggested that training to acquire a nursing qualification should be upgraded from a diploma to a bachelor's degree (Lusk et al., 2001). A subsequent target was set for all nursing programmes in the higher education sector to reach degree level by 1992, which was achieved in 1994 (Ralph et al., 2015). Thus, within Australia, all entry to practise nursing programmes are offered via the tertiary education sector. It is the education department within government that oversees the sector and there needs to be close interaction between departments of health and education for this system of education and training to work effectively.

Contemporary issues in Australian nursing education

Australian nursing education is faced with similar challenges to other countries. Along with grappling with wicked social and healthcare issues within the community, such as the rising prevalence of non-communicable diseases related to life-style, dementia and mental health problems (Hannigan & McAllister, 2019), there are problems affecting nursing which remain unresolved: gender inequity, horizontal and vertical violence, burnout, time students spend in clinical placement, cost of clinical placements and the ideological divide between tertiary providers and health organisations (Huston, 2013).

Specifically, the long-standing challenges of the ageing workforce and workforce shortage require urgent and thoughtful discussion. There are also issues impacting Australian nursing education, leadership, resilience, marginalisation of speciality nursing workforces and the readiness to engage with the digital revolution impacting healthcare.

Ageing workforce and workforce shortages

Australia has an ageing nursing workforce. We also have a shortage in workforce that has been described as severe. By 2030, the shortfall is projected to be 130,000 (HWA, 2014). Nurses, employers of nurses and education organisations need to consider two contemporary debates: the Australian Government considering increasing the general retirement age in 2035 to 70 and the fact that two in every five Australian nurses are aged over 50 (Australian Institute of Health, 2016). An ageing workforce is cause for concern because these workers themselves are at risk of injury (to staff and patients) and because the profession is deprived of a young workforce that offers vitality and growth.

At the same time, when older nurses eventually retire, they take with them many years of nursing knowledge and practical experience, thus affecting skill mix. In 2012, Health Workforce Australia recommended employers work to retain the existing older nurse workforce, thereby reducing predicted nursing shortages by 82%. Innovations to support older workers include reducing their workload and introducing flexible working hours (Duffield et al., 2015).

Employers of older nurses and nursing education providers need to work together to ensure older nurses are able to work to their full scope of practice, have access to appropriate professional development and are supported to remain physically and mentally fit and healthy. Recruitment and retention of older nurses in geographically diverse communities are also essential to supply experienced nursing staff able to work independently and in isolation (Warburton, 2016). Employment, education and utilisation of assistants in nursing and multidisciplinary teams to balance a skilled healthcare workforce should also be considered. Combining these strategies could potentially reduce the severity of the nursing shortage.

The digital revolution in health

Across the world, technological solutions to health and healthcare issues are being avidly pursued, and richly funded, by governments, businesses and private individuals. These include robotics, artificial intelligence, genetic engineering, nanotechnology and virtual reality. While these developments bring the promise of new and more effective ways to understand, manage and prevent diseases and disorders (Mesko, 2018), there are barriers to its uptake because gatekeepers are afraid of technology, poorly trained in its use, or not willing to supervise and control its uptake (Boys et al., 2016). There is, therefore, a need for ongoing education at universities, within the workplace and to the public to address concerns and increase familiarity with robots.

As the use of robots increases within healthcare, there is the potential for the development of dehumanised and depersonalised workplaces, where empathy, ethics, compassion, diplomacy and personal considerations may be overlooked in favour of automation and efficiency (Krol & Lavoie, 2014). Given that dehumanised environments are already of concern in today's highly technical healthcare environment, it is vital that these issues be given serious consideration, for the presence of robots is likely to exacerbate this perception (Gionet, 2017). Ethical concerns and safety also need to be considered in relation to non-human-to-human relationships between nurses, patients and robots as they become more common (Fuji et al., 2011). In the future students may find themselves tending more to machines than to patients (Gionet, 2017) – although, arguably, this is already the case. As Barnard and Sandelowski (2001), argue, the responsibility is on nurses to articulate an ethic of care that integrates technology as a basic part of nursing work. It needs to be sensitively and safely incorporated into patient care. If robots were to malfunction, then nurses need to be prepared and competent to respond promptly (Fuji et al., 2011). A future for nursing in which robotics and technology work become routine will require the revision and rewriting of nursing competency standards.

Leadership

Constraints that stand in the way of nurses providing safe and effective patient care, causing moral distress and burnout and being ignored at the policy table, could be overcome if nurses develop and practise expert leadership skills as students. Clinical leadership skills are important for all nurses to learn, because they often lead or participate in small clinical teams. Thus, all students need to learn how to draw upon clinical expertise and knowledge to drive and lead reform (Stanley, Blanchard, Hohol, Hutton, & McDonald, 2017). Cleary, Horsfall and Jackson (2013) suggest that the curriculum should emphasise leadership skills such as: self-reflection, lateral and critical thinking, public speaking and writing, technological and systems competence, ability to engage with diverse people and system networks, mentorship and global awareness.

Resilience

Stress and experiences of adversity are unfortunately common in nursing, and these issues appear to be rising as the nature of healthcare becomes more complex, and resources tighter (Khamisa, Peltzer, & Oldenburg, 2013). An important asset for nurses in being prepared for challenging health environments, not just for themselves but for the benefit of patients who may also be overwhelmed by their surrounds, is the concept of resilience. Resilience is the positive adjustment to adversity and is characterised by the ability to tolerate stress, use flexible coping styles, to think optimistically and to find ways to transcend suffering (McAllister & Brien, 2019).

Consequently, an important responsibility for educators is to develop nursing students' knowledge of resilience, as well as professional and personal strengths, so that they are equipped with strategies to share resilience with patients and colleagues. Developing a confident, proud identity can build self-belief and a calm demeanour under stress (King, Newman, & Luthans, 2016). Therefore, discussions of positive role models in nursing, and inclusion of nursing history so that students can see how far nursing has developed and what obstacles have already been overcome, can develop a sense of social connectedness and belonging. Asking students what they believe in, what their aims are and what they intend to contribute to the world are all strategies to develop a sense of professional commitment and optimism.

It is also vital that students are responsibly prepared for the reality of the stressors and potential for adversity that are common within complex health systems. One way to do this is to include resilience in the curriculum and to engage students in reflection-for-practice. This involves prompting students to consider and brainstorm questions such as the following:

1. What strengths and supports can I draw upon to help me during stressful times at work?
2. What coping skills have I used effectively in the past to cope with stressful situations? How can I extend my repertoire?
3. What am I likely to encounter in hospitals and health centres that I need to be prepared for?
4. What can I do when I am on clinical placement that may help to contribute to a happy, collaborative atmosphere amongst the team?

Rather than think of resilience as the ability to bounce back to where you once were when faced with adversity, resilience can be thought of as a set of skills that include cognitive flexibility, optimism, stress hardiness and group connection.

Providing high-quality access to healthcare for all within Australia

Another contemporary issue facing countries like Australia is the goal of providing quality healthcare for all, despite geographical and other barriers. This is a main reason for the introduction of the nurse practitioner (NP) role in Australia as well as other specialty roles, such as breast-care and palliative care nurses.

The NP movement, which began in the United States in the 1960s, was introduced in Australia in the 1990s (Australian College of Nurse Practitioners, 2019). It is designed to fill a service gap, particularly the medical practitioner shortages in rural and remote Australia, and to meet the demands for a required specialised and advanced practice nursing workforce (Gardner & Gardner, 2005). NPs complete higher education to allow them to work independently to diagnose people of all ages, implement appropriate therapeutic interventions, prescribe medications and order diagnostics. Introduction of the role has been gradual and challenging because originally access to subsidised health funding for patients was restricted and community awareness-raising strategies to introduce the benefits and scope of the role were slow to be implemented. Now the role is gaining more popularity, mainly in part to the introduction of legislation in 2010 to overcome restrictions to practise. A recent Australian Government initiative aims to further support uptake of the role through raising Australian healthcare consumers and professionals' awareness of the benefits and capabilities of NPs (Boase, 2019).

Another sub-speciality that is developing in Australia is breast care nurses (BCNs).

Breast care specialist nurses

BCNs were introduced in Australia to care specifically for women diagnosed with breast cancer. Ahern and Gardner (2015) studied the role and reported positive valuations from women for timely and appropriate referrals; BCNs are welcomed because they understand a woman's perspective; BCN can offer specific treatment options. Despite these positive evaluations the authors noted service-users reported inconsistent access and few consumers and healthcare providers were aware of the capabilities of a BCN. BCNs were intended to work in urban, rural, remote and geographically diverse areas in Australia; however, few studies were set in geographically diverse locations. Lack of evidence may place this essential role at risk, at great loss to rural and remote communities.

Palliative care nurses are another developing speciality, partly because the role will soon require change.

Palliative care nursing

In June 2019, Australia legislated the first voluntary assisted dying bill, causing inevitable challenges to health organisations and nursing education providers. Evidence from other countries demonstrates an increase in the need for nursing palliative care services following introduction of voluntary assisted dying laws (O'Connor, 2017). Currently the legislation provides no formal guidelines for palliative care nurses, and the general nursing population, around responsibilities for providing care to patients who meet criteria for a voluntary assisted death. It is now urgent that nursing education providers and health organisations develop and offer ethical, moral, humane and compassionate undergraduate and postgraduate learning around voluntary assisted dying (Schroeder & Lorenz, 2018). It is important to remember all tiers of Australian nurses will need to access this education.

Renewed support for enrolled nursing

An important cost-saving approach for maintaining the workforce within health is the use of assistants-in-nursing (AINs). This level of nursing was originally introduced into aged care nursing. Now AINs are employed in a variety of healthcare organisations. ENs, the second tier of Australian nurses, provide another solution to the workforce shortage. In higher-acuity healthcare settings, ENs are trained to provide bedside nursing care, under the guidance and supervision of registered nurses. In other settings ENs practise in advanced roles such as independently performing wound care (Nankervis, Kenny, & Bish, 2008).

Currently recruitment of ENs is hampered by costly course fees that are often required up front. This impost stands in the way of resolving the severe nursing workforce shortage, and denies the reality that the gendered nature of nursing means that most students will carry the burden of family care, study and then a career that is not highly paid.

An issue that may assist in the resolution of this crisis is that nurse–patient ratios have become impossible to ignore (NSWNMA, 2018).

Nurse–patient ratios

Thanks to the sustained work of Aiken et al. (2010), there is global evidence to clearly show that a ratio of one nurse to four patients is associated with patient safety, staff retention and reduced burnout. Aiken's work indicates that, when nurses are allocated two patients less than other nurses, they report greater satisfaction with their work, and managers reported reduction in patient mortality. A later study demonstrated that a 7% reduction in patient mortality occurred from a 10% increase in employment of nurses with a degree (Aiken et al., 2014). This is an important contemporary discussion.

Nurse patient ratios range from 1:4 or 1:7 in most Australian states and are mandated for public hospitals and some aged care facilities, with other organisations adopting profit-driven care models (Olley, Edwards, Avery, & Cooper, 2019). Olley et al. (2019) recommend that more research that is country- and context-specific is required.

Conclusion

While developments in Australian nursing have paralleled those in Britain and the USA, there have been significant developments that have uniquely shaped the profession. The national transfer of nursing education from hospitals to the tertiary sector that occurred in the 1990s heralded a paradigm shift. National bodies exist that separate regulation, registration and quality control of the nursing curriculum. Global advancements, such as the emergence of the NP, and nurse–patient ratios, have been acknowledged and appropriated within Australia to suit needs. Australia is also not immune from global problems, including healthcare inequities that particularly impact upon vulnerable communities and the nursing shortage. Contemporary challenges such as the digital revolution, violence, managerialism and ongoing marginalisation of nursing are some of the pressing concerns facing Australian nursing education. Despite these challenges, the nursing profession has solidified its position within the healthcare industry and will continue to develop to meet the ever-changing needs of society to ensure the provision of high-quality care.

References

Ahern T & Gardner A (2015) Literature review: An exploration of the role of the Australian breast care nurse in the provision of information and supportive care. *Collegian* 22(1): 99–108.

Aiken L, Sloane D, Cimiotti J, Clarke S, Flynn L, Seago J … Smith H (2010) Implications of the California nurse staffing mandate for other states. *Health Services Research* 45(4): 904–921.

Aiken L, Sloane H, Bruyneel DM, Van den Heede L, Griffiths K … Sermeus W (2014) Nurse staffing and education and hospital mortality in nine European countries: A retrospective observational study. *Lancet* 383: 1824–1830.

Australian College of Mental Health Nursing (2016) *A national framework for postgraduate mental health nursing education.* Accessed at: www.acmhn.org/images/stories/Resources/NationalFramework2016.pdf

Australian College of Nurse Practitioners (2019) History of nurse practitioners. Accessed at: www.acnp.org.au/history

Australian Institute of Health and Welfare (2016) *Nursing and midwifery workforce 2015.* Accessed at: www.aihw.gov.au/reports/workforce/nursing-and-midwifery-workforce-2015/contents/who-are-nurses-and-midwives.

Barnard A & Sandelowski M (2001) Technology and humane nursing care: (Ir) Reconcilable or invented difference? *Journal of Advanced Nursing* 34(3): 367–375.

Bessant B (1999) Milestones in Australian nursing. *Collegian* 6(4): i–iii.

Boase L (2019) Nurse practitioners - Transforming health care across Australia. *The Journal for Nurse Practitioners* 15(1): 146.

Boys J, Alicuben E, Demeester M, Worrell S, Oh D, Hagen J & Demeester S (2016) Public perceptions on robotic surgery, hospitals with robots, and surgeons that use them. *Surgical Endoscopy* 30(4): 1310–1316.

Cleary M, Horsfall J & Jackson D (2013) Commentary: Professional mental health nursing bodies: Issues relevant to leadership within and beyond. *Contemporary Nurse: A Journal for the Australian Nursing Profession* 43(2): 257–259.

Duffield C, Graham E, Donoghue J, Griffiths R, Bichel-Findlay J & Dimitrelis S (2015) Workforce shortages and retention of older nurses. *Australian Nursing and Midwifery Journal* 22(7): 18–19.

Fuji S, Date M, Nagai Y, Yasuhara Y, Tanioka T & Ren F (2011, November) Research on the possibility of humanoid robots to assist in medical activities in nursing homes and convalescent wards. *(NLP-KE) 7th International Conference on Natural Language Processing and Knowledge Engineering*, 459–463.

Gardner A & Gardner G (2005) A trial of nurse practitioner scope of practice. *Journal of Advanced Nursing* 49(2): 135–145.

Gionet K (2017). Nurses of the future must embrace high-tech. *The Conversation.* November 20.

Godden J (2006) *Lucy Osburn, a Lady Displaced: Florence Nightingale's Envoy to Australia.* Sydney: Sydney University Press.

Godden J & Helmstadter C (2009) Conflict and costs when reforming nursing: The introduction of Nightingale nursing in Australia and Canada. *Journal of Clinical Nursing* 18(19): 2692-2699.

Hannigan B & McAllister M (2019) The wicked global problems facing nursing. In M McAllister and D L Brien (Eds.) *Empowerment Strategies for Nurses: Developing Resilience in Practice.* New York: Springer. 43-57.

Health Workforce Australia HWA (2014) *Australia's Future Health Workforce – Nurses.* Accessed at: www.health.gov.au

Huston C J (2013) *Professional Issues in Nursing: Challenges and Opportunities.* Philadelphia: Lippincott Williams & Wilkins.

Khamisa N, Peltzer K & Oldenburg B (2013) Burnout in relation to specific contributing factors and health outcomes among nurses: A systematic review. *International Journal of Environmental Research and Public Health* 10(6): 2214–2240.

King D D, Newman A, & Luthans F (2016) Not if, but when we need resilience in the workplace. *Journal of Organizational Behavior* 37(5): 782–786.

Langton M (2018) *Welcome to Country: A Travel Guide to Indigenous Australia.* Melbourne: Explore Australia.

Lusk B, Russell R, Rodgers J & Wilson-Barnett J (2001) Preregistration nursing education in Australia, New Zealand, the United Kingdom, and the United States of America. *Journal of Nursing Education* 40(5): 197–202.

McAllister M & Brien D (2019) *Empowerment Strategies for Nurses: Developing Resilience in Practice.* New York: Springer.

McDonald L (2010) *The nightingale system of training.* Conference paper, American Association for the History of Nursing and European Nursing History Group. Accessed at: www.uoguelph.ca/~cwfn/nursing/nightingale-system-of-training.htm

Mesko B (2018) Health IT and digital health: The future of health technology is diverse. *Journal of Clinical and Translational Research* 3(Suppl 3): 431.

Nankervis K, Kenny A & Bish M (2008) Enhancing scope of practice for the second level nurse: A change process to meet growing demand for rural health services. *Contemporary Nurse* 29(2): 159–173.

New South Wales Nursing and Midwifery Association [NSWNMA] (2018) *Projected nursing shortages must be taken seriously.* Accessed at: www.nswnma.asn.au

O'Connor N (2017) Voluntary assisted death: A poignant clinical dilemma. *Australian Nursing and Midwifery Journal* 25(5): 33. Accessed at: www.anmf.org.au

Olley R, Edwards I, Avery M & Cooper H (2019) Systematic review of the evidence related to mandated nurse staffing ratios in acute hospitals. *Australian Health Review: A Publication of the Australian Hospital Association* 43: 288–293.

Pascoe B (2018) *The Little Red Yellow Black Book: An Introduction to Indigenous Australia* (4th Ed). Canberra: Aboriginal Studies Press.

Ralph N, Birks M & Chapman Y (2015) The accreditation of nursing education in Australia. *Collegian* 22(1): 3–7.

Schroeder K & Lorenz K (2018) Nursing and the future of palliative care. *Asia-Pacific Journal of Oncology Nursing* 5(1): 4–8.

Stanley D, Blanchard D, Hohol A, Hutton M & McDonald A (2017) Health professionals' perceptions of clinical leadership. A pilot study. *Cogent Medicine* 4(1): 1321193.

Warburton J (2016) Extrinsic and intrinsic factors impacting on the retention of older rural health care workers in the north Victorian public sector: A qualitative study. *Rural Remote Health* 14(3): 2721.

Yuginovich T (2000) A potted history of 19th-century remote-area nursing in Australia and, in particular, Queensland. *The Australian Journal of Rural Health* 8(2): 63.

3

HISTORY OF NURSING EDUCATION IN THE UNITED STATES

Sandra B. Lewenson and Annemarie McAllister

Introduction

This chapter begins with the start of the modern nursing movement when the first Nightingale-influenced training schools opened in the United States in 1873. It then explores the development of professional nursing organizations that sought control of both the practice and the education of nurses during the first half of the twentieth century. The early efforts to move nursing education from under the auspices of hospitals and the need for specialized courses for administrators, teachers, and public health nurses led to the introduction of nursing education at Teachers College, Columbia University in New York City. Since 1899, Teachers College graduates have contributed to the development of nursing education around the world. This chapter also includes the ongoing struggle of black nurses to break down racial barriers they faced both in the south by law and in the north by customary practice. The rise of black schools of nursing and the historically black institutions of higher learning adds to this history.

Of importance to the history of nursing education includes the early twentieth-century to mid twentieth-century nursing reports. The report, *Nursing and Nursing Education in the United States* (Goldmark, 1923/1984). published in 1923, commonly referred to as the Goldmark Report, focused on public health nursing and then all of nursing education. The *Future for Nursing: A Report Prepared for the National Nursing Council* (Brown, 1948), commonly referred to as the Brown Report, followed in 1948 and recommended changes to the way nurses were educated in the US and the assurance of the quality of these schools through an accreditation oversight. The Brown Report called for an increase in the diversity of nurses, including more men and women of color, as well as moving nursing education out of diploma training schools affiliated with hospitals into universities and colleges.

By 1952 nursing reorganized the structures of the professional organizations strengthening nursing's resolve to assure a better-educated nurse workforce reflective of a growing diverse population. Nursing leaders like R. Louise McManus, Chair of the Department of Nursing Education at Teachers College, and Mildred Montag, who designed an educational model for a two-year associate degree program, led a tsunami-like change in the way nurses were and still are educated. They took nursing programs out of the hospital and into community colleges throughout the United States. The time following World War II was ripe for change and nursing was poised to make that change.

This chapter continues through the 1960s when nursing responded to the changing social, political, and economic environment over the years. Civil rights and the women's movement of the 1960s and early 1970s impacted nursing practice and subsequently its educational format. The 1960s, a hallmark of social change in America, led to increasing numbers of baccalaureate degree programs, the origination of the nurse practitioner movement, and master's and higher degree programs. This chapter, although it ends around the 1960s, includes a final section on the state of nursing education today and what we might see in the foreseeable future.

The modern nursing movement in the United States

The history of nursing education in the United States often begins with the opening of Nightingale-influenced training schools in 1873. This post-Civil War history renders a starting point for a more complicated and nuanced history of women, work, and the development of a caring profession. Prior to the influence of Florence Nightingale, the Woman's Hospital of Philadelphia, for example, had opened to care and provide health education for women in need and to provide the training experiences on the wards for nursing and medical students (D'Antonio, 2010).[1] Graduates of this program provided the foundation for the Nightingale-influenced schools that opened in 1873 at Bellevue Hospital in New York City, New Haven Hospital in Connecticut, and Massachusetts General Hospital in Boston, Massachusetts. Trained nurses were needed to work with physicians in applying the science of the day to clinical practice. D'Antonio (2010) argues that "modern nursing was born in the mutually constructive process of women seeking medical knowledge and physician seeking knowledgeable women" (p. 3). Another one of the earliest pre-Nightingale-influenced training schools to open was the New England Hospital for Women and Children in 1872. Notable graduates from this early school of nursing included Linda Richards (1841–1930), who became the first president of the American Society of Superintendents for Training Schools of Nurses, and Mary Mahoney (1848–1962), considered one of the first black graduates of a training school for nurses (Lewenson, 1993; American Association for the History of Nursing Website, 2019).

Florence Nightingale (1820–1910) achieved worldwide fame that spread from England to the United States. Her work in the Crimean War (1853–1856), where she provided care to wounded soldiers and improved the poor sanitary conditions found in the military hospitals, provided a framework for her future vision in nursing. Her use of statistical pie graphs demonstrated the decrease in morbidity and mortality rates of the soldiers after instituting her vision of nursing care. Following her success, she returned to England, where she received a hero's welcome and funding to start the St. Thomas School of Nursing. This school of nursing served as a model that later influenced nursing education throughout the world, including the United States. Nightingale's (1859/1946) well-received publication of *Notes on Nursing: What it Is, and What it Is Not* expanded on her work in the Crimea and linked the high morbidity rates of hospitals with the lack of sanitary conditions. Trained nurses, she conceived, would alter these conditions and provide a safer place for those who entered. While not alone in her thinking, Nightingale's biographer Sir Edward T. Cook (1913) wrote that she was "the founder of modern nursing because she made public opinion perceive, and act upon the perception, that nursing was an art, and must be raised to the status of a trained profession" (p. 445).

31

Nightingale-influenced training schools

One of the first Nightingale-influenced training schools to open was at New York City's municipal hospital, Bellevue. Louisa Lee Schuyler (1837–1926), noted for her work during the Civil War (1861–1865), organized a Visiting Committee, which was a subcommittee of the New York Charities Aid Association, to study the conditions at Bellevue hospital (Roberts, 1954). Witnessing the overcrowding and poor conditions at Bellevue, the Visiting Committee recommended a school of nursing be established to improve hospital conditions. W. Gill Wylie, a physician at Bellevue, wrote on behalf of the Visiting Committee to Nightingale seeking advice about starting such an enterprise. Unable to travel due to illness, Nightingale's detailed letter to Wylie speaks to women – specifically nurses – to be responsible for training other women (The Alumnae Association of the Bellevue School of Nursing, 1989). Her recommendations shaped the development of this early training school in the United States, making it one of the premiere diploma schools of nursing in the US until it was phased out in 1967 to make way for a baccalaureate degree in nursing program (Lewenson, 2013).

Throughout the country, hospitals saw the value that nurse-training schools brought to their institutions, making them safer places for physicians to practice. Two other schools that opened in 1873 were the Connecticut Training School for Nurses at the New Haven Hospital in New Haven, Connecticut and the Boston Training School for Nurses at Massachusetts General Hospital in Boston. Schools of nursing opened rapidly, as hospitals saw the economic value of staffing the wards with students. Large hospitals with a variety of cases could offer greater educational opportunities for student nurses in these institutions. But hospitals with fewer beds could not provide sufficient variety in the kinds of cases treated, and as a result left nurses' training lacking in depth and breadth. The inconsistency of training, along with the lack of standards as to who could call themselves a nurse, created a dilemma for the early nursing leaders.

Nursing organizations

Between 1873 and 1893, nurse-training programs opened in hospitals throughout the country. The purpose of educating these women in a profession, however, was often subsumed by the hospitals' need for workers. Hospitals replenished the staff with new students each year, leaving the graduates to find employment as private duty nurses and later as public health nurses. In addition, anyone could call themselves a nurse without ever graduating from a training program. This created problems for both the nurse and the public. Economically, nurses wanted to protect their jobs from uneducated nurses and they wanted to protect the public from those who called themselves a nurse without the training. To address the misuse of these nurses, nursing organizations formed to develop standards for nursing education and practice. Four professional organizations that started between 1893 and 1920 were the American Society of Superintendents of Training Schools for Nurses, the Asosociated Alumnae of the United States and Canada, the National Association of Colored Graduate Nurses (NACGN), and the National Organization of Public Health Nurses (NOPHN). Each organization served as a vehicle in which the constituents could collate power to facilitate the change they sought (Lewenson, 1993). The next sections briefly describe each of these organizations and its purpose.

The American Society of Superintendents of Training School for Nurses

In 1893 a group of 18 superintendents of nursing schools attended the international Nurses Congress, which was a subset of the Hospital and Medical Congress, at the World's Columbian Exposition in Chicago. Isabel Hampton Robb (1860–1910), then superintendent of the Johns Hopkins Hospital in Baltimore, chaired the Nurses Congress and proceeded to organize the American Society of Superintendents of Training Schools for Nurses (ASSTSN). Hampton and the others wanted to assure the quality of both student nurses and the training they would receive. Hospital schools of nursing provided cheap labor for these institutions by using the students as staff (Lewenson, 1993). The ASSTN addressed the education of nurses, renaming itself in 1912 the National League of Nursing Education (NLNE) and then finally in 1952 the National League for Nursing (NLN). It took on the role of developing standards for nursing education reflecting the scientific progress that had taken place to date. Organizing gave nurses a collective voice in which to advocate for the emerging profession of nursing. Sophia Palmer (1853–1920), one of the early pioneer superintendents, spoke to the newly formed membership at their second annual convention in 1895, urging the other schools to establish alumnae associations, as "organization is the power of the age. Without it nothing great is accomplished" (Palmer, 1897/1985, p. 55).

The Associated Alumnae of the United States and Canada

In its early years, the ASSTSN saw the need to protect the practice of the working nurse and urged schools of nursing to form alumnae associations. These associations would become the structure for the second national organization called the Associated Alumnae of the United States and Canada in 1896. Public health nurse and suffragist Lavinia Dock (1858–1956) participated in structuring this organization, fostering the development of school alumnae associations, state associations, and a larger national structure. The Associated Alumnae became the American Nurses Association (ANA) in 1911 and has remained as such throughout its history. Since its inception, the ANA concerned itself with issues relating to professionalizing nursing. This organization focused on developing ethical standards, elevating nursing education, seeking nurse registration legislation in each state, informing the public of the work of nurses, and encouraging collegiality among nurses (Lewenson, 1993).

The National Association of Colored Graduate Nurses

Two other nursing organizations that formed during the first part of the twentieth century were the NACGN in 1908 and the NOPHN in 1912. Each of these organizations grew out of specific needs of nurses. The NACGN addressed similar concerns about education and practice as the NLN and the ANA. Due to the overt and covert racism that pervaded the United States, black nurses found themselves excluded from membership in the ANA in those southern states that prohibited membership in the state nursing associations. Historian Darlene Clark Hine (1989) wrote, "The denial of membership in the national professional nursing association was the most blatant affront to black nurses' self-esteem" (p. 94).

The NACGN formed to respond to the needs of black nurses who were omitted from the organizations forming at the national level, excluded from nurse-training schools, barred from state registration as a result of certain states' discriminatory practices, banned from serving in the American Red Cross (until the end of World War I), and facing unequal pay with their white counterparts. Early nursing leaders like Adah Belle Samuels Thoms (1870–1943), Martha Minerva Franklin (1870–1968), and Mabel Keaton Staupers (1890–1989) fought to raise the standards of the nursing profession while raising the status of the black nurse. Black nurses fought for equal pay and standing as their white counterparts. Educational standards were a high priority and one that led to standards being set in the black training schools of nursing in hospitals and universities. Overcoming racism, a key focus of this organization, led to political advocacy for the rights of black nurses (Hine, 1989; Lewenson, 1993; Threat, 2015). In 1951 members of the NACGN felt they had accomplished many of their goals and voted to dissolve their organization following a vote by the ANA calling for the elimination of discriminatory practices in their organization. Simultaneously the NACGN transferred their membership to the ANA.

The National Organization of Public Health Nurses

The NOPHN organized in 1912 to address the growing needs of the growing specialization known as public health nursing. Lillian Wald (1867–1940), the founder of the Henry Street Settlement on the Lower East Side of New York and the visionary behind the American Red Cross rural nursing service, participated with other nursing leaders, including Lavinia Dock (1858–1956), Mary Sewall Gardner (1861–1971), and Jane Delano (1862–1919), in organizing the NOPHN. This professional organization rose to meet the rapid growth of public health nursing in the United States, and the increasing recognition to provide access to healthcare in the home and community settings. Through a joint committee of the NLN and the ANA, the idea for the NOPHN was born. This organization extended its membership beyond nurses to all parties interested in public health and nursing and permitted black nurses to individually join at the national level (Hine, 1989; Lewenson, 1993). Concern for the education of nurses in this field of nursing was central to their membership. The NOPHN sought to establish postgraduate programs in public health nursing and sought support from the ANA and the NLN leadership to develop these educational programs. Teachers College at Columbia University was one of the first universities to educate nurses at the behest of nurse leaders. It was at Teachers College that one of the early post-graduate programs in public health began in 1910.

Like the other organizations that formed during this period, the NOPHN focused its work on improving educational and professional standards for all public health nurses whether in visiting nurse services, health departments, school nursing, tuberculosis nursing, or occupational health-type settings. The field of public health was expanding, as were the opportunities for nurses to work in these settings situated outside of traditional hospitals and private duty experiences.

Teachers College, Columbia University

Nursing leaders in the NLN, ANA, and NOPHN participated in the development of nursing programs at Teachers College, Columbia University. Mary (M.) Adelaide Nutting (1858–1948), considered to be the first nurse to hold the rank of professor within a university, served on the education committee of the newly formed ASSTSN along with other notable superintendents, including Isabel Hampton Robb (1860–1910) and Linda

Richards (1841–1930). The committee recommended that a year-long course in hospital economics be established within Teachers College to augment the education of graduate nurses. (Graduate nurses were graduates of the two- or three-year diploma hospital-based programs.) They met with Dean James Russell at Teachers College and convinced him of the "seriousness" of their intention to educate nurses to teach and to administer. He agreed a "small experimental group of nurses be admitted to the college, on the condition that the committee should select the students and be responsible for supplying all the instruction dealing directly with nursing and hospital problems" (Stewart, 1931, p. 2). The first class of two students entered in 1899 where they studied household arts as well as the sciences. Additional coursework in psychology and the philosophy of education were added. Lectures were given by members of the Superintendents Society as well as the faculty at Teachers College (Stewart, 1931). The course expanded to a two-year program in 1905 and by the fall of 1907 it became part of the Department of Household Administration. M. Adelaide Nutting administered this department and received the title of professor of domestic education (also referred to as professor of institutional administration). In 1910, her title changed to professor of nursing education as the department became the Department of Nursing and Health. Nutting retired from her position in 1925 after successfully achieving international renown preparing nursing leaders around the world. Nutting had helped make Teachers College a mecca for nursing leaders in education and administration throughout the world. As the next leader of the Department of Education, Isabel Maitland Stewart (1878–1963) wrote that the program had over 578 students enrolled as of the fall 1930 and "an additional 418 enrolled during the summer session" (Stewart, 1931, p. 1)

Lillian Wald, founder of the Henry Street Settlement in 1893, played an important role at Teachers College developing curriculum for a post-graduate program in public health nursing. Wald was the first president of the NOPHN and was interested in the additional education that public health nurses needed, especially those who would serve in rural communities. As early as 1910, Wald along with other public health nurses at the District Nurse Association of Northern Westchester and the Henry Street Settlement on the Lower East Side of New York developed a curriculum for such a program. Enrolled students took courses in both rural and public health nursing, practical sociology, municipal and rural sanitation, and public health nursing along with a practicum (Post Graduate Courses for Red Cross Town and Country Nursing Service Candidates, 1914–1915). This four-month course later extended in length and others that followed were required by nurses applying to become a rural public health nurse in the American Red Cross Town and Country Nursing Service. The Town and Country was a rural nursing service that began in 1912 and lasted until 1948 (Lewenson, 2015). Nurses in this role required the specialized coursework following the hospital-based programs they had attended. The curriculum would provide the skills that these nurses would need to bring public health nursing into these isolated settings.

Health teaching became a big part of this course in public health nursing and, as Stewart (1931) writes, "even before the term 'preventative medicine' was coined, health teaching had been recognized as an important function of the nurse in the home" (p. 2). Stewart also reflects upon the clinical facilities that nurses needed to combine both theory and practice. Wald's curricular ideas included clinicals at the Henry Street Settlement on the Lower East Side for urban experiences and the Northern Westchester Visiting Nurse Association for rural experiences (Lewenson, 2015). By the 1920s clinicals included the East Harlem Nursing and Health Service, or rural settings outside of the metropolitan area – all depending on the area in which students were studying (e.g., school nursing, mental hygiene for children, nutrition) (Stewart, 1931). By 1930, under Stewart's leadership, Teachers College offered bachelor's, master's, and doctoral degrees.

Stewart herself had entered Teachers College in 1908. She hailed from Canada, and received financial support from the then ASSTSN. In one year she received a certificate from Teachers College hospital economics course. She earned a bachelor's degree in 1911 and a master's degree in 1913 (Donahue, 1988, p. 299). Stewart became a faculty member and worked closely with Nutting until 1925 when she assumed the leadership position of division of nursing. Stewart, like Nutting, Robb, Wald, and Dock, participated in the development of the professional nursing organizations. Stewart actively worked with the curriculum committee of the NLNE (formerly the ASSTSN) in developing three of the standard curricula guides that were to be published (1917, 1927, and 1937). Her research related to time and motion studies – specifically in regard to nursing and non-nursing functions (Donahue, 1988). In 1961, an Isabel Maitland Stewart Professional Chair in Nursing Research at Teachers College was established and continues today.

Teachers College served as a model in universities throughout the country for post-graduate education in nursing (Goldmark, 1923/1984). The goal of such education beyond the diploma program was to develop leaders for the future of nursing in education and practice.

> The student should learn not only teaching methods and material, not only the principles of administration, but the breadth of vision which shall envisage the nurse's training and its problems as a whole, and govern its new adjustments and expansions. From this standpoint, the prime service of such college courses is perhaps the student's emancipation. They rescue her from the isolation and parochialism of her nursing school, and make her realize herself and her training as part of the educational system of the country.
>
> *(Goldmark, 1923/1984, p. 559)*

From the early inception of the professional nursing associations, moving nursing education out from under the auspices of the hospital and into colleges and universities was central to the education of nurses. In 1954 Mary M. Roberts (1877–1959) reflected on the question of training versus the education of nurses. Roberts, long-time editor of the *American Journal of Nursing* for over 30 years beginning in 1921, includes a whole chapter on this quandary in her seminal history of nursing, *American Nursing: History and Interpretation*, written in the mid twentieth century. Roberts (1954) wrote, "Before the first decade of the new century … leaders in the movement for the education of nurses, rather than apprentice training on the job, believed that institutions called schools should be expected to have definite educational standards and objectives" (p. 62).

Collegiate schools of nursing open

Early attempts of taking nurses training outside of the hospital apprenticeship model began in the early part of the twentieth century. Economic reasons, as well as the need for theoretical education coupled with practical experience, were vigorously debated by the members of the NLNE. Agnes Brennan, superintendent of Bellevue Training School for Nurses in 1897, argued that "theory fortifies the practical, practice strengthens and retains the theoretical" (Brennan, 1897/1991, p. 25). Yet, education outside of hospitals was slow to take hold. One of the earliest university-based programs in nursing was the University of Minnesota in 1909. Richard Olding Beard, Professor at the University of Minnesota, described this new program at a meeting held by the American Federation of Nurses in 1909. (The

American Federation of Nurses was a short-lived affiliation among the NLNE, ANA, and the NOPHN that was organized to represent American nursing at the International Council of Nursing.) This new program was designed as a training school for nurses in conjunction with the university hospital service whereby the school existed for the purpose of educating nurses and not providing hospital service (Beard, 1910, p. 119). Each student would be an integral part of the university; this in itself was unique. This educational advancement faced opposition from reactionaries in the medical profession, claiming that the graduate nurse "of to-day knows too much, assumes too much by way of position and privilege and lays too large a levy for her service upon her clientele" (Beard, 1910, p. 122). The question of how much nurses needed to know and how they should be educated continued throughout the twentieth century, challenging nurse educators to find new solutions.

In the mid twentieth century, when the associate degree program in nursing was expanding, Bridgman (1953) wrote that less than 5% of nursing students enrolled in schools of nursing were educated in colleges or universities that accepted the full educational responsibility of educating nurses. Those programs, housed in institutions of higher education, typically offered the liberal arts and sciences, leaving nursing instruction to the apprenticeship models in hospital settings. In the closing words of her 1953 book, *Collegiate Education for Nurses*, Bridgman made it clear that "society requires the establishment by higher education of an effective system of appropriate types of preparation for diversified nursing functions and the maintenance of standards that will assure competence. Only a high quality of education will serve the need" (p. 197).

Racism in nursing education

During the early part of the twentieth century most nurses were native-born white women (Reverby, 1987). Brooks Carthon (2017) notes the percentage of non-white women in nursing in 1910 was 4%. Few opportunities existed for black women to enter the newly formed schools of nursing that served mostly white populations. The lack of access to healthcare coupled with exclusion of black women from existing schools of nursing led to the opening of black institutions – hospitals, nurse-training schools, medical schools, and universities – that served the black population. Hospitals and schools of nursing opened in both the north and south to fill the void in education and healthcare (Hine, 1989). Former Executive Secretary and President of the NACGN, Mabel Keaton Staupers (1961) wrote, "'Black codes' were set up by law in the South and by custom in the North, where they were observed just as relentlessly" (p. 3). With few exceptions, like the New England Training School where Mary E. Mahoney had graduated in 1879, black women entered the newly opened black schools of nursing. Hine (1989) emphasized that "political and educational institutions in both the North and South adopted and perpetuated the dogmas of racial segregation and white supremacy" (p. 3). To meet the increasing morbidity and mortality rates within black communities, philanthropists John D. Rockefeller and Laura Spelman Rockefeller established the Atlanta Baptist Female Seminary, in 1881. This was considered the first school of nursing for black women in the US and became known as Spelman College. A few years later, in 1886, Spelman College, now an academic institution, opened a department of nursing offering a two-year diploma in nursing outside of a hospital setting (Hine, 1989). Additional funding by Dr. Malcolm McVicar was obtained in 1901, providing a 31-bed hospital for students to practice the art of nursing as well as to serve as an infirmary for the school.

Hospitals and training schools for black nurses opened throughout the late nineteenth and early twentieth century. Schools opened in northern and southern cities, including Chicago, Illinois; Philadelphia, Pennsylvania; Hampton, Virginia; Washington, DC; New York City; New Orleans, Louisiana; Raleigh and Durham, North Carolina; Nashville, Tennessee; and Charleston, South Carolina. These hospitals and schools of nursing both provided educational training for black women and also provided much-needed access to healthcare to the black community (Kenney, 1919). In an article published in the *Journal of the Medical Association*, Kenney (1919) optimistically concluded that:

> The Negro nurse through efficiency of the nurse training schools scattered all over the country, has come to take her place in the world's work, and as we regard the future so far as the health and mortality of the race is concerned, we are assured that it will be much improved and the race through its physicians and nurses physically will meet the demands of the communities where we are located, either in large or small numbers.
>
> *(p. 68)*

Hine (1989) described over 25 schools of nursing and 200 black hospitals opened by the mid-1920s, with some of these institutions supported by local governments. This number, however, dwindled by the 1940s when only 110 of these black hospitals and only 20 black schools of nursing survived. Funding for these schools was offered by philanthropists who were altruistic and pragmatic, in that improving the health of the black population would also impact the health of the white population.[2]

The post-graduate programs in nursing that were required for advancement into teaching, administrative, and public health positions for the most part also discriminated against black women. Teachers College at Columbia University was one of the only programs to admit black students. Frances Elliot Davis, a graduate of Freedman's School of Nursing in Washington, DC, in 1912 and considered the first black nurse to be admitted into the American Red Cross Town and Country in 1917, attended the post-graduate program in public health. As the researcher Rockefeller hired to study the status of Negro women in nursing, Ethel Johns (1925) opined in her unpublished report that, although some post-graduate programs in northern universities typically admitted black students, their welcome was, she said, "far from enthusiastic" (p. 7). In 1920, nurse educator Anne H. Strong at Boston's Simmons' College post-graduate program in public health responded that Simmons makes "no restriction as to race or color" (letter from Anne H. Strong to Katherine Holmes, September 20, 1920). Yet, when it came to placement of black nurses in clinical settings and in the dormitories, black students, she said, faced greater challenges than their white counterparts. Johns' (1925) report gave credence to the racism that existed, even in schools that accepted black students. Johns wrote that her report "emphasizes, or seems to emphasize, the serious racial disabilities which weigh so heavily on the negro nurse" (Johns, 1925, p. 1). She continued, that while it was not "the intention to make too much of these, but they exist and they cannot be ignored" (Johns, 1925, p. 1).

Black institutions of higher learning

With nursing leaders advocating the education of nurses outside of hospital-based schools and into colleges and universities – especially with the founding of the Association of Collegiate Schools of Nursing in 1935 – leaders within the NACGN responded with concern for the black nurse. Florida Agricultural and Mechanical University in Tallahassee, Florida, offered bachelor's degrees in nursing and Howard University had established such a degree in 1922 (although it was short-lived); few black institutions of higher learning provided this kind of education of black women. Recognizing the too few opportunities in typically white institutions of higher education, the call for additional black schools of higher education was heard. The 1940s saw the opening of bachelor's degrees in nursing at several institutions, including Dillard University in New Orleans in 1942; Hampton Institute in Hampton, Virginia, in 1944; Meharry College in Nashville, Tennessee, in 1943; and then Tuskegee Institute in Alabama offered this higher degree in nursing (Hine, 1989, p. 65). Throughout the twentieth century, the move towards collegiate education in historically black schools of nursing prevailed and post-graduate programs for black students also opened.

Independent studies that identified priorities for the nursing profession in the United States

Over the course of the twentieth century, the nursing profession in the United States has achieved some success in increasing the number of educated, licensed nurses in practice and is recognized as a major component of the healthcare system. The progress was the result, in part, of the multiple reports on the status of nursing with recommendations for nursing, nursing policy, and nursing education (McAllister, 2012). Two reports in particular, *Nursing and Nursing Education in the United States: Report of the Committee for the Study of Nursing Education*, commonly referred to as the Goldmark Report (Goldmark, 1923/1984), and *Nursing for the Future*, commonly referred to as the Brown Report (Brown, 1948), bear examination.

The Goldmark Report

The Goldmark Report was commissioned to define the training that was necessary for public health nurses. Nurse leaders Annie Goodrich (1866–1954), the first Dean at Yale University, noted public health nurse and the founder of the Henry Street Settlement on the Lower East Side of New York City, Lilian Wald, and M. Adelaide Nutting, the first director of the nursing education program at Teachers College, Columbia University, were on the committee. Josephine Goldmark was the primary author and a Bryn Mawr-educated feminist and social reformer. The recommendations of the Goldmark Report included the improvement of the basic education of nurses which then took place in the hospital-based training schools, firm financing of the institution that educated nurses, and the development of a less educated nurse, "a subsidiary worker" to care for the less acutely ill in both hospitals and in the home (Goldmark, 1923/1984, p. 16).

The Brown Report

Esther Lucile Brown, a social scientist, was asked to assess the needed quantity of nurses as well as the quality of the education in 1948, when the US was emerging from World War II. There was a rapid growth of hospital construction during this timeframe as the result of the Hill–Burton Act which provided funding for the construction of hospitals all across the US (Lipscomb, 2002) and this rapid growth fueled the need for an adequate nursing workforce. Brown was unflinching in her determination that,

> by no conceivable stretch of the imagination can the education provided in the vast majority of the 1,250 schools be conceived of as professional education. In

spite of improvements that have been made in most schools over the years, it remains apprenticeship training.

(Brown, p. 48)

Brown was the Director of the Russell Sage Foundation's Department of Studies in the Professions. This landmark report, with Brown's call for the current schools to be replaced by college-based programs, gave energy to the efforts of nurse leaders that were already in progress. When Brown died in 1990, the *American Journal of Nursing* called her "one of nursing's staunchest allies and admirers who saw nursing's worth before nurses themselves seemed to see it" (N.A., 1990).

Ultimately the Brown Report echoed the recommendations noted previously in the Goldmark Report, with the notable addition of the call to increase the diversity of the nursing workforce by increasing efforts to recruit more men and minorities into the profession (McAllister, 2012). At this time in the US women of color and men were marginalized and institutional racism prevented many in these groups from entry into schools of nursing.

Post World War II and the movement of nurse training into the system of higher education

The 1950s was a productive time in the world of American education as the US emerged from World War II. New York City was considered by many to be the center of the world of nursing and home to the "country's most prominent postgraduate educational program at Teachers College" (D'Antonio, 2010, p. 60). During this timeframe, most nurse training took place in the hospital-based diploma programs and was "rule based, activity oriented, and relied heavily on the repetition of procedures rather than scientific or social theory based decision making" (Fairman, 2008, p. 41). At this time, new models of education were introduced as nurse leaders sought to emphasize science-based learning. Gradually, nursing education moved away from the hospital diploma programs and into the nation's colleges and universities (Tobbell, 2014).

The post-World War II years precipitated some of the fastest-moving changes in nursing education in the US as educators at New York City's Teachers College, Columbia University department of nursing education put forth a two-year curriculum for nursing that would take place at the country's fledgling community colleges. The proposal, the result of Teachers College doctoral student Mildred Montag's dissertation, was developed under the supervision of R. Louise McManus, who was the director of the department of nursing education at Teachers College from 1947 to 1961 and a well-known nurse leader. The curriculum, which would result in an associate degree upon completion, was in keeping with nurse leaders' long-held desire to move nursing out from the apprenticeship model of the diploma programs in the nation's hospitals and into the system of higher education. It shortened the time period and would address the needs of society to provide adequately educated nurses in a sufficient quantity to care for the growing population.

There were also multiple societal changes that took place in the US after the war which impacted nursing leadership's ability to institute changes in nursing education. Innovations in surgery and an increase in available healthcare dramatically increased the need for trained nurses (Orsolini-Hain & Waters, 2009). Advances in healthcare arising from wartime experiences in surgery as the result of battlefield injuries occurred. The use of antibiotics changed an infection to a treatable malady rather than the death sentence it was previously and as a result people were living longer. Chronic illnesses such as cancer and cardiac conditions required a change in care as well as an increase in education for public health nurses.

Many assumed that the nurses who returned home after the war would return to work but many stayed home and began families, which resulted in the baby boomer generation (Waters, 1995). Hospital construction flourished as a result of government funding via the Hill–Burton Act of 1946, increasing hospital beds in some of the poorest areas of the country where healthcare previously was unavailable. This worsened an already serious nursing shortage (Dolan et al., 1983).

It was also during this timeframe that health insurance became more common. In 1946 only a third of Americans had access to health insurance (Lynaugh, 2008). As employers began to offer health insurance as a benefit, there was an increase in the number of people who could now afford healthcare. This, along with hospital construction, increased the demand for nurses.

During this timeframe President Truman ordered an examination of the educational system in the US. In 1946, the Truman Commission published its report, *Higher Education for American Democracy*. At this time, only one-sixth of the nation's youth attended college, and less than half completed high school. The recommendations included that all young people should graduate from high school and complete an additional two years after high school for a total of 14 years of education (Havighurst, 1952). The Commission focused on the nation's fledgling community colleges, then called junior colleges. As a result, these colleges started to receive much attention and support (McAllister, 2012). It was during this timeframe and in this context of major societal changes that nurse leaders at Teachers College put forth the idea that nurses could be educated at the nation's community colleges.

The associate degree model for the education of nurses

The development of the associate degree model of nursing (ADN) education occurred rapidly in the early 1950s. It was proposed, initiated, and evaluated in less than 10 years and was developed from the work of the nursing faculty at Teachers College, Columbia University in New York City. It was a direct response of the faculty and staff of the Division of Nursing Education to the needs of society in the years after World War II. The ADN model was a radical change in the way that nurses were educated in the United States. It resulted in a movement away from the apprentice model of nursing education in the hospital schools of nursing. It is firmly established as an educational model and currently the most common entry route into the nursing profession. The unintended consequences of the success of the ADN as a method to educate nurses is a controversial issue for the profession today as nurse leaders seek to require a baccalaureate degree as the minimum requirement for entry into the profession (McAllister, 2017).

Mildred Montag (1908–2004), sometimes referred to as the architect of ADN, is the person most frequently associated with the development of the ADN model and she has taken the blame for the unintended consequences of its success. It was her dissertation topic, *Education of Nursing Technicians* (Montag, 1950), at Teachers College that outlined a two-year curriculum plan that would take place in the nation's burgeoning community college (then called junior college) system. This movement away from the apprenticeship model in hospital diploma schools and into the system of higher education was in keeping with the long-held desire and efforts of nurse leaders from the beginning of the modern nursing movement. Montag's work was presented as experimental and was the only educational model based on research, experimentation, and evaluation (Montag, 1959). In addition to the ability to educate nurses in a shorter timeframe and based on education and not service as in the diploma schools, community college education opened the door for those previously excluded from nursing. People of color, men, and older women were suddenly able to enroll in these programs. The call for a more diverse nursing workforce (Brown, 1948) was being answered.

The experiment: the Cooperative Research Project

A year after the completion of her dissertation, Montag's work was published almost verbatim (Montag, 1951). The publisher, Asa Elliot at Putnam & Sons, worked on the premise that publishers had an obligation to publish a book that would not enjoy widespread circulation but was none the less worthy (Schorr & Zimmerman, 1988). A book review of Montag's work in the *Journal of the American Medical Association* ironically revealed the opinion that the book would have virtually no effect on the education of nurses (Book review, 1951).

Montag had written a detailed study of nursing in the post-World War II era and conceptualized a curriculum for a nursing program at the two-year colleges. The multiple societal changes, the increasing demands for nursing services, the changing functions of the nurse as carer became more complex, and the fact that the needs of society were not being met all impacted the ability of nurse leaders to move forward with this new model. It was the perfect storm.

The power and reputation of Teachers College also influenced the success of the experiment. The Teachers College milieu was notable in the fact that many of the nurse leaders of the time were educated there given their status as the first graduate program for nurses. R. Louise McManus, then the director of the Nursing Education Department, and a notable nurse leader in her own right, was Montag's dissertation advisor. Montag always credited McManus with the idea of the two-year program.

McManus noted that a break in the traditional apprenticeship model as well as a different curriculum than the usual basic school of nursing program was notable in that Montag's proposal outlined previously tested principles of technical education already in use in the community colleges. The two-year timeframe would reduce the cost of the education. In addition, barriers to education long associated with diploma programs, such as the social isolation of the students, would be removed by placing nursing schools in the college community where they were treated as students and not workers. Married students, minorities, and men normally excluded in diploma schools could enroll, thus attracting students who would have been lost to the profession. McManus threw her wholehearted support behind the proposal and strongly suggested that all nursing educators carefully consider this new model of nursing education (Montag, 1951).

When an opportunity to garner funding for the experimental project, called the Cooperative Research Project (CRP), arose, McManus, an ardent fundraiser, remembered reaching into her desk drawer for the draft of what "remained for some time with the other sample projects in the bottom drawer of my desk" (Safier, 1977, p. 200). Others recalled Mrs. McManus' bottom drawer, including Montag, stating, "she saw possibilities in what was going on and she would project it in a written form as a project. That's how the Associate Degree Programs in junior colleges really began" (Interview with Dr. Mildred Montag, 1983, tape 1).

Funding was obtained in the amount of $110,000 from what was first an anonymous donor but later revealed to be Mary Rockefeller, a supporter of nursing, and then the wife of Nelson Rockefeller, then Governor of New York who later became the Vice President of the United States. Mary Rockefeller was a good friend of McManus' and on the board of the Bellevue and Mills School of Nursing. She questioned McManus about what plans were in progress at Teachers College to address the nationwide nursing shortage (Speakman, 2006). McManus responded with the curriculum for the ADN.

Rockefeller's donation and the formation of a committee enabled the work of the CRP. The purpose of the project was to "find a shorter and better method of preparing young men and women to carry out the functions that are usually associated with registered nurses" (Montag, 1955, p. 45).

Six colleges across the nation were chosen from a large group of institutions that expressed an interest in the project and by the end of the five-year project there were more programs outside of the CRP than in it. In 1959, Montag published the results of the CRP. In it she notes the findings include that the graduates of these new programs are able to "pass the licensing exam and … able to carry on the nursing functions as well or better than graduates of other types of nursing programs" (Montag, 1959, p. 339). The associate degree model for the education of nurses was off and running and was soon the most common pathway into the profession as the number of diploma programs was reduced and community college growth increased.

The nation's baccalaureate programs never took off the way the community colleges did. They did not receive the support of the government like the community college system did in the Truman Commission Report (Higher Education for American Democracy, 1946) which championed the junior colleges. Nor did they have leaders like Montag and McManus and the power of Teachers College, all of which clearly helped the ADN's success. There was also the lack of one nursing organization that could legitimately claim to represent all of American nursing like physicians do in the American Medical Association (AMA).

All these factors along with the timeframe after World War II and societal changes created the perfect storm of events that propelled the ADN. It was successful in the intent to produce more nurses in a shorter, more economical timeframe but had the unintended consequence of making the degree the most common pathway into the profession, a consequence that the profession has been grappling with ever since. Community college presidents recognized and supported the value of nursing programs and actively supported the development of this new model. They added prestige to the institutions and prepared a viable workforce in the community which was integral to the community college mission.

In 1965, a mere six years after Montag's final report of the CRP, the ANA published its position paper calling for the baccalaureate degree to be the minimum requirement for entry into the profession. That call has continued into the twenty-first century with the publication of the Carnegie (Benner et al., 2010) and Institute of Medicine (2010) Reports, once again outlining priorities for the profession.

Closing of hospital-based diploma programs

The 1960s heralded the increasing interest in nursing science and an educational level responsive to the interdisciplinary nature of the profession (Tobbell, 2018). The ANA position paper calling for a nurse to hold a baccalaureate degree led schools of nursing to reconsider their educational programs. Bellevue School of Nursing that included the Mills School of Nursing that had opened in 1888 for men was already engaged in discussions about the viability of continuing their well-respected diploma program. In 1942 the school had established a relationship with the private New York University and offered the opportunity for Bellevue's students to obtain a bachelor's degree in nursing. While some students took advantage of this option, most did not. This arrangement lasted until 1959 when alternative strategies for nursing education were sought. Yet by the mid-1960s, with the increasing shortage of nurses within the New York City municipal hospital system, the Department of Hospitals (DOH) explored varying levels of skilled nursing care that was needed and the institutions that would educate these nurses accordingly. The DOH planned to close several of the city-run diploma schools of nursing while opening either an associate or baccalaureate degree program. Bellevue was slated for the latter. Bellevue's administrative leadership worked with the DOH as New York City developed a blueprint mapping out the skill sets that the city required to meet the city's nursing needs.

During the same period, Hunter College, part of the City University of New York, planned to expand their nursing program. This program had started in the 1940s with a clinical site at Metropolitan Hospital, another city-run hospital. With the planned phase-out of Bellevue's school looming, classrooms, student dormitories, and labs would become available to Hunter College. Bellevue's school of nursing building, located at East 25th Street in New York, could easily accommodate the city's need for more highly skilled and educated nurses with a bachelor's degree. After months of negotiating with the city, a contract was signed in June of 1967 that expanded Hunter's collegiate program into the Bellevue facility. The closing of Bellevue's school, one that had maintained a prestigious reputation since it had opened in 1873, heralded a change to other diploma programs around the city and elsewhere. In addition, and perhaps most compelling, the closing of this program moved the control of nurses' training away from the DOH and into the Department of Education, a feat that signified a desired change by some of nursing's pioneers and contemporary leaders (Lewenson, 2013).

Master's degrees and higher education

Specialization of nursing – like the nurse midwife, nurse practitioner, nurse anesthetist, and others – adds to the rich history of nursing education in the United States that goes way beyond the scope of this chapter. Yet, these specialties developed to fill a need in healthcare for more educated nurses to fulfill a role. In the 1960s and 1970s the United States was undergoing significant social and political reforms, including women's rights and civil rights, which influenced the nursing profession and its efforts to move nursing education into higher education (Fairman, 2002). Nursing education in universities and colleges demanded nurses to be better critical thinkers and develop new models of care. The American Association of Colleges of Nursing (AACN) (2011) published the master's essentials calling for graduates to fulfill "a variety of roles and areas of practice" (p. 5). New innovative roles continue to be developed as nursing responds to society's needs and the "changes in an evolving and global health care system" (p. 5). The move from hospital-based training into community colleges and university settings allowed graduates to aspire towards programs in higher education.

Along with the challenges of higher education is the persistent call for a more inclusive and diverse student body and faculty in schools of nursing at all levels. In an oral history of African American nursing leader, Bernardine Lacey revealed how she was a product of a segregated diploma program in nursing in 1962, was one of the first black nurses to receive a bachelor's degree from Georgetown University in Washington, DC, and received a master's degree from the historical black institution, Howard University in Washington,

DC, and a doctoral degree from Teachers College, Columbia University in New York City in the early 1990s (Lewenson, 2018). Although retired from a career of leadership in nursing education and practice, where she had to overcome many of the obstacles in her path, Lacey, like the early nursing pioneers, continues to consider ways in which to contribute and spark a conversation about diversity and inclusivity. In this way, studying these histories contributes to the continuing evolution of nursing education in the United States.

Conclusions

The success of the associate degree model for the education of nurses in the post-World War II era in the United States precipitated the unintended consequence of the majority of the nation's nursing workforce educated at associate degree level. Baccalaureate programs existed but were quickly eclipsed by community college growth. The number of diploma schools plummeted as hospitals closed their programs and community college education became the pathway into the profession. Nursing leadership has struggled with this turn of events ever since. While the associate degree model achieved the goal of increasing the nursing workforce and moving the education of nurses into the system of higher education, the call for a more educated workforce has continued, with the baccalaureate degree cited as the minimal requirement for entry into the profession. More recent research (Aiken et al., 2002, 2003, Kutney-Lee et al., 2013; Harrison et al., 2019) in the US has exposed evidence that the higher the number of baccalaureate-prepared nurses employed in a healthcare system, the better the outcomes. This growing body of evidence supports the need for a better-educated nursing workforce. Nursing has been slow to move on this need for a multitude of reasons.

After a more than 16-year effort in the state of New York, legislation was passed in 2017 (Zittel, 2019) requiring all nurses to obtain a baccalaureate degree within 10 years of graduation. New York was the first to make it a law but other states will inevitably follow. The effort, however, took many years and the movement to have the entire nursing workforce obtain a baccalaureate degree to gain entry into the profession may still be decades away.

As history shows, the rapid success of the model and the proliferation of community college nursing programs did result in a reduction in the number of diploma programs across the United States but a continued concern within the profession that baccalaureate education in nursing took a back seat to the associate degree model. In the report of the Surgeon Generals' Consultant Group on Nursing (U.S. Department of Health, Education, and Welfare, 1963), there were 176 baccalaureate programs, 84 associate degree programs established since the model's inception in 1952, and 875 diploma programs. Within 20 years there were 421 baccalaureate programs, 764 associate degree programs, and 281 diploma programs in the United States. By 2008, the number of baccalaureate programs was 681, the associate degree programs were 1,023, and the diploma programs had dwindled to 69 (National League for Nursing, 2008). Even though the number of baccalaureate programs steadily increased, the growth was nowhere near that of the associate degree programs. The decrease in diploma schools is notable and represents the success of efforts by nurse leaders to move the education of nurses from the outdated apprenticeship model of the diploma schools and into the system of American higher education (McAllister, 2012, 2017).

In the US, there are still three pathways into the nursing profession. Three-year diploma programs still exist in some states and the two-year associate degree model is still the most common entry point. Baccalaureate education has shown increases but not as fast as nurse leaders desire. Lynaugh (1980) examined what seems to be the never-ending conflict in nursing, the entry into practice issue, and termed it a social issue and not just "an interprofessional squabble" (p. 266).

Indeed, as we approach the third decade of the twenty-first century, the nursing profession in the United States remains undereducated, understaffed, and underfunded. The multiple pathways for entry into practice remain, and the multiple calls for a better-educated workforce remain uncompleted. Research shows that an inadequate supply of nurses directly affects the quality of care in hospitals and that education levels directly affect morbidity and mortality in hospitalized patients (Aiken et al., 2002, 2003; Kutney-Lee et al., 2013; Harrison, et al., 2019). But increasing the supply and financing the education of the nursing workforce can lead to escalating healthcare costs that may be intolerable to the American public (Bodenheimer & Grumbach, 2009). The enduring issue of the development of nursing education is reflected in the repeated reports in the twentieth century (Goldmark, 1923/1984; Brown, 1948) and the additional twenty-first-century reports (Benner et al., 2010; Institute of Medicine, 2010) that once again identify priorities as nurse leaders still struggle with the goal of the basic requirement of the baccalaureate degree for entry into the profession. The growing body of evidence that a more educated nursing workforce results in better patient outcomes adds urgency and is hard to ignore.

Currently, there are many factors influencing changes in nursing education: the continued increase in knowledge that is the basis for nursing practice, concerns for patient safety, nursing shortages, faculty shortages, and shortages of nurses prepared at the doctoral level. Nursing continues to develop new models such as the Doctor of Nursing Practice (DNP), a clinical doctorate that is in keeping with the requirements of other health professionals like medicine, dentistry, pharmacy, and physical therapy (American Association of Colleges of Nursing, 2019). But the basic preparation of the nursing workforce is still problematic, with no current plans to phase out the diploma and the associate degree pathway (Matthias, 2017). There are multiple programs that allow for the academic progression of these nurses to obtain higher degrees and the numbers of nurses entering the workforce with a baccalaureate degree are increasing, but the associate degree is still the most common entry-level degree (National League for Nursing, 2014). The advent of Magnet models for healthcare institutions which require the majority of the nursing staff to hold the baccalaureate degree has added pressure to the profession and to the students currently enrolled. Academic progression is facilitated by schools with seamless articulation agreements with baccalaureate programs. And the ongoing legislative efforts for more states to require the attainment of the Bachelor of Science in Nursing within 10 years of graduation. like New York, will continue.

Nursing education in the United States has taken a circuitous route on the journey to provide the public with an adequate number of appropriately educated nurses. The rest of the journey remains to be seen.

Notes

1 For the history of nursing education prior to Nightingale-influenced training schools, see D'Antonio (2010): *American Nursing: A History of Knowledge, Authority, and the Meaning of Work.*
2 For a more detailed discussion of the rise of black hospitals and schools of nursing, see the chapter in Hine (1989), Origins of the Black Hospital and Nurse Training School Movement.

References

Aiken L, Clarke S, Cheung R, Sloane D, & Silber J (2003) Education levels of hospital nurses and surgical patient mortality. *Journal of the American Medical Association* 290(12): 1617–1623.

Aiken L, Clarke S, Sloane D, Sochalski J, & Silber J (2002) Hospital nurse staffing and patient mortality, nurse burnout, and job dissatisfaction. *Journal of the American Medical Association* 288: 1987–1993.

Alumnae Association of Bellevue School of Nursing (1989) *The Alumnae Association of the Bellevue School of Nursing*. Reprint of Letter from Florence Nightingale to Dr. W. Gill Wylie, dated September 18, 1872, The Alumnae Association of the Bellevue School of Nursing. Topeka Kansas: Jostens.

American Association for the History of Nursing (AAHN) (2019) *Linda Richards*. Accessed at: www.aahn.org/richards

American Association of Colleges of Nursing (AACN) (2011) *The essentials of master's education in nursing*. Washington, DC: American Association of Colleges of Nursing. Accessed at: www.aacnnursing.org/Portals/42/Publications/MastersEssentials11.pdf

American Association of the Colleges of Nursing (2019) *American association of colleges of nursing fact sheet. Why move to the DNP?* Washington, D.C. Accessed at: www.aacnnursing.org/DNP/Fact-Sheet

Beard R O (1910) The university education of the nurse. In *Fifteenth Annual Report of the American Society of Superintendents of Training Schools for Nurses including Report of the Second Meeting of the American Federation of Nurses held at St. Paul, Minnesota June 7 and 8, 1909*. Baltimore, MD: J. H. Furst Company.

Benner P, Sutphen M, Leonard V, & Day L (2010) *Educating nurses: A call for radical transformation*. San Francisco: Jossey-Bass.

Bodenheimer T S, & Grumbach K (2009) *Understanding health policy: A clinical approach* (5th ed.). New York: McGraw Hill Medical.

Book review (1951) Review of the book *The Education of Nursing Technicians*, by M. L. Montag. *Journal of the American Medical Association* 146(4): 412.

Brennan A (1897/1991) Comparative value of theory and practice in training nurses. In N. Birnbach & S. Lewenson (Eds.). 1991. *First words: Selected address from the national league for nursing 1894-1933* (pp. 23–25). New York: National League for Nursing.

Bridgman M (1953) *Collegiate education for nursing*. New York: Russell Sage Foundation.

Brooks Carthon J M (2017) Minority nurses in diverse communities: Mary Elizabeth Tyler and the Whittier Centre in early 20th-century Philadelphia. In S.B. Lewenson, A. McAllister & K. M. Smith (Eds.). *Nursing History for Contemporary Role Development* (pp. 3–18). New York: Springer.

Brown E L (1948) *Nursing for the future: A report prepared for the National Nursing Council*. New York: Russell Sage Foundation.

Cook E T (1913) *The Life of Florence Nightingale: 1820-1861* Vol. I. London: Macmillan and Company.

D'Antonio P (2010) *American nursing: A history of knowledge, authority, and the meaning of work*. Baltimore, MD: The Johns Hopkins Press.

Dolan J A, Fitzpatrick M L, & Herrmann E K (1983) *Nursing in society: A historical perspective* (15th ed.). Philadelphia: W.B. Saunders.

Donahue P (1988) Isabel Maitland Stewart (1878-1963). In V.L. Bullough, O.M. Church, & A. P. Stein (Eds.). *American nursing: A biographical dictionary* (pp. 298-301). New York: Garland Publishing.

Fairman J (2002) The roots of collaborative practice: Nurse practitioner pioneers' stories. *Nursing History Review* 10: 159–174.

Fairman J (2008) *Making room in the clinic: Nurse practitioners and the evolution of modern health care*. New Brunswick, New Jersey: Rutgers University Press.

Goldmark J (1923/1984) *Nursing and nursing education in the United States: Report of the committee for the study of nursing education*. New York: McMillan. Reprinted by Garland Publishing.

Harrison J M, Aiken LH, Sloane DM, Brooks Carthon JM, Merchant RM, Berg RA, McHugh MD (July, 2019). In hospitals with more nurses who have baccalaureate degrees, better outcomes for patients after cardiac arrest. Health Affairs 38(7): 1087–1094.

Havighurst R J (1952) Social implications of the report of the President's Commission on Higher Education. In G. Kennedy (Ed.). *Education for democracy: The debate over the report of the President's Commission on Higher Education* (pp. 62–67). Boston: Heath.

Higher Education for American Democracy (1946) *A report of the President's Commission on Higher Education*. New York: Harper.

Hine D C (1989) *Black women in white: Racial conflict and cooperation in the nursing profession 1890-1950*. Bloomington, Indiana: Indiana University Press.

Institute of Medicine (2010) *The future of nursing: Leading change, advancing health.* Washington, DC: National Academies Press.

Interview with Dr. Mildred Montag (1983) Tape 1 and 2. Interview by Louise Fitzpatrick. [Videotape recording]. Archives of the Department of Nursing Education, Gottesman Library, Teachers College, Columbia University, New York. Available at http://pocketknowledge.tc.columbia.edu/home.php/viewfile/103389

Johns E (1925) A study of the present status of the Negro woman in nursing. Rockefeller Foundation, Record Group 1.1, series 200, Box 122, Folder 1507, 1–43, Exhibits A-P, Appendixes I and II). New York: Rockefeller Archive Center.

Kenney J A (1919) Some facts concerning Negro nurse training schools and their graduates. *Journal of the National Medical Association* 11(2): 53–68.

Kutney-Lee A, Sloane DM, & Aiken LH (2013) An increase in the number of nurses with baccalaureate degrees is linked to lower rates of post-surgery mortality. *Health Affairs* 32(3): 579–586.

Lipscomb CE (2002) Lister Hill and his influence. *Journal of the Medical Library Association* 90(1): 109–110.

Lewenson S B (1993) *Taking charge: Nursing suffrage, and feminism in America, 1873-1920.* New York: Garland Publishing.

Lewenson S B (2013) "Nurses" training may be Shifted" The story of Bellevue and Hunter College, 1942-1969. *Nursing History Review* 21: 14–32.

Lewenson S B (2015) Town and country nursing: Community participation and nurse recruitment. In J. C. Kirchgessner and A. W. Keeling (Eds.). *Nursing rural America: Perspectives from the early 20th century* (pp. 1–19). New York: Springer.

Lewenson, S.B. (2018). Oral History of Bernardine Lacey. Unpublished raw data.

Lynaugh, J. E.(1980). The "entry into practice" conflict: How we gor where we are and what will happen next. *American Journal of Nursing* 80(2): 266–270.

Lynaugh J E (2008) Nursing the great society: The impact of the Nurse Training Act of 1964. *Nursing History Review 16*: 13–28.

Matthias A D (2017) Educational pathways for differentiated nursing practice: A continuing dilemma. In S.B. Lewenson, A. McAllister & K.M. Smith (Eds.). *Nursing History for Contemporary Role Development* (pp. 121–140). New York: Springer Publishing.

McAllister A (2012) *R. Louise McManus and Mildred Montag put forth the Associate degree model for the education of nurses: The right leaders, the right time, the right place: 1947-1959.* Unpublished doctoral dissertation.

McAllister A (2017) "On such teachers rests the future of nursing": Preparing faculty for associate degree programs at the mid-20th century. In S.B. Lewenson, A. McAllister & K.M. Smith (Eds.). *Nursing history for contemporary role development* (pp. 141–160). New York: Springer Publishing.

Montag M L (1950) *Education of nursing technicians. A report of a type B project.* Unpublished doctoral dissertation, Teachers College. New York: Columbia University.

Montag M L (1951) *The education of nursing technicians.* New York: Putnam.

Montag M L (1955) Experimental programs in nursing. *American Journal of Nursing* 55(1): 45–46.

Montag M L (1959) *Community college education for nursing: An experiment in technical education for nursing.* New York: McGraw-Hill.

N.A. (1990) Esther Lucille Brown, Nursing's Champion, Dies at 92. *American Journal of Nursing* 90(9): 112.

National League for Nursing (2008) *Basic RN programs and percentage change from previous years by type of program 1981 to 1985 and 2002 to 2008.* NLN Dataview. Accessed at: www.nln.org/research/slides/pdf/AS0708_T01.pdf

National League for Nursing (2014) *Proportion of basic RN programs, 2014.* Accessed at www.nln.org/docs/default-source/newsroom/nursing-education-statistics/proportion-of-basic-rn-programs-2014-(pdf).pdf?sfvrsn=0

Nightingale F (1859/1946) *Notes on nursing: What it is and what it is not.* London: Harrison (Bookseller to the Queen). Philadelphia: Reprinted by Lippincott.

Orsolini-Hain L, & Waters V (2009) Education evolution: A historical perspective of associate degree nursing. *Journal of Nursing Education* 48(5): 266–271.

Palmer S (1897/1985) Training school alumnae associations. *Annual conventions, 1893-1899. First and Second Annual Conventions of the American Society of Superintendents of Training Schools for Nurses* (pp. 52–60). New York: Garland Publishing.

Reverby S (1987) *Ordered to care: The dilemma of American nursing, 1850-1945*. Cambridge, MA: Cambridge University Press.

Roberts M M (1954) *American nursing: History and interpretation*. New York, NY: The Macmillan Company.

Safier G (1977) *Contemporary American leaders in nursing: An oral history*. New York: McGraw-Hill.

Schorr T M, & Zimmerman A (1988) *Making choices, taking chances: Nurse leaders tell their stories*. St. Louis, MO: Mosby.

Speakman, E. (2006). The elephant in our living room: Associate degree education in nursing. In L. C. Andrist, P. K. Nicholas, & K. A. Wolf (Eds.), *A history of nursing ideas* (pp. 363–372). Sudbury, MA: Jones and Bartlett.

Staupers M K (1961) *No time for prejudice: A story of the integration of negros in nursing in the United States*. New York: the Macmillan Company.

Stewart I M (1931) Three decades of nursing education at Teachers College - Columbia University. *Reprinted from – Pocket Knowledge, Nursing Education, Reprinted from Methods and Problems from Medical Education, 21st Series, Rockefeller Foundation: New York City*, 1–20.

Threat C J (2015) *Nursing civil rights: Gender and race in the army nurse corps*. Urbana, Chicago, and Springfield, IL: University of Illinois Press.

Tobbell D (2014) "Coming to grips with the nursing question": The politics of nursing education reform in 1960s America. *Nursing History Review* 22: 37–60.

Tobbell D (2018) Nursing's boundary work theory development and the making of nursing science, ca. 1950–1980. *Nursing Research* 67(2): 63–73.

U.S. Department of Health, Education, and Welfare (1963) *Report of the surgeon general's consultant group on nursing. Toward quality in nursing: Needs and goals*. Washington, DC: United States Government Printing Office.

Waters V (1995) Second annual Mildred Montag excellence in leadership award: The founding directors of the first associate degree nursing programs. In P. Bayles & J. Parks-Doyle (Eds.). *The web of inclusion: Faculty helping faculty* (pp. 3–6). New York: National League for Nursing Press.

Zittel B (2019) *Advancing the education of registered professional nurses to the baccalaureate degree: New York's journey*. Guilderland, New York: The Foundation of NYS Nurses, Inc.

Letter from Anne H. Strong, School for Public Health Nursing, Simmons College and the Instructive District Nursing Association, to Katherine Holmes, Assistant Director, Red Cross Bureau of Public Health Nursing, September 20, 1920). Shared with author by the ARC volunteer Jean Shulman who obtained this material at the American Red Cross Archives, National Headquarters: Washington, DC. These archives are no longer open to the public. Most of the ARC archives are in the National Archives and Record Administration II in College Park, MD.

Post Graduate Courses for Red Cross Town and Country Nursing Service Candidates (four months course) (1914–1915) Pocket Knowledge, Department of Nursing and Health, American Red Cross Town and Country Nursing Service, published 1899–1961, uploaded 6/15/2009 by Pocket Masters, Archives of the Department of Nursing Education, 0397.pdf file, p. 2.

4

THE DEVELOPMENT AND CURRENT CHALLENGES OF NURSING EDUCATION IN HONG KONG

Shirley Siu-yin Ching, Kin Cheung and Yim Wah Mak

Introduction

Nursing is a caring profession that aims to assist people to obtain optimal levels of health. Education is the bedrock of professional nursing development. Nursing education in Hong Kong has undergone a great deal of transformation over the past decades in response to local and global changes. Similarly to the global trend, Hong Kong has had a steadily aging population over the past four decades. Although Hong Kong citizens nowadays suffer less from infectious diseases, non-communicable diseases such as heart disease and strokes, cancers, diabetes, and chronic respiratory diseases have accounted for half of deaths (Food and Health Bureau & Department of Health, 2018). Furthermore, high service demands, increasing patient expectations, and changes in service models are some of the major challenges faced in the healthcare system in Hong Kong (Hospital Authority, 2017). Strategies to strengthen professional accountability, specializations, and career aspirations in the nursing professions are ways to deal with these challenges, with the goal of providing quality patient care. These strategies include the implementation of a three-tier Nurses' Career Progression Model, which stipulates clearly the professional responsibilities of registered nurses, advanced practice nurses, and nurse consultants (Chan, 2014), and led to the establishment of nurse clinics in 2008 (Lee, 2017). As well, the international trend of having nursing education in higher education, a greater diversity of pedagogies in teaching and learning, and changes in students' learning dispositions have been driving forces in moving nursing education forward. The purpose of this chapter is to review the development of undergraduate and post-graduate education and continuing education opportunities in Hong Kong, examine the emerging pedagogies, and discuss the current challenges in nursing education in Hong Kong.

Development and progress of nursing education in Hong Kong

The rankings of the government-funded universities offering bachelor degree nursing programs in Hong Kong have been raised significantly from "not on the list" to within the top 45 of the

QS World University Rankings (2019). This is one of the indicators of the excellent achievements in nursing education in Hong Kong. The achievement, however, has been the result of a long journey. In the old days, pre-registration nursing education was offered mainly by nursing schools affiliated with some hospitals. Since 1990, universities have offered pre-registration nursing programs at bachelor levels. In the past two decades, alternative routes have emerged for students to pursue nursing careers. In response to the development of nursing specializations and professionalization, master and doctoral programs were launched. The progression from hospital-based training to undergraduate and post-graduate nursing programs and continuing nursing education opportunities in Hong Kong are elaborated in this section.

Hospital-based nursing training

Formal nurse training in Hong Kong was established by a British nurse sent from the London Missionary Society to the Alice Ho Memorial Hospital in 1893. The first nursing school, affiliated to a government hospital (i.e., Queen Mary Hospital), recruited students in 1905 (Hong Kong Society for Nursing Education (HKSNE), 2002). In the early days, nursing training followed the apprenticeship system of the British model (Chan & Wong, 1999). Training was on a "time-release basis" in which the students worked in the hospitals and were released to attend lectures in the school. In the 1950s, the "Study Block System" was introduced. Students were withdrawn from ward duty at regular intervals for one to two months to attend lectures and demonstrations in the school. This enabled them to concentrate on learning without the distraction of their responsibilities for patients in the wards (Anonymous, n.d.).

Before 1968, obstetric nursing training was an integral component of basic nursing training and students studied for four years before becoming registered nurses. Then, with the establishment of a midwifery school, the duration of training was reduced to three years (HKSNE, 2002). Before the 1970s, there was no formal clinical supervision/mentoring. Until the 1980s and 1990s, clinical instructors were appointed to teach students on the ward, and the concept of total patient care was introduced in the curriculum (HKSNE, 2002).

Following the British system, students were required to pass the licensing examination conducted by the Hong Kong Nursing Board (renamed the Nursing Council of Hong Kong (NCHK) in 1997), which consisted of written and practical components. In the late 1980s, continuous clinical assessment was introduced (HKSNE, 2002) and students were required to take several practical examinations during the three years of study and sit for a licensing examination before graduation. The entrance requirement for the hospital-based diploma was the Hong Kong Certificate of Education Examination after completion of five years of secondary school study. There were about 13 hospital-based nursing schools in 1999 (Chan & Wong, 1999).

However, apprenticeship training had its limitations, including the emphasis on rote learning and following instructions. As well, learning was directed more to the achievement of specific skills than to the learner's needs, and the quality of learning in clinical areas was jeopardized by the heavy workloads and overcrowded environments in most public hospitals (Chan & Wong, 1999). Nurse education at that time was focused on skill and knowledge acquisition. Students were often required to perform low-complexity tasks repeatedly instead of engaging in nursing care corresponding to their learning (HKSNE, 2002).

Undergraduate nursing education for secondary school graduates

The undertaking to raise basic general nursing training to university level started in the late 1980s. This momentum to reform nursing education came partly from the international arena, such as the international development of nursing education in tertiary institutions (i.e., United States in the early 1900s, Australia in the 1940s, United Kingdom in 1960) (Shield & Watson, 2007), and the local preparation of other healthcare professionals such as physiotherapists and occupational therapists in university. Furthermore, the increasing complexity of care demanded higher levels of knowledge as well as critical thinking and clinical decision-making abilities. Locally, the government's Medical and Health Department was replaced by the Hospital Authority in 1990, which emphasized evidence-based practice and professional accountability (HKSNE, 2002). This was another driving force to the reform. The first pre-registration nursing degree program leading to a registered nurse qualification was a four-year program offered by the Hong Kong Polytechnic University in 1990. The entrance requirement for university-based education was the Hong Kong Advanced Level Examination qualification, which was higher than that for hospital-based programs. The class size was 40 in the first intake. With the unity of nursing associations, nurses, and educators, the government announced, in a policy address, a plan to increase the number of nursing degree places to 200 in 1993. By 1995, three local government-funded universities were offering pre-registration nursing degree programs (HKSNE, 2002).

Compared with apprenticeship training, the baccalaureate degree program not only equipped nurses with professional knowledge, but also with critical thinking and problem-solving skills, as well as cultivating creativity (Chan & Wong, 2005), all of which helped to prepare nurses with autonomous and accountable nursing practices upon registration (Chan & Wong, 1999). In addition to life and behavioral sciences and nursing therapeutics, subjects such as clinical decision making, caring concepts, nursing research, informatics, dissertation, and co-curricular activities provided additional support for the students' personal and professional development during the transition from hospital-based training to baccalaureate education in the universities in the 1990s. Clinical practice is an indispensable component of pre-registration nursing education. NCHK stipulates clinical training in medical, surgical, pediatric and adolescent, obstetric, gerontological, mental health, community, and accident and emergency nursing. Traditional Chinese medicine has a profound influence on health maintenance and treatment of disease conditions in Hong Kong. Chinese medicinal nursing was introduced to the undergraduate nursing programs in the 2000s. There were additional refinements made to the curricula in individual universities because of emerging health needs of local and international societies, such as infection control after the outbreak of severe acute respiratory syndrome in 2003, disaster nursing in the late 2000s, and primary healthcare in 2012. Mechanisms of continuous clinical assessment were introduced by NCHK in 2012 to replace the one-off assessment so that students practiced skills in each placement, with continuous feedback from supervisors bringing about improvement. At present, the minimum hours of theoretical and clinical requirements are 1,250 and 1,400 respectively, including several night-shift duties (NCHK, 2016). Upon regular accreditation of the bachelor nursing programs by NCHK to ensure the standards, levels of educational and pedagogical practices, and professional conduct (NCHK, 2017), students who fulfill the graduation requirements of the bachelor program satisfactorily can apply directly for registration with the NCHK.

In response to the 3+3+4 education reform in Hong Kong in 2012, the duration of secondary school study was reduced from seven to six years (i.e. 3+3) and students received one more year of higher education. The pre-registration nursing degree program was lengthened from four to five years. In general, the new university curriculum emphasizes broadening students' knowledge base. Subjects such as general education, physical education, life-long learning, leadership, intrapersonal development, service learning, cultural studies, and electives have become elements of the undergraduate curriculum for university students (University Grants Committee (UGC), 2012). The UGC is the non-statutory body which advises the Hong Kong Government on the strategic development of higher education. It promoted an outcome-based approach in its funded universities (Stone, 2005). In response to this change, the nursing curriculum was revised to include a clear articulation of intended learning outcomes and the design of various outcome-based teaching, learning, and assessment methods.

In 2019, the three UGC-funded universities and three self-financing universities are generally providing five-year nursing programs. These nursing programs are subject to accreditation by the offering university and the Hong Kong Council for Accreditation of Academic and Vocational Qualifications (HKCAAVQ) (mainly for self-financing universities) to ensure quality assurance. Owing to the need to meet the shortage of nurses in healthcare sectors and to encourage young people to enter into nursing, the student intake numbers have been increased to about 200 in each class (UGC, 2019). Moreover, transfer students in associate degree or higher diploma graduates (referred to as senior-year places admitted students in Hong Kong) with credit transfers have been admitted from 2015. The number of freshmen entrants (referred to as first-year first-degree intake admitted students in Hong Kong) by the three UGC-funded universities was 625 in 2017–18 (Benitez, 2018), while the number of first-year transfer students from community colleagues was about 120 in 2019.

Closing and re-opening of nursing schools affiliated to hospitals

With the transition of nursing education from hospital-based to university training and a steady decline in the turnover rates of nurses, the Hospital Authority announced the suspension of hospital-based nursing training in 1999. All the schools of general nursing closed after the graduation of the last batch of students in 2002 (HKSNE, 2002). However, because of the nursing shortage in the following years in the social services sector (Chan, 2010), three nursing schools were re-opened in 2008 (School of General Nursing, TMH, 2019). In order to improve the pathway to higher education, the qualification title of "hospital-based diploma" was changed to "higher diploma," accredited by the HKCAAVQ. Currently, three hospitals under the Hospital Authority provide a three-year higher diploma in nursing, with a registered nurse qualification. Clinical training is often provided by the affiliated hospital.

Pre-registration master degree for non-nursing degree graduates

As well as admitting graduates from secondary schools, associate degrees, or higher diplomas to bachelor degree nursing programs, another pathway was established in 2008 to prepare graduates of non-nursing first degrees to pursue nursing careers. Two UGC-funded universities offer a three-year full-time self-financed Master in Nursing for non-nursing degree graduates. This is a fast-track program which was developed in North America (American Association of Colleges of Nursing, 2019). Building on the previous learning experience, students normally complete this program in three years. The curriculum includes theoretical input and practicum of the undergraduate nursing program and additional post-graduate components such as concepts of advanced and professional nursing practice, and leadership and management in healthcare. Graduates from the pre-registration master nursing program bring their previous education and working experiences to the nursing service and are valued members of their healthcare teams.

Post-registration nursing education

To equip nurses with advanced knowledge in the areas of practice, education, management, and research, universities also offer master and doctoral programs. Students are required to complete core subjects (e.g., concepts of advanced nursing practice, advanced research methods, advanced health assessment, philosophy of nursing, healthcare management), choose elective subjects covering a wide range of nursing specialties (e.g., critical care nursing, gerontological nursing, infection control, nursing education), and complete a capstone project which often includes writing a dissertation after a research study or clinical practicum project. Overseas attachment or exchange is an integral part of some programs. As an alternative to these mainstream post-graduate nursing programs, a master program in Chinese medicinal nursing was launched in 2015 in a self-financed university with the aim of enabling nurses to apply the principles of traditional Chinese medicine in their clinical practice. Master programs usual take one to 1.5 years full-time or two to 2.5 years part-time to complete. Doctoral programs are more in-depth in terms of theoretical input and dissertation requirements. They usually take three years full-time or four years part-time to complete.

Master of Philosophy (MPhil) and Doctor of Philosophy (PhD) programs are offered by universities to nursing graduates who have bachelor's or master's degrees and would like to develop their research expertise and scholarship. The normal durations of full-time MPhil or PhD programs are about two and three to four years respectively. Students who choose to study in part-time mode may take one more year to complete the program. In addition to the requirement of coursework on research knowledge and skills, and ethics, students are required to prepare a proposal, complete a final thesis, and pass an oral examination under the supervision of nursing faculties. Teaching in university is an additional component of the research degree program, to prepare candidates for an academic career.

Continuing nursing education opportunities

Continuing nursing education, another important aspect, is defined as any post-registration educational experience with an aim to enrich nurses' contribution to quality healthcare and help them in their pursuit of professional goals (NCHK, 2011). Since the mid-1980s, tertiary institutions in Hong Kong have provided education opportunities to registered nurses by offering diploma programs in nursing, nursing education, and nursing administration/management. The Institute of Advanced Nursing Studies (IANS), an integral part of the Nursing Services Department of the Hospital Authority Head Office, was inaugurated formally in July 1995. It offers Specialty Nursing Certificate courses, enhancement programs, and e-learning programs (Hospital Authority Institute of Health Care, 2018). In addition short-term or long-term education programs, talks, workshops, and professional certificates/diplomas in specialties are offered by tertiary institutions, hospitals, and professional organizations (e.g., Hong Kong Academy of Nursing (HKAN), HKSNE). Nurses can earn continuing nursing education points, a requirement for nursing practice as stipulated by NCHK (2011). The completion of continuing nursing education programs, especially the Specialty Nursing Certificate courses offered by IANS and master programs offered by universities, is often a pre-requisite for registered nurses employed by the Hospital Authority to advance their careers.

Emerging teaching and learning methods

The advancement of technology has created the digital era, with the current generation typically good at using electronic technology (Chicca and Shellenbarger, 2018). With the aim of enabling today's students to develop higher-order thinking capacities, parts of the traditional instruction-centered approaches have been replaced by student-active pedagogies in the past two decades in Hong Kong. A Google search was conducted on the effects of pedagogies used in nursing education in Hong Kong using the key words "nursing education" and "Hong Kong." The results indicated that, from 2002, pedagogies such as problem-based learning, inter-professional education, and technology-assisted approaches have gradually been employed in nursing education in Hong Kong. The development of these pedagogies is summarized briefly in the following sections.

Problem-based learning (PBL)

PBL originated at the McMaster School of Medicine in Canada in 1965 (Berkson, 1993). It is a student-centered approach that enables students to work cooperatively in small groups to seek solutions to situations or problems. Students are presented with a problem in a clinical scenario. They are required to apply their previous knowledge and acquire new knowledge to solve the problem. Learning takes place in small groups. In response to the need to develop critical thinkers who are able to deal with the increasingly complex healthcare context, PBL was first incorporated as a pedagogical strategy in the pre-registration nursing curriculum in 2000 in Hong Kong (Pang et al., 2002). This team reported that overall positive results were found after adopting PBL for two semesters. Improvements were found in students' learning outcomes, and self-learning in terms of preparing and studying information, acceptance of criticism, and willingness to change their perceptions about new information. They were also more willing to give feedback to other group members. However, on the other hand, some students had experienced group difficulties, found it time consuming to gather information, and felt they had not received adequate guidance before self-study (Mok & Wong, 2002; Pang et al., 2002; Tiwari et al., 2006a; Wong et al., 2001). When compared with traditional lectures, another team of researchers found that PBL was more effective in fostering critical thinking skills (i.e., overall critical thinking skills, and sub-skills such as truth seeking, analytical skills, and self-confidence). However, the overall scores for critical thinking disposition before and after the intervention did not reach the cut-off score, which indicated a weak critical thinking deposition (Tiwari et al., 2006b). In applications of PBL to clinical nursing education for undergraduate nursing students, they improved significantly on deep learning approaches. Students also perceived that the approaches were useful for motivating them to learn; self-directing their learning; facilitating active, and interactive and student-centered learning. They also said that the overall learning experience was rather enjoyable, but no significant change was found to their original surface learning approaches (Tiwari et al., 2006b). In summary, PBL can improve students' learning in both classroom and clinical settings.

Inter-professional education (IPE)

IPE is defined as "occasions when two or more professions learn with, form and about each other to improve collaboration and the quality of care" (Centre for the Advancement of Inter-professional Education (CAIPE), 2019). Since the 1970s, many IPE initiatives have been developed in western countries and have become a part of official government policies in some countries due to their benefits, in terms of better quality of services and improved outcomes (CAIPE, 2019). The first IPE involving nursing students in Hong Kong was launched in 2005, with students from social work (Chan et al., 2010). These students were encouraged to learn from each other's disciplines in the ethical decision-making process and caring practice through a case scenario on elder abuse. Each seminar lasted about three hours. At the end of the four inter-disciplinary seminars, the students reported an increased awareness of each other's professional values, disciplinary knowledge, and their roles. They also expressed an appreciation of the opportunity for mutual learning.

More recently, a large-scale inter-professional team-based learning program (IPTBL) involving nursing students and another five undergraduate health and social care programs (biomedical sciences, Chinese medicine, medicine, pharmacy, and social work) from two universities in Hong Kong was conducted in the academic year 2015–16 (Chan et al., 2017; Wong et al., 2017). The program consisted of three instructional units including anticoagulation therapy, multiple drugs and complementary therapies, and developmental delay, each of which lasted for about four hours on a Saturday. Throughout the program, the students were encouraged to work together in solving clinical problems, and to learn about the roles, responsibilities, and limitations of the different health professions. The results of the program revealed a significant improvement in students' readiness to prepare themselves for collaborative practice, including improved interactions among the students for teamwork and collaboration, increased positive professional identity, and increased awareness of their own roles and responsibilities and those of the other professions. The students also reported a reduced negative professional identity. Team-based learning approaches are still very new in Hong Kong. Evaluations of the effects on students' skill performances and patient outcomes, in addition to students' attitudes toward other professions, are warranted in the future.

Technology-assisted approaches

A wide variety of technology-assisted teaching has been employed increasingly in nursing curricula in the past 10 years. These pedagogies have included the use of simulators (Fong, 2013), flipped classrooms (Kwan, 2017), video-taped vignettes (Chau et al., 2001), and mobile learning (Li et al., 2019). Those pedagogies have had positive effects in enhancing students' learning skills/intellectual gains and personal growth and clinical reasoning skills (Chan et al., 2016). Each is described in more detail below.

Simulation-based learning

High-fidelity simulators are employed in nursing curricula because of the multiple advantages that simulation offers. Simulation is a rich, active, and learning-centered approach that has been found to increase students' motivation and interest, and allows them to learn and practice in a safe environment with no harm to patients (Feingold, Calauce, & Kallen, 2004). The first study examining the effects of human patient simulation in nursing education was conducted in the United States (Ravert, 2008). In Hong Kong, a patient simulator was first introduced into nursing education in 1999. A mixed-method design was employed to examine the effects of four-hour high-fidelity human simulation training on nursing students' self-confidence in learning and the development of critical thinking. The participants were found to have improved both self-confidence in learning and critical thinking after the training (Fong, 2013).

Flipped-classroom approach to teaching

Blended learning is an approach whereby students learn in part face to face, and in part by doing learning activities through the internet. Students can choose to learn in different places at their own time (Osguthorpe & Graham, 2003). Of the many different models of blended learning in practice, the use of the flipped-classroom approach has become increasingly popular in higher education (Garrison & Kanuka, 2004), particularly in nursing education (Sung, Kwon, & Ryu, 2008). In Hong Kong, this approach was initiated recently in nursing education (Kwan, 2017). Kwan and his team employed the approach in two groups of 40 nursing students enrolled for a Bachelor of Nursing program in 2016 and 2017 to improve their academic performance and learning. In their study, links to YouTube video clips, short readings, and online/in-class quiz testing were provided to the students to pre-view before class. The overall participation rates were 46% and 81% in 2016 and 2017 respectively. Most of the participants found the pre-class activities had helped them to achieve the subject learning outcomes. A similar approach was employed by Tiwari and her team (2016) with a group of post-graduate students enrolled in a family violence course. Both teams found that the pre-class on-line materials were useful to provide fundamental information that facilitated face-to-face interactions in class.

Video vignettes

Chau and her colleagues compared the use of four video vignettes across 13 weeks to enhance critical thinking in undergraduate nursing students. They used a pre-and-post study design with no control group (Chau et al., 2001). No statistical differences were found between the pre- and post-intervention scores. Low doses of the intervention may have contributed to the min-imal effect on critical thinking. The results suggested that the web-based approach was compar-able to a traditional classroom approach since there are no significant differences in effects by using the two approaches.

Mobile learning in the clinical practicum

A recent study examined the effects of mobile apps on the learning motivation, social inter-action and study performance of nursing students (Li et al., 2019). Quantitative data col-lected from surveys revealed that the students had relatively high levels of motivation to use the apps, but reported low satisfaction and self-efficacy with mobile learning. Nevertheless, findings from 20 students via focus group interviews found that the students actively used the mobile apps to study supplementary materials as well as participating in in-class activities and clinical assessments.

Although technology-assisted approaches are a trend, studies to evaluate their effective-ness in nursing education are limited in Hong Kong. The results of recent studies serve as a foundation for further research in this area.

Current challenges of nursing education in Hong Kong

Conflicting views about diverse pathways in nursing education

In addition to the retention strategies employed in clinical settings, diverse pathways of pre-registration programs are being used to tackle nursing shortages in overseas countries and in Hong Kong (as discussed earlier). While diverse pathways have the advantages of admitting students with diverse educational backgrounds, they can also lead to confusion and conflict-ing views. There is a continuous debate about whether the bachelor degree should be the entry level into the profession instead of the higher diploma in Hong Kong (Chan, 2010) or associate degree in the United States (Smith, 2017). The increased complexity and demands on the nursing role nowadays are driving a call for advancements in nursing education.

In addition, the articulation from a higher diploma or an associate degree to a pre-registration or non-nursing first degree to a pre-registration master degree is another issue. Similar to transfer students in other countries, it is a challenge to enhance their learning since most of the university resources are allocated to freshmen entrants (Blaylock & Bresciani, 2011), with the assumption that these transfer students are mature enough to navigate their new university learning and social environments (Cheung, 2015; Cheung et al., 2015). "Transfer shocks" (Flaga, 2006) and "feeling of demotion" (Townsend, 2008) are some of the phenomena that describe the experiences of students transferring from community colleges to universities. Similar experiences might be encountered by other pathway students. More research should be conducted to learn what is needed to enhance the transition process.

Supporting continuous professional development of graduated nurses

The nursing profession in Hong Kong has developed rapidly in the past decade. In 2011, HKAN was established with the aim to strive for excellence in achieving safe and quality healthcare that can benchmark with international standards (HKAN, 2019). In the report of the Institute of Medicine (2011) on *The Future of Nursing: Leading Change, Advancing Health*, one of the recommendations for transforming the nursing professions was having nurses achieve higher levels of education and training through an improved education system that promotes seamless academic progression. NCHK encourages nurses to engage in continuing nursing education (NCHK, 2011). In order to support the advancement of the profession, nurses should be encouraged to pursue master and doctoral degrees to support their evidence-based practices. It has been suggested that the major factors hindering Hong Kong nurses' active participation in continuing education are time, finances, and family commitments (Lee et al., 2005). Flexible or self-paced studying scheduled with the adoption of e-learning pedagogies is recommended to allow nurses to access learning without the constraints of time and place. Moreover, within the nursing arena, there have been recommendations put forward for advanced, specialty-focused, and award-bearing education programs with professional organizations (e.g. HKAN), universities/tertiary institutions, and involving nurse consultants and advanced practice nurses. Patient care involves multi-disciplinary approaches, and the inter-professional/inter-disciplinary education and simulations adopted in undergraduate nursing education have shown promising results (Chan et al., 2017; Wong et al., 2017). Their applications in post-registration or continuing education programs are warranted.

Adopting new pedagogies in nursing education

As stated, common pedagogies such as PBL, inter-professional learning, and technology-assisted approaches have been employed gradually over the past 20 years to promote active learning in nursing students in Hong Kong. Current, albeit limited, studies on these pedagogies in Hong Kong have found that students, teachers, or both benefited to some extent from the pedagogies. These results are promising and encouraging. Future studies should improve the methodology used for evaluating new pedagogies in nursing education. Longitudinal study designs involving nursing students in all year groups should be implemented. For example, Tiwari et al. (2006b) found that overall scores for critical thinking disposition, both before and after a one-year PBL intervention, failed to reach the instrument's cut-off score of 40, indicating a weak critical thinking disposition (Tiwari et al., 2006b). Intervention with longer duration may be required to bring about positive change (Carter, Creedy, & Sidebotham, 2016). Further assessment should also be considered to examine whether a flipped-classroom approach can foster learning attention over a longer period of time (Kwan, 2017). Recent research on the use of videos in Hong Kong has focused on effectiveness, efficiency, and usage of videos, but no attention has been given to the quality of the video materials (Chau et al., 2001). There is a need for additional research in the area since the quality can affect students' learning outcomes. The use of e-learning has also been exposed to a number of challenges. For example, technological issues have caused frustration for both teachers and students. Teachers are content experts but they might not be familiar with the many different types of technologies. Thus, there is a need for support and training in the use of these technologies. Furthermore, students' performances in clinical practice have not yet been evaluated from a research perspective (Li et al., 2019).

Another area in which there is a need for further research is for more country-specific studies, particularly in Asian countries. The learning approaches of western and Asian students might be different. In Asian countries, didactic models of teaching are still predominant, students seldom question those in authority, and these practices tend not to foster independent thinking (Chan et al., 2011; Lim et al., 2009). While these practices are often led by the view that Hong Kong Chinese students are rote learners, Watkins and Biggs (2001) found that they scored higher than western students on deep learning strategy scales and lower on surface learning strategy scales. Hong Kong students also do better than western students in international assessments, such as the Program for International Student Assessment (PISA) that assesses how well students can apply what they learn in school to real-life situations; and Third International Mathematics and Science Study (TIMSS) that assesses students' science literacy (HKSAR, 2019). In short, effective methods to facilitate the learning of Chinese students should be further explored.

Meeting the demand for nursing manpower

The nursing shortage is a global issue, and Hong Kong is no exception. Of all healthcare professionals in Hong Kong, nurses contribute the most manpower (7.3 per 1,000 population), 3.8 times more than physicians (Food and Health Bureau, 2019), to serve a population of 7.48 million (Census and Statistics Department, 2019). It is projected that, by 2030, there will be a shortfall of over 1,600 nurses and 1,000 doctors in Hong Kong (The Government of the Hong Kong Special Administrative Region (HKSAR), 2017). Moreover, the number of nurses per 1,000 population in Hong Kong is lower than in Singapore and Japan (Research Office, 2018). The nurse-to-patient ratio for night shifts has been recorded as 1:24, much higher than the international standard of 1:6 (as cited in HKSAR, 2018). Nursing shortages may lead to decreases in safe and quality patient care as well as access to healthcare (American Association of Colleges of Nursing, 2019). A further potential problem is the well-being of the nurses themselves (Santos, Barros, & Carolino, 2010). It is a challenge to sustain an adequate nursing workforce. The numbers of places for nursing degrees in the government-funded universities are manpower-driven. The government has also encouraged the launching of self-financed nursing programs and provides subsidization (HKSAR, 2018). The Hospital Authority needs to conduct a comprehensive evaluation of the effectiveness of the current retention measures. Collaboration with university researchers could be one way to develop specific local strategies with reference to international guidelines.

Nurturing personal development of nursing students to cope with nursing work

It is well known that the demanding nature of nursing work may result in high levels of stress (Santos et al., 2010) which pose challenges to nurses' mental and psychological health. In Hong Kong, a study found that it was not only nurses, particularly those working in public hospitals, who were more stressed, depressed, and anxious (Cheung & Yip, 2015), but also that nursing students experienced considerable stress from many aspects. Although nursing students in Hong Kong have moderate levels of compassion and satisfaction, they have also been found to have moderate to high levels of burnout (Ching & Cheung, 2019), stress, and psychological morbidity (Watson et al., 2008). As discussed, nurses have a high patient load in Hong Kong, so it is not surprising to have nurses and nursing students with high levels of stress. There is a need to review nursing curricula to enhance students' coping mechanisms (Timmins et al., 2011) and promote well-being. In addition, an academic community has a responsibility to facilitate nursing students to transit into nurses with the capability of handling the rigors of the profession (Reeve et al., 2013). Thus, building resilience through promoting reflection and application to give students strength, focus, and endurance should be a component of pre-registration nursing curricula (McAllister & McKinnon, 2009). Strategies that nurture reflective learning, emotional literacy, empathy, and self-awareness (Grant & Kinman, 2013) should be developed in both nursing education curricula and clinical staff development programs.

Conclusion

In this chapter, we have described the development of nursing education in Hong Kong from hospital-based training to university higher education; from apprenticeship to schooling; from a single-point of entry to multiple pathways; from diploma to bachelor, master, and doctoral degrees; from teacher- to student-centered teaching approaches; from instruction-centered to active pedagogy; and from classroom to electronic learning. This development has occurred in response to global, national, and local changes, particularly the aging population, complex health conditions, healthcare system reforms, education reforms, the advancement of technology, generational diversity, and many other driving forces. To recap, the purpose of nursing education is to educate nursing students to become competent, caring, and professional nurses, and to provide post-graduate studies and continuing nursing education to enable them to attain academic or clinical advancement. In this digital era, technology-assisted teaching and learning pedagogies are still flourishing. Further methodologically rigorous studies should be conducted, particularly in evaluating the effectiveness of nursing education pedagogies.

References

American Association of Colleges of Nursing. (2019). *Accelerated baccalaureate and master's degrees in nursing.* Retrieved from www.aacnnursing.org/Nursing-Education-Programs/Accelerated-Programs.

Anonymous. (n.d.). *History of school of general nursing QMH.* Retrieved from www3.ha.org.hk/qmh/qmhnaec/Resource/Files/Home/doyouknow/History_of_School_of_General_Nursing_QMH.pdf.

Benitez, M. A. (2018, May 31). Student intakes ramped up as Hong Kong grapples with chronic shortage of doctors, nurses and dentists. *South China Morning Post.* Retrieved from www.scmp.com/news/hong-kong/health-environment/article/2148653/student-intakes-be-boosted-hong-kong-tackles.

Berkson, L. (1993). Problem-based learning: Have the expectations been met? *Academic Medicine, 68*(10, Suppl), S79–S88.

Blaylock, R. S., & Bresciani, M. J. (2011). Exploring the success of transfer programs for community college students. *Research & Practice in Assessment, 6,* 43–61.

Carter A. G., Creedy D. K., Sidebotham M. (2016). Efficacy of teaching methods used to develop critical thinking in nursing and midwifery undergraduate students: A systematic review of the literature. *Nurse Education Today, 40,* 209–218. doi:10.1016/j.nedt.2016.03.010.

Census and Statistics Department. (2019). *Population size.* Retrieved from www.censtatd.gov.hk/hkstat/hkif/index.jsp.

Centre for the Advancement of Interprofessional Education (CAIPE). (2019). *What is CAIPE?* Retrieved from www.caipe.org/about-us.

Chan, A. W. K., Sit, J. W. H., Wong, E. M. L., Lee, D. T. F., & Fung, O. W. M. (2016). Case-based web learning versus face-to-face learning: A mixed-method study on University nursing students. *Journal of Nursing Research, 24*(1), 31–40. doi:10.1097/jnr.0000000000000104.

Chan, E. (2014). Advancing nurses contribution through a clinical career pathway [PowerPoint slides]. Retrieved from www.cnhk.org.hk/eng/Files/1.%20Dr.%20Eric%20Chan.pdf.

Chan, E. A., Chi, S. P. M., Ching, S., & Lam, S. K. (2010). Interprofessional education: The interface of nursing and social work. *Journal of Clinical Nursing, 19*(1–2), 168–176. doi:10.1111/j.1365-2702.2009.02854.x.

Chan, K., & Wong, A. M. (2005). The advancement of nursing in Hong Kong: Reflections of the principal nursing officer. Hong Kong Society for Nursing Education *(HKSNE). Newsletter, 2005,* 5–7.

Chan, L. K., Ganotice, F., Wong, F. K. Y., Lau, C. S., Bridges, S. M., Chan, C. H. Y., … & Chu, J. K. P. (2017). Implementation of an interprofessional team-based learning program involving seven undergraduate health and social care programs from two universities, and students' evaluation of their readiness for interprofessional learning. *BMC Medical Education, 17*(1), 221. doi:10.1186/s12909-017-1046-5.

Chan, M. F., Creedy, D. K., Chua, T. L., & Lim, C. C. (2011). Exploring the psychological health related profile of nursing students in Singapore: a cluster analysis. *Journal of Clinical Nursing, 20*(23–24), 3553–3560. doi:10.1111/j.1365-2702.2011.03807.x.

Chan, S., & Wong, F. (1999). Development of basic nursing education in China and Hong Kong. *Journal of Advanced Nursing, 29*(6), 1300–1307. doi:10.1046/j.1365-2648.1999.01015.x.

Chan, S. W. C. (2010, May). From Hong Kong to Singapore - A personal reflection on nursing education. *HKSNE Newsletter, 2010,* 5–8.

Chau, J. P. C., Chang, A. M., Lee, I. F. K., Ip, W. Y., Lee, D. T. F., & Wootton, Y. (2001). Effects of using videotaped vignettes on enhancing students' critical thinking ability in a baccalaureate nursing programme. *Journal of Advanced Nursing, 36*(1), 112–119. doi:10.1046/j.1365-2648.2001.01948.x.

Cheung, K. (2015, April). Academic advising & support for senior year admitted students. *Paper presented at the towards effective academic advising – Academic advising symposium 2015,* Hong Kong.

Cheung, K., Lai, P., Yick, K.L., & Chan, S.W. (2015, May). Perception of the teaching-learning environment and learning approaches on the academic results of senior-year admitted (SYA) students. *Paper presented at the international conference: Assessment for learning in higher education 2015,* Hong Kong.

Cheung, T., & Yip, P. S. F. (2015). Depression, anxiety and symptoms of stress among Hong Kong nurses: a cross-sectional study. *International Journal of Environmental Research and Public Health, 12,* 11072–11100. doi:10.3390/ijerph120911072.

Chicca, J., & Shellenbarger, T. (2018). Connecting with generation Z: Approaches in nursing education. *Teaching and Learning in Nursing, 13*(3), 180–184. doi:10.1016/j.teln.2018.03.008.

Ching, S. S. Y., & Cheung, K. (2019). Resilience of nursing students in Hong Kong. Manuscript in preparation.

Feingold, D. E., Calauce, M., & Kallen, M.A. (2004). Computerised patient model and simulated clinical experiences: Evaluation with baccalaureate nursing students. *Journal of Nursing Education, 43*(4), 156–163.

Flaga, C. T. (2006). The process of transition for community college transfer students. *Community College Journal of Research and Practice, 30*(1), 3–19. doi:10.1080/10668920500248845.

Fong, W. C. K. (2013). *Nursing students' satisfaction and self-confidence towards high-fidelity simulation and its relationship with the development of critical thinking in Hong Kong.* Doctoral dissertation. Chinese University of Hong Kong. Retrieved from. https://core.ac.uk/download/pdf/48545624.pdf.

Food and Health Bureau. (2019). *Table 1. Health care resources. Table 2. Population and vital events.* Retrieved from www.fhb.gov.hk/statistics/en/health_statistics.htm.

Food and Health Bureau & Department of Health. (2018). *TOWARDS 2025: Strategy and action plan to prevent and control non-communicable diseases in Hong Kong (Summary Report).*Retrieved from www.chp. gov.hk/files/pdf/saptowards2025_summaryreport_en.pdf.

Garrison, D. R., & Kanuka, H. (2004). Blended learning: Uncovering its transformative potential in higher education. *The Internet and Higher Education, 7*(2), 95–105. doi:10.1016/j.iheduc.2004.02.001.

Grant, L., & Kinman, G. (2013). *The importance of emotional resilience of staff and students in the 'helping' professions: Developing an emotional curriculum.* Retrieved from www.heacademy.ac.uk/system/files/emotional_resilience_louise_grant_march_2014_0.pdf.

Hong Kong Society for Nursing Education. (2002). *The transition of nursing duration in HongKong.* Hong Kong: Author.

Hospital Authority. (2017). *Innovating for better care: Strategic plan 2017-2022.* Retrieved from www.ha. org.hk/haho/ho/ap/HA-SP_1.pdf.

Hospital Authority Institute of Health Care. (2018). *Institute of advanced nursing studies*. Retrieved from www.ihc.ha.org.hk/en/About/IANS.

Institute of Medicine (US). Committee on the Robert Wood Johnson Foundation Initiative on the Future of Nursing. (2011). *The future of nursing: Leading change, advancing health*. Washington, DC: National Academies Press.

Kwan, R. Y. (2017, October). Use of flipped classroom teaching to promote students' active learning. *Paper presented at the 44th biennial convention*, Indianapolis, IN, USA. Retrieved from https://sigma.nursin grepository.org/bitstream/handle/10755/623205/Kwan_R_86804_1.pdf?sequence=1&isAllowed=y.

Lee, A. C., Tiwari, A. F., Hui Choi, E. W., Yuen, K. H., & Wong, A. (2005). Hong Kong nurses' perceptions of and participation in continuing nursing education. *Journal of Continuing Education in Nursing, 36*(5), 205–212.

Lee, S. (2017). HA nurse clinics [PowerPoint slides]. Retrieved from www3.ha.org.hk/haconvention/hac2017/proceedings/downloads/PS3.3.pdf.

Li, K. C., Lee, L. Y. K., Wong, S. L., Yau, I. S. Y., & Wong, B. T. M. (2019). The effects of mobile learning for nursing students: An integrative evaluation of learning process, learning motivation, and study performance. *International Journal of Mobile Learning and Organisation, 13*(1), 51–67. doi:10.1504/IJMLO.2019.096471.

Lim, C. C., Chua, T. L., Creedy, D. K., & Chan, M. F. (2009). Preliminary study of stress in undergraduate nursing students in Singapore. *Asia-Pacific Psychiatry, 1*(2), 74–80. doi:10.1111/j.1758-5872.2009.00019.x.

McAllister, M., & McKinnon, J. (2009). The importance of teaching and learning resilience in the health disciplines: A critical review of the literature. *Nurse Education Today, 29*(4), 371–379. doi:10.1016/j.nedt.2008.10.011

Mok, E., & Wong, F. K. Y. (2002). The issue of death and dying: Employing problem-based learning in nursing education. *Nurse Education Today, 22*(4), 319–329. doi:10.1054/nedt.2001.0708.

Osguthorpe, R. T., & Graham, C. R. (2003). Blended learning environments: Definitions and directions. *Quarterly Review of Distance Education, 4*(3), 227–233.

Pang, S. M., Wong, T. K., Dorcas, A., Lai, C. K., Lee, R. L., Lee, W. M., … & Wong, F. K. (2002). Evaluating the use of developmental action inquiry in constructing a problem- based learning curriculum for pre-registration nursing education in Hong Kong: A student perspective. *Journal of Advanced Nursing, 40*(2), 230–241. doi:10.1046/j.1365-2648.2002.02365.x.

QS World University Rankings. (2019). *The QS world university rankings by subject 2019: Nursing*. Online accessed on February 28, 2019 www.topuniversities.com/university-rankings/university-subject-rank ings/2019/nursing.

Ravert, P. (2008). Patient simulator sessions and critical thinking. *Journal of Nursing Education, 47*(12), 557–562.

Reeve, K. L., Shumaker, C. J., Yearwood, E. L., Crowell, N. A., & Riley, J. B. (2013). Perceived stress and social support in undergraduate nursing students' educational experiences. *Nurse Education Today, 33*(4), 419–424. doi:10.1016/j.nedt.2012.11.009.

Research Office, Legislative Council Secretariat. (2018, November 2). *Healthcare workforce*. Retrieved from www.legco.gov.hk/research-publications/english/1819issh05-healthcare-workforce-20181102-e.pdf.

Santos, M.C., Barros, L., & Carolino, E. (2010). Occupational stress and coping resources in physiotherapists: A survey of physiotherapists in three general hospitals. *Physiotherapy, 96*, 303–310. doi:10.1016/j.physio.2010.03.001.

School of General Nursing, Tuen Mun Hospital (TMH). (2019). *School of general nursing*. Retrieved from www3.ha.org.hk/tmh/en/healthcare_pro/03_03.asp.

Shield, L., & Watson, R. (2007). The demise of nursing in the United Kingdom: A warning for medicine. *Journal of The Royal Society of Medicine, 100*, 70–74. doi:10.1258/jrsm.100.2.70.

Smith, A. A. (2017, Dec 22). Debate continues on nursing degrees. *Inside Higher ED*. Retrieved from www.insidehighered.com/news/2017/12/22/battle-over-entry-level-degree-nursing-continues.

Stone, M. V. (2005, December). *Symposium on outcome-based approach to teaching, learning and assessment in higher education international perspectives*. Retrieved from www.ugc.edu.hk/eng/ugc/about/press_speech_other/speech/2005/sp171205.html.

Sung, Y. H., Kwon, I. G., & Ryu, E. (2008). Blended learning on medication administration for new nurses: Integration of e-learning and face-to-face instruction in the classroom. *Nurse Education Today, 28*(8), 943–952. doi:10.1016/j.nedt.2008.05.007.

The Government of the Hong Kong Special Administrative Region (HKSAR). (2017). *LCQ17: Manpower of healthcare professionals.* Retrieved from www.info.gov.hk/gia/general/201707/12/P2017071200517.htm

The Government of the Hong Kong Special Administrative Region (HKSAR). (2018). *LCQ19: Healthcare manpower.* Retrieved from www.info.gov.hk/gia/general/201804/25/P2018042500725.htm

The Government of the Hong Kong Special Administrative Region (HKSAR). (2019). *International study shows Hong Kong students' continued outstanding performance in reading, mathematical and scientific literacy.* Retrieved from www.info.gov.hk/gia/general/201612/06/P2016120600679.htm.

The Hong Kong Academy of Nursing Limited. (2019). *Home.* Retrieved from www.hkan.hk/main/en/.

The Nursing Council of Hong Kong. (2011). *Manual for continuing nursing education system.* Retrieved from www.nchk.org.hk/filemanager/en/pdf/continue_e.pdf.

The Nursing Council of Hong Kong. (2016). *A reference guide to the syllabus of subjects and requirements for the preparation of registered nurse (general) in the Hong Kong Special.* Retrieved from www.nchk.org.hk/filemanager/en/pdf/sf04.pdf.

The Nursing Council of Hong Kong. (2017). *Handbook for accreditation of training institutions for pre-enrolment/pre-registration nursing education. Hong Kong*: Nursing Council of Hong Kong. Retrieved from www.nchk.org.hk/filemanager/en/pdf/Accreditation_Handbook.pdf.

Timmins, F., Corroon, A. M., Byrne, G., & Mooney, B. (2011). The challenge of contemporary nurse education programmes - perceived stressors of nursing students: Mental health and related lifestyle issues. *Journal of Psychiatric and Mental Health Nursing, 18*, 758–766. doi:10.1111/j.1365-2850.2011.01780.x.

Tiwari, A., Chan, S., Wong, E., Wong, D., Chui, C., Wong, A., & Patil, N. (2006a). The effect of problem-based learning on students' approaches to learning in the context of clinical nursing education. *Nurse Education Today, 26*(5), 430–438. doi:10.1016/j.nedt.2005.12.001.

Tiwari, A., Cheung, D. S. T., & Li, W. (2016). Flipped classroom teaching. In Mak, Y.W., Chiang, C. L.V & Fung, W.M.O. (Eds.), *Enhancing patient safety through quality nursing education: The challenges and solutions from a multi-disciplinary perspective* (pp. 58–65). Hong Kong: Hong Kong Society for Nursing Education. ISBN 9-789628-662623.

Tiwari, A., Lai, P., So, M., & Yuen, K. (2006b). A comparison of the effects of problem-based learning and lecturing on the development of students' critical thinking. *Medical Education, 40*(6), 547–554. doi:10.1111/j.1365-2929.2006.02481.x.

Townsend, B.K. (2008). Feeling like a freshman again: The transfer student transition. *New Directions for Higher Education, 144*, 69–77. doi:10.1002/he.327

University Grant Committee. (2012). *The "3+3+4" new academic structure.* Retrieved from www.ugc.edu.hk/minisite/eng/ugc/report/figure2011/d001.htm

University Grant Committee. (2019). *General statistics on UGC-funded institutions/programs.* Retrieved from https://cdcf.ugc.edu.hk/cdcf/statEntry.action?language=EN.

Watkins, D., & Biggs, J. B. (2001). *Teaching the Chinese learner: psychological and pedagogical perspectives.* Hong Kong: Comparative Education Research Centre, The University of Hong Kong.

Watson, R., Deary, I., Thompson, D., & Li, G. (2008). A study of stress and burnout in nursing students in Hong Kong: A questionnaire survey. *International Journal of Nursing Studies, 45*(10), 1534–1542. doi:10.1016/j.ijnurstu.2007.11.003.

Wong, A. K. C., Wong, F. K. Y., Chan, L. K., Chan, N., Ganotice, F. A., & Ho, J. (2017). The effect of interprofessional team-based learning among nursing students: A quasi-experimental study. *Nurse Education Today, 53*, 13–18.

Wong, F. K. Y., Lee, W. M., & Mok, E. (2001). Educating nurses to care for the dying in Hong Kong: a problem-based learning approach. *Cancer Nursing, 24*(2), 112–121.

5

A HISTORY OF NURSE EDUCATION IN THE BAILIWICK OF GUERNSEY

Tracey McClean

Introduction

The Bailiwick of Guernsey is populated by nearly 66,000 people, including those inhabiting the islands of Guernsey, Alderney, Sark, Herm, Brecqhou and Jethou. Guernsey is the largest island, spanning 24 square miles with a population of over 60,000. The Bailiwick consists of three sub-jurisdictions which independently govern the islands; these are the States of Guernsey, the States of Alderney and Sark Chief Pleas, all of which have independent powers of primary legislation (Ministry of Justice 2013; States of Guernsey 2018).

Health and social care within the islands is funded through a mix of compulsory insurance and taxation supported with private out-of-pocket payments for some services such as primary and emergency care. The States of Guernsey Committee for Health and Social Care (HSC) is the main provider of health and social care across the Bailiwick, employing 2,000 staff, 1,100 of whom are unregistered nurses, registered nurses and midwives (HSSD 2013; Winterflood 2016). Nurses and midwives working within the Bailiwick are expected to be registered with the Nursing and Midwifery Council (NMC); they are also admitted to a local register, along with other health and social care professionals working in the islands (States of Guernsey 2006).

Despite serving a small population HSC provides a wide range of health and social care services across Guernsey and Alderney. These have expanded over the years to the point where Guernsey hospital services are commensurate with those provided by a UK district general hospital delivering care to a much larger population (HSSD 2011). Although Alderney residents access hospital services in Guernsey, including maternity services, Alderney has a 22-bedded community hospital which provides a mix of long-term, acute and urgent care together with a community outreach service. Whilst technological advances have aided the communication between the island care providers and specialist services in the UK (HSC 2017), the geographical isolation remains a challenge when an island resident requires physical transfer to these specialist centres.

The recruitment and retention of appropriately skilled nursing staff on the islands are problematic. One solution which was first mooted in the mid-1940s was for Guernsey Health Services to "grow their own" workforce. A review of Guernsey hospitals in 1946 supported the idea of having a training school on island as a means of developing a local workforce (Bourne et al. 1946). However, it wasn't until 9 December 1966, 20 years later, that the General Nursing Council (GNC) Enrolled Nurses Committee gave provisional approval for Guernsey to have its own training school (Briggs 1966b). The first cohort of seven pupil nurses began their training on 20 February 1967 (Craig 1968). The training school has evolved over the past more than 50 years from an establishment which employed one sister tutor to an institute validated and endorsed to run under- and postgraduate programmes, delivered by 14 lecturers from a range of health and social care backgrounds.

This chapter will provide a scholarly account of nurse education in the Bailiwick of Guernsey and in so doing will include the following:

- a history of nurse education on the island, analysing the exciting and transformational journey from "Nursing School" to "The Institute" as it is today;
- a critical analysis of the challenges of providing nurse education to prepare nurses to work within a small-island context;
- a critical evaluation of how these challenges have been addressed and the plans and options for future provision

Nurse education in Guernsey – a transformational journey

According to Gallienne (1999), prior to 1887 "Professional nursing was almost non-existent; the nursing staff generally being untrained" (p. 47). The formation of the St Peter Port Nursing Corps in early 1887 brought together women who had been trained in first aid and nursing through the St John's Ambulance Association. Dr E. Robinson was instrumental in forming the Nursing Corps and providing additional training for them. His intention was to develop a cottage hospital in Guernsey, where patients would be treated with modern equipment and provided with good nursing care. The Victoria Cottage hospital, which opened in 1888, proved to be a more favourable alternative than the two establishments which existed under the control of the Poor Law Board: the Town Hospital (founded in 1741) and the Country Hospital (founded in 1751), both serving to shelter the poor and destitute as well as the old, infirm, inebriated, orphaned, mentally ill and those with learning disabilities. In addition, the King Edward Sanatorium was built in 1903 to treat patients with infectious diseases and became an isolation hospital.

Records indicated that in the years leading up to the first World War there was "considerable" staff turnover at the Town Hospital, where "nurses and assistants come and go at alarming regularity" (Lenfesty 1999, p. 33). It is unclear whether it was this turnover which acted as a trigger to provide a more formal qualifying certificate for assistant nurses. These individuals were required to undergo 3 years of lectures delivered by doctors and practical instruction facilitated by "Sister"; they also sat exams and were awarded a certificate on completion.

The Second World War instigated further change when the Country Hospital was converted into an emergency hospital to deal with war casualties, as well as serving the 23,000 islanders who chose not to evacuate to England. Patients from the Victoria Hospital and the Maternity Home were relocated at the Country Hospital. The German occupying forces took over the Victoria hospital in 1940 and the newly built "modern mental hospital" the Vauquiedor Hospital, as military hospitals (Tough 1999).

There was no formal training for nursing staff during the war period, with all ward nurses beneath the rank of "Sister" being unqualified. However, records indicate that these nurses were required to attend lectures after their shift which covered subjects such as "anatomy and physiology, cookery, nutrition, personal hygiene and first aid" (Birchenall 1997, p. 1315). Birchenall goes on to state that most of the training involved "sitting with Nellie", with the ward nurses learning their skills from the three matrons and ward sisters who themselves were "fully qualified". Beryl Ozanne's account of being a surgical ward nurse during the Occupation talks openly about being "thrown in the deep end", by being asked "to do things [she] hadn't done before" (Ozanne 1994, p. 53). This included scrubbing for a theatre case and giving an injection without prior training.

The end of the war and German Occupation of Guernsey marked a turning point in the delivery of hospital-based services and the subsequent education of nursing staff in Guernsey. Following reports of the poor conditions within the Emergency Hospital, the then States of Guernsey Board of Health requested a review of Health and Hospital Services. The report produced by Bourne et al. (1946) confirmed that the Emergency Hospital was not fit for purpose and that "the acute sick must have claim upon a modern building" (p. 14). The Vauquiedor Hospital, as a modern building, was identified as a sound alternative site to develop a general hospital. The report went on to suggest that it would be worth exploring with the GNC the feasibility of developing the island's General Hospital into "a complete training school". The same report recommended that the Victoria Hospital become a maternity hospital and, once a resident obstetric officer was appointed, to seek approval as a Part II training school for midwives. Correspondence between the GNC and the President of the Board of Health supported this intention (Henry 1948a, 1948b, 1948c; Symons 1948a, 1948b, 1948c). However, in 1949 the newly named Princess Elizabeth Hospital finally opened (Seth-Smith 1999) but the desire to seek approval for nurse training on the island seemed to cease in 1948. A letter from the President indicated that approval would not be sought until the new nurses' home had been built in 18 months' time (Houghton 1948a, 1948b; Symons 1948d).

The 1960s saw a slow but fruitful effort to develop a training school to deliver enrolled nurse training. This was driven by Emma Ferbrache, a retired nurse turned politician and elected member of the Board of Health (States of Guernsey 1959), who suggested that the provision of training on the island would reduce the need to fill nurse vacancies with agency nurses (Anon, undated notes). Miss Briggs, on behalf of the GNC, visited the island hospitals in 1964 to review their suitability to support enrolled nurse training. Although she granted provisional approval at this time, she did highlight 14 recommendations which needed to be implemented to bring the Princess Elizabeth Hospital and teaching facilities up to standard (Briggs 1964a). In addition, she made 11 recommendations to bring the Town Hospital to the required standard "to provide a minimum of three months and a maximum of six months geriatric nursing in a scheme of training for pupil nurses to be based at the Princess Elizabeth hospital" (Briggs 1964b, p. 4). Some of the practices in need of improvement included checking of patient medication for more than one patient at a time without a prescription and the sluicing of foul linen on the ward by the nursing staff prior to sending it to the laundry.

This review was a powerful tool in affecting change, resulting in investment to improve the estate, and the establishment of a nursing procedures committee to drive change in nursing practice. In addition, a high-level Education Committee, consisting of political and senior professionals from health and education to oversee the development and management of the school, was convened (Grut 1965; Sarre 1965a, 1965b). A further approval visit, in 1966, demonstrated that improvements had been made, but some practices were still unacceptable, including the sluicing of foul linen on the wards (Briggs 1966a). However, this did not prevent Miss Briggs from presenting her report to the GNC Enrolled Nurse Committee, who in turn granted provisional approval for 2 years for enrolled nurse training to take place on island but insisted that unsatisfactory practices required eradication in the next 6 months (Briggs 1966b; GNC 1967).

The first intake of seven pupil nurses entered the newly built "school" on 20 February 1967 and the "school" was officially opened on 20 March 1967 (Grut 1967). Sister Craig, a qualified nurse tutor, managed the 2-year training programme which offered two intakes of 7–8 pupils per year (Craig 1968). A second tutor was appointed in1968 (Sarre 1968). The educational entry requirements at the time were "a good general education and those without GCE or CSE English language and Arithmetic would be "asked to sit a simple educational test" (Bell undated). The pupil nurses also received a salary which varied from £365 to £545 per annum; the higher salary was given to those who were over 21 years of age.

In light of the fact that the provisional approval to run the enrolled nurse training course was for just 2 years, the GNC announced that they would be visiting the hospitals in the training schemes in early 1970 (Briggs 1969). In the period leading up to the visit there is a written document detailing a conversation with Sister C around the degree to which the recommendations made by the GNC in 1966 had been addressed by the organisation (unknown author, 1970). The language used demonstrates the frustration she was experiencing in implementing and sustaining change in practice. She was "horrified" to find unlocked drug cupboards and "mystified" as to why sterile dressing packs were not available. More worrying was her statement that "in spite of all that has gone before some Doctors still order drugs over the telephone" (p. 2). Despite these concerns the GNC approved the training school, acknowledging that much had been done to improve the service, as demonstrated in the correspondence between the hospital administrator and the GNC (Sarre 1967, 1969) However Ms Radway felt further improvements were required and made 11 recommendations (Radway 1970).

It is interesting to note that one of the recommendations being made was to reduce bed numbers in the island's geriatric hospital, the Town Hospital (Briggs 1964b; Radway 1970). The political response to this request was that the "GNC were pursuing an ideal whereas the first need must be to give the best possible service to patients in need of hospital treatment" (Grut 1971). Despite this political pushback it was agreed to reduce bed numbers. In 1972, the Matron of the town hospital was concerned about the impact on the training school when she was required to accept an additional 10 male patients who were being transferred from a condemned building. The GNC were consulted and were apparently reasonable about this need for emergency action and this temporary solution. The document detailing this course of events notes that the hospital administrator was unable to understand Matron's apparent "flap" (Sarre 1972a). Unfortunately, the GNC visited a few months later and withdrew approval for placements at the Town Hospital due to over-crowding, despite the subsequent written protestations from the same administrator (Briggs 1972a, 1972b; Sarre 1972b, 1972c).

Unfortunately, the records kept during the 1970s and 1980s are not as detailed but some of the key milestones include the renaming of the Training School to the Emma Ferbrache School of Nursing (EFSoN) in 1977 to mark the 10th anniversary of its opening. Also, in 1987, because of the declining interest in enrolled nurse training in the UK and the move to a single level of registered nurse who is prepared in a higher education setting (The Institute for Employment Studies 1997) significant changes affected the provision of nurse education on island (Winterflood 1987). Firstly, the EFSoN was approved by the English National Board, which replaced the GNC for this function, to run a course to convert enrolled nurses to staff nurses. The first cohort began their course in 1988 in the larger relocated premises based on the Princess Elizabeth Hospital campus (Howell 1989).

Secondly, discussions took place in earnest to run the new Project 2000 course to enable locally based students to undertake registered general nurse training on Guernsey (Courtney 1988). The first cohort of three students began their course in September 1991 through a collaborative partnership between the newly named Emma Ferbrache Nurse Education Centre (EFNEC) and Portsmouth Polytechnic. An audio bridge was used to enable students to link into teaching sessions being delivered on the UK site, substantially reducing the time they needed to spend in Portsmouth (Howell 1992). The course proved to be successful, with intakes every 18 months and 20 students undertaking the common foundation programme and adult branch by 1995. The number of staff at this point had increased from one in 1967 to 12 staff, including a librarian and two administrators.

The turn of the millennium saw what could be considered a paradigm shift in the way nurse education and the on-going professional development of staff were delivered on the island. In 1999 the EFNEC went out for tender to partner with a university to deliver pre-registration nursing, adult and mental health branch and to provide a post-qualifying higher education pathway to degree level. Sheffield University won the tender by offering the opportunity for the EFNEC to become an institute validated to design its own curricula, rather than rely on a franchise model of delivery (Fuller 2003). This exciting initiative resulted in EFNEC being validated by the university, leading to yet another change of name, the Institute of Health Studies (IHS), and a move to larger refurbished premises to cope with the increased volume of activity.

The partnership with Sheffield saw the first group of mental health and adult branch nurses graduating with a Diploma in Higher Education in 2003. Approximately half of the total cohort at the time were entering via a vocational route, having been nursing auxiliaries in a previous role (Fuller 2003). This was an attractive option in that staff members could progress their career and remain on the same salary; this fully embraced the concept of "growing our own". It is interesting to note that only three of this cohort no longer work in Guernsey. The post-qualifying programme was also buoyant, with the first graduates graduating in 2006 (Martel 2006).

This period also saw a change in the way nurse education was regulated with the emergence of the NMC and the demise of the English National Board (ENB). The Nursing and Midwifery order (UK Government 2001) also brought with it a new approval process for programmes being delivered outside of the UK. Endorsement is a process by which the NMC is assured that NMC programmes approved to be delivered by a UK higher education institute are implemented in a comparable way in the offshore islands of the British Isles and for the British Forces Health Services (NMC 2006). This had an impact on the delivery of pre-registration nursing programmes in Guernsey. Firstly, the requirement for the IHS to deliver a comparable pre-registration programme to that being delivered to the peer group of students in the UK took away some of the autonomy the Guernsey lecturing staff had experienced previously. Secondly, there was no longer a designated reviewer allocated to Guernsey as there had been with the ENB. The NMC reviewers did not gain the same level of understanding of the context within which nurse education takes place in Guernsey; visits required lengthy explanations of the differences in healthcare provision, legislation and the complexities of the economies of scale.

Following a review of the machinery of government in Guernsey, health and social services were integrated in 2004 (States of Guernsey 2003). This triggered another name change to the Institute of Health and Social Care Studies, shortened to 'The Institute'.

In 2008 a change in partner university provided pre-registration nursing students the opportunity to exit with either a degree or a diploma in higher education depending on their performance in year two. The entry gate was still wide, with cohorts consisting of students representing both vocational entry as well as the more traditional A-level route. However, this was set to change with the proposals for an all-graduate route for nurse education (NMC 2010). The entry requirements for the course narrowed considerably and the last 8 years have seen the profile of students becoming more homogenous and more likely to be a school leaver than a mature applicant. This has proved challenging in terms of recruitment to the course, even though students are given a salary and so can "earn as they learn". In addition, the recruitment pool has been confined to individuals who hold the qualifications to be resident on the island; without this permit they are unable to apply for the course, thus narrowing the applicant population further.

The Institute moved to purpose-built premises in November 2009 and for the first time was housed in an environment to be proud of. The seven classrooms contained new furnishings and teaching equipment. There was a designated practical room and IT training room. The library was a bright airy space conducive to study and a video-conference suite added another dimension for communicating with partners off island.

The next 9 years in the Institute's history have been eventful in many ways. A new Master's programme was validated by Middlesex University which, in turn, became the main partner university for pre- and post-qualifying provision, including non-medical prescribing and the new Nursing Associate course, the latter two being an important new addition in 2018 to the portfolio of programmes offered by the Institute. The profile of the team has also changed during this period to accommodate a more interprofessional approach to learning and includes 14 lecturers, two administrators and one librarian.

A less positive event was the suspension of the pre-registration nurse training programme following the extraordinary Midwifery Review in 2014 (NMC 2014), which identified several organisational failings around the governance of services, including the practice of taking verbal orders for medication. The three student groups at the time were phased back into their training programme over a 1-year period. The NMC was in close contact with the organisation for 2 years whilst an extensive action plan was completed and "signed off" in November 2016. The last group of students affected by the suspension have now completed their programme and the Institute welcomed its biggest intake of pre-registration nursing students in September 2018.

Having reviewed the historical perspective, it is evident that several themes re-emerge from time to time. The first is the drive to deliver a pre-registration nursing course on island to address recruitment and retention problems. The second is the challenge the organisation faces in meeting the standards required by the regulatory body, and the third is the apparent power of the regulatory body to effect change in an organisation, by virtue of its quality assurance function for pre-registration nursing programmes.

The challenges of providing nurse education in the Bailiwick

This section will analyse more specifically the challenges of delivering nurse education on the island along with a critical evaluation of how these challenges have been met. The challenges can be grouped into three key areas: (1) the island infrastructure supporting health and social care; (2) maintaining a quality student experience; and (3) student nurse recruitment.

The island infrastructure supporting health and social care

The infrastructure supporting the delivery of health and social services on the island has several key differences when compared to the UK context. Firstly, the Bailiwick of Guernsey has the infrastructure to develop its own primary legislation and as such UK law has no legislative power within the jurisdiction (Ministry of Justice 2013; Ogier 2005). There is no compulsion to adopt UK policy; The States of Guernsey can set the policy agenda for the island, including that related to health and social care. Whilst all registered health and social care professionals are required to be registered with the relevant UK regulatory body to practice on island (States of Guernsey 1987), organisational policy, guidelines and standards are developed locally by HSC.

Secondly, most of the services are delivered by the public sector and are funded through compulsory insurance and taxation. However, general practice (GP) services or primary care are delivered by private GP practices which are predominantly funded by out-of-pocket payment or private insurance. Secondary care is delivered by the public sector and is free at the point of delivery, except for emergency care which attracts a charge (Institute of Economic Affairs 2017). In addition, hospital-based services are predominantly led by consultant-level medical staff who, in the main, are part of the Medical Specialist Group which is contracted by HSC to provide medical care (The Medical Specialist Group 2018).

Finally, the provision of health and social care within the Bailiwick has expanded to the point where the breadth of services within the hospital setting alone compares favourably with a UK district general hospital serving a larger population (HSSD 2011). Whilst this provides good access for the island community, the limitations in available resources have impacted on the way the workload is organised. The development of specialist units, as seen in large urban trusts, is not sustainable in a smaller setting; for example, there is no access to a stroke unit on the island. The consequence of this is such that the standards set nationally for the delivery of health services cannot always be achieved (Academy of Medical Royal Colleges 2016; National Quality forum 2015). In addition, registered professionals are often placed in a situation where they are caring for people with a wide range of needs; for example, there is just one acute mental health facility and one paediatric ward available to address the needs of those service users. Whilst there is the option for islanders to access specialist services in the UK, including long-term placements for people with highly complex mental health problems and learning disability needs, there is an increasing trend to support these individuals on island to contain costs (HSSD 2012; SLAWS Working Party 2016).

These differences in infrastructure have impacted the nature of the roles that registered professionals hold within the field of health and social care. In line with other small, rural and remote contexts, these roles, by necessity, are broad and require a wide set of generalist skills to match the demands they face in practice (Academy of Medical Royal Colleges 2016; McClean 2016). In addition, the absence of junior doctors within the hospital requires registered nurses to extend the boundary of their role to "fill the gap" (Nuffield Trust 2016). This is not an uncommon feature of small, remote and rural working and is often perceived as an attractive aspect of the role, bringing with it an opportunity to develop into a highly skilled professional (MacVicar and Nicoll 2013).

As stated previously, the programmes endorsed by the NMC need to be delivered in a comparable way to the programmes being offered to peer groups based in the UK. The curriculum has been designed in partnership with key stakeholders, including representatives from UK trusts, to ensure the programme not only complies with the standards set by the NMC (NMC 2010) but also meets the needs of the organisations that will be employing the students completing the course. The current curriculum therefore fits more closely with the UK context, rather than the local one. This has created a problem in that students become well versed in policy and legislation related to the delivery of healthcare in the UK and, more specifically, England, but are less familiar with the local legislation, policy agenda and strategic direction impacting on the health services they will be working in. Whilst there is some flexibility in the programme to accommodate these differences, they have not always been made explicit to the students. In remedying this issue there is also an opportunity to highlight that the four countries which make up the UK have variations in their own healthcare agenda (The Nuffield Trust 2011) and that the developers of local policy and legislation can look to all four jurisdictions for guidance and not just England. For example, elements of children's law (SoG 2008) and mental health legislation (SoG 2016) are based on Scottish law.

In addition, there have been calls for students to access practice-based experiences in the UK to enable them to gain a broader perspective of healthcare provision. This is possibly fuelled by the widely held perspective that specialist services delivered within large urban settings are the gold standard and as such the smaller generalist environment is somewhat second best (Brevetti et al. 2007). However, the fact that the students can meet all their practice-based competencies in Guernsey suggests that an off-island placement is unnecessary. Student nurses educated on the island are given the opportunity to develop a broad range of skills through their placements which provide a wider more generalist experience in the context they will be working in, rather than a potentially narrower more specialist one in a different healthcare system.

Maintaining a quality student experience

It is acknowledged that the learning context is different for the student nurses based in Guernsey compared to their peers in London, for example, and as such it is questionable as to whether the experiences are comparable and of the same quality. Whilst the students in Guernsey have access to a purpose-built facility, this is not the same as a large university environment catering for many different student groups undertaking courses covering different disciplines. However, the university experience is not just about the environment (Kandiko and Mawer 2013); it is about the ability to foster critical thinking and the development of the independent learner (QAA 2014) and in the case of a pre-registration nursing course, a professional who is fit for admission to the NMC register. The curriculum design, the development of study skills and the ability to facilitate interactive classroom-based sessions due to the small group size go some way to achieve this. The lecturing staff liaise closely with their counterparts in the UK and utilise the same learning resources to deliver the curriculum. The ability to communicate agilely is essential and as such relies heavily on electronic modes of communication, including e-mail, teleconferencing and use of a virtual learning environment. The small cohorts enable the lecturing staff to gain supportive links with the students, and to identify quickly if they are not achieving. This level of support is mirrored in the practice setting where students receive one-to-one mentorship and sometimes the allocation of an associate mentor.

It could be argued that this level of support both by the lecturing staff and the practice mentors will not foster independence or resilience in the learner. However, the use of university guidelines for the support of students by lecturers and mentors ensures that the approaches used are comparable; this is further evaluated through the annual monitoring review (The Institute 2017) and endorsement events (Middlesex University and NMC 2016).

The lack of junior doctors provides the students with a wealth of opportunity for not only clinical learning from the consultants but also gaining confidence to communicate with them directly. By the time they qualify they have observed how more experienced nurses are able to gather the essential information about a patient prior to contacting the consultant. They would have seen how this information is communicated and the plan of care agreed. However, as highlighted above, registered nurses working in small, remote and rural settings are required to extend the boundary of their role to meet service needs (Nuffield Trust 2016). In so doing there is a danger for nurses to feel compelled to practise outside the scope of their licensure (Vukic and Keddy 2002) – the acceptance of verbal orders is an example of this. In addition, it is not clear to what extent an organisation can deliver services which do not conform to national standards due to being "small" with limited resource. This creates a dilemma of what acceptable practice "looks like" within the local context.

Since the NMC review in 2014 (NMC 2014), the clinical governance infrastructure has matured and includes an educational component which provides the opportunity for educationalists and service colleagues to review the quality of placement learning (NMC 2015a, 2015b), highlighting any risks and issues related to the learning experience. In addition, all students and mentors have been made aware of the "raising concerns policy" and the importance of using it to highlight areas of concern (Middlesex University and NMC 2016).

Whilst the organisation looks to the UK to guide best practice, there is no external regulatory scrutiny of health and social services from bodies such as the Care Quality Commission (CQC) to assure best-practice standards are followed (States of Guernsey 2017a). The organisation does request external reviews of specific services from time to time from UK experts; in much the same way that Bourne et al. were commissioned to review hospital services in 1946. This does provide a dilemma where the people reviewing the services are viewing them through the lens of the delivery of healthcare in the UK, where resources and infrastructure are quite different to those available on an island, and as a result may make recommendations which are difficult to implement (SoG 2017a). However, it is acknowledged that having "fresh eyes" to review the provision of services is essential to avoid the tolerance of unsafe practice. It could be argued that the presence of student nurses in the workplace can be a source of "fresh eyes" by asking the naïve question and challenging practice which deviates from the expected standard. In addition, placement reviews or audits are completed by an academic from the university in partnership with lecturing staff in Guernsey, adding another tier of scrutiny. The fact that the pre-registration nursing programme has been endorsed by the NMC to be delivered in Guernsey and is subject to annual monitoring review by the university in line with the quality assurance framework (NMC 2018a) gives some reassurance. However, in terms of student experience the current evaluative and feedback mechanisms do not capture how their experience differs from their UK peers, where they receive added value and most importantly how far they feel prepared to work as a registered nurse in Guernsey; this is an area for further exploration.

The recruitment of students

The recruitment and retention of registered nurses remain problematic with the organisation experiencing high turnover and a vacancy rate of 18% in 2017 (States of Guernsey 2017a). The recruitment of registered nurses from off island is costly and, as demonstrated by the turnover, not an effective long-term solution. As identified already, this appears to be an old problem and one that is commonly experienced in underserved or remote and rural contexts (Grobler et al. 2009). At the same time the dwindling recruitment pool across the globe continues to compound the problem (States of Guernsey 2017a).

Since the inception of enrolled nurse training in 1967, pupil and then student nurses have always received some form of salary as a means of attracting recruits, especially the more mature applicant. This has enabled a successful stream of enrolled and registered nurses to emerge and join the local workforce. The fact that the education of nurses on island has been in place for over 50 years and nearly 300 registered nurses have been educated locally since 2000 demonstrates the success of the project.

The Institute has been commissioned to increase student numbers from 15 a year to 25 a year to help meet the deficit in the current workforce. This is going to be very challenging as the recruitment has, to this point, been from the local population which totals 63,000. The island has virtually zero unemployment (1.2%) amongst its working population, with 21% being employed by the finance sector, which offers competitive salaries (States of Guernsey 2017b). The fact that England has made the decision to remove student nurse bursaries and fee waiver from 2017 (Department of Health and Social Care 2017) influenced the decision to enable UK residents to apply to train in Guernsey. From 2018 UK residents who apply and are accepted on the local course will receive a permit to live in Guernsey for 3 years of their training and will be required to work for HSC for a further 2 years. In exchange they will have no fees to pay and will receive a bursary of £19,000. The local residents will also receive this bursary and be required to work for HSC for 2 years to avoid the requirement to pay back fees (HSC 2018).

It is noted that the removal of bursaries has had a significant impact on the number of applicants for nursing in England, with a fall of 12% in 2018 compared with 2017, with a slight rise in applicants in Wales and Scotland, where a bursary system is still in place (UCAS 2018). It will be interesting to see if the Guernsey offer has the desired attraction. So far, the numbers of enquiries from UK applicants has been low, which could be due to the lack of web presence, no identified resource or expertise for marketing, the requirement to relocate to the island and the fact that applications are sent directly to the Institute and not through the Universities and Colleges Admissions Service (UCAS).

It is perhaps slightly reassuring that many providers are experiencing problems in recruiting student nurses and in response to this NHS England has launched an £8 million campaign to boost nursing as a career (NHS England 2018). This, together with plans to launch a new website and develop a marketing strategy to raise the profile of the Institute to the UK candidate, may result in greater success.

Plans for the future

The only certainty for the future is that there will be more change; increased demand on health and care services has prompted an extensive review of the delivery of these services on island. A Partnership of Purpose (SoG 2017a) policy paper details the proposals for remodelling health and care to provide an infrastructure which meets the needs of the population. This will result in the channelling of resources into the community and the promotion of health and well-being through preventative healthcare. In addition, there is a commitment to good governance which provides clear boundaries between the commissioning, provision and regulation of services. The latter will be a model that is "risk-based" and proportionate to the size of the Bailiwick, with consideration being given to the appointment of a health ombudsman.

In terms of the provision of nurse education on the island, there will be continued competition with other sectors to attract the right candidates to undertake the pre-registration nursing programme. A new website is about to be launched to raise the profile of the Institute and the services it offers. This will be a good platform for disseminating the availability of the pre-registration nursing programme and the benefits being offered to applicants. In terms of marketing, the Institute is becoming better known from the local perspective, but there is much to do to raise the profile in the UK. A targeted marketing strategy is needed to alert the UK applicant to the tempting package being offered, which not only provides an excellent learning experience in a unique context but also offers the opportunity to earn as they learn.

On a positive note, the Institute is actively engaged with the university in the design of the new pre-registration nursing programme in line with the revised standards (NMC 2018b), with the intention that has been endorsed for delivery in Guernsey from September 2019. The new standards are ambitious, in terms of the type of registrant that will be produced after 3 years. Although the fields of practice still exist as options, the student will be a more rounded professional with high-level generic skills suited to the complexity of contemporary healthcare practice. Arguably the practice context in Guernsey will fit well with the new programme and will provide a practitioner who is better prepared to practise in Guernsey.

Alternative models of provision for mental health, children's and learning disability nursing need to be considered due to the low cohort numbers and limited placement experience. The opportunity to share the learning experience between the UK and Guernsey is an option to ensure that the student achieves the outcomes of the course but gains experience of the Guernsey context at the same time.

Finally, assuring a quality student experience will continue to be a challenge, with plans to bring together three organisations currently delivering post-16 education into one college of further and higher education. Whilst this move began in 2016 with the Institute becoming part of the Committee for Education, Sport and Culture, the Institute has remained situated on the Priincess Elizabeth Hospital campus (*CfESC* 2018). As the plans for post-16 education come to fruition the Institute team will relocate to a new building on a different site. This move will be a timely one, as it will be in tandem with the implementation of the new model of health and care delivery, which is moving from a hospital-centric service to a more community-based one. However, despite so much change there is one certainty for the future, and that is the commitment to providing high-quality nurse education which prepares registered nurses for the purpose of caring for our island community.

References

Academy of Medical Royal Colleges (2016) *Acute Care in Remote Settings: Challenges and Potential Solutions*, London: Nuffield Trust.

Anon (undated) *Notes of Recollections from Emma Ferbrache*, Guernsey: Emma Ferbrache Nurse Education Centre.

Bell G (undated) *Enrolled Nurse School*, Guernsey: Princess Elizabeth Hospital.

Birchenall P (1997) Nursing in war-time Guernsey: A preliminary review. *British Journal of Nursing*, 6 (22), pp. 1315–1322.

Bourne G F, Grundy & Beardsall J (1946) *Hospital Services of the Island*, Guernsey: States of Guernsey.

Brevetti G, Oliva G, Giugliano G, Schiano, V, De Maio J and Ciarello M (2007) Mortality in peripheral arterial disease: A comparison of patients managed by vascular specialists and general practitioners. *JGIM*, 22, pp. 639–644.

Briggs M (1964a) *Report on First Visit to Hospital (PEH, July 1964)*, London: General Nursing Council.

Briggs M (1964b) *Report on First Visit to Hospital (The Town Hospital, July 1964)*, London: General Nursing Council.

Briggs M (1966a) *Report on Second Visit to Hospital (PEH, November 1966)*, London: General Nursing Council.

Briggs M (1966b) *Letter from the GNC Ref: BNF/MRB/CM*, London: General Nursing Council.

Briggs M (1969) *Letter from the GNC 6th November*, London: GNC.

Briggs M (1972a) *Letter from the GNC Ref MRB/EMB*, London: GNC.

Briggs M (1972b) *Letter from the GNC 11th October*, London: GNC.

Committee for Education, Sport and Culture (2018) *Secondary and Post-16 Education: The Alternative Model: A Proposal for Opportunity and Excellence*, Guernsey: SoG.

Courtney D (1988) *Guernsey to Use New Training Plan*, The Guernsey Press, 7th June, 1 and 3.

Craig J (1968) *Tutor's Report*, Guernsey: Princess Elizabeth Hospital.

Department of Health and Social Care (2017) *Policy Paper NHS Bursary Reform* available from file:///C:/Users/User/Desktop/NHS%20bursary%20reform%20-%20GOV.UK.html accessed 09/09/18.

Fuller A (2003) *Media Release: Award Ceremony-Diploma of Nursing Studies*, Guernsey: IHS.

Gallienne W (1999) Chapter 4: The Victoria hospital (Amherst). in *One Hundred Years of Health: The Changing Health of Guernsey 1899-1999*, Guernsey: Guernsey Board of Health.Jeffs, D. (ed.).

General Nursing Council (1967) *The 488th Meeting of the General Nursing Council for England and Wales (January 27th)*, London: GNC.

Grobler L, Marais S, Marindi P, Reuter H and Volmink J (2009) *Interventions for Increasing the Proportion of Health Professionals*. www.cochranelibrary.com/cdsr/doi/10.1002/14651858.CD005314.pub2/media/CDSR/CD005314/rel0002/CD005314/CD005314_abstract.pdf accessed 28/06/19.

Grut A (1965) *Training School for the Roll of Nurses and New Board of Health Offices*, Guernsey Board of Healt.

Grut A (1967) *Letter to the Bailiff*, Guernsey: Board of Health.

Grut A (1971) *Extract from Board of Health Minutes 17th November 1971*, Guernsey: Guernsey Board of Health.

Health and Social Services Department (HSSD) (2011) *2020 Vision: A Strategic Framework*, Guernsey: HSSD.

Health and Social Services Department (HSSD) (2013) *2020 Vision: Progress Report and Next Steps*, Guernsey: HSSD.

Henry M (1948a) *Letter from General Nursing Council Registrar ref: MH/IG/OFA*, London: General Nursing Council.

Henry M (1948b) *Letter from General Nursing Council Registrar ref: MH/IG/VM*, London: General Nursing Council.

Henry M (1948c) *Letter from General Nursing Council Registrar ref: MH/IG/JMW*, London: General Nursing Council.

Houghton M (1948a) *Letter from General Nursing Council Education Officer ref: MH/IG*, London: General Nursing Council.

Houghton M (1948b) *Letter from General Nursing Council Education Officer ref: MH/IG/JMW*, London: General Nursing Council.

Howell L (1989) *Precis of Annual Report for Award Ceremony*, Guernsey: Emma Ferbrache School of Nursing.

Howell L (1992) *Award Ceremony 1992: Precis of Annual Report*, Guernsey: Emma Ferbrache Nurse Education Centre.

HSC (2017) *A Partnership of Purpose: Transforming Bailiwick Health and Care*, Guernsey: HSC.

HSC (2018) *Funding for Pre-Registration Nursing Students: Terms and conditions*, Guernsey: SoG.

HSSD (2012) *Mental Health and Wellbeing in Guernsey and Alderney; A Research Report*, Guernsey: States of Guernsey.

The Institute for Economic Affairs (2017) *Healthcare: Lessons from Guernsey*, available from https://iea.org.uk/healthcare-lessons-from-guernsey/accessed 04/09/18.

The Institute for Employment Stu.dies (1997) *Enrolled Nurses: A Study for the UKCC*, Brighton: IES.

The Institute of Health and Social Care Studies (2017) *Annual Monitoring Report*, Guernsey: IHSCS.

Kandiko C B. and Mawer M (2013) *Student Expectations and Perceptions of Higher Education*, London: King's Learning Institute.

Lenfesty G (1999) Chapter 3: The story of the Town Hospital 1900-1987. in *One Hundred Years of Health: The Changing Health of Guernsey 1899-1999*, Guernsey: Guernsey Board of Health.Jeffs, D. (ed.).

MacVicar R and Nicoll P (2013) *NHS Education for Scotland: Supporting Remote and Rural Healthcare*, Scotland: NHS Scotland.

Martel N (2006) *Health Institute has its First In-house Graduates*, The Guernsey Press, 18th December, 14.

McClean T (2016) *An Exploration into the Professional and Personal Challenges Facing Migrant and Overseas Generalist Registered Nurses Working and Living in Two Small Island Communities*, Guernsey: University of Bath.

The Medical Specialist Group (2018) available from www.msg.gg/accessed 05/09/18.

Middlesex University and NMC (2016) *Confirmed Validation and Endorsement Report*, London: Middlesex University.

Ministry of Justice (2013) *Background Briefing on the Crown Dependencies: Jersey Guernsey and the Isle of Man*, available from www.justice.gov.uk/downloads/about/moj/our-responsibilities/Background_Briefing_on_the_Crown_Dependencies2.pdf accessed 22/02/18.

National Quality Forum (2015) *Performance Measurement for Rural Low-Volume Providers*, London: Department of Health.

NHS England (2018) NHS launches multi million pound TV advertising campaign to recruit thousands of nurses in landmark 70th year, available from www.england.nhs.uk/2018/07/nhs-launches-multi-million-pound-tv-advertising-campaign-to-recruit-thousands-of-nurses-in-landmark-70th-year/accessed 10/09/18.

NMC (2006) *Revision to NMC Circular 5/2005, Endorsement of NMC Programmes Approved in the UK for Delivery in Specified Locations Outside the UK*, London: NMC.

NMC (2010) *Standards for Pre-Registration Nurse Education*, London: NMC.

NMC (2014) *Extraordinary LSA Review: Princess Elizabeth Hospital, Health and Social Services Department, Guernsey 01-03 October 2014*, London: NMC.

NMC (2015a) *Extraordinary LSA Follow Up Review Guernsey*, London: NMC.

NMC (2015b) *Review of Pre-registration Nursing Guernsey*, London: NMC.

NMC (2018a) *Quality Assurance Framework for Nursing, Midwifery and Nursing Associate Education*, London: NMC.

NMC (2018b) *Future Nurse: Standards of Proficiency for Registered Nurses*, London: NMC.

Nuffield Trust (2016) *Reshaping the Workforce to Deliver the Care Patients Need*, London: Nuffield Trust.

Ogier D (2005) *The Government and Law of Guernsey*, Guernsey: The states of Guernsey.

Ozanne B (1994) *A Peep Behind the Screens: 1940-1945*, Guernsey: The Guernsey Press Co. Ltd.

QAA (2014) *UK Quality Code for Higher Education: Part A: Setting and Maintaining Academic Standards*, Gloucester: QAA.

Radway J (1970) *Report of Hospital Visit May 1970*, London: GNC.

Sarre J (1965a) *Education Committee for Pupil Nurse Training School*, Guernsey: Board of Health.

Sarre J (1965b) *Letter to Miss Briggs, GNC Ref: FAV/IG/PB*, Guernsey: Board of Health.

Sarre J (1967) *Letter to GNC Ref: BNF/MRB/CM*, Guernsey: Board of Health.

Sarre J (1968) *Memo: Enrolled Nurses' Training School- Appointment of Second Tutor*, Guernsey: Board of Health.

Sarre J (1969) *Letter to GNC Ref: RL/JB*, Guernsey: Board of Health.

Sarre J (1972a) *File Note*, guernsey: Board of Health.

Sarre J (1972b) *Letter to GNC 26th October*, Guernsey: Board of Health.

Sarre, J (1972c) *Letter to GNC 10th November*, Guernsey: Board of Health.

Seth-Smith B (1999) Chapter 10: The Post-war Period. In *One Hundred Years of Health: The Changing Health of Guernsey 1899-1999*, Guernsey: Guernsey Board of Health.

SLAWS Working Party (2016) *Research Report for the Supported Living and Ageing Well Strategy (SLAWS)*, Guernsey: States of Guernsey.

States of Guernsey (1959) *Index to the Billet D'Etat, Volume XLIV – 1958*, Guernsey: States of Guernsey.

States of Guernsey (1987) *The Nurses, Midwives and Health Visitors Ordinance, 1987*, Guernsey: States of Guernsey.

States of Guernsey (2003) *Billet D'Etat*, Guernsey: States of Guernsey.

States of Guernsey (2006) *The Registered Health Professions Ordinance*, Guernsey: States of Guernsey.

States of Guernsey (2008) *Children (Guernsey and Alderney) Law, 2008 (the 'Children Law')*, Guernsey: States of Guernsey.

States of Guernsey (2016) *The Mental Health (Transfer of Patients) (Guernsey and Alderney) Ordinance, 2016*, Guernsey: States of Guernsey.

States of Guernsey (2017a) *Guernsey Facts and Figures*, Guernsey: States of Guernsey.

States of Guernsey (2017b) *A Partnership of Purpose: Transforming Bailiwick Health and Care*, Guernsey States of Guernsey.

States of Guernsey (2018) *Guernsey Annual Electronic Census Report*, available from https://gov.gg/CHttpHandler.ashx?id=111829&p=0 accessed 22/02/18.

Symons A (1948a) *Letter to Miss Henry, Registrar, GNC (Feb 1948)*, Guernsey: Guernsey Board of Health.

Symons A (1948b) *Letter to Miss Henry, Registrar, GNC (March 1948)*, Guernsey: Guernsey Board of Health.

Symons A (1948c) *Letter to Miss Henry, Registrar, GNC (June 1948)*, Guernsey: Guernsey Board of Health.

Symons A (1948d) *Letter to Miss Henry, Registrar (July 1948), GNC*, Guernsey: Guernsey Board of Health.

Tough K (1999) Chapter 9: Health in the Occupation. in *One Hundred Years of Health: The Changing Health of Guernsey 1899-1999*, Guernsey: Guernsey Board of Health.

UCAS (2018) *Cycle Applicant Figures* available from www.ucas.com/corporate/data-and-analysis/ucas-undergraduate-releases/2018-cycle-applicant-figures-june-deadline accessed 09/09/18.

UK Government (2001) *The Nursing and Midwifery Order 2001*, London.available from https://www.legislation.gov.uk/uksi/2002/253/contents/made accessed 12/09/19

Unknown author (1970) *Conversation with Miss Craig re GNC report -16th April*, Guernsey: Guernsey Board of Health.

Vukic A and Keddy B (2002) Northern practice in a primary healthcare setting. *Journal of Advanced Nursing*, 40(5), pp. 542–548.

Winterflood H (1987) *Boost for Training of Nurses in Island*, The Guernsey Press, 9th February, 1 and 3.

Winterflood S (2016) *HSC Nursing and Midwifery Skill Mix Review*, Guernsey: HSC.

6

HISTORICAL DEVELOPMENT OF NURSING EDUCATION IN AFRICA

Kwadwo Korsah

Background

In many African countries, traditional healthcare systems continue to operate. Western influences, which commenced around the late nineteenth century to provide healthcare to the colonial people, are evident in the cities and towns of sub-Saharan Africa (Klopper and Uys, 2013).

Christian missionary-based healthcare facilities and some public health agencies served the healthcare needs of the local people but these were inadequate. Overall, Christian missionaries had an oversight role on health and education, whereas economic activities, for instance, were placed in the hands of business firms and companies. The colonial authorities limited their powers to upholding and preserving law and order, instituting and raising taxes and building infrastructure such as roads and the railway system (Klopper and Uys, 2013).

As African countries started gaining independence, the influence of the colonial powers from Europe started to dwindle. This led to a new era whereby indigenous African people began to marshal their own governments and other essential institutions such as hospitals and nursing schools, to draw new policies to augment self-rule. Demand for the establishment of new nursing schools, hospitals and similar institutions required the training of experts and the need for skilled labour and personnel such as nurses to staff the healthcare institutions.

Africa faces particular challenges in its provision of healthcare. Most of the countries in Africa are located in tropical regions where infectious tropical diseases are prevalent, and continue to account for the highest death rates globally. After many African countries gained independence they were soon confronted with acute skills scarcity and deficiency as European people departed. For instance, in French-speaking colonies, there were no universities and a limited number of secondary schools. In relation to developing a health workforce, colonial front-runners initiated plans to work with African healthcare officers to train nurses through apprenticeship programmes in most cities and towns across Africa (Klopper and Uys, 2013).

Whilst this was the general process of development of nursing education across Africa, there were also unique approaches taken by specific independent countries. Country-specific developments in nurse education are presented below, taking into consideration three cardinal periods, namely pre-colonial, colonial and post-colonial eras, commencing with nurse education in Botswana and drawing predominantly on the work of Klopper and Uys (2013) as a definitive guide.

Nursing education in Botswana

As with other African states, nursing education and hospitals in Botswana were established by the missionaries (Selelo-Kupe, 1993; World Health Organization, 2010). In most of the large cities and towns, such as Mochudi in Kenya, nursing schools were affiliated to local hospitals and used the apprenticeship training model of enrolled nurses (ENs), registered nurses (RNs) and midwives. In other cities and towns, the Protectorate Government also set up nursing schools to train ENs and midwives. Through these programmes, students were allowed to be trained as both midwives and nurses and thus most candidates were able to attain the dual status of nurse and midwife.

The apprenticeship nursing programme in Botswana was discontinued in 1970 (Klopper and Uys, 2013). At about 1990, it was recognized that there were overlaps in the curriculum for ENs and RNs and thus a restructuring between the diploma and degree programmes was undertaken under the auspices of the Kellogg Foundation Consultancy services in Botswana (Selelo-Kupe, 1993). Following the committee's recommendations, enrolled nursing in Botswana was discontinued, with request made for the minimum entry level for nursing practice in Botswana to be an RN holder. Following this, all existing enrolled nursing certificate holders were given "top-up" training via a special curriculum, which allowed them on completion to practise as RNs from 1995 onwards. The ENs who did not undertake the conversion course were permitted to practise pending superannuation or death. The committee also noted the need to coordinate the convergence of all basic diploma nursing programmes to the bachelor of nurse education (Selelo-Kupe, 1993; WHO, 2010).

The University of Botswana has subsequently examined nursing programmes in Botswana to reveal gaps, overlaps, similarities and differences. Recommendations saw the establishment of four categories of nursing: (1) a basic diploma in general nursing available for secondary school graduates for a period of 3 years; (2) a post-basic diploma in nursing, which is open to registered diploma holders and bachelor's degree holders who are trained to acquire nursing specialty skills in community health, family health practice, mental health and nurse anaesthetics; (3) a bachelor's degree in nursing; and (4) postgraduate programmes.

The bachelor's degree was first introduced by the University of Botswana in 1978 as a means of training nurse educators and administrators for nursing schools and hospitals (Klopper and Uys, 2013). Admission requirements included possession of the Cambridge School Certificate in addition to 2 years' work experience as a practical nurse.

Postgraduate programmes in nursing commenced in Botswana in 1996. They included a master's in adult health, mental health, community health and midwifery. In addition to the four specialty areas at postgraduate level, the opportunity to specialize in a family health nurse practitioner programme was introduced by the University of Botswana in 2003 at the request of the Botswanan Ministry of Health.

National accreditation needed to deliver nursing programmes in Botswana was traditionally given by the South African Nursing Council. However, nursing examinations were moderated by the National Examinations Board of Botswana, Lesotho and Swaziland. Accreditation responsibilities were taken over by the National Council for Nursing and Midwifery in Botswana in the middle of 1970. In recent years, the Ministry of Education has set up the Tertiary Education Council, which has overall responsibility for accreditation and quality assurance in all tertiary institutions in Botswana (Klopper and Uys, 2013). The regulation of nursing and midwifery practice in Botswana is performed by the Nursing and Midwifery Council of Botswana, which receives support and funding from the Ministry of Health. In association with the Botswana Nurses and Midwives Association, the council influenced the establishment of the Nurses and Midwives Act of Botswana in 1995 (Klopper and Uys, 2013). The umbrella association of nurses and midwives in Botswana is the Nurses Association of Botswana, which is a recognized member of the International Council of Nurses – in other words the oversight body for nursing and midwifery.

The next section considers nursing education in Nigeria.

Nursing education in Nigeria

As previously stated, nursing education in Africa emerged principally through three stages, pre-colonial, colonial and post-colonial eras, responding to unique country healthcare needs. Much information about pre-colonial nursing in Nigeria is not known. However, much like other countries, nursing in Nigeria was initiated to meet the needs of the sick and the wounded in the African community, particularly in areas where there were significant inter- and intra-tribal conflicts (Adejumo and Lekalakala-Mokgele, 2009). Over the years, the Nursing and Midwifery Council in Nigeria has worked to develop nurses who can function self-sufficiently to enhance the health of the populace in Nigeria, and to preserve and promote excellence in nursing practice and education, in line with the local and global canons (Adejumo and Lekalakala-Mokgele, 2009).

Nursing and midwifery professions in Nigeria were considered highly important by the British during its colonization in 1914 because of nursing's significant contribution to the health of the colonial masters, their families, the members of the army, the colonial administrators and the public at large (Adelowo, 1988). In view of this, the British Government set about instituting reforms to nursing in Nigeria, to be in line with the standards of nursing in Europe that had changed dramatically following the Crimean War. As the influence of Florence Nightingale with respect to nursing gained momentum in Europe, it flowed through to the African colonies. As British rule officially took control in Nigeria in 1861, a European perspective was brought to bear on nursing in Nigeria (Klopper and Uys, 2013).

The formal training and education of nurses and midwives commenced in 1930 in Nigeria, typically in the mission hospitals as well as government hospitals similar to that pertaining to other African countries (Adelowo, 1988). At that time nursing and midwifery training programmes were regulated by the Nursing and Midwifery Board of Nigeria. The Board was recognized by the Ordinance of 1930 and inducted in 1931. This paved the way for the establishment of the School of Nursing under the University College Hospital in Ibadan in 1952, under the leadership of a premier principal from London, a former student from Nightingale's School of Nursing at St Thomas' Hospital, London. Secondary graduates who met the minimum full completion requirements qualified to be enrolled into the nursing programme. However, there were flexibilities in the entry requirements compared with the other government schools, probably due to the limited number of applicants into nursing programmes. Generally, candidates with Standard VI as well as Government IV grades were accepted on to nursing programmes (Adelowo, 1988). Upon successful completion of a nursing programme, graduates were awarded with the state registered nurse (SRN) certificate by the Nursing Council of England and Wales. The University College Hospital in Ibadan was later permitted to offer the State Registered Nursing programme (Koyejo,

2008). Many nursing schools were established in Nigeria during the post-colonial era in the 1960s, working within the remit of the established principles and policies of the well-established schools, for example, the University College of Ibadan School of Nursing. Among the new nursing schools were those established by Lagos University Teaching Hospital and Ahmadu Bello University and the Department of Nursing at the University of Ibadan in 1965 (and other similar departments to produce tutors and administrators to meet the growing needs of nursing schools in Nigeria and in the sub-region). Nursing programmes were extended to other public and private universities in Nigeria, which offered the Baccalaureate/Bachelor of Nursing based on the requirements set by the National Universities Commission (NUC) (Dolamo and Olubiyi, 2013).

The Nursing and Midwifery Council of Nigeria is the regulatory government body in charge of nursing and midwifery practice and education. The roles and functions of the Nursing and Midwifery Council of Nigeria are enshrined in the Nursing and Midwifery Council of Nigeria Act, Section 1, established in 1992. Over the years nursing standards have changed, requiring reforms to the training of nurses and midwives, which paved the way for the award of RN certificate following 3½ years of training. Midwifery and other post-basic nursing courses were 18 months in duration (Nursing and Midwifery Council of Nigeria, 2009).

In Nigeria, the national policy on education established in 1981 requires Nigerians to be trained towards the achievement of effective skills and competencies deemed to be on a par with the international standards and required by the Federal Ministry of Education (Dolamo and Olubiyi, 2013). In 1993, 2001 and 2006 revision of nursing and midwifery education was considered, minded towards new trends in health and diseases locally, additional to the international requirement for the achievement of five credits, including English language and mathematics at the West Africa School Certificate and the General Certificate Ordinary Level as entry minimum requirements. However, in the 2006 revision, candidates with more than two attempts at the West Africa School Certificate and General Certificate Ordinary Levels were not considered for enrolment in nursing programmes. The requirement for the admission to the degree nursing programme was however based on the general requirement for admission into the university in addition to nursing-specific requirements, including the registered nursing certificate and five credit passes in sciences, mathematics and English and not more than two sittings for professional nurse applicants for a 4-year duration. In contrast, applicants with Senior High School Certificate or Senior Secondary School Certificate enter the university with five credit passes, including science, English and mathematics and not more than two sittings, in addition to a pass in the university entrance examination for a nursing programme spanning 5 years (Dolamo and Olubiyi, 2013).

Post-basic nursing programmes in Nigeria include mental health and psychiatric nursing programme, midwifery as well as peri-operative and critical care nursing. The development of the general nursing programme and post-basic components has acknowledged the need to embrace student learning needs at all levels, which centre on cognitive, psychomotor skills and affective modes of student development, while at the same time recognizing societal needs and the concepts of nursing (Olanipekun, 2007).

The next section considers the development of nursing education in Ghana.

Nursing education in Ghana

In Ghana, information about nurse education between 1957 and 1970 is limited. However, interviews with key individuals as well as analysis of specific letters and published papers have uncovered a limited history of nurse education in Ghana (Opare and Mill, 2000). Between the period examined, nursing education in Ghana was associated with dramatic changes and growth, primarily influenced by external experts providing advice on health matters. During this period, policy was formulated to ensure that nurses were trained locally. Nurses were encouraged to pursue further education in order to hold specific positions in nurse education in addition to administration and practice, which emphasized the need to prepare for the practice area and the health system, which was itself a remnant of colonialism. Within this time frame, nurse education in Ghana was exposed to a number of challenges, including economic issues, which the nursing leaders at that time recognized and were instrumental in overcoming in order to aid the growth of the nursing profession (Opare and Mill, 2000).

Ghana was the first country in Africa to gain independence and subsequently the initiatiors in developing nursing education in Africa. The first diploma programme in nursing in Ghana was commenced at the University of Ghana in 1963 to train teachers and nurse administrators for nursing schools and hospitals respectively (Chittick, 1965). Professional nurse education in Ghana prior to independence was part of the structural organization of healthcare services in general by the colonial masters.

Around the nineteenth century, Ghana was known as the British Gold Coast and colloquially considered the *white man's grave* (Hart, 1904) because of the high prevalence of infectious and usually fatal tropical diseases such as malaria and yellow fever (Addae, 1997; Hart, 1904). Thus, enhancement of healthcare during this period was of great importance to the British Government.

The colonial powers had a vested interest in improving the healthcare system because the Gold Coast was rich in mineral deposits that the British were keen to mine. Because of political priorities, limited resources and logistics, the focus for medical staff was restricted to the care of the colonial masters and their families and the African soldiers and civil servants. Healthcare policy was also directed towards preventive care, including vaccination, water and sanitation (Patterson, 1981). Even so, only about 2% of the people of African origin in this region had access to healthcare provided by the government (Kay, 1972). The colonial powers over time identified the need to offer healthcare services to the indigenous African population, which led to the staffing of "male orderlies" to support in the delivery of healthcare services to the native Africans (Akiwumi, 1971; Osei-Boateng, 1992). Males, according to local customary duties and rituals, were allowed to give healthcare services to their family members, while females were prohibited, which led to the training of male orderlies (Twumasi, 1979). However, by the year 1899, nursing sisters from Britain started to fill appointment positions in the Gold Coast on a systematic basis (Addae, 1997). Later, women were trained as nurses in addition to their male counterparts as a direct result of the arrival of nursing sisters from Britain (Akiwumi, 1992). The British nursing sisters were given additional duties. These included teaching student nurses human anatomy, physiology, medical and surgical nursing and first aid. On successful completion of this special training by the nurses, students were awarded the Director of Medical Services Certificate and were recognized as "second division nurses" in the colonial ranking (Akiwumi, 1988). In Accra, a new hospital built to offer maternity services commenced recruitment of women to undertake a midwifery course in 1928, which was in line with the traditional and customary roles of women in the Africa context (Akiwumi, 1971). In 1931, the Midwives Decree or Ordinances was formed, which led to the establishment of the Midwives Board to supervise the Order with respect to the training, examination, registration as well as midwifery practices in the Gold Coast epoch (Akiwumi, 1988).

Most senior nursing positions, including tutorial staff prior to 1945, were colonial nursing sisters. However, from 1945 the situation changed (Akiwumi, 1971). A prototype of British nurse education was commenced by Isobel Hutton, who arrived in Ghana in 1945 with a remit to train SRNs. Hutton was located in Kumasi, the Ashanti regional capital. However, the school was relocated to the city of Accra around the Korle-Bu Hospital (Boahene, 1985; Kisseih, 1968; Osei-Boateng, 1992). Hutton noted that nursing professionals at that time were males and was instrumental in ensuring that new recruits admitted into the new nursing college were females. Historical and indigenous explanations are not readily available to explain the cultural shift from the male-dominated norm towards the recognition and acceptance of a female nursing workforce. However, it is likely due to the influence of the British system of nurse education and the predilection for favouring the British system, promulgated by the arrival of Hutton in Ghana (Addae, 1997; Patterson, 1981).

Nursing programmes in Ghana, which adhered to course structures similar to those designed by the British General Nursing Council (GNC) of England and Wales, ensured that Ghanaian nursing students, upon successful completion, were eligible for international registration and recognition in Britain, and were also able to pursue post-basic nursing programmes overseas and be able to take over the affairs and roles of the colonial tutorial as well as the nursing staff (Kisseih, 1968). Alongside the training of SRNs the qualified registered nurse (QRN) qualification was established in the Gold Coast, which was equivalent to the EN programme in the United Kingdom. In fact, the QRN was a higher-level qualification than the EN programme (Rose, 1987).

Nursing education in Ghana during the post-independence era in 1957 was characterized by important landmarks in which the training of the SRNs was officially offered in the two major cities in Ghana, namely Accra in the south and Kumasi located in the middle belt of Ghana. However, the schools in Cape Coast, Sekondi-Takoradi and Tamale offered nurse education for QRNs. Mission hospitals such as the Seventh-Day Adventist Hospital situated in Kwahu in the eastern region of Ghana also augmented the training of QRNs as well as midwives (Risk, 1966). The nursing training courses were consistent with the content for the training of nurses prepared by the GNC of England. However, programmes did not develop in tandem with the trends in health and illness locally and globally. In 1952, the GNC curriculum was updated in the United Kingdom, whereas the training modules for nursing in Ghana in 1957 remained the same without any meaningful revision, remaining relatively unchanged from UK programmes offered by the GNC in 1925 (Rose, 1987).

The government of the day decided to train doctors locally at the University of Ghana, which called for an expansion and transformation of the Korle-Bu Hospital to a training hospital, which influenced the development and progression of nursing training as well as nursing practice in the country. Skilled manpower was needed at this time, therefore SRNs were sponsored to pursue specialized nursing courses in the United Kingdom, including orthopaedic, paediatric and genitourinary nursing, as well as courses in central sterilization processes in order to ensure nurses were able to function efficiently within the teaching hospital. In addition, there was a need to increase the nursing, nurse educator and nursing manager workforce during the post-independence period in order to staff nursing schools and colleges adequately (Rose, 1987). In 1961, Marjorie Houghton, an active past member of the GNC, was invited and tasked to assess programmes, and thus recommended a 4-year nursing course, with an entry requirement (the West African School Certificate), and that the Pre-Nursing Course be discontinued. In addition, student nurses were designated as having a support role for hospital ward-based staff (Rose, 1987). Houghton also instigated a discussion around the efficacy of the tutor's course at the University of Ghana, which involved tutors and clinical instructors.

The progress of nurse education in Ghana occurred in 1963 when the first university nursing programme at the University of Ghana was created under the guidance of Dorcia Kisseih. The establishment of the nursing programme at the University of Ghana was under the agreement between the government of Ghana, the World Health Organization (WHO) and the United Nations International Children's Fund (UNICEF) (Kisseih, 1968). Kisseih was the first Ghanaian to become a chief nursing officer in Ghana following the separation of the colonial nursing masters from Britain. The subsequent nursing programme was a 2-year post-basic diploma in nursing programme established with a remit to prepare nurse tutors, and nurse managers, as well as nurse instructors and drew on the work of Dr Rae Chittick, a Canadian WHO staff member who acted in a consultancy role (Akiwumi, 1976). Though, it was preferable by the University of Ghana at that time to train nurses as degree holders it is worth noting the limited number of applicants who met the admission criteria and thus who were able to commence the programme at the time of post-independence, which added to the challenge of recruitment (Akiwumi, 1976).

The WHO provided financial support for the post-basic diploma programme at Ghana's premier university, the University of Ghana. Five major positions were established, including the director's position and four other tutorial staff positions. The director position was held by Dr Rae Chittick, a product of a nursing programme in the United States, while the other four nursing positions were given to individuals who had undertaken their nurse education at McGill University. However, Dier (1992) reported, several Canadians were also employed by the WHO around that time, as they were considered to be well trained and subsequently were readily accepted to undertake training, although their attitude towards nursing training and education was in general a complete departure from the British model of nurse education and/or training. Logistics in general as well as the purchase of library materials and means of transport were provided by UNICEF (Chittick, 1965). One of the two buses provided by the UNICEF programme at that time was in use up to 1999 (J. Laryea, personal communication, 1999, former tutor of the then Department of Nursing, Legon). Later, most Ghanaian nurses who had trained outside Ghana returned to take up teaching appointments at the University of Ghana, Department of Nursing, which coincided with the end of the WHO initial establishment of the project. One of the pioneer nurses, Ayodele Akiwumi, who held a senior lecturer position around the mid-1960s before she retired from active service in 1995, was very instrumental in nurse education in Ghana during the post-independence period, and very influential as an "agent of change".

Disparities in the educational system by the WHO nurse educators and British system brought numerous challenges to nursing training at this time. Whereas the British system promoted "rote learning", the programmes offered by the WHO nurse educators on the other hand sought to develop problem-solving skills in students. Several critiques of the British system of nurse education were noted; among them was that by Chittick (1965), which centred on the fact that the British education system lacked a scope or specific patterns for the training of nurses to work efficiently in a tropical setting or environment. It was obvious that there was a significant tension between the British nurse education and the one introduced by the WHO. Rose (1987) reported that the British nurse educators who were working in Ghana around that time were welcomed by other healthcare professionals better than the WHO nurse educators.

Future developments ensured that, in the late 1960s, the WHO was once again contacted by the Ghana Government for support to come up with a wide-ranging diploma programme for the SRNs, which included courses in social sciences, public health, psychiatry and obstetrics as well as the basic nursing programme (Osei-Boateng, 1992). This ensured that nurse education in Ghana shifted from hospital-based administration to a classroom-based nursing institution, including nursing in community settings. The general idea was to expand the nursing programme to include all clinical specialty courses. The nurses who had the opportunity to be trained within the new programme had new positions in the new hospitals and new community health settings and situations.

The Africanization of nurse education in Ghana

Nurse education during the post-independence period continued to be beset by serious challenges for both students and the faculty, including financial and logistics as well as teaching materials, including books and other resources (Rose, 1987). The effects of tropical diseases such as malaria and similar conditions also resulted in student absenteeism. There were also tensions between hospital matrons who were the clinical supervisors of students and the tutors due to role conflicts, which put students in restricted positions in terms of their supervisory roles and activities (Rose, 1987). Within a short period following independence, the Government of Ghana introduced the concept of Africanization, a form of revolution which replaced all white colonial staff in all sectors, including nurses, in which the appointments of most of the nurses were not renewed (Rose, 1987), which resulted in opportunities for most Ghanaian professional nurses to rise to occupy the positions of the expatriate nurses. Of course, this took some time for the nurses to rise to that level. History records that Africanization around the time provided a significant force as a form of revolution or reformation for the nurse education and profession in the post-independence era in Ghana (Rose, 1987).

The Nurses Ordinance as well as the Statutory Board were established in 1946 to supervise nursing activities and to regulate the education of nurses, including nursing examinations, registration and the general practice of nursing. In 1948, the premier registration of nurses was logged and midwifery was separated from nursing and obtained its own registration and set-up decree (Kisseih, 1968; Rose, 1987). Separate registers were created for female nurses and tutors, male nurses, mental health nurses, paediatrics, public health nurses and medical nurses respectively (Kisseih, 1968). The Ghana Registered Nurses Association (GRNA) was established in 1960 as a "voice" for nurses in Ghana and in the subsequent year, Ghana officially became a member of the International Council of Nurses (Bridges, 1967). The training of nurses as enshrined in the colonial healthcare system, i.e. to be trained to offer curative care in the hospital-based format, was gradually transformed for nurses to be trained to work in different healthcare settings, additional to hospital settings.

In Ghana, the present nursing curriculum was introduced in 2015. The plan for the revision of the nursing curriculum, which had been used more than a decade earlier, was based on the decision by the WHO to adopt common global standards for initial training of professional nurses as well as midwives around the world (WHO, 2009). Currently, nursing and midwifery training in Ghana is delivered by both public and private institutions at different levels, including basic, post-basic, undergraduate and postgraduate levels. In addition, there are auxiliary nursing programmes, for example, the health assistant clinical (HAC) course, as well as community health nursing (CHN) (MOH, 2018). The basic nursing programmes include the registered general nursing, registered mental nursing, registered midwifery (for females only) and registered community health nursing programmes, which are 3-year programmes for senior high school or senior secondary school graduates in nursing training institutions (Ministry of Health, Ghana (MOH), 2018). The post-basic nursing programmes are peri-operative and critical care nursing, public health nursing, post-basic midwifery, ophthalmic nursing and anaesthesiology (Ministry of Health, Ghana (MOH), 2018). Both the public and private nursing training schools are involved in the training of nurses and midwives, albeit under the supervision of the Nurses and Midwives Council of Ghana, which is the regulatory body for nursing in Ghana. The bachelor of nursing and mid-wifery programmes are offered by public and private universities, which are available for direct-entry applicants from the senior high schools or senior secondary schools or their equivalents and also for nurses and midwives with the basic nursing and midwifery backgrounds, such as those with the registered general nursing and registered midwifery qualifications, respectively.

Currently, the master's programmes in nursing are only offered by Ghana's public universities. The School of Nursing at the University of Ghana offers both the master of philosophy in nursing and master of science in nursing. None of the universities in Ghana have commenced the doctorate programme in nursing. The National Accreditation Board (NAB) is the governmental body responsible for authorization to establish any educational programme in Ghana and also to ensure that permission is given to educational institutions for renewal of a licence to operate. Nursing schools in the country renew their licences from time to time with the NAB. The permission to continue to operate as an institution is based on the satisfaction of the NAB upon their inspection and evaluation of the institution in question. As part of the regulatory policy in the training of nurses in Ghana, the public and private nursing training schools'/university colleges are affiliated with the full public universities until such institutions are able to independently shoulder their own administrative issues and affairs. For instance, some of the public nursing schools/colleges are affiliated with the Kwame Nkrumah University of Science and Technology (KNUST) and the University of Cape Coast (UCC). Similarly, some of the private nursing schools/colleges are also affiliated with the University of Ghana, Legon. Ghana Registered Nurses Association and the Ghana Registered Midwives Association are the peak bodies for nurses and midwives.

Conclusion

This chapter has outlined the historical background of nursing education in Africa. The chapter focused on the developments in three specific countries – Botswana, Nigeria and Ghana – and explained how colonial influence shaped the development of nursing education generally in Africa. Historical events specific to the three countries were considered, highlighting how nurse education was shaped by both external and internal forces. Comparative analysis shows that, in most African countries, nursing care and healthcare began as a means to provide care for expatriates, but developed gradually over time to focus on indigenous populations through a period of Africanization.

References

Addae S (1997) *History of Western medicine in Ghana: 1880-1960.* Edinburgh and Scotland: Dur-ham Academic Press.

Adejumo O and Lekalakala-Mokgele E (2009) A 2-decade appraisal of African nursing scholarship. *Journal of Nursing Scholarship* 41(1): 64–69.

Adelowo E O (1988) *The nursing profession in Nigeria. Lagos*: Lantern Books.

Akiwumi A (1971) *Higher education for nurses.* An inter-faculty lecture delivered at the University of Ghana, Legon, December, 1, 1970. Accra and Ghana: Ghana Universities Press.

Akiwumi A (1976) Degree for nurses. *Ghanaian Nurse* 9(1): 5–7.

Akiwumi A (1988, December) Nurse education in contemporary Ghana. Keynote address to the *10th Annual Conference of the Nurse Education Group*, Accra and Ghana.

Akiwumi A (1992) Roles, competencies and qualities of the nurse in Ghana in the 21st century. In A Akiwumi (Ed.), *Nurse education in Ghana for the 21st century*. Accra and Ghana: Woeli Publishing Service.

Boahene A (1985) Appraisal of the comprehensive nursing program. *Nurse Educators Bulletin* 3: 13–16.

Bridges D. C. (1967). A history of the international council of nurses 1899-1964. Philadelphia: J. B. Lippincott.

Chittick R (1965) Post-basic nursing in the University of Ghana. *International Journal of Nursing Studies* 2: 39–42.

Dier K A (1992) Nursing practice in international areas. In A J Baumgart & J Larsen (Eds.), *Canadian nursing faces the future*. 2nd ed. (pp. 200–217). Scarborough and Ontario: Mosby Year Book.

Dolamo B L and Olubiyi S K (2013) Nurse education in Africa: South Africa, Nigeria, and Ethiopia Experiences. *International Journal of Nursing and Midwifery* 5(2): 14–22.

Hart F (1904) *The gold coast: Its wealth and health*. London: Ereckson's.

Kay G B (1972) *The political economy of colonialism in Ghana, a collection of documents and statistics, 1900-1960*. Cambridge: Cambridge University Press.

Kisseih DAN (1968) Developments in nursing in Ghana. *International Journal of Nursing Studies* 5: 205–219.

Klopper H.C. and Uys L.R. (2013)The State of Nursing and Nursing Education in Africa. Cape Town: A Country-by-Country Review. Sigma Theta Tau Inter-national Honor Society of Nursing.

Koyejo K O (2008) Overview of nurse education in Nigeria. A paper presented at the *2008 Annual Conference of Principals of Schools of Nursing, Midwifery, Psychiatry and Post Basic Nursing Programmes*. Katsina, Katsina State and Nigeria.

Ministry of Health, Ghana (MOH) (2018) Admission requirements for nursing programmes in Ghana. Available at: https://nursinginghana.com/admission-requirements-nursing-programmes-moh/

Nursing and Midwifery Council of Nigeria (NMCN) (2009) Curriculum for general and post basic nurse education.cited in B L Dolamo & S K Olubiyi *Nursing education in Africa: South Africa, Nigeria, and Ethiopia experiences International Journal of Nursing and Midwifery* 5(2): 14-21, March 2013.

Olanipekun OA (2007) Nurse education reforms in Nigeria: The journey so far. Paper presentation at *2007 Nurse' Leaders Conference*. Lokoja, Kogi State and Nigeria.

Opare M and Mill J E (2000) The evolution of nurse education in a post-independence context – Ghana, from 1957 – 1970. *Western Journal of Research* 22(8): 936–944.

Osei-Boateng M (1992) Nursing in Africa today. *International Nursing Review* 39(6): 175–180.

Patterson K D (1981) *Health in colonial Ghana: Disease, medicine, and socio-economic change, 1900-1950*. Waltham, MA: Crossroads.

Risk J A (1966) Graduation service in Ghana. *Nursing Mirror* 122(5): ix.

Rose H (1987) Teaching nursing in Ghana, 1957 to 1964: A personal experience. *Bulletin of History of Nursing* 2(3): 4–18.

Selelo-Kupe S S (1993) *An uneasy walk to quality: The evolution of black nurse education*. Battle Creek, MI: W K Kellogg Foundation.

Twumasi P A (1979) A social history of the Ghanaian pluralistic medical system. *Social Sciences and Medicine* 13(4): 349–365.

World Health Organization (2009) *Global standards for the initial education of professional nurses and midwives*. Geneva: WHO.

World Health Organization (2010) *Botswana factsheets of health statistics 2010*. Geneva Africa World Health Organization. Available at: www.afro.who.int/index.php?option=com_content&view=article&id=1017&Itemid=2043&lang=en

7

CROSSING BORDERS IN EDUCATION

A conceptual and contextual approach

Teresa Stone and Margaret McMillan

So no matter who you are working with or whether that person comes from, you should begin any relationship with the desire to understand what is specific and unique to that individual. Don't assume that you can determine anything specific about how they will think or behave from what you know about their cultural background.

Yet the culture in which we grow up has a profound impact on how we would see the world. In any given culture, members are conditioned to understand the world in a particular way, to see certain communication patterns as effective or undesirable, to find certain arguments persuasive or lacking merit, to consider certain ways of making decisions or measuring time as "natural" or "strange."

(Meyer, 2014, p. 252)

Introduction

Educators are increasingly working transnationally or offshore (Gribble & Ziguras, 2003) and require a frame of reference for their interactions with those from other cultures. Graduates and educators need cross-cultural proficiencies to be able to work in today's globally interconnected world (Stone et al., 2014). In this chapter we will argue that consideration of principles for practice and education are critical and clinical and theory should be integrated. Practice-informed education is the optimal way to approach facilitation of learning and practice development in different contexts and cultures to bring about change that is consistent with the best possible outcomes for the population served. With this in mind we posit principles that underpin conceptual frameworks for practice-informed education relevant to educators regardless of context. These centre on the need for both better-integrated elements within care processes and education and promoting best practices for alignment of practice and education, i.e. integration of processes and outcomes within learning events that prepare health professionals for practice, irrespective of the situations demanding their responses.

We will first explore the essential elements informing practice-informed education and integrated care as a basis for discussing principles for working across cultures and contexts derived from the American Psychological Association (APA) and World Health Organization (WHO) (Van Lerberghe, 2008) before focusing on curriculum design. To illustrate these elements we provide some reflections on personal experiences of working in a range of contexts of practice and with peers from diverse cultures.

A global perspective

The WHO (2016) is itself a catalyst for capacity building reliant on transnational expertise. The WHO argues for a greater orientation towards more integrated care if aspirations for more person-centred care are to be realized. They suggest a more strategic "all encompassing" approach in a change agenda in which nurses feature as the key coordinators within service provision that reflects the need to:

- put people and their needs first
- re-orient the model of care
- reorganize the delivery of services
- engage patients, their families and carers
- rearrange accountability mechanisms
- align incentives
- develop human resources for health
- uptake innovations
- partner with other sectors and civil society
- manage change strategically (World Health Organization, 2016).

Any or all of the concepts and issues cited above are part of deliberations within transnational activities in situations in which professionals (clinicians and/or educators) engage. The choices about approaches to professional development within transnational initiatives are best served by principles and frameworks that are able to accommodate practice development irrespective of the challenge of situations that are represented within learning events that acknowledge the impact of context and culture.

Challenges in contextualizing curriculum development and implementation

Irrespective of the goals and thus the choices in stimulus material or learning activities, certain beliefs about curriculum design and implementation are universal if one is to provide the learner with optimal learning outcomes. In the past educational theories and practices have been imported from the West with little consideration for the host culture's heritage (Nguyen, Terlouw, & Pilot, 2006). The development of a suite of abilities that will serve learners well, irrespective of their context of practice, will assist in preparing them for an unpredictable and ambiguous future (Waters, Rochester, & McMillan, 2012). These abilities are often framed as graduate attributes or qualities and include "critical thinking, intellectual curiosity, problem-solving, logical and independent thought, communication and information management skills, intellectual rigour, creativity and imagination, ethical practice, integrity and tolerance" (Bath, Smith, Stein & Swann, 2004, p. 313).

Of importance is the articulation of the relationship between practice and the conceptual frameworks that are informed by practice. There is a clear relationship among beliefs, thoughts, judgements and actions of health professionals. We assert that knowledge follows experience and is not its antecedent. If one accepts that professional nurses all over the world, given the nature of their practice, are "action-based thinkers" who confront and are confronted by different and sometimes novel contexts of practice, client situations, circumstances, health status and protocols, it follows that educators must rely on frameworks as conceptual maps for both *integrated practice and education*, to enable interrogation of the nature and scope of practice situations (Australian College of Mental Health Nurses (ACMHN), 2016). This means encouraging the learner to begin and continue to question the issues under interrogation. This implies that the stimulus material should represent common contextual and cultural factors (reflected above), particularly those that impede the achievement of desirable learner and client outcomes.

However, the context of care is a crucial moderator of the manner in which health professionals respond to demands on their skill sets. The world of work is complex – measures of safe and therapeutic practice differ across settings and cultures and contexts vary in response to differing clientele; there are different capacities and levels of competence within professional and inter-professional groups; and different approaches to managing well with available resources within a variety of structures and processes. However, we also assert that, universally, health professionals such as nurses are well placed to respond to pressing issues such as:

- demographic, environmental, political and social changes and the impact of these trends on health education and practice
- access and less than optimal education for healthcare
- balancing healthcare and education quality, effectiveness and efficiency
- ways of growing and sustaining the future healthcare workforce.

It is a universal ambition for health professionals working in any field across the world to have the necessary access to contemporary evidence-based knowledge and know-how if they are to influence care delivery processes; they need to pursue initiatives that lead to optimal patient outcomes and facilitate greater assurance of quality and safety for their consumers and peers. How best to develop professional capability around greater integration of services and processes for education and care must be informed by answers to the right questions. The blueprint for education and an approach to training and education around professional development should lead to outcomes that have relevance for the learner and the practice setting. Further to this, it is important to acknowledge that values and beliefs that are not evidence-based will impact the nature of care processes and outcomes. Interrogation of commonly held values and beliefs is an essential part of education also influenced by context and culture. This is summarized in Figure 7.1.

Curricula for contemporary practice irrespective of context

Curriculum design and delivery should be responsive to local offshore policies, practices and procedures (Melano, Bell, & Walker, 2014) as well as cultural values. As discussed above, professional development aligned to capacity building should cause the educator to think about appropriate curriculum frameworks but also approaches to working within different contexts and cultures. Of critical importance is the need to operationalize particular concepts that are relevant and meaningful to the audience of clinicians and learners and to decide what the key elements are in the process of globalization that are likely to affect education and healthcare and which of these elements can be used as part of the core strategy for curriculum planning (Nguyen et al., 2006). Integrated and service learning in an international

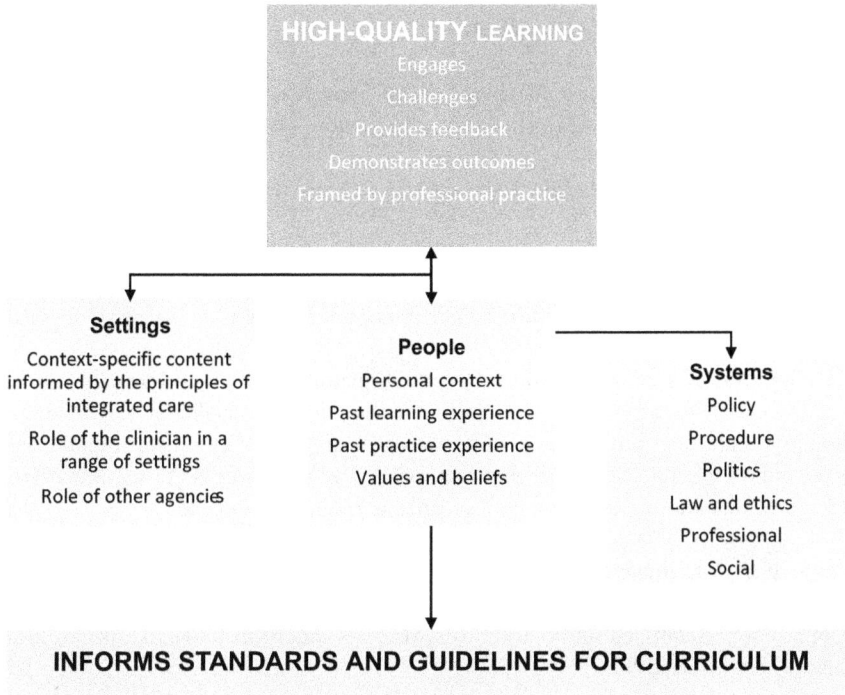

HIGH-QUALITY LEARNING
Engages
Challenges
Provides feedback
Demonstrates outcomes
Framed by professional practice

Settings

Context-specific content
informed by the principles of
integrated care

Role of the clinician in a
range of settings

Role of other agencies

People

Personal context

Past learning experience

Past practice experience

Values and beliefs

Systems

Policy

Procedure

Politics

Law and ethics

Professional

Social

INFORMS STANDARDS AND GUIDELINES FOR CURRICULUM

Figure 7.1 A conceptual model for curriculum development (adapted from Conway, Little, & Fitzgerald, 2011).

context of practice can be evaluated across two dimensions – that of service, assessed as whether learning materials meet the real needs of the local context, and integration, that is, the extent to which learning is clearly integrated with knowledge, skills and values of the educational institution (Jeong & McMillan, 2015). Educational materials must represent contextual variables such as:

- specific local needs
- predisposing factors to health and/or health breakdown
- demographics, ethnicity and social relationships, family relationships
- patterns of health service utilization
- beliefs, attitudes, values and knowledge about health and well-being
- cultural norms, political systems and processes.

The desired outcomes statements (abilities for competent and confident practice), the skills of the facilitator, the meaningfulness of the frameworks for integrating and interrogating practice and the value of the stimulus material will contribute to optimal learning results and thus changes in behaviours and practices.

The media/platforms for learning will influence choices of activities, but in the Asian context, the questions developed by Little (Conway et al., 2011, pp. 359–360) provide useful universally applicable stimuli for learning processes.

Examples of questions might include

- Situation/analysis or decision making – What information do I have? What further information do I need? Can I justify this action (lawfully, ethically, effectively, theoretically)?
- The learning process – What do I already know? How do I know it? What do I need to know?
- Perceptions – What are my feelings? What are my beliefs about the situation? How have I derived these beliefs/assumptions? How do my feelings/beliefs affect my response? Why do I hold this belief/assumption? What are alternative beliefs/assumptions?
- These are examples of broad, culturally neutral questions that allow learners to envisage their own contexts of practice. The questions also allow the facilitator to ask additional probing questions to provide answers to the question, "How could this be otherwise?" In our view, sharing with colleagues is a useful way to reflect on critique experiences and approaches and build on the pool of suitable resources available.

If one is invited to facilitate building capacity for translation of curricula from a traditional to a more process-oriented design, there is a need for cultural sensitivity at a range of levels. Nurses in a newly established university in the Maldives sought to undertake major curriculum renewal that featured the

- movement from vocational to tertiary-level qualifications
- expansion of roles and functions within their scope of practice
- need for curriculum development based on a design that reflected international standards for practice and education
- orientation to processes of learning with the student at the centre of learning activities.

An experiential approach to the enrolment of 10 registered nurses in master's-level studies ensured that curriculum development was a central feature of all their own postgraduate student experiences. Key features of the learning activities included the flexibility in sequencing of subject offerings to accommodate local commitments to Muslim holy days, building capacity in the use of information technology and the need to introduce and then incrementally add new concepts across the entire programme. All reflective pieces centred on ascertaining an appreciation of the meaningfulness of learning outcomes to their context of practice and culture. Individualized projects enabled students to focus on the application of their graduate abilities from coursework to higher levels of evidence-based practice in settings in which they chose to specialize. The latter were also areas of need for the country's population.

By taking this approach we demonstrated that context was the crucial moderator of features of curriculum design and implementation. All stimulus material featured the local context and culture; we made no assumptions about how these members of a moderate Islamic country interpreted features of their daily life. We thus developed a sense of trust in the processes and stronger relationships in which questioning of new concepts was encouraged. The enhancement of resources through capacity building in the use of information technology meant that a vast range of evidence-based material became available to these health professionals. The country was already immersed in information technology that supported a robust tourism industry.

The Higher Education Research and Development Society of Australasia (HERDSA) guide (Melano, Bell, & Walker, 2014) is an excellent resource for educators teaching off-shore at a partner institution and includes a checklist of considerations to ensure that transnational teaching is coordinated and effective.

Principles informing integrated care

Globally developing and sustaining a more integrated approach to both education and practice is an important strategy to manage the care required to manage people with long-term and complex health conditions (ACMHN, 2016). Integrated care is a means for "improving accessibility, affordability and the quality of health care, especially for people with complex needs" (Valentijn et al., 2015) and its relevance for any discussion of health professional education is that the model includes consideration of "how clinical, professional, organisational and system integration efforts act at several levels (micro, meso and macro) and can be defined from multiple stakeholder perspectives (patients, professionals, managers and policy-makers)" (Valentijn, 2016). Educators working overseas can use this framework to understand and explore health in settings unfamiliar to them. For example, education about the impact of HIV is enriched by context and consideration of the perspective of an adolescent living as an HIV-positive teenager in northern Thailand in a rural area also demands an exploration of cultural beliefs, organizational and system issues.

Principles for working across cultures and contexts

The ACMHN (2016) has an excellent example of a framework informed by a set of principles agreed upon by the professional body and demonstrative of values that reflect integrated practice and education. Those most relevant to becoming a citizen of the global educational and capacity-building environment are as follows:

- Partnerships in learning generate and frame learning outcomes for individual students across a range of contexts of practice settings.
- Learning events are constructed in a way that respects individual worldviews but enhances critical thinking to challenge students' assumptions in a manner consistent with curriculum goals and objectives and consumer needs.
- The learning process is designed to capitalize on the shared knowledge and experiences of the learners and teachers, consumers, their families and significant others.
- The learning processes are conducted in such a way (ethical, legal, professional) that the safety and well-being of students and consumers are maintained.

Such frameworks could be used to explore the complexities of working as an educator in any context and as a yardstick for healthcare professionals to examine health service and education processes across diverse and rapidly changing contexts and cultures.

The APA's multicultural guidelines assert that cultural competence involves more than cultural knowledge (American Psychological Association, 2003). The importance of knowledge of differences is highlighted, but so too is the recognition that we may hold attitudes and beliefs that can detrimentally influence perceptions about and interactions with others who are ethnically and racially different from us. Health professionals are "cultural beings" and thus represent an important aspect of our cross-cultural work in research and clinical practice. There is a need for an "acute lens" to assess the cultural world, but also for a heightened awareness of "the lens itself and its tendency to focus and bend images based on his or her own cultural beliefs and values" (p. 283).

Acquisition of knowledge for developing an appreciation of every culture is challenging, if not impossible (APA, 2003). Few clinicians or academics will have had experience with more than a few cultural groups outside of their own. Cultural competence has been seen as having the cognitive flexibility to move between two cultural perspectives; competence should be demonstrated at organizational and system level to engage in actions or create the conditions that maximize the optimal development of the healthcare recipient (Sue & Torino, 2005; Whaley & Davis, 2007). It involves having a high level of personal insight and acceptance of diversity. Universities in Asia, perhaps most markedly in Japan, have faced many problems with internationalizing (Tsuneyoshi, 2005), including a great deal of reluctance to do so, and host institutions should demonstrate organizational commitment by providing resources such as translator to the educator and prioritizing cultural competence in the curriculum (Cox, 2011).

The distinct way *nurses* have of relating and interrelating with consumers and their families particularly distinguishes them in their practice; as professionals they offer a high level of coordination that leads to greater integration, irrespective of the country or cultural context in which they are working. Therefore, certain principles can contribute to the development of conceptual frameworks for practice in a range of contexts and situations, aspiring to greater integration in nursing care and culturally sensitive and process-oriented learning events that are:

1   … influenced by "service to others" and "on the ground" interaction with their consumers and their families
    Rationale: In integrated care and education this facilitates a person-centred focus (for the client and the student) that is intimately in tune with the person's culture and beliefs, that is, their life needs as well as their health needs in usual and crisis situations.
2   … determined by the nature of the clientele and the health professional's worldviews and testing of beliefs that are based on evidence-informed knowledge acquisition
    Rationale: The nurse/educator is committed to delivering broad, flexible, achievable realistic care/education that often goes beyond health and professional paradigms to individual commitment to consumer-generated care and student-directed learning.
3   … consistent with outcomes that are facilitated by acknowledging and responding to consumers' (clientele and students) needs
    Rationale: The nurse/educator takes the time to generate and nurture a special collaboration with consumers/students and others that results in mutual benefits; the nurse/educator maintains an ongoing relationship and consumers/students are able to set and realize their own realistic goals for health improvement/learning.
4   … is collaborative, co-constructed with students/consumers and their family
    Rationale: The distinctive contribution by integrated care/education is characterized by a partnership approach that is committed to a rehabilitative and recovery-oriented approach that results from the special way in which nurses view, relate and respond to an individual's needs and are active, information-fluent and committed to lifelong learning.
5   … is conducted in such a way (ethical, legal, professional, non-discriminatory) that the safety and well-being of consumers/students are maintained
    Rationale: Personal growth, recovery and rehabilitation are contingent upon a sense of respect for individuals' worldviews even though assumptions and beliefs are being challenged.

6   ... is underpinned by contemporary evidence that informs care processes and tests the validity of outcomes

Rationale: A critical examination of sources of evidence and their efficacy is central to nursing practice, learning and consumer outcomes.

7   ... is considerate of the nature and extent of contextual and cultural influences (social, political, economic and organizational) but does not constrain options and aspirations for learning

Rationale: Collaborative engagement within the partnerships for practice and learning will lead to collaborative critical reflection on the competing tensions within situations and issues raised.

To illustrate the application of the principles outlined above, what follows is a collection of exemplars of the authors' experiences in working in South-East Asia and their reflections on the manner in which they responded to situations that demanded transcultural under-standings and sensitivities.

The perspective of the educator

As a nursing academic working as a professor in Japan, there were no other West-erners working in nursing at that time and hence there was little opportunity to form a network to support change. My Japanese peers were pessimistic about making any change to the broader system given the resistance to change in Japan in general and nursing in particular.

As a response to this situation I modelled ways of encouraging faculty members to incorpor-ate new ideas into their teaching and ways to encourage learners to interrogate the situation and:

* justify what nurses can and should do for their clientele
* view themselves as among the key professionals in their context of practice
* assume a voice in formulating new ways to deliver care
* examine ways to manage practice more effectively
* explore options for testing the evidence base for their traditional ways of providing care.

At times, working in another culture presents the educator with two equally difficult alter-natives: to accept what cannot be changed within a particular situation or to attempt as an outsider to make changes.

I have been teaching postgraduate students mental health in China for a few years and was increasingly aware that, although I was positively affecting the students' attitudes towards those with mental health problems that it was likely that students would be unable to translate this change into practice as most had no clinical experience in any setting.

I organised a visit to a mental health unit and community facility with classes of students to run an activity of painting masks. My own and the students' learning was profound. Whilst I had done a reasonable job of assisting the students to talk one on one with clients and in so doing conduct an assessment what was missing was their ability to be sensitive to the milieu. The novelty of the activity rapidly drew more and more people to the room and no one seemed to be aware of the potential safety issues until I asked nurses to close the doors as numbers swelled over 60. The debriefing included a discussion on this and that many of the "patients" were in fact relatives and even other staff. We discussed the pros and cons of having relatives constantly with the patients as is the norm in China. On the next visit with the students it was patients only with the students. I had underestimated the anxiety that the relatives felt at the separation and they gathered five deep to gaze in at the door to the activity room. I asked several students to join me and we started a discussion with them about their experiences of looking after someone with a mental health problem and eventually the students were able to invite them into another room.

For me it was an eye opener. It is one thing to understand the importance of extended family in China but another to really experience the power of the bond. This was the first chance the students had been given to discuss the strong negative feelings they had about people with mental health problems and how to include families in care.

The perspective of the learner

People in Asia are unlikely to give honest feedback on performance to either faculty or students. Students are frequently treated like children to be nurtured at whatever cost and students reciprocally hold teachers in high regard (Xu & Davidhizar, 2005). It is their task to understand the teacher rather than the teacher's to make the material understandable and they are reluctant to ask for clarification (Cox, 2011). They are also unused to being asked to do readings and coursework or demonstrate the achievement of objectives through formal assessment (Tsuneyoshi, 2005).

> Students are accustomed to delivery that is largely via lecture to large numbers of students and there is little interaction between learners and the educator. Students are frequently expected to take notes and uncritical notice of the expert and acquire details of the content verbatim.
>
> It is a mistake to think that this method is without any advantage for acquisition of credentials. In Japan and Korea, students have to sit for a national licencing examination which comprises short answer and multiple-choice questions and pure knowledge acquisition is remarkably effective at short term memorizing to prepare students to pass an examination that consistently tests a limited range of content.

Despite this view, which is often mooted to justify a directive style of teaching, we have not yet found a student from any context whose preference has been for teacher-centred learning over active learning. A group of students in China summarized it thus:

> we hate content-heavy lectures with overloaded slides, being given answers instead of posing questions, a lot of useless homework, being "tested only on memory level" and most of all "using only one method to teach such as talking, talking and talking and then class is over".

The knowledge acquired from teacher-centred learning, if retained even for a short timeframe, is lacking a contextual set of principles for application to novel situations. This can be accommodated in part by immersing the relevant details in scenarios. In this way some context is available to students and practice at the examination techniques can be achieved at the same time as other outcomes achieved through more process-oriented approaches.

Great care needs to be taken not to overburden the students. As always, the design of the situation-based learning activities is of great importance.

The reluctance to question teachers means that one has to honestly evaluate one's own work and find other ways of inviting feedback. Students frequently expect to gain high marks and are disappointed with constructive feedback or poor marks. The view is often that they have worked hard to enter university and the role of the teacher is to instruct and support them and poor marks are a sign that they are not doing so.

The curriculum designer's perspectives

The propensity for thinking critically is not necessarily a feature of the repertoire of abilities that health professionals bring to their teaching and has been recognized as lacking in the intercultural–global competencies required for contemporary practice, along with communication, problem solving, leadership, self-regulation, and cultural, creative and reflective thinking (Esterhuizen & Kirkpatrick, 2015, p. 209).

> It would be a mistake to think that introducing critical thinking and problem solving would be unproblematic in any environment, let alone in classrooms that foster passive approaches.

Bringing critical thinking into the classroom requires long-term commitment (Park, Conway, & McMillan, 2016). Nursing is still dominated by physicians and it is unlikely that independent critical thinkers would be welcomed in hierarchical workplaces. Individual leaders will also have long histories within their professional roles and might not readily adapt to new ways of thinking about curricula. However, many simple strategies can be introduced to shift the balance from the educator to the student and encourage a more critical stance (Hiler & Paul, 2005). From time to time, it is worthwhile causing the academics who are comfortable in their beliefs about learning and teaching to reflect on what they intend to achieve in respect to student learning and the extent to which they actually test these goals in assessment tasks, especially around critical thinking (Park et al., 2016).

One needs to be constantly working with curriculum design and implementation processes that are considerate of the following issues that need to be embedded in situation-based stimulus material for learning:

- The nature of person-centred care and the manner in which this can be developed in countries with a medical model and its effects on teaching and curricula. For nurses, negotiating the hierarchical terrain is best managed through stimulus material that embeds the nursing role and response.
- The existence of strong stigma about particular differences in Eastern and Western orientations in organization of care. Given the global imperative for movement away from curative to preventative ideals, there is a need to address the social determinants of health and health breakdown through intra- and inter-sectoral action that promotes public health and health promotion (Ferrer & Goodwin, 2014).

For the professional bodies and institutions

While there are international forums where professional and regulatory bodies share knowledge about trends in curriculum design, implementation and evaluation, there is an extensive timeline from conceptualization of ideas to change and policy development. Many South-East Asian countries have outdated nursing legislation and curricula are reliant on a medical model, content-heavy and are not concept-based. In Japan, for example, the core curriculum is regulated by two government ministries and universities have discretion only to add additional requirements. Curricula frequently lack focus on therapeutic skills and holistic care (physical, socio-economic, mental and emotional wellness) (Ferrer & Goodwin, 2014).

Through the efforts of The International Foundation for Integrated Care (2017) confirmation of the strong theoretical foundations for practice and education is emerging, the evidence base has been tested and the emerging frameworks are underpinned by principles and values which ensure that care processes and treatment are therapeutic (helpful and salient).

Environment: societal influences

Religious beliefs

As educator I was asked to critically appraise a doctoral research proposal. The context was an Islamic university in Indonesia, the requirement by the university is that all research should include teaching from the Quran. The researcher planned to implement a sex education program for 12 year olds based on Islamic principles and asked advice on how to do this. I am not Muslim and do not share the same worldview. At this point I could have declined to comment saying that I disagreed with Islamic teaching and pointing out all the difficulties with this approach.

Both the researcher and educator could have missed an important opportunity for exchange about this situation. Critical thinkers can deal with contextual variables; instead the researcher used a process of exploratory questions including revisiting the purpose of the research, which was concern about rising numbers of teenage pregnancies and where she ultimately wanted to publish. This collaborative and respectful process enabled the researcher herself to explore the tensions between her beliefs, the research objectives and philosophical basis and the demands of contemporary evidence-based practice.

Ethics

Developing countries are at various stages in establishing internationally credible ethical approval systems for both education and research.

While working alongside local faculty to raise awareness of appropriate ethical requirements to establish committees and processes is the ultimate goal there are times when the educator needs to more assertively establish a "bottom line". A colleague witnessed clinical nurses practising cannulation techniques on unconscious or incapacitated patients in preparation for a national competition and acted immediately to stop this happening.

It is not unusual for student nurses to practise invasive techniques on each other and in many countries, there is little understanding of the principles of informed consent. It is however possible to introduce situations that involve techniques that at best inform the client around the processes and some notion of choice.

Scholarly activities and plagiarism

For the newcomer to scholarly activities there is little understanding of what constitutes plagiarism in both undergraduate and postgraduate studies. In many countries, including China, Indonesia and Japan, plagiarism software is not used to check student work.

> Assignments are often submitted in hard copy and change little from year to year and students are not taught how to reference or paraphrase. Assessments are frequently designed to capture recall and it is not surprising that students do not realise the importance of correctly attributing sources.

As well as discussing the principles of ethics clearance in academic pursuits at all levels of student education, designing assignments which tap into students' ability to apply and create and promote discovery and evidence informed practice helps to avoid these problems. To do this it is important to design assessments that foreground the structure and concepts rather than isolated facts and emphasize depth of learning rather than breadth (Biggs & Tang, 2009).

Political influences: freedom of speech

Person-centred care is "endowed with rights and responsibilities – that all citizens should expect, exercise and respect" (Ferrer & Goodwin, 2014), but this presents challenges in managing spontaneity in expression of beliefs that might be confronting to others.

> Educators in China, including overseas educators, are digitally recorded–without their permission or knowledge. These tapes are scrutinised to ensure that discussion is uncritical of the Communist Party. Discussion of human rights is forbidden and students have to report weekly on their own thoughts and behaviours to Party members.

Unwilling to compromise my own standards, I ground discussion firmly in the situations that pose contradictions or discomfort. For example, in discussion of what constitutes mental health and mental disorder we discuss whether sexual, political beliefs and practices constitute a mental illness. I use an unfamiliar and non-threatening example of the Flat Earth Society to explore the difference between delusion and belief.

Implications for education and practice

There is an enormous difference between teaching learners from a different cultural context in one's own environment and teaching overseas in a context different to one's own. The shift in thinking can be likened to the need to accommodate differences when moving between hospital-based and community nursing – consideration of the nature and extent of the impact of context for both client and health service provider.

Solutions to situations within particular contexts cannot be imposed from outside a culture. Instead we suggest the need for encouraging thoughtfulness around ways for enabling them to adopt the tools to fashion their own strategies. In this way we are not offering stimulus material for learning that cannot be applied in their own clinical or managerial context. It is important to consider how best to ensure that learning outcomes are meaningful and that new ideas are transferred to local people in a manner that ensures they are enabled, not disabled by the intervention of foreign "experts". Central to cross-cultural interactions is trust; openness to new ideas arises from deliberations that reflect deliberating in context and moving beyond simply being polite. Disagreements should arise from responses to stimulus materials that cause the learners to identify issues and provide resolutions with consideration of their place in their world.

Communicating in context is critical. Advocacy for the primacy of primary health care has long been espoused by the WHO but only recently the Chinese media outlined new policy directions to the public on particular population health matters. Now there needs to be a lot more work on health promotion and education; nurses are well placed in developing countries to assume a key role in preventive health measures.

The concept of empowerment demands a facilitative approach supporting people to manage and take responsibility for their own health (Ferrer & Goodwin, 2014) and learning. For us it is important to first empower nurses on how to use facilitative techniques in classrooms, clinical and parallel processes of discovery. Teaching styles and learning styles can cross borders but one might need to abandon some of the myths around fully transformative styles of teaching. It is preferable for the learner to assume responsibility for discovering alternative ways of setting and achieving realistic personal and professional goals.

Contextualizing nurse education within national, international and global health challenges reminds us that there are particular context-specific issues that demand greater focus; for example, disaster preparedness, developments around genetics and climate change need to move to the fore in choices of stimulus material.

Health beliefs and cultural differences demand respect if we are to avoid damage to people's dignity, social circumstances and cultural sensitivities. However, searching for evidence to support beliefs should be governed through shared accountability for information literacy.

The maintenance of personal well-being when teaching overseas is critical to the success of the venture and the learning outcomes and dealing with expectations. Critical and constructive feedback on one's effectiveness may not be forthcoming and it is important to critically examine one's own performance using models such as Cox (2011) suggests. Teaching people who have English as an additional language and working with translators demands a level of trust and use of all the senses in spaces and places beyond the formal education environment. Often one can better appreciate the personal requirements for overseas faculty from informal interactions.

> Any list of personal requirements for working for any length of time overseas should include four essentials – adaptability, self-awareness, curiosity and resilience. Living and teaching overseas means that you have to give up a lot of control and go with the flow accepting what can and needs to be changed in the work environment and what cannot be changed. Self-awareness allows us to examine our own culture and beliefs and remain empathic and respectful of differences. Curiosity is essential to explore, observe, enjoy, learn about and understand cultural differences as is resilience to withstand the stresses and sense of being different.

Discussing cultural adaptation and our ability and knowledge about which of our behaviours we use, Molinsky (2013: p. 174) has six key takeaway points:

> In this situation 1) Directness: How straightforwardly am I expected to communicate? 2) Enthusiasm – How much positive emotion and energy am I expected to show to others? 3) Formality: How much deference and respect am I expected to demonstrate? 4) Assertiveness: How strongly am I expected to express my voice? 5) Self promotion: How positively am I expected to speak about my skills

and accomplishments? 6) Cross-cultural adjustment involves the knowledge of which behavior to execute or suppress in given situations and the ability to effectively actualize this understanding.

Conclusion

The culture of my country has a strong character that was totally invisible to me when I was in it and part of it.

(Meyer, 2014)

We hope that this chapter has provided readers with some ideas about frameworks and processes to use in any context of learning as well as offering food for thought for those working in an overseas context; we have provided tools and frameworks to inform and reflect on practice. Developing the next generation of healthcare professionals whatever their context to deliver integrated healthcare means impacting learners' knowledge, skills and attitudes (Stein, 2016) but also demands of the educator working in an overseas context to be reflective of their own knowledge, skills and attitudes. Implications for their work with respect to future directions for nurse education are both process-oriented and demanding of more personal reflection on learning activities and outcomes.

Educators need the humility not to see the West as the wellspring of all that is good in education and practice and need to avoid ethnocentric interpretations of other cultures and practices. In addition, educators need to practise flexibility and the ability to discern what can and cannot be changed, promotion of greater independence in learning, role modelling cultural sensitivity, collaboratively building capacity at all levels (from micro to macro) and most of all encouraging curiosity in students for accommodating worldviews beyond that with which they are most familiar. The central concern for those working transnationally is to build capacity to enable health professionals to address contemporary issues in an integrated way. As always one should build relationships with transnational peers and students with the assumption that the culture in which each of us grew as a person has a profound impact on how we see the world. However, each of us is also challenged to embrace the need for generational changes in responses to our context and culture. There is an imperative for greater global dexterity.

References

ACMHN (2016) A national framework for postgraduate mental health nursing education. Retrieved from www.acmhn.org/images/stories/Resources/NationalFramework2016.pdf

American Psychological Association (2003) Guidelines on multicultural education, training, research, practice, and organizational change for psychologists. *American Psychologist, 58*(5), 377.

Bath D, Smith C, Stein S, & Swann R (2004) Beyond mapping and embedding graduate attributes: Bringing together quality assurance and action learning to create a validated and living curriculum. *Higher Education Research & Development, 23*(3), 313–328.

Biggs, J., & Tang, C. (2009). *Teaching for Learning at University*. University Press. Maidenhead.

Conway J F, Little P, & Fitzgerald M (2011) Determining frameworks for interprofessional education and core competency through collaborative consultancy: The CARE experience. *Contemporary Nurse: A Journal for the Australian Nursing Profession, 38*(1/2), 359–360.

Cox K R (2011) Evaluating the effectiveness of intercultural teachers. *Nursing Education Perspectives, 32*(2), 102.

Esterhuizen P & Kirkpatrick M K (2015) Intercultural–global competencies for the 21st century and beyond. *The Journal of Continuing Education in Nursing, 46*(5), 209–214.

Ferrer L & Goodwin N (2014) What are the principles that underpin integrated care? *International Journal of Integrated Care, 14*(4). https://www.ijic.org/articles/10.5334/ijic.1884/

Gribble K & Ziguras C (2003) Learning to teach offshore: Pre-departure training for lecturers in transnational programs. *Higher Education Research & Development, 22*(2), 205–216. doi:10.1080/07294360304115

Hiler W & Paul R (2005) *Active and Cooperative Learning.* Dillon Beach, CA: The Foundation for Critical Thinking.

The International Foundation for Integrated Care (2017) The International Foundation for Integrated Care (IFIC) Retrieved from https://integratedcarefoundation.org/our-work

Jeong S & McMillan M (2015) Work integrated learning (WIL): Integrating frameworks for education and practice. *Journal of Problem-Based Learning, 2*(1), 1-10.

Melano A, Bell M, & Walker R (2014) *Transnational Teaching and Learning.* Milperra: Higher Education Research and Development Society of Australasia (HERDSA).

Meyer E (2014) *The Culture Map: Breaking through the Invisible Boundaries of Global Business.* PublicAffairs. USA.

Molinsky A (2013) *Global Dexterity: How to Adapt Your Behaviour across Cultures Without Losing Yourself in the Process.* Boston, MA: Harvard Business Review Press.

Nguyen P M, Terlouw C, & Pilot A (2006) Culturally appropriate pedagogy: The case of group learning in a Confucian heritage culture context. *Intercultural Education, 17*(1), 1–19.

Park M Y, Conway J, & McMillan M (2016) Enhancing critical thinking through simulation. *Journal of Problem-based Learning, 3*(1), 31–40.

Stein K (2016) Developing a competent workforce for integrated health and social care: What does it take? *International Journal of Integrated Care, 16*(4), 9.

Stone T E, Francis L, van der Riet P, Dedkhard S, Junlapeeya P, & Orwat E (2014) Awakening to the other: Reflections on developing intercultural competence through an undergraduate study tour. *Nursing & Health Sciences, 16*(4), 521–527. doi:10.1111/nhs.12139

Sue D W & Torino G C (2005) Racial-cultural competence: Awareness, knowledge, and skills. In *Handbook of Racial-Cultural Psychology and Counseling: Training and Practice*, Vol. 2, 3–18.

Tsuneyoshi R (2005) Internationalization strategies in Japan: The dilemmas and possibilities of study abroad programs using English. *Journal of Research in International Education, 4*(1), 65–86.

Valentijn P (2016) Rainbow of chaos: A study into the theory and practice of integrated primary care. *International Journal of Integrated Care, 16*(2).

Valentijn P, Boesveld I, van der Klauw D, Ruwaard D, Struijs J, Molema J, & Vrijhoef H (2015) Towards a taxonomy for integrated care: A mixed-methods study. *International Journal of Integrated Care, 15*(1)., e003.

Van Lerberghe W (2008) *The World Health Report 2008: Primary Health Care: Now More than Ever.* World Health Organization. TSL Geneva.

Waters C D, Rochester S F, & McMillan M A (2012) Drivers for renewal and reform of contemporary nursing curricula: A blueprint for change. *Contemporary Nurse, 41*(2), 206–215.

Whaley A L & Davis K E (2007) Cultural competence and evidence-based practice in mental health services: A complementary perspective. *American Psychologist, 62*(6), 563.

World Health Organization (2016) Lessons from transforming health services delivery: Compendium of initiatives in the WHO European Region. Retrieved from www.euro.who.int/en/health-topics/Health-systems/health-services-delivery/publications/2016/lessons-from-transforming-health-services-delivery-compendium-of-initiatives-in-the-who-european-region-2016

Xu Y F & Davidhizar R (2005) Intercultural communication in nursing education: When Asian students and American faculty converge. *Journal of Nursing Education, 44*(5), 209.

8

COLLABORATIVE ONLINE INTERNATIONAL LEARNING (COIL): A NEW MODEL OF GLOBAL EDUCATION

Teddie Potter and Helga Bragadóttir

Introduction

Ideally, nursing education is a collaborative interplay between students, faculty, and clinicians. Collaborative Online International Learning (COIL) is a new way of transforming nursing students and nurses into global thinkers and leaders. The core of COIL is collaboration and partnership across cultures and nations, where mutual respect and trust are components of success. Shishani et al. (2012) point out the important role of nurses regarding global health issues and for future nurses to be able to practice to their full potential requires them to be true global thinkers. This underscores the importance of incorporating internationalization and global leadership in nursing education. Investing in the globalization of the nursing workforce should therefore be a prioritization for nursing education (Shishani et al., 2012).

In this chapter, we introduce COIL as an optimal way of promoting global thinking skills and cultural competence in nursing. We discuss the need for nurses to have a global perspective and why traditional global education does not go far enough to address this competency. COIL, a new model of global education, is introduced along with its process, and how to successfully use COIL in healthcare education. The main benefits and challenges of COIL for students and faculty are introduced, as well as the benefits of COIL for global nursing education. Future directions for COIL and global nursing education are also discussed. A global perspective helps us understand that local health is global, and global health is local (Shishani et al., 2012). Nursing and healthcare become *glocal,* indicating the interdependence of local and global health (Rosa, 2017). COIL is an excellent way to effectively reach the goal of globalizing nursing and healthcare.

The need for nurses to have a global perspective

Every year the globe gets a little smaller. Cultures and nations that we would never have encountered in the past are now at our fingertips via the Internet. Healthcare challenges and threats are also moments away. Global travel and immigration have brought people with new infectious diseases to our clinics and emergency departments. Global is now local, requiring nurses to be educated to have a global perspective. Technology opens doors to relationships with people from different parts of the world, but we still need to develop the intercultural skills required to make those relationships work.

Until recently, many considered global health to be the same as international health. Koplan et al. (2009) clarify the difference. International health "focuses on health issues of countries other than one's own, especially those of low-income and middle-income" whereas global health "focuses on issues that directly or indirectly affect health but that can transcend national boundaries" (p. 1994). International health therefore tends to be unilateral, whereas global health is concerned with health equity issues that span the globe. "The global in global health refers to the scope of problems, not their location. Thus – like public health but unlike international health – global health can focus on domestic health disparities as well as cross-border issues" (p. 1994). This perspective is now being called "glocal" in the literature (Beck et al., 2013).

In order for nurses to lead global health initiatives, they must first have a shared definition of global health and global nursing. A global advisory panel synthesized the literature and developed a consensus statement on the following definitions:

Global health

Global health refers to an area for practice, study and research that places a priority on improving health, achieving equity in health for all people and ensuring health-promoting and sustainable sociocultural, political and economic systems. Global health implies planetary health which equals human, animal, environmental and ecosystem health and it emphasizes transnational health issues, determinants and solutions; involves many disciplines within and beyond the health sciences and promotes interdependence and interdisciplinary collaboration; and is a synthesis of population-based prevention with individual holistic care.

(Wilson et al., 2016, p. 1536)

Global nursing

Global nursing is the use of evidence-based nursing process to promote sustainable planetary health and equity for all people. Global nursing considers social determinants of health, includes individual and population-level care, research, education, leadership, advocacy and policy initiatives. Global nurses engage in ethical practice and demonstrate respect for human dignity, human rights and cultural diversity. Global nurses engage in a spirit of deliberation and reflection in interdependent partnership with communities and other health care providers.

(Wilson et al., 2016, p. 1537)

When planning curriculum, healthcare educators frequently ask themselves, "Is this content essential, nice to know, or not necessary to know?" Unfortunately, given the current rise of care and treatment complexities, many faculty have determined that global issues and global education must be relegated to "nice to know" status. Some faculty even believe that global health and transcultural competence only belong in the public health curriculum and are not pertinent to all care and all treatment. Therefore, they feel that development of a global perspective is "unnecessary" content. The authors propose that global perspective and transcultural relationships are germane to every area of health education. Like inclusivity and diversity, they are every healthcare professional's everyday work. They also reflect a lifelong process of professional development. We are never experts or fully competent but instead, we are on a journey toward enhanced understanding and cultural humility.

One issue that underscores the need for nurses to have a global perspective is the global refugee crisis most recently witnessed when millions of Syrians fled their country in the face of civil war and overwhelmed health infrastructures in Europe. In response to this refugee crisis and others, the International Council of Nurses (ICN) (2018) revised its policy statement on the *Health of Migrants, Refugees and Displaced Persons* (MRDPs), which stresses that "Care of MRDPs is complex and nurses must be supported through education, ongoing training and with adequate resources in order to provide high-quality, culturally competent care" (p. 1).

We are beginning to understand that the health and even survival of all life on the planet is deeply connected to cross-border issues such as population, water and land use, and social system stability. The most challenging global health issues require global thinking and effective intercultural relationships. Nurses educated with a global perspective and intercultural relationship skills can make a significant contribution to global and planetary health. Having universal definitions of global health and global nursing allows nurse educators to design an effective curriculum to educate global nursing leaders.

Traditional global education often fails to promote development of a global perspective

Global perspective and intercultural competence should be required competencies for all levels of nursing education. The sustainability and quality of nursing and healthcare services are dependent on healthcare professionals being culturally skilled global thinkers. The nursing profession has always honored equity and human justice and from early on the International Council of Nurses (ICN) identified the importance of nursing education to be aligned with the Universal Declaration of Human Rights. Nursing services should be universal and nursing practice unrestricted by nationality, race, creed, color, politics, or social status (ICN, 1969). This declaration however underscores the need for nurses to be educated with intercultural competence and global thinking. Nurses and nursing need to become global. Global nursing is not about working internationally or participating in projects abroad, but a shift of awareness and consciousness on how the work of nurses applies to all sectors and levels of healthcare and society as a whole, by providing clinical care but no less by being an active voice in policy-making, education, economy and environmental issues. The transformation is crystalized in the identified themes of global nursing. To reach the goals of the United Nations 2030 Agenda, which entail reducing poverty, ensuring food security, improving health, and fighting climate change, nurses need to become global citizens (Wilson et al., 2016, in Rosa, 2017). As identified by Koplan et al. (2009), global health overlaps with international health and public health.

Throughout the centuries the way for students to get exposed to intercultural education has been by traveling abroad spending time in another country or in recent years by participating in online courses across countries. However, traditional online global education is limited as it includes only the theory of internationalization and cultural competence without any skills training or practice. Traditional intercultural programming has also often been based on a domination model (Marginson, 2004), which implies inequity of cultures and nations, with one school playing the role of the superior providing the teaching while the others play a subservient role as receivers.

Furthermore, previous models of global learning posed a "have and have not" dichotomy. Those with sufficient money and time assets were able to travel abroad and develop their intercultural competencies through engaging people living in different nations. Students with limited resources such as insufficient funds, family responsibilities, and medical or visa travel restrictions, on the other hand, could not benefit from travel to a different land.

In recent decades, the growing opportunities of the Internet have offered additional options. However novel the intentions may be, the tendency toward a domination mindset is evident. Examples of this paradigm can be seen in Supercourse, a global library of over 5,100 public health and medical lectures and a network of over 56,000 public health professionals in 174 countries of the world. The focus of the Supercourse platform is to empower local educators by giving them access to high-quality teaching materials (Shishani et al., 2012). The notion that some give while others are primarily or entirely recipients indicates power inequality and lack of partnership and mutuality. The lack of emphasis on global perspective and intercultural skills is evident in the fact that major policy papers published in the past failed to mention the need for or requirements of internationalization and cultural competence of nurses (WHO, 2009, 2015).

Recently the World Health Organization (WHO) published *Nurse Educator Core Competencies* (2016), acknowledging that nursing education and practice are changing. The competencies confirm that the nursing profession must practice, lead, and adapt to new evidence, increasingly diverse populations and changing needs and that education is an important starting point for change. The paper also points to the fact that appropriate use of technology can help to expedite such changes (WHO, 2016). The aim of the *Nurse Educator Core Competencies* is for nurse educators to gain increased proficiency in assisting nursing students to acquire all the knowledge, skills, and attitudes necessary to practice nursing effectively in the twenty-first century (World Health Organization [WHO], 2016). COIL not only advances nursing student competencies in multiple ways; it is also an optimal way to meet the WHO *Nurse Educator Core Competencies* (World Health Organization [WHO], 2016) and enhance the professional development of involved faculty (Bragadóttir and Potter, in press). COIL is based on and requires a cross-cultural dialogue with a global dimension as well as critical intercultural reflection of both faculty and students. To prepare and start a COIL initiative the State University of New York (SUNY) COIL Center recommends three basic steps and a number of important facilitating issues (Center for Collaborative Online International Learning [COIL], n.d.). In Table 8.1 we have summarized the COIL steps and facilitators with important issues to address for developing a COIL initiative with descriptions on how we did it.

A new model of global education: Collaborative Online International Learning

The previous section discussed gaps in the current methods to prepare globally ready nurses. We suggest that COIL can promote the development of a global perspective and prepare nurses to address global health challenges using advanced intercultural skills. The Center for Collaborative Online International Learning was established in 2006 at SUNY (Center for Collaborative Online International Learning, n.d.). As mentioned before, previous models of online international learning have been unidirectional, meaning the faculty from one country create and teach the material to students in another country. COIL, however, is based on the premise that the most effective online international learning is co-created and co-taught by two or more faculty from different nations. COIL promotes the "creation of co-equal learning environments where instructors work together to generate a shared syllabus based on solid academic coursework emphasizing experiential and collaborative student learning" (SUNY, n.d.a.).

A COIL approach allows all students to have an international experience regardless of personal constraints or economic challenges. COIL supports equality in the classroom so that all future nurses can practice with a global perspective. Commitment to equity was the driving force behind adoption of the COIL method for intercultural coursework by the University of Minnesota (UMN) and the University of Iceland (UI). The UMN School of Nursing and the UI Faculty of Nursing have had a decades-long relationship. In response to the emerging need for all nursing leaders to be able to demonstrate intercultural skills, faculty from both schools made a commitment in 2015 to develop and implement a COIL course to educate nursing leadership students to have a global perspective.

COIL courses are taught in many disciplines, from clothing design to international policy. Currently SUNY lists nearly 40 Global Partner Campuses (SUNY, n.d.b.), but these represent only the formal relationships with SUNY. There are other universities across the globe starting to implement this methodology. The course taught by faculty from UI and UMN appears to be the first application of COIL in nursing and perhaps even healthcare in general.

Koplan et al. (2009) compared and contrasted global health, international health, and public health. They acknowledge an emerging shift from patterns of one nation dominating another nation (international health) to an "attitude that emphasizes the mutuality of real partnership, a pooling of experience and knowledge … Global health thus uses the resources, knowledge, and experience of diverse societies to address health challenges throughout the world" (p. 1995). The COIL methodology facilitates the development of nurses who think in terms of partnership rather than superiority when working with people from other cultures and nations. COIL therefore prepares nurses to work collaboratively on health and health equity issues that are universal.

The COIL process

COIL involves two or more schools from at least two different countries co-teaching parallel courses, using online technology and co-created learning objectives. The courses have a determined timeframe, preferably a number of weeks to several months, where students follow comparable course content, communicate, and critically discuss their ideas and thoughts, and work on shared assignments. The core of COIL is partnership of faculty and students within and between schools. The commitment to partnership ensures mutual teaching and learning (Eisler and Potter, 2014). The driving goal of COIL is to develop the global perspectives and cultural competence of students and faculty (Wahls et al., 2017).

COIL requires equal commitment of both parties and solid preparation. The following are essential components of the COIL process: (1) the objectives and extent of the project need to be determined; (2) the content and timing of the common assignments need to be designed; (3) the website or online platform for the COIL course needs to be established; (4) the evaluation and grading of the common assignments need to be determined; (5) the technology that the students will use needs to be decided; and (6) there needs to be agreement about evaluation of the knowledge, growth, and partnership of the involved students and faculty (Center for Collaborative Online International Learning [COIL], n.d.; Starke-Meyerring and Andrews, 2006).

There are at least three main components to COIL: the course material being taught, the process of transcultural collaboration, and the method of using online computer technology for creating a learning community. During the implementation of the COIL course the role and responsibilities of each faculty need to be clear. Unexpected events should be anticipated. The process in itself as well as all occurring events, whether expected and planned or unexpected, should be seen as learning opportunities for students; the *process* of COIL has as much educational value as the *content*. COILing is a perfect match to the Nurse Educator Core Competencies identified by WHO (2016), which are the minimum competencies that a qualified nurse educator should possess. Application of COIL methodology particularly supports Nurse Educator Core Competency 2, which encourages educators to develop curricula based on innovative teaching and learning strategies and best evidence.

The *Guide for Collaborative Online International Learning* (Center for Collaborative Online International Learning [COIL], n.d.) is an essential tool for any faculty designing a COIL course. In addition to the process established by SUNY, the authors have found it very important to approach the entire relationship and initiative from a partnership perspective (Eisler and Potter, 2014). Faculty may collaborate but if the relationships are hierarchical, where one person has more power or influence then the other, the true potential of COIL cannot be attained. Partnership creates an environment where educational outcomes are greater than anything that could have been accomplished by one faculty alone.

Potter and Bragadóttir both teach nursing leadership and administration for graduate nursing students. One of their shared core competencies is global nursing leadership. They both agreed that COIL offers an innovative approach to help all of their students expand their global perspective. Designing their COIL course involved all of the steps in Table 8.1. Throughout the planning and implementation process, careful attention was given to mutual respect and shared creation. A partnership approach gives students a template for intercultural and international relationships that may be different from what they see in the news or read about in textbooks.

Implementation of the COIL steps recommended by the SUNY

COIL steps cited from Center for Collaborative International Learning (COIL, n.d.)

With COIL, global partners co-create new models of global learning with shared contributions by the global partners and co-creation of curriculum to enhance a global perspective (Starke-Meyerring, 2010). COIL is an optimal way of breaking down the global hierarchy, giving all nurses the opportunity to become global nurses.

Benefits and challenges of COIL for faculty and students

Benefits

There are both benefits and challenges for students and faculty participating in COIL courses. Everyone participating in a COIL course is a "student", and therefore experiences the same benefits and challenges. The shared learning experience is a fundamental contribution of COIL. The main benefits of COIL from our experience are listed in Figure 8.1. Through the COIL experience participants realize that nursing and healthcare are global, that the two countries have more in common than not, and it teaches them what different healthcare systems have in common. COIL helps participants recognize the importance of cultural competence in healthcare and may correct their bias and change their way of thinking. COIL encourages students to get acquainted with healthcare and healthcare professionals in other countries.

Challenges

COIL may provide several challenges for students as well as faculty. Participants should anticipate technical challenges as individuals' technical competence varies and common computer programs may differ between schools. Also there will be cultural and linguistic

Table 8.1 Partnership-based global perspective

COIL Steps	Important issues to address	How we approached this step
Step 1: Determining your content and institutional resources	- Decide what part(s) of your course can be modified to be "COILed" - Identify what institutional resources are needed - Identify required technical resources - Identify other resources - Assess your own readiness to teach a technologically enhanced course - Identify administrative support at your institution	Leadership in nursing and healthcare was a focus we shared and we both wanted our students to become global leaders. We believe that leadership is an issue that can be taught in numerous ways which makes it an ideal subject to modify for COIL. Both of us were looking for collaboration abroad, as we had the common belief that international collaboration would increase the value of our education as well as help us develop as competent teachers. Later, when preparing the COIL course, we collaborated with an intercultural specialist who analyzed and compared each of our syllabi to identify commonalities and difference in content and assignments. This feedback allowed us to determine the best sections of our courses to COIL. We consulted technical support at both universities to see whether there was a common learning platform that could be used. Administrative support was evident, as the deans in both our schools were the ones to suggest we work together
Step 2: Finding and developing your partnership	- Identify key criteria a partner needs to meet - Identify potential partners	Criteria important to both of us were a common language (English), a common semester, and all students being at a graduate level. The long-standing research collaboration between the UI and UMN led us together. Starting by looking into possibilities with those you already know may be wise

Step 3: Beginning negotiation	- Decide on a timeline for the COILing
	- Identify the common:
	
	  • goals
	  • content
	  • assignments
	
	- Be aware of differences in:
	
	  • time zones
	  • languages
	  • culture
		We decided to COIL a semester-long course from January to April. Our first COIL assignment is at the beginning of our course; the second one is in February–March; and the third one is towards the end of the course in April.
		The shared goal in both of our courses is that upon completion students will become culturally sensitive global leaders in healthcare.
		We decided to use the same main textbooks and some other readings, but we each also had additional readings that were specific to our own courses. However, students were

(Continued)

Table 8.1 (Cont).

COIL Steps	Important issues to address	How we approached this step
	• technology competence - Identify possible computer program options and ways of communication (synchronous vs. asynchronous)	informed and had access to the reading material in the other school. Due to time differences in our countries and technical issues, we only required asynchronous discussions between the students
Facilitators		
1: Arrange a face-to-face meeting with your partner, if possible	Preferably meet or at least arrange for a face-to-face collaboration online if traveling is not possible	Faculty from the UMN secured a travel grant to bring the UI faculty to Minnesota for a week six months before the COIL course was first implemented. This face-to-face time proved invaluable as it fostered a shared vision and promoted co-created assignments
2: Foster honesty and open communication	1. Clearly state all expectations 2. Seek first to understand 3. Resist being judgmental 4. Don't assume that what was meant was understood (and vice versa) 5. Don't take things personally. Or in other words, assume positive intent	The UI and UMN faculty worked closely with a UMN intercultural specialist. The specialist listened to dialog between the two faculty and was able to discern differences that, left unrecognized, could have impacted desired outcomes. We each had implicit biases about our courses and our students' learning needs that needed to be illuminated before we could create a shared learning experience
3: Get a real commitment from your partner and your institution	Define expectations and true commitment in writing	Given the nature of our long-standing relationship, it was not necessary to formalize our agreement in writing
4: Envision your COIL enhanced course as a forum for developing intercultural competence	Both teachers and students need to be prepared for new challenges and lessons from the intercultural communication	Both of us made a point in our syllabi and during orientation to our courses that intercultural experiences offer rich learning opportunities as well as challenges to overcome. We acknowledged that unexpected situations were likely to arise and together we would collaborate to find solutions
5: Develop lesson plans	Co-develop a clear lesson plan	The lesson plan details, including shared assignments and due dates, were determined during the face-to-face planning session
6: Test the technology	Check and double check; however teachers and students should be prepared to encounter technical challenges	Moodle was the online learning platform that we had in common. It was important for us to have information technology assistants in both countries who could help students troubleshoot online enrollment and platform navigation

(Continued)

Table 8.1 (Cont).

COIL Steps	Important issues to address	How we approached this step
7: Engage students with icebreaker activities to get to know each other	Foster relationship building between students with fun activities	The second week of class we asked students to create a 90-second online video that briefly introduced themselves, their nursing specialty, why they were in graduate school, and what they hoped to learn through COIL
8: Have at least one cross-border collaborative assignment	COIL includes not only teaching but also training, so there needs to be at least one collaborative assignment with at least one common goal that relies on the interdependence of the teachers and students	The goal is to create an assignment that prompts an "Aha" experience – one where students gained insights because they learned about the experiences and encountered the views of students from another nation. Our shared assignment involved interviewing a recent immigrant about his or her experiences of healthcare in the adopted country
9: Provide the opportunity for critical reflection	Students need to critically reflect on what they learned about themselves in working across differences, as well as what they learned from their peers	Once the students had interviewed a recent immigrant, they wrote a paper and shared their observations in a COIL chat discussion space on Moodle
10: Expect the unexpected	Teachers and students need to be prepared to positively and constructively use every opportunity as a learning experience	Again, the spirit of innovation as well as patience was fostered from the beginning by the faculty setting the tone during orientation

COIL, Collaborative Online International Learning; UI, University of Iceland; UMN, University of Minnesota.

challenges as well as logistic ones. There may be an imbalance regarding language as one school may be using their native language while the other one may have to use a second language, or both schools may be using a third language. The main challenges of COIL we identified are listed in Figure 8.2.

Benefits of COIL for global nursing education

COIL allows nursing faculty to ensure that all students have the same opportunity to engage and learn from global faculty and students. Prior to COIL, students with financial challenges, family or work commitments, or travel restrictions were not able to participate in a global experience. COIL ensures that all students have an opportunity to learn and grow. Similarly, COIL affords all nursing faculty an opportunity to be involved in global nursing education. In some colleges and universities only a select few are invited or permitted to teach global courses. In the COIL paradigm, any course can be "COILed" as long as faculty have a willing partner in another country.

- New learning experience

- Exposure to new views

- Promotion of new ideas

- Involvement of a larger number of students

- Increased student diversity

- Increased faculty diversity

- Opportunity to learn about different healthcare delivery models

- Asynchronous classes

Figure 8.1 Benefits of Collaborative Online International Learning (COIL).

Best practices in nursing education indicate that students benefit most when they are able to see their faculty demonstrate or apply the skills they are reading about in a textbook (Benner, 2010). In COIL courses students have an opportunity to observe faculty demonstrate the application of a global perspective and use intercultural relationship skills to foster a positive and effective learning environment. COIL can therefore be one of the most effective approaches to ensure all students experience global nursing education.

The COIL approach also makes it possible for global nursing education to occur anywhere there is Internet access and faculty willing to co-create and co-facilitate shared coursework. That means that developing nations that may have been previously left out of global nursing education experiences can participate as full partners. This will benefit nursing education globally and global healthcare as a whole. Countless global health issues are emerging, and their complexity requires that solutions involve intentional and strategic global partnerships. Nursing education can no longer relegate global nursing to the sidelines. Global nursing must become a core competency that is threaded through the entire curriculum. COIL facilitates this shift in nursing education priorities.

- Technology differed from one campus to another

- Cultural subtleties that challenged communication

- Different languages

- Different time zones

- Course complexity; one course had different versions for odd and even years

- Logistics such as enrolment

- Different healthcare systems

- Asynchronous classes

Figure 8.2 Challenges of Collaborative Online International Learning (COIL).

Conclusion and implications: future directions for nurse education

The diverse demands and increasing urgencies related to global health require nursing education to adapt in order to meet these growing complexities. At the same time new technologies and new pedagogical methodologies facilitate this adaptation. COIL is one of these emerging methodologies and it has much to offer global nursing education. In addition to preparing nurses with a global perspective, there are opportunities for COIL to promote interprofessional education and collaborative practice (IPECP). Nursing faculty can engage faculty from other health professions in other nations and co-create IPECP learning modules for their students. This is particularly important for schools and colleges that are not part of a university system that has multiple health profession programs.

COIL courses also facilitate international network opportunities. Students from both schools can continue to support one another and even collaborate on initiatives long after the COIL course has been completed. For example, one Icelandic student and one Minnesota student, both managers in the operating rooms of their hospitals, plan to co-author a paper on the differences and similarities of care for operating room patients. If they had not had the COIL experience, they would have continued to only see practice with the lens of nurses in their country. Now they are able to compare and contrast surgical patient care, moving forward toward global best practice.

Nursing by definition is a relationship-oriented profession and therefore well suited to the COIL methodology. Nursing is also a global profession, therefore this methodology is perfect for building cross-border relationships. COIL equips nurses to lead international healthcare initiatives as well as leading local actions from a global perspective. With COIL nurses can become glocal.

References

Beck D. M., Dossey B. M., & Rushton, C. H. (2013). Building the Nightingale initiative for global health – NIGH – Can we engage and empower the public voices of nurses worldwide? *Nursing Science Quarterly, 26,* 366–371. doi: 10.1177/0894318413500403.

Benner, P., Sutphen, M., Leonard, V., & Gay, L. (2010). *Educating nurses: A call for radical transformation.* Stanford, CA: Carnegie Foundation for the Advancement of Teaching.

Bragadóttir, H., & Potter, T. (in press) Educating global nursing leaders with Collaborative Online International Learning (COIL). *Nordic Journal of Nursing Research 0*(0), 1–5. doi: 10.1177/2057158519856271

Center for Collaborative Online International Learning [COIL]. (n.d.). *Guide for collaborative online international learning course development.* New York, NY: State University of New York.

Eisler, R., & Potter, T. M. (2014). *Transforming interprofessional partnerships: A new framework for nursing and partnership-based healthcare.* Indianapolis, IN: Sigma Theta Tau International.

International Council of Nurses [ICN]. (1969). ICN statement on nursing education, nursing practice and service and the social and economic welfare of nurses. *American Journal of Nursing, 69*(10), 2177–2179.

International Council of Nurses [ICN]. (2018). Position statement: Health of migrants, refugees and displaced persons. Retrieved from www.icn.ch/sites/default/files/inline-files/ICN%20PS%20Health%20of%20migrants%2C%20refugees%20and%20displaced%20persons.pdf

Koplan, J. P., Bond, T. C., Merson, M. H., Reddy, K. S., Rodriguez, M. H., Sewankambo, N. K., & Wasserheit, J. N. (2009). Towards a common definition of global health. *Lancet, 373,* 1993–1995.

Marginson, S. (2004). Don't leave me hanging on the Anglophone: The potential for online distance higher education in the Asia-Pacific region. *Higher Education Quarterly, 58*(2/3), 74–113. doi: 10.1111/j.1468-2273.2004.00263.x.

Rosa, W. (2017). *A new era in global health: Nursing and the United Nations 2030 agenda for sustainable development.* New York, NY: Springer.

Shishani, K., Allen, C., Shubnikov, E., Slman, K., Laporte, R., & Linkov, F. (2012). Nurse educators establishing new neues in global nursing education. *Journal of Professional Nursing, 28*(2), 132–134.

Starke-Meyerring, D., & Andrews, D. (2006). Building a shared virtual learning culture: An international classroom partnership. *Business Communication Quarterly, 69*(19), 25–49. doi: 10.1177/1080569905285543 (n.d.).

Starke-Meyerring, D. (2010). Globally networked learning environments: Reshaping the intersections of globalization and e-learning in higher education. *E-Learning and Digital Media,* 7(2), 127–132. Doi: doi.org/10.2304/elea.2010.7.2.27

State University of New York [SUNY]. (n.d.a). About COIL. Retrieved from http://coil.suny.edu/page/about-coil-0

State University of New York [SUNY]. (n.d.b). Global partner network. Retrieved from http://coil.suny.edu/page/global-partner-network

Wahls, N., Méndez-Betancor, A., Brierley, M., Ariza Pinzón, V., Matsunaga, Y., Bocanegra, N., & Burns Vidaurrázaga, M. (2017). Collaborative learning in global online education using virtual international exchanges. *Educausereview.* Retrieved from https://er.educause.edu/articles/2017/9/collaborative-learning-in-global-online-education-using-virtual-international-exchanges

Wilson, L., Mendes, I. A. C., Klopper, H., Catrambone, C., Al-Maaitah, R., Norton, M. E., & Hill, M. (2016). 'Global health' and 'global nursing': Proposed definitions from The Global Advisory Panel on the Future of Nursing. *Journal of Advanced Nursing, 72*(7), 1529–1540. doi: 10.1111/jan.12973.

World Health Organization [WHO]. (2009). *European Union standards for nursing and midwifery: Information for accession countries* (2nd ed.). Copenhagen and Denmark: World Health Organization.

World Health Organization [WHO]. (2015). A guide to nursing and midwifery education standards. Nasr City, Cairo and Egypt: World Health Organization.

World Health Organization [WHO]. (2016). *Nurse educator core competencies.* Geneva and Switzerland: World Health Organization.

SECTION 2

Pedagogy in Nurse education

Foreword: Sue Dyson

Nurse education is a value-laden, political activity with multiple social meanings. In this context pedagogy in and for nurse education is vital in shaping the future of the profession. Transformative pedagogies are essential if nurses are to develop critical consciousness, in other words an in-depth understanding of the world and the knowledge and skills needed to oppose oppressive structures, wherever and whenever they occur. This section is premised on the belief that it is incumbent upon nurse educators to have knowledge of and the perquisite skills to prepare nurses for the challenges of contemporary nursing practice and to do so through exploration and consideration of transformative, innovative pedagogies for nursing.

The section begins with a chapter by Margaret McAllister and Colleen Ryan who present a viable alternative to the transmission mode of teaching, which they argue remains the prevailing model of teaching in many academic settings and one where communication flows from expert teacher to the receiving, passive student. Transformational learning, according to the authors, operates differently by emphasizing transaction, and promoting perspective change in learners. Learners thus come to fully appreciate issues affecting global nursing, such as global health inequities and global social injustices.

Helen Allan and Karen Evans argue in their chapter while the relationship between theory and practice has been extensively covered in the nursing literature, populist thinking tends to criticize the gap, rather than consider it a potentially productive relationship, resulting in a devaluing of either practice or theory, and of nursing as professional project as a whole. The authors suggest the lens of re-contextualization focuses attention on processes involved in successfully moving knowledge from disciplines and workplaces into a curriculum, from a curriculum into successful pedagogic strategies and learner/employee engagement in educational institutions and workplaces.

Colleen Ryan's chapter discusses the complexities of clinical teaching. She suggests theories for developing the role of the clinical teacher, emerging clinical teaching practices, and a number of innovations to support professional development. Clinical teaching, she says, is a recognized subspeciality, which should be developed through scholarship and workplace support.

Leeanne Heaton, Kerry Reid-Searl, and Rachelle Cole discuss simulation as an effective and efficient teaching strategy. When utilized appropriately the authors suggest simulation enables learners to link theory to practice. Whilst common within the clinical teaching environment, simulation is an evolving tool that, in order to maintain its effectiveness, must remain contemporary to ensure that learners obtain all the benefits of this positive teaching technique.

The final chapter in this section comes from Trish Hafford-Letchfield, Kate Leonard, and Wendy Couchman and looks at some of the arguments put forward as to why the arts are considered to be helpful to the caring professions. The authors provide a review of some of the key empirical evidence in relation to arts-based pedagogies (ABP). ABP, according to the authors, facilitates the integrative and social model of health, and has opened the space for creative arts activities in healthcare education. The chapter considers and discusses the potential for introducing and engaging with ABP in nurse education.

9

TRANSFORMATIVE LEARNING

Global approaches to nurse education

Margaret McAllister and Colleen Ryan

Introduction

All across the world nurses work in complex healthcare systems, based not only on medical treatment and cure, but also on enabling individuals and communities to adapt to their health issues and engage in more effective self and community care. Students of nursing about to practice in these complex environments need to have a strong nursing identity: one that differentiates itself from other health disciplines, so that they can work skillfully, strategically, and collaboratively with patients and colleagues, and also so that they can rethink problems affecting their nursing work with vision and creativity.

There are many modes of teaching and learning that can prepare students for the world of nursing, including narrative pedagogy, feminist pedagogy, and structural competence. An overarching term for these pedagogies is transformative learning (TL).

TL is defined as learning experiences in which students' assumptions, biases, or lack of knowledge, which impede productive clinician–patient relationships, are revealed and where new ways of thinking and relating, that are more liberal, respectful, and empowering, are developed – or transformed (McAllister, 2012a). There is wide variation in approaches, but the common features in this learning are that it engages students in reflection on current and taken-for-granted practices, and discussion of alternatives to become a catalyst for change. The aim of this chapter is to argue the need for TL approaches, outline global health inequities about which nurses could be playing a more active role, explain approaches to transformational teaching and learning, and show examples of TL in action.

Globalization requires awareness of health inequities and transferable skills

According to Wilson et al. (2016), contemporary healthcare workers need a different skill set than 30–50 years ago for various reasons. The sheer breadth and depth of healthcare procedures, including medical and surgical treatments and their monitoring, have vastly grown. Similarly, disciplinary knowledge emanating from other sciences, including psychology, exercise physiology, nutrition, robotics, information technology, as well as sociology, has made service delivery options more sophisticated and targeted. Consumers are more health-literate and have expectations of involvement in decision making, value for money, and accountability. Thus, students of nursing need to study many applied sciences and to be able to operationalize person-centered care and interprofessional communication adeptly. More-over, the contexts of care have expanded and thus nursing graduates need to have the ability to work in and adapt to issues arising because of globalization.

Globalization is a process of interaction and integration among the people, companies, and governments of different nations. The process is driven by a desire to trade, travel, and invest internationally and is facilitated by the ease with which people can communicate and transact online and through high-speed, affordable transportation (Ralston Saul, 2005). Glo-balization has impacted the world tremendously – in positive and negative ways. Countries and people are less isolated and more aware of other nations and cultural practices. Globalization offers the potential to raise standards of living and promote exchange of knowledge, skills, and culture, but it has also led to unintended consequences of pollution, trade and financial tensions, over-migration, refugee mistreatment, and nations becoming defensive of their identities and borders.

Globalization is affecting healthcare delivery significantly. Communities are multicultural, requiring nurses to have an understanding of many cultures, languages, and beliefs. Vast numbers of people requiring healthcare may be refugees who are fleeing deprivation and thus have significant unmet physical and mental health needs. Climate change, pollution, fires, droughts, and floods are all exacerbated due to globalization, and often lead to healthcare crises that require the mobilization of nurses and others. International exchange also means that nurses can study and work in many foreign contexts – including providing humanitarian nursing or working in countries with very different standards of nursing and work conditions. Increasingly, too, students of nursing are able to access clinical placement experiences in developing countries, and thus educators need to be able to cultivate appropriate cultural competence and humility in students (Hanson, 2010).

In all of these situations, nurses need to have a clear sense of what global nursing means. Wilson et al. (2016) suggest that it means nurses should be advocates for worldwide sustainable health and equity. To do this, nurses need to gain an understanding of world problems. A major issue that globally prepared nurses need to understand is that health and social inequities are rising, not reducing (WHO, 2018). An estimated 15 million people between the ages of 30 and 69 die from non-communicable diseases annually and people living in low- and middle-income countries are disproportionately affected. Health gaps between the average person and the worse-off person and between genders and age are widening. Indigenous and low-socioeconomic groups live shorter lives and experience more preventable non-communicable diseases. Non-communicable diseases fall into five categories: cancer, cardiac disease, chronic kidney disease, diabetes, and chronic respiratory diseases. Diagnoses such as sun cancers, obesity, type 2 diabetes, respiratory diseases related to smoking and living in mold-infested environments, pneumonia preventable by antibiotics, and malnutrition, as examples, are preventable.

Compounding this challenge is the reality that nursing is not playing a big enough role in the resolution of inequities (Mechcatie, 2018). For nurses to take effective action they need to know about the issues, be moved to care about them, and be politicized and skilled to lobby for change. These actions are difficult to take when a nurse is working within a bureaucratic system that is busy, directive, and controlling. It is all too easy for individual nurses to simply work within a service and not to engage in what is happening on the world stage. It would be a mistake, however, to believe that global events have no influence on daily life. Indeed, conflict between nations and political leaders may well serve as a model for interpersonal behavior. Similarly, apathy towards the needs of people in crisis is leading to what some writers call a pervasive empathy deficit – this deficiency within healthcare systems has been responsible for numerous healthcare scandals, where patients have suffered or died from preventable situations (Campling, 2015).

An empathy deficit exists in nursing at several levels: at the bedside, when nurses may not be sufficiently responsive or sensitive to the needs of vulnerable patients; between nurses, where the phenomenon of lateral violence which involves displacing anxiety, frustration, and hostility on to each other is undertaken without regard for dignity and compassion; and at the level of educator and student when insufficient awareness of power differentials leads to hurt. Conversely, being able to think empathically about another person, a precursor for ethical practice, requires a healthy self-identity and respect for difference. TL intentionally aims to develop empathy and promote transformation in perspective.

Transformative learning

A common metaphor used to explain transformation is a chrysalis turning into a butterfly. The metamorphosis takes time, and the butterfly cannot turn back into a worm. While this is a vivid image, students rarely make dramatic change as the imagery suggests. But students do change from being hampered by ill-fitting emotions or opinions to being enlightened and more aware of how professional values should replace lay values. For example, there was a student who was convinced that he would hate working in mental health because he believed it would be a violent place where no real change would be seen. At completion of a three-week placement, that same student was so confident working in that context that he intended to make mental health nursing his career! Throughout his placement he began to appreciate that many clients in the service were not just "ill" but hampered by social inequities. Particular clients he worked with lived in unstable housing, had no meaningful employment and thus experienced poverty, boredom, and social isolation. The strategies the team put into operation were holistic – the patient's psychosis was settled with medication and a quiet environment, and the student played an important role in facilitating new and sustainable community-based social connections. The student regularly engaged in reflection. He shared his admiration for staff who remained optimistic even though many patients lacked self-belief. The student realized that holism was not just a theoretical term but of great relevance in this field. Each member of the multidisciplinary team had different and complementary aims. Ultimately, the student admitted that his old ideas about mental illness were borne of ignorance and that his placement experience had really opened his eyes not just to mental distress, but to effective mental health nursing care.

This anecdote illustrates the aims of TL – where a student engages in learning designed to uncover biases or lack of knowledge that can impede mutual relationships between clinician and patient, and establishes new ways of thinking and relating that are more liberal, respectful, and empowering (McAllister, 2015).

Origins and developments

Transformative education is grounded in critical social theory and the belief that social inequalities are human constructions and they can be addressed and resolved. Whilst power and ideology are at the root of domination, they are also the sources for freedom (Giroux, 2000). Once people in positions of power stop oppressing and make room for vulnerable people to have their own agency, then change is possible.

In relation to health professionals, the goals in this model of teaching are for learners to begin to recognize the social and cultural practices that support dominating systems of healthcare in society and to reflect on *their* role in perpetuating injustice or facilitating agency. Without preaching at students or frightening them with tragic stories, it is possible to awaken them so that they see their role in making a positive difference.

TL can be traced back to the late 1970s when Jack Mezirow outlined a series of ten steps in rational development that lead to a transformation in learner perspective (Mezirow, 1991). Since Mezirow's articulation of transformed perspective, educational scholars have continued to build on his ideas (Table 9.1).

A disorienting dilemma

The enduring concept that Mezirow (2000) introduced is that the trigger for TL is the presentation of a disorienting dilemma. This becomes the object for new learning and may result in a new awareness of a paradox or something unfair, or the knowledge that old ways of approaching the problem have been insufficient or inadequate. Through the teaching and learning process, the situation is examined (objectively and subjectively), ways of thinking about it are interrogated, reflection is encouraged, and novel solutions supported. Disorienting dilemmas are likely to occur the most when someone is moving from one life position to another – for example, when a child moves into adulthood, or a student moves into working life. It is at these junctures when old ideas may not hold as useful or true in different or more complex contexts (see example in Box 9.1).

Table 9.1 Branches of transformational learning (TL)

Theme	Example scholar	TL perspective
Cognitive	Jack Mezirow (1991)	A cognitive perspective, which emphasizes the development of rational logical thinking in a step-wise fashion to achieve perspective change. The goal is personal transformation
Aesthetic/ emotional	Patricia Cranton (1994)	Aligned with the rational perspective, Cranton considered the notion that individuals learned and might "see the light" using different learning styles, depending on their personality and powers of imagination
Power/ change	John Dirkx (1997)	In this more transcendent view, Dirkx argues that not all learning is rational and individuals may have their perspective changed through immersion in emotion, imaginal, unconscious, spiritual, and inner world such as are triggered through the creative arts
	Stephen Brook-field (2005)	In this explicitly political view, change can be impeded or facilitated through power relationships and if learners experience what oppression, marginalization, or inequity may be like, they may grow in understanding and be driven to create change

---

Box 9.1 An example of a disorienting dilemma

A young man entering nursing had never noticed sexism occurring. His female friends all seemed outspoken and strong and he had a view that sexism was made up by a small minority of radical feminists. On his first clinical placement, he was assigned to care for a young woman who had been walking home from a movie and was raped and assaulted by a stranger. He learned that this was the sixth such case the hospital had seen in little more than a month. From that day on, he realized his views were mistaken, he listened to how his mentors supported the patient, and worked to lobby for street safety. He knew that he had to play a part – in his personal and professional life – in promoting equality.

The transformative educator will create learning environments that encourage learners to be curious about the issue and engage in collaborative thinking to examine the situation from many angles and use new cognitive tools to interrogate it and to generate new ways of looking at it and new ways of acting. Collaboration is key for this to occur as students need to practice learning new cognitive strategies and developing the confidence to practice new skills in a world where the old habits remain commonplace (Dirkx et al., 2006).

Beginning to teach transformatively

It is important for teachers to *prepare* to teach transformatively because the method is intentional, not laissez-faire. Just like the student, teachers need to consider how they have been socialized, to look again at common-place practices that may have become naturalized and taken for granted – such as the tendency to fill the class time with delivery of content or assume the role of expert when students too may have expertise. Educators who are sensitive to the problems of domination and control can set the tone for an inspiring, exciting, critical environment where new ideas and optimism for change prosper. See McAllister et al. (2013) for more detailed information on how to prepare for this novel teaching role. including engaging students in a productive learning relationship, and introducing new cognitive and affective skills to help students build a better world. As mentioned previously, educating to transform is all about taking the time to engage and sensitize students to issues that need changing, but which may have become embedded, taken for granted, not noticed, or perhaps something one feels helpless to change. Change doesn't have to be monumental. One small step, one ripple can have huge effects.

Not every class that nursing students experience needs to have a transformative aim. Learning techniques for practice, such as blood glucose monitoring, is an example. But when perspective change and clarity is required, TL could work well. Perspective is the lens through which we view the world, and altering this lens can be confronting and emotional, and may generate defensiveness or resistance, particularly if those views are fixed or unconscious. Thus, educators need to take care, and be gentle and supportive. The advantage of working with nursing students in perspective transformation is that most are novices in the discipline and this opens up the opportunity for offering them new ways of thinking and working. The challenge is to cultivate an excitement for new learning, and a trusting safe environment. Revealing students' old perspectives, without judgment, and encouraging testing and development of new ideas until confidence is produced is the intention of TL (McAllister et al., 2013). This introduces the idea of learning thresholds, and the educator's role in supporting students experiencing learning thresholds.

Create learning thresholds

A threshold is the space between one land or boundary and another (Meyer & Land, 2003). The apse in a church marks the threshold space between the secular and spiritual spaces of a community. Foyers too are threshold spaces because the architectural design is deliberate so that the person coming in has some space between the outside world and the inner space. In this little hallway – be it foyer or apse – something profound is happening. People shake off the rain and the busy-ness of the outside world and take some time to acclimatize to the inside. Transformative classrooms need to be similarly designed (McAllister et al., 2013). This is done simply by acknowledging the change of space. The educator might say "You are entering a nursing classroom now, so some of the old ideas you may have personally believed may be replaced as you learn about and take up professional values."

When in this new space students can be presented with a disorienting dilemma, which requires them to use critical thinking skills and which leads them to transform from lay person to a nursing professional (McAllister, 2013). Strategies to use include those that present the subjective and unique experience of a health problem that has been hard to resolve. Testimonials or re-enactments made through film, novel, or biography are examples, and the educator could ask students to describe the dilemma.

When transformative educators join students in the inner space, they can expect to engage with students who may not be confident in the new world, where old knowledge isn't certain any more, or is no longer relevant for the new land of nursing. Transformative educators will need to support students as they traverse between old and new lands and learn to transform old perceptions. This is known as the learning threshold because, essentially, students come in one door, and they leave through the other, thinking in new ways, ready to be with people in more effective ways (McAllister, 2010).

Becoming non-judgmental

One important learning threshold to pass through as a nurse is that of becoming open, non-judgmental, and equitable – to treat people fairly. In the personal world, it may be acceptable for some to hold on to biases and preferences in wanting to associate with one group of people over another. School leavers, for example, who are in their late teens may be more attracted to conversing with people their own age, and at the same time, find interaction with people who are aging difficult because worldviews and experiences are so different. Students may feel uncertain about how to relate. Working with people who are aging is a common part of nursing work, and so learning to step over this threshold is well suited to a TL lesson plan. Personal ideas and biases, drawn from prior experiences about what old age may mean, may impact knowledge of how old age constitutes a vulnerable life stage, and the prevalence of older consumers being marginalized and treated inequitably in the healthcare system. If biases do exist, then a process of unlearning, followed by new learning, including developing new perceptions, ways of knowing, and transferring to more effective nursing actions, needs to occur (Dirkx et al., 2006).

Moderating own emotions

Another important learning threshold is that of being able to moderate one's own emotions, such as anxiety, frustration, and anger. All healthcare contexts carry with them a certain level of anxiety – this could be because patients are anxiously waiting for their diagnosis or feeling stressed about discomfort and other issues. Anxiety could also be generated by new staff members, such as students, who are unaware of the routine, and perhaps fear being out of their depth. Within healthcare there are many contexts that evoke anxiety, or which are off-putting and result in strong emotions. But when paired with issues of political unrest, scarce resources, short staffing, or other uncertainties, emotional reactions may be amplified and exacerbated. In this environment, emotional distress can be contagious and clinicians and students may unconsciously mirror patient anxiety, thus fueling distress. Learners who are aware of their own emotions and are able to contain and suppress them so that they don't interfere with patient care will experience self-efficacy, an important lesson in how to care for others.

Ensuring that important lessons are enriched with imagery, emotion, context, and complex scenarios helps to reinforce the reality that students will need to learn how to problem-solve and be of service, even in the context of tense situations and uncertainties.

In other situations, showing emotional reactions may be forbidden and students may need to suppress, disguise, or hide their true feelings. When emotions are stifled in these situations this may create inner conflict and lead to stress build-up. Consider, for example, the student who feels horrified when she sees a suppurating wound. She may know enough to hide her reaction for fear of upsetting the patient. Later, this may lead to the nursing student avoiding the patient, or other patients like this, for reasons she no longer recognizes. In this situation, TL may be relevant for preparing the student to understand emotions, to uncover previously suppressed emotions and to be more conscious of the benefits of facing upsetting feelings at a later stage.

Caring about vulnerable people

Within healthcare there are many endemic problems that are seemingly intransigent, and about which individual clinicians, on their own, may feel helpless or unable to make positive change. It is in these very sites that a liberating approach is vital; that is, where education has the potential to liberate and transform the outlook of the helpers, healers, and leaders so that they have a course of action to take which can lead to change. Rather than the view to the future being fatalistic or pessimistic, because opportunities are created to discuss ideals and give students the faith that they can make a difference, transformational learners are more likely to look ahead with optimism and self-efficacy.

Various educational research projects have produced evidence of positive effects on learners. In the context of media literacy, several studies have shown that it can produce measurable results in learners' ability to analyze, critique, and produce media messages (Hobbs & Frost, 2003; Quin & McMahon, 1991). In the context of health professional learning, TL approaches enhance empathy and understanding and prompt critical thinking, as well as the generation of alternative solutions to entrenched problems

Model a discourse where uncertainty, curiosity, and possibility are useful

In conventional didactic teaching, there is a tendency for a discourse of certainty to be modeled (Brodkey, 1987). Discourses of certainty make the world seem as though things can be either right or wrong. Learners may believe that nursing simply involves the memorization of these facts and procedures. Students may experience helplessness and surrender because knowledge comprising facts and procedures is not always helpful in providing solutions to problems they face. Within nursing and medicine, discourses of certainty are supported by a focus on the one-way transmission of biomedical facts and procedures. Giroux (2000) argues for learning experiences to include discourses of uncertainty as well as certainty. Facts can be discussed and taught, but examining exceptions to rules and offering challenges for which there is no right or wrong perception can also make for legitimate subject matter.

For example, students could be presented with scenarios where patients choose to uphold their right of refusal of care, against medical advice. Encourage discussion and dialogue to promote a solution-focused way of approaching the problem. Students will benefit from learning to advocate for their rights as professional nurses as well as advocating for the patient's right to refuse.

Find opportunities for students to interject their own voice

Parker Palmer (1998) once said that good teaching is "an act of generosity" in that it takes a willingness to share, a lot of patience, and persistence. Palmer writes so eloquently about the craft of teaching that readers are urged to find his books and articles and savor his wisdom directly. Parker talks of patience and persistence because many students prefer to sit on the sidelines in silence. Understandably, speaking up takes courage; there is a risk that others will criticize or even denigrate our ideas, yet when learners find their voice they also find power and influence. Ways to help students find their voice begin with issues that connect directly with their life and sparking learners' interest so that they *want* to speak (McAllister, 2010).

For example, rather than teach the mechanics of the heart via diagrams and talk, students could be instructed to undertake a brief period of cardiac exercise, such as running, and asked to notice what changes were occurring in their body. Excerpts from film, television, music, literature, or poetry can be used to ask students to describe what they have just observed (McAllister et al., 2015, 2016). Being able to describe is a relatively easy task. Gradually though the task needs to become more challenging by teaching a cognitive skill such as synthesis to break the story down and rebuild it up or asking students to interrogate the text, to look beyond the written words and try to understand the real meaning the author is wanting to share with the audience.

Palmer's idea when difficult topics arise is to give students cards and ask them to each write a few lines expressing a personal opinion on the issues (Palmer, 1998). The cards are collected and redistributed so that no one knows whose card he or she is holding. Then students are asked to read that card aloud and take a minute to agree or disagree. In this way, the issue is aired, diversity has been exposed, the unspeakable may have been spoken, and a foundation for real conversation has been laid. This brings us to the notion of generating dialogue rather than discussion.

Generate dialogue

Many authors have argued that dialogue is preferable to discussion in generating critical thinking and new insights (Daft, 2007; Freire, 1972; Senge, 1994) as discussion merely achieves the statement of position and can meander without direction, whereas dialogue can reveal feelings and explore assumptions such that common ground and shared meanings are built. Yet discussion is the way most people communicate. It is also a common aim in lesson plans. In the transformative classroom, however, communication works best when it is used with conscious intent. Conscious intent is applied when we learn to pause and think about what the intention is of the spoken word in discussion. Discussion can be transformed into dialogue by helping students to communicate with conscious intent. The conscious intent is to be heard and understood rather than communicating to be right or to voice an opinion (Freire, 1972).

For example, students could be encouraged to understand the power of silence, to pause and think before speaking, and to listen deeply to each other. And students can be explicitly taught ways to consider an issue from many angles. Dialectical critique, searching for the thesis and the antithesis in an argument, is one way to do this. Students could be asked to consciously try to doubt the facts they are being presented and play the devil's advocate and defend the opposite side. Then move to the believing stance and weigh up which arguments were most persuasive.

Transformational educators facilitate effective dialogue through ensuring everyone has a chance to contribute; students learn to suspend their assumptions and see each other as equal team members, and students learn to really listen and communicate with intent. Releasing imagination too is important if students are to be transformed through education.

6 Encourage students to be creative in their solutions to dilemmas

To prepare for TL experiences the transformative educator will have a goal of arousing the learner's imagination. Imagination by its nature is about the uncertain. It invites people to reach beyond themselves and to create new and different happenings (McAllister, 2012a). When learners' imagination is awakened, they become engaged, and educators can then encourage learners to become critical and to create new solutions and arrive at new knowledge. When learners begin to see that they have the skills to critique and reinvent, learner transformation occurs.

Frida Kahlo's (cf. Herrera, 1991) paintings are a rich source for imagination exercises. Kahlo's *The Little Deer* can be used to evoke discussion on what it might be like to be marginalized, wounded, in pain, and in need. It can also invite thinking on what the role of the engaged, committed, health professional could be in that encounter. When asked to imagine what the health professional could do in this image, students offer suggestions such as reorienting the deer so that it is turning towards the light and so able to see a way forward (see McAllister, 2012b).

Using film is also valuable in stimulating learner engagement by releasing imagination in various teaching sessions (McAllister et al., 2016).

Teach constructive thinking

Critical thinking involves two aspects: deconstructing a problem and reconstructing. Deconstruction is a process of dismantling an issue so that its components are open to scrutiny and its triggers are revealed. Constructive thinking involves reconstruction – a process where social problems are not just revealed, but solutions generated.

Assisting learners to release their imagination is one way to inspire constructive thinking – a skill that is slightly different from, and complementary to, critical thinking (Thayer-Bacon, 2000). Critical thinking has historically emphasized rational thinking – that which is dispassionate, deductive, and science-based. Constructive thinking attempts to correct the imbalance in thinking about knowledge by arguing that human beings know things also through imagination, emotion, and intuition and that deep thinking about an issue can be assisted through these artistic lenses. Thus, in a TL classroom, the objective is not to reject critical thinking, but to *augment* it, through constructive thinking exercises, such as those found in metaphor activities, poetry analysis, and so on, where the learner is assisted to imagine new ways of operating other than those that have been critiqued.

For example, students discussing ethical principles in research could view the film *Fog in August* (Wessell, 2016). It is based on the true story of one of the child victims of Nazi "euthanasia." The film prompts thinking on unethical healthcare practice. When students remember this film, the four fundamental principles of ethics are cemented into memory, including that patients were treated unjustly, with some being categorized as deserving of care, and others labeled as incurable, and their lives were intolerable and therefore they should be killed; the provision of good care was not the intent of the healthcare providers; maleficence, which should not have occurred, was present; and patients had no autonomy and decision-making power.

Clarify vision and values

Students about to enter a health profession, or perhaps reflect on their place within it, can benefit from reflection on who "we" are (as opposed to "I"), what we stand for, and what we don't. As a member of a profession, identity is shared rather than simply personal, and thus there is value in spending time coming to know, feel, and practice the shared values. Human development theories have shown that positive self-identity is strongly correlated with well-being, happiness, self-efficacy, internal locus of control, and stress hardiness (Luthar, 2003). These are all characteristics of resilience. A focus on resilience, rather than our weaknesses and troubles, may assist in strengthening nursing identity.

Interrupt gently

As has been explained, the process of socialization within general society and the professional culture leads to the uptake and absorption of norms and ways of seeing the world that over time become deeply engrained and taken for granted. These tools of thinking are used often out of habit, rather than with conscious intent. When they are used inappropriately or ineffectively, the transformative educator's role can be to interrupt them so that, firstly, they cannot occur without notice; and secondly, an alternative way of thinking can be fostered (McAllister et al., 2007).

An effective way to interrupt a student without the individual taking offence or losing face is to gain permission for this strategy in the forming stage of the teacher–student relationship. For example, you could say, "If I hear or see things that could be challenged, scrutinized, or replaced, I will try to interrupt these with you. Is that OK?", and "At what times will it not be OK?" Teacher–student rules such as these encourage transformation through invitation of the student voice (Taylor, 2007).

Rethink assessment: produce tangible products of that voice

For voice and dialogue to have meaning, it is useful – indeed, important – to set assessment and other learning activities that have a purpose larger than the mere testing of knowledge. Good assessment actually serves two purposes: it provides an opportunity to give guidance and feedback to the learner; and it provides a means to ensure that minimum standards of entry to a profession are maintained (Dolin et al., 2018). Essays, clinical reports, journaling, posters, and tutorial presentations and other commonly used assessment items remain useful in the transformative context, especially when they are designed to directly contribute to the professional/social world, be personally engaging, and stimulate reflection.

An example is provided by Taylor (2007, p.182) in what he calls creating "artifacts of mind." This involves setting activities that produce tangible products wherein ideas that stem from the learning experience are made available for others. The assessment thus becomes a social communication activity and a potential change project. In this way, assessment activities, like the student–teacher relationship, contribute to the transformational experience.

Use inspirational stories that spark optimism for change

The use of memorable story-telling can also be transformative. There are many stories the reader could access to share in a TL classroom. Some, such as the collected stories of Kroth and Cranton (2014), are in book collections; others can be found in digital media sources such as YouTube and blogging sites (Ryan et al., 2017). McAllister et al. (2016) provide examples around accessing stories from the arts, poetry, and film. Students too, once orientated to TL, will have stories that the transformative educator may elicit, either in the written or spoken word, and students could be encouraged to share their stories for purposes of encouraging transformation. Other stories worth sharing may require a creative approach to sourcing them, such as this Australian story about transformation that aired on a radio station (Cohen, 2017) (see Box 9.2).

Box 9.2 An Australian story of transformation

Katherine Hospital in the Northern Territory of Australia serves a majority population of Australian Indigenous people. Many of the people accessing the hospital live traditional lives – they are semi-nomadic, speak traditional languages, and are very poor. Diabetes, kidney disease, obesity, alcohol misuse, and untreated communicable and non-communicable diseases were occurring because of poverty, and lack of trust in Western medicine and white people. Culturally, Australian Indigenous people value courtesy and are shy and often will walk away from a white nurse or doctor, rather than explain their concerns. Western medicine and hospitals constrain Indigenous peoples, forcing separation of patients from family and making patients feel lonely, bored, useless, and burdensome. In 2011, Katherine Hospital had a poor reputation. There was rapid staff turnover causing patients to repeat their stories to new staff on many occasions. One in four patients would walk out of the hospital before they were well enough.

In 2017, less than 5% of patients discharge before care is complete. The transformation came about because the predominantly white medical and nursing staff learnt to listen and share stories with local Indigenous people to help them to learn about and respect Indigenous culture, and find better ways of communicating with Indigenous peoples, and understand the value of Indigenous medicine. Staff learnt, for example, there are no words for cancer or fungus in the local people's language, so instead now the words "weeds" and "mushrooms" are described as "growing inside them" to help patients better understand the cancer disease process.

Patients still doubt the benefit of white-man's medicine. Rather than creating an impasse, clinicians are encouraged to respect this view and encourage the contributions that bush medicine and witch doctors can make to complement the white medicine. Witch doctors visit the hospital. Walkabout is an Indigenous cultural activity that may see Indigenous peoples going for a walk and not returning for a lengthy period. Now, a patient intending to go walkabout are offered a supply of medications, in case they don't make it back that night.

This story emphasizes the social health inequities in an Australian community and is valuable in offering students a TL experience in a twenty-first-century nursing curriculum. Issues in this story are also relevant to global health concerns.

Conclusion

This chapter has provided a rationale for a viable alternative to the transmission mode of teaching that unfortunately remains the prevailing model of teaching in many academic settings, and one where communication flows from the expert teacher to the receiving, passive student. Transformational learning operates differently: by emphasizing transaction, it places the lens of inquiry squarely on to issues of inequity and marginalization, it emphasizes the need for change not just understanding, and argues that, whilst technical skills need to be practiced, so too does the language of possibility, for it is here that constructive ideas for the future will emerge. TL then promotes perspective change in learners so they may learn to work in ways informed by knowledge linked to action, so that consumers feel heard and respected and nurses can understand the need for change from being illness care workers to facilitators of well-being, social connection, and freedom. Because of its origins in critical education nursing graduates of curricula embracing TL will learn to fully appreciate issues affecting global nursing such as: global health inequities; global social injustices; the need for nurses to be empathetic and practice ethically; and the impact of consumerism and emerging technologies. In this way, nursing graduates will be well placed to bring positive change to global health.

References

Brodkey L (1987) Postmodern pedagogy for progressive educators. A review of literacy: Reading the word and the world. *Journal of Education* 169(3): 138–143.

Brookfield S D (2005) *The Power of Critical Theory Liberating Adult Learning and Teaching.* San Francisco: Jossey-Bass.

Campling P (2015) Reforming the culture of healthcare: The case for intelligent kindness. *British Journal of Psychology Bulletin* 39(1): 1–5.

Cohen H (2017) Katherine hospital: Back from the brink. *Radio National, Australian Broadcasting Commission.* Accessed at: October 22 2017 at www.abc.net.au/radionational/programs/backgroundbriefing/2017-03-26/8360398

Cranton P (1994) *Understanding and Promoting Transformative Learning: A Guide for Educators of Adults.* San Francisco: Jossey-Bass.

Daft R (2007) *The leadership experience (4th ed).* Hampshire: Thomson.

Dirkx J (1997) Nurturing soul in adult learning. In P. Cranton (Ed.), *Transformative learning in action: Insights from practice* (New directions for adult and continuing education, No. 74) (pp. 79–88). San Francisco, CA: Jossey-Bass.

Dirkx J, Mezirow J & Cranton P (2006) Musings and reflections on the meaning, context, and process of transformative learning: A dialogue between John M. Dirkx and Jack Mezirow. *Journal of Transformative Education* 4(2): 123–139.

Dolin J, Black P, Harlen W & Tiberghien A (2018) Exploring relations between formative and summative assessment. In *Transforming Assessment* (pp. 53–80). New York: Springer.

Freire P (1972) *Pedagogy of the Oppressed.* Harmondsworth: Penguin.

Giroux H (2000) *Impure Acts: The Practical Politics of Cultural Studies.* New York: Routledge.

Hanson L (2010) Global citizenship, global health, and the internationalization of curriculum. A study of transformative potential. *Journal of Studies in International Education* 14(1): 70–88.

Herrera H (1991) *The Little Deer. in Frida Kahlo: The Paintings.* London: Bloomsbury, 189.

Hobbs R & Frost R (2003) Measuring the acquisition of media-literacy skills. *Reading Research Quarterly* 38: 330–355.

Kroth, M., & Cranton, P. (2014). *Stories of transformative learning.* New York: Springer.

Luthar S (2003) *Resilience and Vulnerability: Adaptation in the Context of Childhood Adversities.* New York: Columbia University.

McAllister M (2010) Awake and aware: Thinking constructively about the world through transformative learning. In T. Warne & S. McAndrew (Eds.), *Creative Approaches to Health and Social Care Education* (pp. 157–170). UK: Palgrave MacMillan.

McAllister M (2012a) Star: A transformative learning framework for nursing education. *Journal of transformative education* 9: 42–58.

McAllister M (2012b) Positive skills, positive strategies: Solution focused nursing. In de Chasney & B. Anderson (Eds.), *Caring for the Vulnerable: Perspectives in Nursing Theory, Practice and Research* (3rd ed.) (pp. 153–167). MA: Jones & Bartlett Learning.

McAllister M (2015) Exploring transformative learning and the courage to teach a values-based curriculum. *Nurse Education in Practice* 15(6): 480–484.

McAllister M, Lasater K, Stone T E & Levett-Jones T (2015) The reading room: Exploring the use of literature as a strategy for integrating threshold concepts into nursing curricula. *Nurse Education in Practice* 15(6): 549.

McAllister M, Levett-Jones T, Petrini M A & Lasater K (2016) The viewing room: A lens for developing ethical comportment. *Nurse Education in Practice* 16(1): 119–124.

McAllister M, Oprescu F, Downer T, Lyons M, Pelly F & Barr N (2013) Evaluating STAR–A Transformative Learning Framework: Interdisciplinary Action Research in Health Training. *Educational Action Research* 21(1): 90.

McAllister M, Tower M & Walker R (2007) Gentle interruptions: Transformative approaches to clinical teaching. *Journal of Nursing Education* 46(7): 304–312.

Mechcatie E (2018) The WHO Highlights Nurses' Role in Reducing Noncommunicable Diseases. *AJN The American Journal of Nursing* 118(9): 16.

Meyer, J., & Land, R. (2003). *Threshold concepts and troublesome knowledge: Linkages to ways of thinking and practising within the disciplines* (pp. 412–424). Edinburgh: University of Edinburgh.

Mezirow J (1991) *Transformative Dimensions of Adult Learning*. San Francisco, CA: Jossey-Bass.

Mezirow J (2000) *Learning as Transformation*. San Francisco: Jossey-Bass.

Palmer P (1998) *The Courage to Teach*. San Francisco: Jossey Bass.

Quin R & McMahon B (1991) *Media Analysis: Performance in Media in Western Australian Government Schools*. (excerpted for Media Literacy Review, Media Literacy Online Project, College of Education) Oregon: University of Oregon. Accessed at: http://interact.uoregon.edu/MediaLit/mlr?readings/articles/standard.html

Ralston Saul J (2005) *The Collapse of Globalism: And the Reinvention of the World*. Toronto: Penguin.

Ryan C, Heidke P, Blunt N, Williamson M Brien D (2017) Blogging: A strategy to engage final year nursing students in reflective practice. *TEXT Special Issue 38: Illumination through narrative: Using writing to explore hidden life experience*. Accessed at: www.textjournal.com.au

Senge P (1994) *The Fifth Discipline: The Art & Practice of The Learning Organization*. New York: Double Day.

Taylor E (2007) An update of transformative learning theory: A critical review of the empirical research (1999-2005). *International Journal of Life long learning* 26(2): 173–191.

Thayer-Bacon B (2000) *Transforming critical thinking: Thinking constructively*. New York: Teachers College Press.

Wessell K (2016) *Fog in August*. [motion picture]. Berlin: Collina Films.

Wilson L, Mendes I A C, Klopper H, Catrambone C, Al-Maaitah R, Norton M E & Hill M (2016) "Global health" and "global nursing": Proposed definitions from the global advisory panel on the future of nursing. *Journal of Advanced Nursing* 72: 1529–1540.

World Health Organization WHO (2018) *Time to Deliver: Report of the WHO Independent High-level Commission on Noncommunicable Diseases*. Accessed at: http://apps.who.int/iris/bitstream/handle/10665/272710/9789241514163-eng.pdf?ua=1

10

REINTEGRATING THEORY AND PRACTICE IN NURSING

Knowledge and theories of practice learning

Helen Allan and Karen Evans

Introduction

While the relationship between theory and practice has been extensively covered in the nursing literature (Clark & Holmes, 2007; Monaghan, 2015), it is argued in this chapter that populist thinking tends to criticise the gap, rather than consider it a potentially productive relationship. This has resulted in a devaluing of either practice or theory, and of nursing as professional project as a whole (Fealy, 1999; Smith & Allan, 2010; Laiho & Ruoholinna, 2013). Perceiving difference between theory and practice in nursing as a gap that must be closed constitutes a lack of understanding that students learn across contexts, including academic, clinical and self-directed, and a lack of support for students' learning holistically.

If nurse lecturers and students could understand the potential for learning across settings, they could articulate a more meaningful theory for practice and inform theory from practice. Fawcett (1992: p. 224) describes the "reciprocal relationship between conceptual models (theories) and practice". She sees this as (more or less) a one-way street with theory informing practice as the dominant partner; practice may have some feedback to theory but, essentially, theory should guide practice in her view.

The view put forward in this chapter is that the relationship can be a more symbiotic one which is based on *knowledge* rather than (nursing) theory, as Fawcett and others argue. Nurse educators need to be quite clear that some nursing activities, such as dressing wounds, require theoretical knowledge. Other nursing activities are not underpinned by evidence and rely instead on knowledge; which could be empathic knowing, aesthetic knowing or knowledge about how to reflect and learn. As Allmark (1995) suggests, the type of knowledge associated with nursing practice should not be taught through theory, nor is it well represented in theoretical terms. The knowledge of the practitioner is not theory, but something else.

Rather than proposing ways of bridging the gap, a new way of thinking is proposed to enable students to integrate their learning in what is currently a disintegrated learning context. This builds on writing on practice-driven theory and different forms of knowledge in nursing. The focus here is on *knowledge* rather than theory. In so doing two studies into practice learning in nursing are drawn on: the General Nursing Council-funded Leadership for Learning (Allan et al., 2008) and the Academic Accreditation and Recontextualising Knowledge (AaRK) project (Magnusson et al., 2014). Data from these studies are used to illustrate arguments put forward in this chapter.

Allan's earlier empirical work into practice learning showed that there are several forms of knowledge – experiential, emotional, practical and theoretical – which nursing students struggle to integrate (Allan, 2011; Allan et al., 2011; Hatlavik, 2012). In addition to being faced with different forms of knowledge and learning, as Dyson suggests in this volume, we do not give students the skills or time to understand how to integrate learning in the curriculum and prepare them for practice. Hatlavik (2012) proposes that this is because we do not know enough about how different forms of knowledge and knowing are integrated. She advocates the use of reflective skills to integrate theoretical knowledge and practical skills. Maben et al. (2006) argue that students need to be supported in their transition to practice, to retain their values in the face of disparities between what they've been taught and what they observe in practice. These disparities frequently mean they must compromise their values. Özyazıcıoğlu et al. (2011) argue that to improve learning and teaching we should use lecturers who .are able to role model with confidence grounded in current practice-based knowledge

In an integrative literature review of clinical education in nursing, Forber et al. (2016) suggest that there are three main models of clinical learning which underpin current nursing programmes. These are the: traditional or clinical facilitator model delivered via block or rotational placements; the preceptorship or mentoring model; and the collaborative education unit model where the majority or all student placements occur in one healthcare organisation and all staff engage in teaching and support. Various limitations and strengths were identified for each model. They identified four common elements across the models: the centrality of relationships; the need for consistency and continuity; the potential for variety of models; and the viability/sustainability of the model.

Evans' work in other fields (Evans et al., 2006) shows that this concern for integrating practice-based forms of knowledge is not unique to nursing; it happens in a range of other disciplines and occupations. Most higher-education degrees and diplomas that aim to prepare participants to work in a particular profession or occupational field now incorporate placements or periods of practice-based learning as part of the learning programme. Work-based learning components have proliferated with the expansion of new degrees and diplomas in areas such as agricultural technology and digital forensics. Sometimes essential periods of practice-based learning take place after the programme as the graduates take up positions that enable or require further workplace–based learning. For example, for legal careers, firm-based "training contracts" offer periods of recognised practice-based training that are requirements for full entry to the profession; and, in commercial firms, structured internships in graduate training schemes often fulfil this function. In fields as diverse as aircraft engineering, finance, glass industry, media practice and public administration, the challenges of theory–practice gaps have become evident, as students, teachers, mentors and supervisors struggle to put the different forms of knowledge developed within and beyond the degree or diploma to work in new and changing contexts, as exemplar cases in Evans et al. (2009) have shown. Previous and current conceptualisations of the theory–practice gap in nursing fail to examine the nature of knowledge in a practice discipline. In so doing, they do not resolve the problematic relationship between knowledge, curriculum, learning and practice. In nurse education, it is typical for questions to focus on how learning can be "transferred" from one setting to another, relating the assumed "abstract" nature of theory to the assumed "real" nature of practice. This is often seen as a single movement, as encapsulated in the term "from theory to practice".

Interestingly, the Nursing and Midwifery Council (NMC) in the UK has recently published its new standards for registered nurses and for preparatory nursing programmes. These standards use words such as thinking critically and self-reflection to describe learning but not learning itself. There are references to demonstrating and applying knowledge and a list of different forms of knowledge, including (as you would expect) physiology, psychology, policy, politics. But there is no description of what nursing knowledge might be or how it might be taught or learnt apart from through evidence-based knowledge for practice (NMC 2018a, 2018b, 2018c). In Standard 1.0 (Learning Culture) (NMC 2018b) there is no reference to knowledge transfer at all. Reading the new Standards, it is as if not only is the theory–practice gap reinforced, but there is a structural divide between practice and theory.

The approach developed by Evans et al. (2009) concentrates on different forms of knowledge that students learn from and the ways in which these are contextualised and "re-contextualised" in movements between different sites of learning in colleges and workplaces. The original research was carried out in a range of professional fields outside nursing, but the arguments put forward by the authors were found to be relevant to continuing debates within nursing around the theory–practice gap (Evans et al., 2010). The aim of this chapter is to explore how the different forms of knowledge developed through the subject-based and work-based aspects of a curriculum or learning programme can articulate with one another more effectively, both before qualification and in the "newly qualified" early career period. The potential of the "re-contextualisation" approach for nurse education is outlined as well as a discussion of how learning in re-contextualising knowledge can be supported by mentors and peers.

The relationship between theory and practice in nursing

Laiho and Ruoholinna (2013) suggest that theory and practice are vague terms which are nevertheless formulated in terms of a theory–practice distinction (Nieminen, 2008). Underpinning this distinction is the belief that education and work are significantly different learning contexts and it's from here that the theory–practice gap arises. The theory–practice gap in professional education depends heavily on a belief that education and work are significantly different learning contexts (Smeby & Vågan, 2008a, 2008b). Laiho and Ruoholinna (2013) argue that the theory–practice gap is an expression of the issues and problems that arise in connection with the expectations of the professional fields towards "their" sciences. This is not made any easier in nursing because we draw on such a wide range of knowledge and learn in many different learning environments and contexts. Theory applicable for one context is unlikely to be appropriate for all other contexts in which nursing is practised.

The theory–practice gap manifests itself in many different ways in nursing. It has been described as a *mismatch* between nursing as taught and nursing as practised (Gallagher, 2004). Allan et al., (2011) describe it interfering in the partnership between universities and clinical context. And it can also be manifested in the difficulties of integrating nurse education into higher education, especially in the traditional university (Spitzer & Perrenoud, 2006a; Smith & Allan, 2010). Heggen (2008) argues that, in some disciplines, including nursing, academic knowledge has a relatively low value or status. Social work and primary school teaching value academic knowledge in a similar way. She suggests that this is because their practice is inherently social. They are professionals who act in the social field – meet other people with their intentions and opinions – and therefore cannot apply theoretical knowledge to predict or explain exactly what is happening when they work. Theories which aim to predict are likely to fail in these disciplines and as a consequence be devalued by the professionals in practice in these disciplines.

Before discussing the relationship between theory and practice in nursing, it is necessary to examine how theory and practice are taught to nurses as this is likely to be student nurses' first encounter with nursing theory or knowledge. It is important to note the distinction between evidence for nursing practice (taught as introduction to research or evidence for practice) and nursing theory (frequently introduced as grand nursing theories or models). In the UK, nursing students may be presented with a nursing theory textbook such as Aggleton and Chalmers' (2000) *Nursing Models and Nursing Practice* on the basis that nursing practice is underpinned, informed by and predicated upon nursing theory derived from nursing research. However there are some fundamental flaws in this assumption which have been commented on over some considerable time by (amongst others) Wimpenny (2002), McCrae (2012) and Yancey (2015).

Alternatively, students may be introduced to grand nursing theories. These orientate a student to one dominant view of the patient, family, health, environment and the nurse's role but are largely normative (Allmark, 1995; Murphy & Smith, 2013). While there is nothing wrong per se in getting students to think philosophically about the nature of nursing, the nature of being a patient and health, it can seem remote from the practice nursing students witness in clinical placements. Grand nursing models can also seem overprescriptive as they assume one theory applies in all nursing contexts.

Several questions arise immediately. For example, where is the student nurse's disciplinary knowledge and is it possible for practice which is determined by an employer to be professional knowledge? One of the most common difficulties for nursing students is helping the student to integrate theory and practice both in practice and in college/university to form a coherent body of nursing knowledge. This is not infrequently an unsatisfactory process as students realise that what has been taught in university is not what is used or seen in practice. Jensen and Lahn (2005) point out that perhaps the student does not feel what has been taught in the university is relevant, or the student is actually told it is not relevant. Perhaps students cannot find evidence for caring activities, for washing or dressing patients, or indeed students are told it is sufficient to be kind and compassionate. Much of the nursing witnessed by nursing students in clinical placements is governed by custom and practice, or by organisational policy which means nurses learn to rely on protocols, which reduce critical thinking and thereby professionalism (Allan, 2007). This is fertile ground for an uncritical acceptance – a reification – of the theory–practice gap, as the knowledge students create in practice goes unrecognised as it falls between the knowledge taught in the university and knowledge learned through practice protocols and from their observations of other nurses.

Students can be taught theory in nursing programmes through introducing them to evidence-based practice and research skills (Billings & Kowalski, 2006); theory from this perspective is thought of as evidence for practice (Kitson, 2002). Learning research skills such as critiquing a research paper, searching the literature and understanding hierarchies of evidence is intended to help students understand the underpinning research evidence behind the nursing they deliver while on clinical placement. It is hoped that nursing students become critical practitioners in future who are able to sift evidence after searching the literature, and weigh possible courses of action from evidence. However, research has shown that research utilisation by practising nurses is low (Kajermo et al., 2000).

The assumptions behind the concept of *hierarchies of evidence* is also strongly disputed generally (Kitson, 2002) and particularly so in nursing where many nursing tasks are orientated to developing relationships between patients, families and nurses and are not supported by or possibly conceptualised as evidence. This is the point above which evidence for practice (theories based frequently in biosciences) is separate from knowledge nurses use in interpersonal relationships with patients, carers and families. The latter are grounded in the psychological and social sciences and may not be used as evidence. Unfortunately, many approaches to teaching theory or evidence-based practice in undergraduate nursing curricula do not articulate this clearly. Kitson (2002) takes this position further and argues that the evidence-based nursing movement is based on assumptions about the nature of nursing which are in tension with – if not in opposition to – person-centred caring and practice theories.

A further difficulty with teaching theory as evidence is that there are different types of theory. Theories of hand washing, pressure area relief, nutrition, wound and bone healing are middle-range theories and (hopefully) reflect what students observe in practice. Kitson (2002) and Rolfe (1997, 1998) among others argue that person-centred theories of nursing are not middle-range theory but practice theories which are, by their nature, local theories created by nurses in teams in local settings. These theories are excluded by a hierarchies-of-evidence approach to nursing knowledge and practice and suggest to students that theorising and knowledge production have no place in clinical nursing.

Students may be taught to integrate theory and practice through the mastery of clinical skills in clinical skills laboratories (Morgan, 2006). These are designed to allow students to *literally* practise in safety with support from their clinical educators or teachers; this enables them to develop their psychomotor skills (Jeffries et al., 2002) and decision making. The acquisition of skills is once again heavily promoted in the UK within the 2018 NMC Standards and in Standard 1.0 (Learning Culture) (2018b), 1.1–1.8 relate entirely to promoting safe learning but do not comment on learning from mistakes or challenging situations.

Teaching theory in clinical laboratories allows theory to be linked explicitly with practice skills in ways that cannot be guaranteed in practice where registered nurses acting as mentors have to balance patient workload and safety with the learning needs for their allocated students (Lee & French, 1997; Dix & Hughes, 2004). Skills labs are used to teach essential skills such as communication, moving and handling as well as more complex skills such as handling equipment and catheterising patients; they are also used for "skills and drills" to learn to react in clinical emergences (Morgan, 2006). Learning in skills labs is predicated upon role play, repeated psychomotor practice, observation and feedback (Haskvitz & Koop, 2004). Nevertheless, caution about how much the skills laboratory resembles real life is required (Morgan, 2006)

Lastly, a word about balance between theory and practice in nurse preparation programmes. Over the years, nurse educators and practitioners have argued for either more theory or more practice (Morgan, 2006; Evans, 2009). The current pre-registration professional preparation programmes in the UK balance learning across the university setting and clinical placements where 50% is taught in university and 50% in practice. Universities and their practice organisations work in well-established partnerships to produce competent and caring registered nurses at all stages of the process, from interview to assessment. As Fealy (1997: p. 1160) suggests, "to practitioners and to educators the concern has tended to focus on efforts to achieve greater theory–practice integration, and more specifically, to promote practices which best express theoretical positions and propositions, principles and prescriptions". This has had two effects. Firstly, where theory is not available, such as in caring practices, these activities have been reframed as nursing's moral enterprise encompassed in the *Compassion in Practice* vision and strategy for nursing, midwifery and care staff (O'Driscoll et al., 2017). Secondly, a concern with evidence has pushed nursing knowledge, along with grand theories of nursing, to the margins and allowed person-centred nursing to be increasingly threatened.

The relationship between theory and practice in nursing

Fealy (1999, citing Carr, 1986) proposes a typology to characterise the theory–practice relationship in nursing, drawing on Carr's assertion that one can describe theory–practice relationships as: the common-sense approach, the applied science approach, the practical approach and the critical approach.

The recognition of different forms of theory and knowledge in nursing has been possible because of a rejection of the technical-rational approach to knowledge and the assumption that theory informs practice rather than there being a symbiotic relationship. Since the 1990s, theorists have been concerned with understanding how nurses theorise in practice (Benner & Wrubel, 1989). Benner (1984) in work over two decades (Benner & Sutphen, 2007; Benner et al., 2009) emphasises that students learn from experience where tacit knowing and intuition become critical skills to acquire expertise and that the acquisition of practical skills is a critical feature of and pre-requisite for professional expertise. Many nurse theorists have argued for the use of critical reflection as a tool with which to create knowledge for practice (Rolfe, 1993; Hatlavik, 2012). This is known as practice-driven theory – theory recoverable from good practice to guide practice. Central to practice-driven theory is *praxis* or the action of learning to change practice (Rolfe, 1997). Through reflecting on practice while in practice, the nurse or team of nurses modify and develop practice. Critical reflection or reflexivity validates the professional judgements of practitioners. And the theory–practice gap disappears as theory is derived from and tested in practice. However, the knowledge and theory utilised in practice are local and situated. While local situated knowledge is valid, this approach to knowledge and practice-driven theory may be too situational, too local (Fealy, 1999). In reality, there is place for both forms of knowledge and different levels of theory (Gortner, 1992; Fealy, 1999): local situated knowledge which informs local practice and theorising; middle-range theory which takes nursing practice beyond the local to inform nursing care such as wound care, pressure area care, mouth care – even grand theory when used appropriately in context. We have argued elsewhere (Allan et al., 2018) that Benner largely overlooks or fails to emphasise enough in our view the emotional side of learning.

Drawing on Fabricius (1999) and Menzies-Lyth (1970), emotional learning within the student as a means to integrate theory with practice has been discussed elsewhere (Allan, 2011). Proposing an approach to understanding emotional learning psychodynamically or learning to work with feelings suggests that feelings shape learning both consciously and unconsciously; they are the fundamental basis of learning for student nurses as they learn from interactions with patients, their families and colleagues. Feelings shape interactions and therefore learning, in other words.

Allan (2011) argued that using a psychodynamic approach in nurse education may address the theory–practice gap for student nurses by allowing them to reflect on the emotional issues arising in clinical placements. She showed how supervision can assist students to integrate theory and practice through guided reflection on feelings arising from their learning in placements in small-group work with a skilled tutor who works psychodynamically. Learning to work with feelings means that, following Menzies-Lyth, the nurse is aware that as well as the clinical dimension of delivering care, there are also social and emotional processes at work in interactions with patients which affect how we feel (Fabricius, 1999). Sometimes we are aware of these feelings and can reflect in action – this means we are able to recognise the patient's feelings and our own responses, and act appropriately. Sometimes we can only reflect on action, i.e. after the event, and learn from that reflection to work differently in similar situations in the future. This approach derives from Freud's theory of pyschodynamics or psychoanalysis (Fabricius, 1991b, 1995). These feelings are frequently buried and, although they shape action, are not processed or learnt from.

Evans (2009) has described the theory–practice gap as a way (in psychodynamic terms) of keeping the messiness of learning through being with the patient under control. The student's learning challenges this control over feeling and messiness and educators and mentors split theory from practice – the theory–practice gap, which splits theory off from having a relationship with practice.

Workplace expectations and disintegrated learning

A feature of the British learning environment or clinical placement for nursing students is that it is also a workplace. People employed by hospitals are expected to work hard and it is recognised that the NHS is not a learning organisation because it struggles to balance its work demands with its teaching and learning demands (Melia, 2005). Indeed, the 2018 NMC *Standards Framework for Nursing and Midwifery Education* make this very plain (2018b); safety of patients, staff and students is considered to be the most important standard. Therefore having a mentor who has realistic expectations of students in busy workplaces and knows the curriculum is important in creating good learning experiences for students (Gray & Smith, 2000). Mentors who have positive attitudes and motivations towards teaching and supporting student nurses' learning in practice (Spouse, 1998b; Hall, 2006) and perceive their mentoring role as part of their personal and professional development as well as contributing to the development of the profession as a whole are a resource for students to succeed in clinical placements. However, mentoring may not be undertaken voluntarily and mentors may fail to connect clinical nursing with academic knowledge explicitly (Cahill, 1996). This is likely to become more complex if, as Fealy (1999) argues, many mentors *believe in* the theory–practice gap and describe it as not being integrated; in this way, mentors may reproduce a disintegrated learning environment for students.

The mentor's contribution to student nurse learning may not always be beneficial and many students learn from negative experiences of being mentored (Pearcey & Elliott, 2004). Brammer (2006) suggests that the mentor may act as a "gatekeeper" (in a positive or negative sense) to learning and the integration of theory and practice in the clinical learning environment while students may perceive the assessment role as interfering with their relationship with mentors. The 2018 NMC Standards for supervision and assessment go some way to addressing this concern by separating out the supervisor and assessor roles.

The hidden curriculum can also be an area where conflict arises between different approaches to learning. Benson and Latter (1998) argue that the theory–practice relationship is shaped by politics in each clinical placement where students are allocated to learn. The political climate across all placements results from the hierarchy between those who have knowledge (staff) and students who need to learn (Cahill, 1996). The students are dependent on staff to learn and to succeed. This hierarchy constructs two curricula, the formal and the hidden, which are opposing experiences that lack integration for both students and their mentors (Field, 2004). One way survival strategies are learned is through clinical role

136

modelling, which socialises neophytes into professional practice and into local political ways of behaving (Allan et al., 2011). The following extract from the Leadership for Learning project shows how successful students become at negotiating learning opportunities. But it is essentially a disintegrated learning which is haphazard, unplanned and unsupervised. Importantly, clinical role modelling also validates students' experiences in practice which the university fails to do (Spouse, 1998a, 1998b; Cribb & Bignold, 1999). Students learn that knowledge and experience gained in practice are professionally valued by their discipline and mentors while academic knowledge and theory are not.

Essentially, students are expected to provide labour as students and on registration are expected to be able to work immediately as fully competent nurses. Expectations of students (Gray & Smith, 2000) and the lack of integration of theory and practice (Fealy, 1999), the lack of preparation for practice and mentors' expectations of students form the learning context where students have to learn to negotiate their status as students in practice. Students have to learn in a disintegrated learning context where opposing values of learning exist. Allan et al. (2011) concluded that students learned despite the learning frameworks rather than because of them.

Brammer (2006) also argues that students are proactive in constructing learning opportunities, as they cannot afford to rely on mentors as they are not the only keys to learning in clinical areas. Understanding the strategies that students use to draw out learning opportunities in clinical areas when mentors might be gatekeeping and not facilitating access is useful in identifying active learning and facilitating such strategies in preparing students for practice areas. Students desire to fit in and want to be accepted by their mentors (Brammer, 2006). Brammer argues that negative experiences do not always reduce learning as some learning can come out of negative experiences; but when learning is negative and the student becomes demoralised, the focus on learning is lost as the feelings become paramount and interfere with learning (Brammer, 2006).

Spouse (2001) argues that practice placements are where professional development is the key activity. A key characteristic of practice placement is the centrality for the student to gain the experience of linking theory to practice.

Jackson and Mannix (2001) contend that practice placements provide nursing students with an opportunity to integrate theoretical knowledge whilst developing clinical skills.

The following extract from the Leadership for Learning project shows what happens when a student works on her own to essentially guide her own learning unsupervised by qualified staff in an emergency unit.

"Putting knowledge to work" –the theory of knowledge re-contextualisation

Evans et al.'s (2009) theory of re-contextualisation provides a way to understand the complexities of the relationship between contexts of learning for students by picking apart *knowledges* which underpin the curriculum, the work placement, the student's internal world and the pedagogic approach. The theoretical approach, developed further in Evans and Guile (2012) and elaborated for post-qualification learning in Evans (2015), reframes knowledge transfer by arguing that knowledge in practice-based disciplines is not merely transferred from theory to practice but re-contextualised in different practice settings. Students and newly qualified practitioners learn actively to change and use knowledge rather than passively take knowledge from one area to another, sometimes finding it useful and sometimes not. This is a dispiriting process where knowledge then appears to be superfluous to practice and only useful for passing examinations. This insight is useful for practice disciplines where theoretical knowledge is not always directly transferable to practice (Evans et al., 2010).

Explaining re-contextualisation

Understanding the flows of knowledge in programmes involving substantial elements of work exposure, such as in nursing and midwifery, goes beyond typologising forms and features of knowledge. This level of understanding works to analyse the knowledge logics that underpin programme flows and how knowledge is changed as it is "put to work" across contexts of learning and practice in universities, colleges and workplaces. All knowledge has a context in which it was originally generated. Contexts are often thought of as settings or places, but contexts in our use extend to the "schools of thought", the traditions and norms of practice, the life experiences in which knowledge of different kinds is generated. For knowledge generated and practised in one context to be put to work in new and different contexts, it has to be re-contextualised in various ways that simultaneously engage with and change those practices, traditions and experiences.

Evans et al. (2009) have argued that re-contextualisation is multi-faceted pedagogic practice, based on the idea that concepts and practice change as we use them in different settings. The original research has drawn on developments of Bernstein's idea that concepts change as they move from their disciplinary origins and become a part of a curriculum (Bernstein, 2000; Barnett, 2006) and on van Oers' (1998) recognition that concepts are interpreted in the contexts of activity and developed through embodied practice. These notions have been substantially expanded to embrace the ways in which learners themselves change as they re-contextualise concepts and practices. Four kinds of re-contextualisation are significant:

1. content re-contextualisation – putting knowledge to work in the programme design environment
2. pedagogic re-contextualisation – putting knowledge to work in the teaching and facilitating environment
3. workplace re-contextualisation – putting knowledge to work in the workplace environment
4. learner re-contextualisation – what learners make of these processes.

Putting knowledge to work in the programme design environment: content re-contextualisation

The theory–practice relationships depend in part upon the ways in which knowledge has been "codified" in accordance with the rules and procedures of the disciplines and schools of thought that inform the field of practice. When curricula are created, this occurs through content re-contextualisation – when knowledge moves from its original context of production (for example, in the academic research community or industry research and development programme) into the formal learning programme offered by a learning provider. This is a process whereby codified knowledge is selected, simplified, recast and made more teachable and learnable for the intended participants, as part of the programme design.

In professional and vocational education, combinations of disciplinary and codified occupational sector knowledge are drawn on and organised to meet the presumed demands of practice and criteria for professional recognition. Different knowledge logics complicate this process, as logical structures that move towards higher levels of abstraction and theoretical understanding differ from knowledge logics that rely on a series of practical, operational connections. These knowledge logics are not easily related to one another. Disciplinary knowledge logics are more amenable to re-contextualisation processes than others because principles for selection and recombination are embedded within them. In contrast, codifications of procedural and work process knowledge offer few principles for selection and combination because codification is largely descriptive. So practitioners involved with curriculum design need to develop a common approach, agreeing criteria to determine how content based on different forms of knowledge should be selected and combined to achieve programme goals. This content re-contextualisation process thus entails the first set of knowledge re-contextualisation practices.

Putting knowledge to work in the teaching and facilitating environment: pedagogic re-contextualisation

When educators approach the recontextualised content in curricula, the focus changes to pedagogic re-contextualisation, the design and organisation of the teaching and learning dimensions of programmes. Pedagogic re-contextualisation takes place as different forms of knowledge are organised, structured and sequenced into learning activities, options and modules, for the purposes of effective learning and teaching. Pedagogic re-contextualisation practices involve teachers, tutors and trainers in making decisions about how much time and emphasis they want to devote to different forms of knowledge, striking a balance between time and freedom to engage with these forms of knowledge in their own terms while progressively focusing attention on knowledge use in specific areas of practice. These decisions are never technical matters; they are often contested. They are inevitably influenced by teachers', tutors' and trainers' assumptions (often unarticulated) about what constitutes good learning experiences and worthwhile learning outcomes, and also by the specifications set by professional or examination bodies. Often, the positions educators take reflect differences in what they believe they are supporting their students to be and become in their chosen profession (Bound et al., 2019). Academic engineers, for example, can disagree with practice engineers about the level and nature of mathematics teaching that new entrants to the profession need to ensure both safe practice and a platform for progression to higher academic levels at a later stage. Similarly, academic nurses and practice-based nurses often disagree about the extent to which students need to engage with nursing theory, with differences in view about the relative importance of investigative learning and foundations for future progression to more senior roles. Reconciling conflicting views entails pedagogical re-contextualisation practices, as practitioners work together to ensure that concepts and general principles are well understood, internalised and enacted as work-based learning provides a series of suitably challenging "test benches" for the use of knowledge in action.

Putting knowledge to work in the workplace environment: workplace re-contextualisation

Workplace environments fundamentally affect how knowledge is put to work, and they vary considerably in the nature, extent and quality of learning experience that they afford (Felstead et al., 2009). Workplace re-contextualisations take place through the workplace practices and activities that support knowledge development, and through the mentorship, coaching and other arrangements that enable new entrants to engage with and learn through workplace environments. These practices and supports are fundamental to undertaking standard workplace activities effectively and to developing the confidence and capability to work with others to change those activities where the situation demands it. They allow learners to experience how individuals and teams "progressively re-contextualise" concepts in activity. This is a form of learning that is often triggered by the activity and the context. Knowledge re-contextualisation takes place when a student or newly qualified practitioner recognises a new situation as requiring a response and uses knowledge – theoretical, procedural and tacit – in acts of interpretation in an attempt to bring the activity and its setting under conscious control (van Oers, 1998). When the interpretation involves the enactment of a well-known activity in a new setting, an adaptive form of re-contextualisation takes place as existing knowledge is used to reproduce a response in a parallel situation. Where the interpretation leads the learner to change the activity or its context in an attempt to make a response, a productive form of re-contextualisation takes place, as new knowledge is produced (Allan et al. 2017). Knowledge re-contextualisations are fundamental to learners and new entrants beginning to enact existing workplace activities; or working with experienced others to modify them in the face of unexpected occurrences or the need to find new solutions. These workplace re-contextualisations are facilitated when workplaces create stretching but supportive environments for working and when learners expect, and are expected, to take responsibility for observing, inquiring and acting on what they learn. Learners, through a series of such knowledge re-contextualisations, come to self-embody knowledge cognitively and practically. This is the start of a long-term process of personal and professional development that is difficult to detect, elusive of measurement and often appreciated only in retrospect.

What the learner/employee makes of it: learner re-contextualisation

Learner re-contextualisation takes place through the strategies learners themselves use to bring together and put to work different forms of knowledge they have gained through the programme, through working with learning partners in college and workplaces and by observing, inquiring and working with more experienced people in the workplace. What learners make of these re-contextualisation processes varies according to their personal characteristics and the scope for action that they have, individually and collectively, in any particular environment. Together with their prior learning and tacit knowledge, opportunities and affordances for learning may be unequally distributed (Evans et al., 2006).

Learner re-contextualisation is critical to the development of a professional identity. The theory–practice relationship is reflected in the interplay of professional and academic identities, and in the longer-term development of the new entrant as a knowledgeable practitioner (Evans, 2015). Thinking and feeling one's way into a professional identity is facilitated by such practices as engaging in "learning conversations", articulating new insights and sharing perceptions of practice with others, being stretched through opportunities to work at the next level. More fundamentally, learners' embodied experiences of becoming a professional in their chosen field can be considered in some respects as diverse re-contextualisations of their own prior experiences and their educators' aims in designing and planning the content and activities of programmes of learning. Integrated practice, which breaks free of dichotomous understandings of knowledge and practice (Bound et al., 2019), lays the foundations for knowledgeable practice. Most importantly, the development of the learner as a knowledgeable practitioner continues beyond qualification; through mentorship, coaching and peer learning; and by reflecting, continuously and critically, on new ideas and experiences accessed through work and through wider professional and personal networks that extend beyond the immediate work environment.

Connecting the four expressions of re-contextualisation

Each of the four expressions of re-contextualisation sheds light on some element of the challenges of connecting theory with practice and relating subject-based and work-based knowledge in the processes of professional learning and practice development. When connected, they offer a framework that can be used to analyse existing programmes, interrogate research and design new approaches.

The framework in Figure 10.1 summarises and provides a simplified representation of the ways in which re-contexualisation processes can combine in learning programmes. Knowledge from disciplinary sources is combined with occupational sector knowledge and codified practice-based knowledge, re-contextualised through context re-contextualisation into the content of the curriculum or learning programme. Teachers and facilitators of learning develop teaching, learning and assessment strategies that re-contextualise the content into activities to generate worthwhile learning processes and outcomes (pedagogic re-contextualisation), connecting directly and reflexively with work-based practice and the affordances of specific work environments through workplace re-contextualisation. Learners draw on their prior disciplinary knowledge and on their prior and current work experiences in the ways in which they engage with the teaching, learning and assessment strategies and eventually their new work roles (learner re-contextualisation). These processes are facilitated

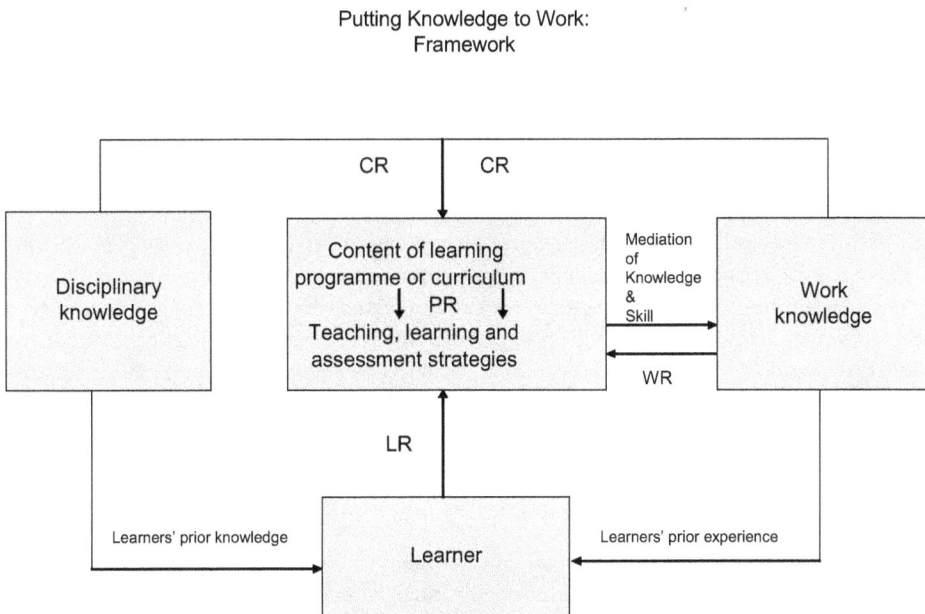

Putting Knowledge to Work:
Framework

Figure 10.1 Putting knowledge to work framework. CR, context re-contextualisation; LR, learner re-contextualisation; PR, pedagogic re-contextualisation; WR, workplace re-contextualisation.

when learners develop meta-cognitive strategies; and when learning partners work together to help the learners, whether students or newly qualified practitioners, to see connections and make sense of the whole process.

This theoretical framework has strong implications for professional practice. The long-standing language of "transfer" hinders rather than facilitates the search for solutions to the "theory–practice" gap. Using the concept of re-contextualisation explains the ways in which all forms of knowledge are tied to context (settings where things are done):

- identifies what actions assist people to move knowledge from context to context;
- identifies how knowledge changes as it is used differently in different social practices (ways of doing things) and contexts;
- identifies how new knowledge changes people, social practices and contexts;
- identifies who and what supports the re-contextualisation process.

Putting knowledge to work to meet educational, sectoral, organisational and learner needs depends on greater use of re-contextualisation practices across all teaching, learning and workplace environments as a way of maximising the integration of subject-based and work-based knowledge and developing strong foundations for knowledgeable practice. For example, the original research (Evans et al., 2009) has shown how the construction of multi-faceted, multi-level partnerships between colleges, organisations and workplace sites can embed knowledge flows in and across programme design, teaching and learning and the facilitation of learning in workplace practices. Re-contextualisation can be assisted by the "gradual release" of knowledge and responsibility to learners over time and in contexts of increasing unpredictability of tasks. Using "industry educators" as knowledge brokers can support the effective use of workplace and professional resources for teaching and learning, and development of new knowledge through learning conversations. Furthermore, pro-gramme structures including coordinated assessment practices can be developed to achieve a critical mass of compatibility between employer, professional body and academic requirements.

Discussion – using re-contextualisation theory in nursing

The ideas that re-contextualisation generates for restoring firstly, the fragmented curriculum in nursing and secondly, disintegrated learning environments for nursing students can be organised according to the four expressions of re-contextualisation. Nursing as a field entails the selection and organisation of subject knowledge for the demands of practice (content re-contextualisation) from social and psychological sciences as well as (predominantly) on medi-cine, pharmacology and microbiology. Some knowledges (e.g. biomedicine) are valued more than others depending on different tutors' preferences and different university tradi-tions; some forms of knowledge are privileged by government policy, e.g. evidence-based practice; and the ascribing of value to knowledge is gendered (Davies, 1995).

Learning outcomes are overtly agreed by both education and practice in the pedagogical re-contextualisation process, but each has different agendas about the learning process during the professional preparation programme and the final outcome on graduation. The clinical areas are very busy in acute areas and therefore the patient takes priority, not the learner. What does "super-numerary" status really mean for learning in these settings? Issues for workplace re-contextualisation follow from these last points. For practice, what is required is a nurse who is ready to work as a registered nurse; for education, while learning outcomes are achieved, this is intended to be built on as newly qualified nurses enter into the workplace as lifelong learners.

The integrative concept of knowledgeable practice, developed by Evans (2015) as an extension to re-contextualisation theory, has strong resonances for nurse education. Knowledgeable practice is characterised by the exercise of attuned and responsive judgement when individuals or teams are confronted with complex tasks and often unpredictable situations at work. The concept of knowledgeable practice facilitates a focus on practices while attending to the knowledge frameworks that underpin the directing of work and the exercise of judgement that is involved in working with others to vary or change practices or products at work. The different forms of knowledge inherent in workplace practice must be kept in view – scientific, procedural, ethical, experiential – together with a recognition that "work process" knowledge, including organisation-specific knowledge embedded in routines, artefacts and protocols, is often used tacitly.

In the workplace, student nurses and newly qualified nurses are assessed in accordance with competence-based criteria that are themselves heavily contested. Socio-cultural theories of learning have problematised these approaches as based on a "product view" that separates learning from the network of relations, including power relations, that constitutes the framework of participation (Hager, 2011), but have themselves not sufficiently attended to the question of what is learned and how knowledge changes as it is put to work in practice. When knowledge is put to work at the point of practice the relationship between discipline-based, practice-based and work-based knowledge often has to be rethought, particularly by newly qualified professional workers. As we have shown (Allan et al., 2016), newly qualified nurses often take a considerable time to "think and feel" their ways into using their knowledge at work (see also Eraut, 2004). Judgement takes time to develop and is a critical capability for nurse involvement in the improvement of care.

Overarching questions remain for the development of nursing curricula: can the student's learning be "progressive", has it ever really been so and is it legitimate to be so in the current climate? (See Spouse, 1998b.) And whose voices are heard in the discipline when these too are fragmented? Arguably, steps can be taken towards restoring the curriculum from its current state of fragmentation and disintegration through the working of re-contextualisation ideas into strategies and pedagogic approaches that move beyond dichotomous understandings of knowledge and practice.

Conclusion

Dyson (2018) argues that the British curriculum is too restrictive to develop critical thinking in nursing graduates. The lens of re-contextualisation focuses attention on processes involved in successfully moving knowledge from disciplines and workplaces into a curriculum, from a curriculum into successful pedagogic strategies and learner/employee engagement in educational institutions and workplaces. Some pedagogic strategies that facilitate these outcomes are "smart" re-workings of long-standing pedagogic practices such as the "gradual release" of knowledge and responsibility. Other strategies, such as the use of distributed mentorship, supplement educational expertise while keeping academic requirements in view. The goals of nurse education are best accomplished when a critical mass of compatibility is established and kept under review between professional body, course and employer requirements. Furthermore, for large-scale public services such as the NHS, putting knowledge to work more effectively may require fundamental shifts in work organisation to foster cultures that embrace and promote knowledge-enhancing practice at all levels.

References

Aggleton P & Chalmers H (2000) *Nursing Models and Nursing Practice.* 2nd ed. Oxford: Macmillan.

Allan H T (2007) The Rhetoric of caring and the recruitment of overseas nurses: the social reproduction of a care gap. *Journal of Clinical Nursing Special Edition* 16(12): 2204–2212.

Allan H T (2011) Using psychodynamic small group work in nurse education: closing the theory–practice gap? *Nurse Education Today* 31: 521–524.

Allan H T, Magnusson C, Evans K, Ball E, Westwood S, Curtis K & Johnson M (2016) Delegation and supervision of healthcare assistants' work in the daily management of uncertain and the unexpected in clinical practice: invisible learning among newly qualified nurses. *Nursing Inquiry* 23(4): 377–385.

Allan H T, Magnusson C, Johnson M, Evans K, Ball E, Horton K, Curtis K & Westwood S (2018) Preceptorship and safe delegation: the key to improved standards in bedside care? *Journal of Clinical Nursing* 27(1-2): 123–131.

Allan H T, Magnusson C, Johnson M, Evans K,, Ball E, Horton K, Curtis K, Westwood S (In press) Putting knowledge to work in clinical practice: Understanding experiences of preceptorship as outcomes of interconnected domains of learning Journal of Clinical Nursing Accepted version online: 12 APR 2017 01:55AM EST | Doi: 10.1111/jocn.13855

Allan H T, Smith P A & Lorentzon M (2007) Leadership for learning: a literature study of leadership for learning in clinical practice. *Journal of Nursing Management* 16 545–555.

Allan H T, Smith P & O'Driscoll M (2011) Experiences of supernumerary status and the hidden curriculum in nursing: a new twist in the theory–practice gap? *Journal of Clinical Nursing* 20: 847–855.

Allmark P (1995) A classical view of the theory-practice gap in nursing. *Journal of Advanced Nursing* 22: 18–23.

Barnett M (2006) Vocational knowledge and vocational pedagogy. In M Young & J Gamble (Eds.), *Knowledge, Curriculum and Qualifications for South African Further Education* (pp. 56-72) Cape Town: HSRC Press.

Benner P (1984) *From Novice to Expert: Excellence and Power in Clinical Nursing Practice.* Menlo Park: Addison-Wesley.

Benner P & Sutphen M (2007) Learning across the professions: the clergy, a case in point. *Journal of Nursing Education* 46: 103–108.

Benner P, Tanner C A & Chesla C A (2009) *Expertise in Nursing Practice: Caring, Clinical Judgment and Ethics.* New York: Springer.

Benner P & Wrubel J (1989) *The Primacy of Caring: Stress and Coping in Health and Illness.* Menlo Park: Addison-Wesley.

Benson A & Latter S (1998) Implementing health promoting nursing: the integration of interpersonal skills and health promotion. *Journal of Advanced Nursing* 27: 100–107.

Bernstein B (2000) *Pedagogy, Symbolic Control and Identity: Theory, Research Critique.* Revised ed. Lanham: Rowman and Littlefield.

Billings D M & Kowalski K (2006) Bridging the theory-practice gap with evidence-based practice. *Journal of Continuing Education in Nursing* 37(6): 248–249.

Bound H, Evans K, Sadik S & Karmel A (2019) *How Non-Permanent Workers Learn and Develop.* Abingdon: Routledge.

Brammer J (2006) A phenomenographic study of registered nurses' understanding of their role in student learning—An Australian perspective. *International Journal of Nursing Studies* 43(8): 963–973.

Cahill H A (1996) A qualitative analysis of student nurses' experiences of mentorship. *Journal of Advanced Nursing* 24(4): 791–799.

Carr W (1986) Theories of theory and practice. *Journal of Philosophy of Education* 20(20): 177–186.

Clark T & Holmes S (2007) Fit for practice? An exploration of the development of newly qualified nurses using focus groups. *International Journal of Nursing Studies* 44(1): 2210–2220.

Cribb A & Bignold S (1999) Towards the reflexive medical school: the hidden curriculum and medical education research. *Studies in Higher Education* 24: 195–209.

Davies C (1995) *Gender and the Professional Predicament of Nursing.* Buckingham, UK: Open University Press.

Dix G & Hughes S (2004) Strategies to help students learn effectively. *Nursing Standard* 18: 39–42.

Dyson S E (2018) *Critical Pedagogy in Nursing: Transformational Approaches to Nurse Education in a Globalized World.* London: Palgrave Macmillan.

Eraut M (2004) *Developing Professional Knowledge: A Review of Progress and Practice.* London: Falmer Press.

Evans K (2015) Developing knowledgeable practice at work. In M Elg. et al. (Ed.), *Sustainable Development in Organizations Studies on Innovative Practices* (pp. 63-81) London: Edward Elgar Publishing.

Evans K (2016) Higher vocational learning and knowledgeable practice. The newly qualified practitioner at work. In S Loo & G Jameson (Eds.), *Vocationalism in Further and Higher Education Policy, Programmes and Pedagogy* (pp. 117–130). Abingdon: Routledge.

Evans K & Guile D (2012) Putting different forms of knowledge to work in practice. J Higgs, R Barnett, S Billett, M Hutchings & F Trede (Eds.), *Practice-Based Education: Perspectives and Strategies*. Rotterdam: Sense Publishers.

Evans K, Guile D & Harris J (2009) *Putting Knowledge to Work: The Exemplars*. Centre for Excellence in Work-Based Learning (WLE Centre) UCL Institute of Education. London: University of London. London. Accessed at: http://discovery.ucl.ac.uk/1527268/

Evans K, Guile D, Harris J & Allan H T (2010) Putting knowledge to work: a new approach. *Nurse Education Today* 30: 245–251.

Evans K, Hodkinson P, Rainbird H & Unwin L (2006) *Improving Workplace Learning*. Abingdon: Routledge.

Evans M (2009) Tackling the theory-practice gap in mental health nurse training. *Mental Health Practice* 13(2): 21–24.

Fabricius J (1991b) Running on the spot or can nursing really change. *Psychoanalytic Psychotherapy* 5: 97–108.

Fabricius J (1995) Psychoanalytic understanding and nursing: a supervisory workshop with nurse tutors. *Psychoanalytic Psychotherapy* 9: 17–29.

Fabricius J (1999) The crisis in nursing: reflections on the crisis. *Psychoanalytic Psychotherapy* 13(3): 203–206.

Fawcett J (1992) Conceptual models and nursing practice: a reciprocal relationship. *Journal of Advanced Nursing* 17: 224–228.

Fealy G (1997) The theory-practice relationship in nursing: an exploration of contemporary discourse. *Journal of Advanced Nursing* 25: 1061–1069.

Fealy G M (1999) The theory-practice relationship in nursing: the practitioner's perspective. *Journal of Advanced Nursing* 30(1): 72–82.

Felstead A, Fuller A, Jewson N & Unwin L (2009) *Improving Working as Learning*. Abingdon: Routledge.

Field D (2004) Moving from novice to expert – the value of learning in clinical practice: a literature review. *Nurse Education Today* 24: 560–565.

Forber J, DiGiacomo M, Carter B, Davidson P, Phillips J, Jackson D (2016) In pursuit of an optimal model of undergraduate nurse clinical education: An integrative review. Nurse Educ Pract. 2016 Nov; 21: 83–92.

Gallagher P (2004) How the metaphor of a gap between theory and practice has influenced nursing education. *Nurse Education Today* 24(4): 263–268.

Gortner S (1992) *Nursing values and science: towards a nursing scientific philosophy*. In L H Nicholl (Ed.), *Perspectives in Nursing Theory* (pp. 176–186, 2nd ed). Philadelphia: J B Lippincott.

Gray M A & Smith L N (2000) The qualities of an effective mentor from the student nurse's perspective: findings from a longitudinal qualitative study. *Journal of Advanced Nursing* 32(6): 1542–1549.

Hager P (2011) Theories of workplace Learning. In M Malloch, L Cairns, K Evans & B O'Connor (Eds.), *The Sage Handbook of Workplace Learning* (pp. 58-73) London: Sage.

Hall A (2006) Mentorship in the community. *Journal Community Nursing* 20(7): 2–6.

Haskvitz L & Koop E (2004) Students struggling in clinical? a new role for the patient simulator. *Journal of Nursing Education* 43: 181–184.

Hatlavik I K R (2012) The theory-practice relationship: reflective skills and theoretical knowledge as key factors in bridging the gap between theory and practice in initial nursing education. *Journal of Advanced Nursing* 68(4): 868–877.

Heggen K (2008) Social workers, teachers and nurses—from college to professional work. *Journal of Education and Work* 21(3): 217–231.

Jackson D & Mannix J (2001) Clinical nurses as teachers: insight from students of nursing in their first semester of study. *Journal of Clinical Nursing* 10: 270–277.

Jeffries P, Rew S & Cramer J (2002) A comparison of student centered versus traditional methods of teaching basic nursing skills in a learning laboratory. *Nursing Education Perspectives* 23: 14–19.

Jensen K & Lahn L (2005) The binding role of knowledge: an analysis of nursing students' knowledge ties. *Journal of Education and Work* 18: 305–320.

Kajermo K N, Nordström G, Krusebrant A & Björvell H (2000) Perceptions of research utilization: comparisons between health care professionals, nursing students and a reference group of nurse clinicians. *Journal of Advanced Nursing* 31(1): 99–109.

Kitson A (2002) Recognising relationships: reflections on evidence-based practice. *Nursing Inquiry* 9(3): 179–186.

Laiho A & Ruoholinna T (2013) The relationship between practitioners and academics – anti-academic discourse voiced by Finnish nurses. *Journal of Vocational Education and Training* 65(3): 333–350.

Lee C & French P (1997) Education in the practicum: a study of the ward learning climate in Hong Kong". *Journal of Advanced Nursing* 26: 455–462.

Maben J, Latter S, MacLeod Clark J (2006) The theory–practice gap: impact of professional–bureaucratic work conflict on newly-qualified nurses. *Journal of Advanced Nursing* 55(4): 465–477.

Magnusson C, Westwood S, Ball E, Curtis K, Evans K, Horton K, Johnson, M and Allan, H T (2014) *An investigation into newly qualified nurses' ability to recontextualise knowledge to allow them to delegate and supervise care (AaRK).* Project Report. University of Surrey.

McCrae N (2012) Whither nursing models? The value of nursing theory in the context of evidence-based practice and multidisciplinary health care. *Journal of Advanced Nursing* 68(1): 222–229.

Melia K (2005) *Nursing in the New NHS: A Sociological Analysis of Learning and Working.* Accessed at: www.researchcatalogue.esrc.ac.uk/grants/R000271191/outputs/read/f513ae62-6f5f-403d-9796-135a576f339f

Menzies-Lyth I E P (1970) *The Functioning of Social Systems as a Defence Against Anxiety: Report on a Study of the Nursing Service of a General Hospital.* London: The Tavistock Institute of Human Relations.

Monaghan T (2015) A critical analysis of the literature and theoretical perspectives on theory–practice gap amongst newly qualified nurses within the United Kingdom. *Nurse Education Today* 35: e1-e7.

Morgan R (2006) Using clinical skills laboratories to promote theory–practice integration during first practice placement: an Irish perspective. *Journal of Clinical Nursing* 15: 155–161.

Murphy F & Smith C (2013) *Nursing Theories and Models Volume 3.* Sage Library of Nursing. London: Sage.

Nieminen P (2008) Caught in the science trap? A case study of the relationship between nurses and "their" science. In J Välimaa & O Ylijoki (Eds.), *Cultural Perspectives on Higher Education* (pp. 127–141). New York: Springer.

Nursing & Midwifery Council. (2018a) *Future Nurse: Standards of Proficiency for Registered Nurses.* Accessed at: www.nmc.org.uk/globalassets/sitedocuments/education-standards/future-nurse-proficiencies.pdf?utm_source=Council+of+Deans+of+Health+Policy+Bulletin&utm_campaign=2c5365ca7f-EMAIL_CAMPAIGN_2018_05_14&utm_medium=email&utm_term=0_7c5e43a9b0-2c5365ca7f-171617605

Nursing & Midwifery Council. (2018b) *Standards Framework for Nursing and Midwifery Education.* Accessed at: www.nmc.org.uk/globalassets/sitedocuments/education-standards/education-framework.pdf?utm_source=Council+of+Deans+of+Health+Policy+Bulletin&utm_campaign=2c5365ca7f-EMAIL_CAMPAIGN_2018_05_14&utm_medium=email&utm_term=0_7c5e43a9b0-2c5365ca7f-171617605

Nursing and Midwifery Council. (2018c) *Standards for Preregistration Nursing Programmes.* Accessed at: www.nmc.org.uk/globalassets/sitedocuments/education-standards/programme-standards-nursing.pdf?utm_source=Council+of+Deans+of+Health+Policy+Bulletin&utm_campaign=2c5365ca7f-EMAIL_CAMPAIGN_2018_05_14&utm_medium=email&utm_term=0_7c5e43a9b0-2c5365ca7f-171617605

O'Driscoll M, Allan H T, Serrant L, Corbett K & Lui L (2018) Compassion in practice—Evaluating the awareness, involvement and perceived impact of a national nursing and midwifery strategy amongst healthcare professionals in NHS Trusts in England. *Journal of Clinical Nursing* 27(5-6): e1097–e1109.

O'Driscoll M, Allan H T, Serrant L, Corbett K, Lui L (2018) Compassion in Practice – evaluating the awareness, involvement and perceived impact of a national nursing and midwifery strategy amongst health care professionals in NHS Trusts in England. *Journal of Clinical Nursing.* 27 (5-6): e1097–e1109 Doi: 10.1111/jocn.14176

Özyazıcıoğlu N, Aydınoğlu N & Ayverdi, D (2011) Commentary on Allan HT, Smith P & O'Driscoll M experiences of supernumerary status and the hidden curriculum in nursing: a new twist in the theory-practice gap? *Journal of Clinical Nursing* 20: 847–855.

Pearcey PA & Elliott B E (2004) Student impressions of clinical nursing. *Nurse Education Today* 24(5): 382–387.

Rolfe G (1993) Closing the theory-practice gap: a model of nursing praxis. *Journal of Clinical Nursing* 2: 173–177.

Rolfe G (1997) Nursing praxis: a zealot speaks. *Journal of Advanced Nursing* 25: 426–427.

Rolfe G (1998) The theory-practice gap in nursing: form research-based practice to practitioner-based research. *Journal of Advanced Nursing* 28(3): 672–679.

Smeby J-C & Vågan A (2008a) Recontextualising professional knowledge—newly qualified nurses and physicians. *Journal of Education and Work* 21(2): 159–173.

Smeby J C & Vågan A (2008b) Caught in the science trap? A case study of the relationship between nurses and "their" science". In J Välimaa & O H Ylijoki (Eds.), *Cultural Perspectives on Higher Education* (pp. 127–141). New York, NY: Springer.

Smith P & Allan H T (2010) We should be able to bear our patients in our teaching in some way' theoretical perspectives on how nurse teachers manage their emotions to negotiate the split between education and caring practice. *Nurse Education Today* 30(3): 218–223.

Spitzer A & Perrenoud B (2006a) Reforms in nursing education across western Europe: From agenda to practice. *Journal of Professional Nursing* 22(3): 150–161.

Spouse J (1998a) Scaffolding student learning in clinical practice. *Nurse Education Today* 18: 259–266.

Spouse J (1998b) Learning to nurse through legitimate peripheral participation. *Nurse Education Today* 18: 345–351.

Spouse J (2001) Bridging theory and practice in the supervisory relationship: a sociocultural perspective. *Journal of Advance Nursing* 33: 512–525.

van Oers B (1998) The fallacy of decontextualisation. *Mind, Culture and Activity* 5(2): 143–152.

Wimpenny P (2002) The meaning of models of nursing to practicing nurses. *Journal of Advanced Nursing* 40(3): 346–354.

Yancey N R (2015) Why teach nursing theory? *Nursing Science Quarterly* 28(4): 274–278.

11

CLINICAL TEACHING AND ASSESSMENT IN NURSING

Colleen Ryan

Introduction

Clinical teaching is concerned with facilitating integration between theory and practice so that students develop, and nurses maintain, fitness for practice. Clinical teachers form a vital part of the team that provides education to nurses but they are also a hidden resource that may not be reaching its fullest potential. The numbers of nurses working as clinical teachers globally are difficult to estimate because in most countries there are no mandatory or specific educational requirements for the role. In Australia as one example, it is estimated more than 6,000 nurses work part-time in education roles (Job Outlook, 2019). The aim of this chapter is to provide an overview of the strengths and challenges of this subspecialty of nursing education.

Challenges

Many nurses believe that clinical teaching as a subspecialty is overlooked (Woods, Cashin & Stockhausen, 2016), evidenced within the profession by the few high-ranking nursing journals and conferences dedicated to the specialty of clinical learning and teaching. Exceptions include the UK *Journal of Nurse Education in Practice* and the Australian National Nurse Educators Conference.

Consequently, the educational preparation and clinical teaching approaches taken by this diverse group are also not fully understood. Working to educate in clinical settings may be different to working to educate in academia (Huston et al., 2018; McAllister & Flynn, 2016); the roles are diverse, thus it is difficult to uncover specific challenges and rewarding aspects experienced by clinical teachers (McAllister et al., 2011; Ryan & McAllister, 2019). One known global challenge is that contemporary education providers now cater for diverse student populations with increasingly diverse learning needs.

The clinical environment is ever changing and is fraught with complexities, making the environment difficult to educate and learn in. In high-acuity settings, where nursing students commonly learn nursing, patient status changes rapidly, requiring students to step back from providing care. Variances in levels of support from education providers and inconsistency between key stakeholders' opinion of clinical practice learning objectives create differences in student learning (Ryan & McAllister, 2019).

Another known challenge is that appointment to the role is often without formal or adequate training and support to teach others, meaning many lack confidence in their teaching abilities (Oprescu et al., 2017). Clinical teachers are mostly multi-tasking professionals – working as clinicians for one employer, and as clinical teachers for education providers – which makes them time-poor and unable to undertake scholarly activities which would see the subspecialty develop. Further, clinical learning pedagogies are not widely developed or shared with clinical teachers. Contemporary healthcare environments are not always conducive to innovation in learning and teaching because of an emphasis on clinical skills development as one way of reducing risk to patients (McAllister, Oprescu & Jones, 2014). Also, clinical teachers mostly deliver learning that situates students as passive rather than active learners (Kell & Jones, 2007). Tredinnick-Rowe (2018) stressed innovation in approaches to learning and teaching are now necessary to facilitate effective learning in clinical learning environments. With this complex picture in mind, this chapter explores clinical teaching, its common challenges and solutions to the problems in ways that will inspire future clinical teachers.

Diversity and clinical teaching

Across the world, most universities have attempted to attract a diverse student body so that principles of equity include students from marginalised backgrounds, and so that the university itself can be profitable. For clinical teachers, this means that the student cohort is diverse and the styles of teaching need to vary. Diversifying university student cohorts produces new income sources, provides a more highly educated and skilled workforce and works towards social fairness. Challenges to overcome are pressure to increase student support services and diversification of learning and teaching materials.

Diverse student populations

Widening participation and access policies have changed global nursing student cohorts. There are various entry points to study. Younger students can complete foundational nursing courses whilst completing high school, learners arrive with prior experience in nursing and some nursing students are graduates from other disciplines. A global "user pays" culture means students are conscious of fees, have an expectation of a "service" provided by university staff and may incur financial burden if they do not succeed in their studies. The widened access to university has also meant that people from a variety of ethnic, indigenous, international, social and psychological backgrounds can access study. Because students are increasingly diverse, there is potential that their needs will not be sufficiently catered for at university. Without sufficient supports students may experience stress, which may exacerbate or lead to mental health conditions.

Wynaden et al. (2014) found that university staff struggle to understand and manage student mental health concerns. Even more concerning, university students and staff remain silent when mental health concerns are identified, perhaps because health professionals presenting with mental health concerns are not always welcomed by healthcare organisations. These attitudes hinder appropriate access and use of supports for students experiencing mental ill health, which only serves to exacerbate their challenges. One solution suggested by clinical teachers was for universities to involve all concerned in exploring and implementing positive outcomes for the student (McAllister et al., 2015). Another solution is to introduce education for clinical teachers and students to develop mental health literacy, for teachers to learn and practise low-intensity counselling skills, such as listening, supporting and easing tension, and for both groups to practise self-care and compassion.

Diversity in nursing student cohorts is affected by the increasing global trend to study abroad. International study enhances student understanding of global health and students benefit through increased cultural awareness, and personal and professional growth (Napolitano & Duhamel, 2017). International students, though, experience culture shock, isolation from social and family networks and language difficulties and many suffer additional pressures from families to do well in their studies. On-campus supports for international students such as after-hours activities, academic learning supports and access to technology to facilitate communication with family members are available; however, they may not be sufficient. Clinical teachers are increasingly requesting support in their work with international students to overcome cultural, language and learning barriers in busy clinical settings. Extending the role of culture brokers, already employed to work with international patients, to also support students on placement; university support workers and clinical teachers working more closely together; and the need for more research to understand clinical teacher experiences have been recommended (Lee et al., 2016).

Many contemporary students expect face-to-face teaching and distance education is one option that is becoming more popular. Preparing clinical teachers to understand nuances of distance education is necessary. Learning to reach out from behind teaching platforms to engage and support students in their learning is an example. Nursing students spend limited time on campus, often only to achieve skills competencies prior to attending clinical learning experiences. This limited time impacts student–teacher relationships and poses difficulties identifying students at risk and referral to necessary supports (McAllister et al., 2015). Student supports will need to be offered in a variety of ways, such as through chat functions, text messaging, user-friendly applications for mobile devices, face-to-face virtual technology and 24-hour access to learning materials to ensure equity. Virtual-reality counselling sessions and smartphone apps to access support are becoming more popular in the wider population – universities could follow suit (Firth et al., 2018).

One overlooked component of clinical learning students may not be prepared for is termination of time in clinical settings. Students may suffer anxieties on terminating newly built relationships or may not be able to come to terms with positive or adverse experiences during the clinical learning experience. McAllister (2008) successfully introduced thank you cards for students to learn how to terminate relationships. This solution doubled as an avenue for students to provide constructive and positive feedback to staff. In another project, blogging assignments set by university clinical teachers assisted students to overcome cultural and learning difficulties during clinical practice (Ryan et al., 2017). Similarly, programmes to support international students in terminating study time abroad and preparing to reconnect with home life are now needed (McDermott-Levy, 2013).

Nursing graduates also need to be equipped with necessary skills to work with diverse patient populations. This is one reason why nursing generally benefits from increased participation from students who speak more than one language and represent minority groups. Engaging ethnic nurse clinical teachers from various ethnic and culturally diverse backgrounds, actively recruiting ethnic students to nursing and encouraging them to maintain their ethnic identities have long been suggested (Yoder, 2001).

More recently a move by universities to assess student and clinical teacher cultural competence knowledge and capabilities has emerged. Smith (2018) suggests clinical teachers might undertake a self-assessment of cultural competence before also quizzing students about their diverse backgrounds and their understanding and awareness of other cultures. This information could then inform meaningful educational activities, before assessing cultural competence. As previously mentioned, host organisational staff are requesting supports for working with diverse populations, indicating there may be a need for universities to design similar professional development to support these clinical teachers.

Clinical teachers need to value diversity in nursing cohorts, including advocating for student learning needs. This creates tensions of another nature. Ryan and McAllister (2019) reported on clinical teacher experiences in which health organisations and clinical staff, who are unfamiliar or doubt the benefit of the clinical teaching role, can sometimes undermine clinical teachers, which in turn creates stress and role conflict. Role complexity in the role is a known long-standing challenge.

Complexity in the clinical teaching role

Clinical teachers multi-task and thus their role is complex. They are often working as clinicians for one employer, and as clinical teachers for sometimes several education providers. Consequently, they are often time-poor, have to be aware of numerous curricula and clinical teaching expectations and are expected to also be lifelong learners (McAllister, Oprescu & Jones, 2014). Clinical teaching takes place in many and diverse learning and teaching environments, including at the bedside, in lecture rooms, corridors, laboratories and online. Not surprisingly, clinical teachers often experience role conflict and overload. There are many demands placed upon them and sometimes these are competing. To succeed in the role, they need preparation, realistic expectations and understanding of how to deal with role challenges.

Addressing role complexities and role stress

Ideally, a clinical teacher of nursing is engaged in two simultaneous pursuits – facilitation of an individual's nursing competence and advancement of the profession. These two aspects of the role are summarised in Table 11.1.

With an appreciation of these two levels of responsibilities the clinical teacher may begin to work towards preventing and resolving role tensions. One way to do this is for the

Table 11.1 Components of the clinical teaching role

Role	Description
Facilitator of learning	Assessor/examiner
	Classroom teacher
	Clinician
	Pastoral carer
	Relationship builder
	Role model
Advancing the discipline	Role model
	Involved in curricula
	Knowledge translator
	Change agent
	Engaged in research

clinical teacher to learn through informal and formal professional development. An example of an informal approach is mentorship by experts in a community of practice (McAllister, Oprescu & Jones, 2014) and an example of formal preparation is for the clinical teacher to study education and educational research.

Articulating a teaching philosophy

In developing realistic expectations of the role, and supporting the likelihood for fulfilments and self-efficacy, clinical teachers benefit from articulating their teaching philosophy. This is a statement about beliefs and practices in the role. Ability to articulate a belief system may provide the clinical teacher with the confidence to guide clinical teaching practice across diverse settings and interactions with students.

There are many philosophies of teaching that have developed over the years. Three belief systems influential in clinical learning drawing from psychology include: humanistic education, applying the work of Carl Rogers; behaviourist education, applying the work of Skinner; and social constructivist education, applying the work of Vygotsky (Elias & Merriam, 2005).

Humanistic approaches to learning prioritise and validate the learner's needs. When students' individual learning objectives are given priority over the learning outcomes of the curriculum and when patients are nursed holistically this is humanism at play. An example of a clinical teacher enacting this philosophy is when he or she finds out who each of the students are, what their goals, needs and strengths are and then works closely with them, with direct and indirect support, to meet those expectations.

Behaviourist education is the belief that learning is enhanced when it is reinforced. An example of this in action clinically is when students are praised for competence and reminded to observe behaviours of role models. Behaviourism is at play when clinical teachers support students to learn and apply principles of asepsis, as in performing wound dressings. Clinical teachers also need to support students to understand their emotions affecting behaviours; for instance, overcoming fear associated with experiencing a patient death for the first time. Behaviourism supports learners to learn when to implement deliberate actions through repetition and desirable outcomes.

Social constructivist learning is when students are supported by clinical teachers and peers to develop knowledge and appropriate action, moving from where they are presently to where they need to go professionally. This can be facilitated by gently interrupting behaviours that are not appropriate from an expert's point of view (McAllister, Tower & Walker, 2007) and when learners are facilitated to grow through a community of practice. In this context, learning is collaborative, peer-led and relies on individuals engaging in social interactions with others in a knowledge community. Online learning communities such as N2E (McAllister, Oprescu & Jones, 2014) are examples.

Because clinical education is experiential, Kolb's (1984) theory of learning in action is relevant. In this model, students are expected to acquire clinical knowledge, take action and then review the effectiveness of that action. In addition, some educators might value the importance of critical reflection (Brookfield, 2005), which involves deeply reconsidering clinical actions in order to bring about change, and not just repetition. Understanding, for instance, that there is tension between a nursing value of nurturing others and a teaching value of making objective judgements about level of competence in the other (as learner) may trigger thinking on ways to resolve this tension by becoming both nurturing and critical.

Two nursing theories of knowledge relevant to enhance a clinical teacher's philosophy are the work of Carper and Benner. Carper (1978) developed the idea that there are four unique ways of knowing in nursing, differentiating personal, empirical, ethical and aesthetic ways of knowing. These provide identity and purpose for nurses. Personal knowing is the knowledge developed from our own life experiences, observation and reflection that help us to know the world. It is important for establishing personal, professional and therapeutic relationships. Empirical knowledge draws upon research and evidence and comprises the science of nursing. Codes of ethics, professional conduct and practice standards help to guide nurses in making everyday moral and ethical decisions. Ethical knowledge then is important in working situations unique to clinical teaching, such as student learning that involves real patients. Aesthetic knowledge refers to how nurses learn and develop empathy, compassion and awareness of individual needs. This is the art of nursing, similar to Habermas' (1968) practical level of knowing, where actions are implemented with a level of sophistication and sensitivity that comes about through observation of expert others, and the application of compassion and empathy.

Patricia Benner's (1984) influential work tracking the development of a nurse, *From Novice to Expert*, is also applicable to clinical learning. Novices may learn through recitation of rules and being challenged to articulate principles prior to action. As they develop in proficiency they move towards a level of expertise, where knowledge, such as timing, sensitivity and compassion, has become engrained and implicit in their actions. To facilitate student clinical learning clinical teachers will also need to understand signature pedagogy.

Signature pedagogies in clinical teaching

Signature pedagogy is a term used to describe fitting teaching approaches specific to a discipline (Shulman, 2005). Signature pedagogies that fit clinical teaching are those that work with the time-sensitive nature of student–teacher interactions, clinical contextual issues such as specific health issues, teams and treatments, relevant patient encounters and ways to reflect just prior to, during and following patient care issues. Long lectures, PowerPoints and lengthy Socratic discussions are not applicable in clinical settings.

Nursing theories to inform pedagogy

Some nursing theories are fitting for a clinical teaching pedagogy. These may include grand theories, such as those that seek to explain the whole of nursing, and middle-range theories, which are those that seek to explain nursing actions in certain contexts and provide students with a theory to guide professional action (Table 11.2).

A contemporary pedagogy that may fit clinical education in multi-faceted healthcare services is solution-focused nursing (McAllister, 2006). This approach was developed specifically for the discipline of nursing and elaborates on a strengths-focused assessment and communication approach, arguing that the nursing role mostly concerns the facilitation of patient well-being and adaptation to illness and thus ways to understand and enhance patient motivation and treatment adherence are paramount. Nurses learn to approach the patient as a whole person and to be inclusive of concerns and situations outside of the presenting problem or diagnosis. For example, a person admitted for acute exacerbation of psychosis may also be a yoga instructor and validation of these personal strengths may assist in rapport as well as creating ease throughout the acute phase. This theory offers nurses a way of working with patients, consumers and clients that values both biomedical treatment and well-being.

Table 11.2 A selection of theories for clinical teaching

Grand theory	Application in clinical teaching
Adaptation model Roy Adaptation Association (2019)	In acute crisis, nurses can assist patients to adapt by focusing on homeostasis, coping and maintaining roles and social supports
Human caring theory Watson (1985)	Ten carative factors implemented by the nurse to help patients to meet their basic and complex needs

Middle-range theory	Application in clinical teaching
Interpersonal relations Peplau (1952)	Therapeutic use of self in communicating with a vulnerable patient
Story Smith and Liehr (2005)	Assisting patients to re-story their lives
ComfortKolcaba (1994)	An important part of nursing is to provide comfort and for nurses to be comfortable providing care
Self-reliance Lowe (2002)	Nurses need to support patients to self-care and become self-reliant
Moral reckoning Nathaniel (2006)	Moral and ethical thinking guards against unfairness and harm and assists nurses to understand individual moral stressors
Solution-focused nursing McAllister (2006)	Nurses assess patients' strengths as well as vulnerabilities to be wellness and illness workers

Nurses who learn to manage and understand their own and others' moral and ethical thinking will experience less moral distress. Involvement in practices that prolong life is an example preventing nurses from adhering to personal moral codes, leading to moral distress. Moral distress has been cited as one reason nurses exit the profession. The theory of moral reckoning (Nathaniel, 2006) could also become a signature nursing pedagogy to teach nurses skills in moral thinking.

Emerging theories

Another relevant and emerging theory that may fit clinical teaching is *patient as teacher*. Tredinnick-Rowe (2018) states that learning with and from patients has many benefits: listening to patient experiences may assist students to become more empathic and compassionate and more person-centred, rather than have an orientation towards the system, the disease or the treatment. In some contexts, this pedagogy is working well. For example, recovery mental health camps, where nursing students participate alongside mental health consumers on an adventure camp, focus on an equal relationship, where consumers are leaders and peers (Perlman et al., 2017). This pedagogy is yet to be fully utilised across all care contexts, perhaps because of the long history of patients being seen as passive recipients of care and because of their vulnerable position within the system.

In situ simulation may also be relevant. This is an advancement on traditional clinical simulations where the simulation experience is offered in workplaces. Advantages have been noted, including an increase of skills mastery, because actors and manikins are replaced by authentic patients. Ability to test and fine-tune equipment in authentic settings is another reported benefit (Schofield, Welfare & Mercer, 2018). However, participant stress increased because of the impromptu nature of the simulations and work pressures determined staff involvement and commitment. Sørensen et al. (2017) urged that practitioners must consider risks to patient care and privacy of information.

Just in time learning (JiTL) is a contemporary learning approach encouraging learners to access information in the moment when knowledge is needed. JiTL relies on smartphones and access to the worldwide web through applications such as QR codes. One disadvantage is privacy and confidentiality: patients and staff must first be convinced learners and staff are using smartphones for JiTL purposes (Jamu, Lowi-Jones & Mitchell, 2016).

Mobile learning makes use of a range of devices and wireless links to the internet. Peer- and teacher-led scholarly discussion forums, accessing course content at all times, ease of participation in group assignments and ability for teachers to simultaneously message student cohorts through short message services (SMS) are advantages. Using devices in real-world settings raises infection control concerns. That not all students will have access to appropriate devices and reliable connectivity to the internet must also be considered (Roberts & Williams, 2017).

Clinical teachers are well placed to determine nursing's clinical teaching pedagogy. The sharing of knowledge to develop and evaluate fitting clinical teaching pedagogies is now necessary to advance the profession. With this in mind, the next section introduces inspiring professional development solutions.

Professional development in clinical teaching

When clinical teachers have been appointed to the role without sufficient training, they may feel tentative in their responsibilities guiding and assessing students and experience a conflict between confidence clinically and educationally (Oprescu et al., 2017). Clinical teachers are often appointed to the role without prior training and professional development rarely covers clinical teaching. Given that there are a range of contexts in which clinical teachers work, there is need for professional development to cover a range of topics. Clinical teaching in mental health, working effectively with diverse and minority groups of learners, knowledge translation and change maker practices are recent innovations in the role that clinical teachers now need to learn. In a small study of regional clinicians and clinical educators, Katsikitis et al. (2013) found that teaching and learning methods were rarely offered as topics for professional development, even though clinical teachers would benefit from exploring this. Similarly, when clinical teachers are asked about professional development they feel pressured to prioritise clinical skill development above teaching knowledge (Ryan & McAllister, 2017). Thus there may be missed opportunities in professional development for clinical teachers.

Towards innovative clinical teacher professional development

Innovative professional development activities include the Nurse to Educator (N2E) project. This approach employed transformative learning principles and a community of practice. McAllister, Oprescu and Jones (2014) developed the peer learning virtual community (N2E) to connect clinical teachers and experienced educators so that craft knowledge could be shared. The site is freely available at www.n2e.org.au. This is one of few published evaluated examples of a professional development solution, appreciated by clinical teachers for easy and in-the-moment access to meaningful clinical teaching supports and resources (Ryan & McAllister, 2017). Another unknown is how many clinical teachers prioritise the time to engage with learning educational know-how in this way. Similar but different resources, found on the worldwide web, offer user-pays access to large collections of information, often not suited to time-poor and part-time clinical teachers. Consideration for future funding by professional bodies of freely available sites, such as N2E, for further development is a more attractive solution.

N2E could be developed to store meaningful resources such as self-assessment tools and also provide access to digital media learning and teaching resources. Innovations such as contemporary and insightful apps could likewise be considered. Validated tools for clinical teachers to self-assess required skills sets are helpful for providing direction for professional development (Bengtsson & Carlson, 2015; McAllister & Flynn, 2016). Podcasts are an ideal source of digital media, to inform and guide development and understanding of educational know-how and relevant learning and teaching theories.

Immersive-style learning is here to stay. Aside from learning through immersive simulations, a popular and validated way of learning in health settings, immersive story-telling is emerging as another powerful and compelling way to learn (Arrow, 2019). Immersive story-telling affords learners first-hand experiences, transporting them to situations and encouraging observer connection with those involved. Three hundred and sixty-degree immersive story-telling videos, depicting clinical teachers working in a variety of ways with students, could be developed and uploaded to N2E.

Gaming is another popular innovation in medical education. Gaming is gaining recognition for enhancing individual and group collaboration and problem-solving ability and encourages development of creative and visionary solutions (Schlegel & Selfridge, 2014). However, accessing digital media and sourcing appropriate games, stories and other meaningful self-directed activities requires intrinsic motivation. Some podcasts, for example, are lengthy and it is time consuming for listeners to search for and find appropriate offerings. Besides there is little evidence of evaluation of these resources. One solution is for clinical teachers to be consulted and included in designing professional development courses to suit their needs.

Emergent studies around clinical teaching professional development suggest professional development for this important group of nurse educators is done well when intended target groups are included. Designing and developing professional development with rather than for intended groups results in more meaningful professional development (McAllister et al., 2013). Education providers could liaise, for instance, with healthcare organisations and clinical teachers to collaborate on the design and development of bespoke clinical teacher professional development curricula. In countries such as Australia, where educational qualifications are not required of clinical teachers, such a curriculum could attract academic qualifications. In other countries where clinical teacher certification is a requirement to work in the role, collaboration could inform more relevant and meaningful curricula. Clinical teachers, globally, then will be recognised and suitably professionally prepared and supported for the vital and important role they undertake in educating the next generation of twenty-first-century global nurses.

Conclusion

The clinical teaching role is complex but rewarding. This chapter overviewed the challenges and suggested theories for developing the role and emerging clinical teaching practices and a number of innovations to support professional development. It is recommended that more innovations to support groups of clinical teachers and to evaluate innovations in the role be conducted and reported. Clinical teaching is a recognised subspecialty within nursing and health and thus it needs to be developed through scholarship and workplace support.

References

Arrow M (2019) Immersive Storytelling is everywhere and there's no going back. *The Guardian* Accessed at: www.guardian.com

Bengtsson M & Carlson E (2015) Knowledge and skills needed to improve as preceptor: Development of a continuous professional development course: A qualitative study part 1. *BioMedCentral Nursing* 14(1): 1–7. 2015.

Benner PE (1984) *From Novice to Expert: Excellence and Power in Clinical Nursing Practice*. Menlo Park, CA: Addison-Wesley Publishing Company, Nursing Division.

Brookfield S (2005) *The power of Critical Theory; Liberating Adult Learning and Teaching*. San Francisco, CA: Jossey-Bass.

Carper BA (1978) Fundamental patterns of knowing in nursing. *Advances in Nursing Science* 1(1): 13–23.

Elias JL & Merriam SB (2005) *Philosophical Foundations of Adult Education* (3rd ed.). Malabar: Krieger Publications.

Firth J, Torous J, Carney R, Newby J, Cosco T, Christensen H & Sarris J (2018) Digital technologies in the treatment of anxiety: Recent innovations and future directions. *Current Psychiatry Reports* 20(6): 1–8.

Habermas J (1968) *Erkenntnis und Interesse*. Frankfurt: Suhrkamp Verlag.

Huston CL, Phillips B, Jeffries P, Todero C, Rich J, Knecht P … Lewis MP (2018) The academic-practice gap: Strategies for an enduring problem. *Nursing Forum* 53(1): 27–34.

Jamu JT, Lowi-Jones H & Mitchell C (2016) Just in time? Using QR codes for multi-professional learning in clinical practice. *Nurse Education in Practice* 19: 107–112.

Job Outlook (2019) Nurse educators and researchers [ANZCOID 2542]. Accessed at: https://joboutlook.gov.au.

Katsikitis M, McAllister M, Sharman R, Raith L, Faithfull-Byrne A & Priaulx R (2013) Continuing professional development in nursing in Australia: Current awareness, practice and future directions. *Contemporary Nurse* 45(1): 33–45.

Kell C & Jones L (2007) Mapping placement educators' conceptions of teaching. *Physiotherapy* 93: 273–282.

Kolb DA (1984) *Experiential Learning: Experience in the Source of Learning and Development*. New Jersey: Prentice-Hall.

Kolcaba K (1994) A theory of holistic comfort for nursing. *Journal of Advanced Nursing* 19: 1178–1184.

Lee C, Marandola G, Malla A & Iyer S (2016) Challenges in and recommendations for working with international students with first-episode psychosis: A descriptive case series. *International Journal of Migration, Health, and Social Care* 12(3): 185–193.

Lowe J (2002) Cherokee self-reliance. *Journal of Transcultural Nursing* 13(4): 287–295.

McAllister M (2006) *Solution Focused Nursing: Rethinking Practice*. New York: Palgrave.

McAllister M (2008) Thank-you cards: Reclaiming a nursing student ritual and releasing its transformative potential. *Nurse Education in Practice* 8(3): 170–176.

McAllister M & Flynn T (2016) The Capabilities of Nurse Educators (CONE) questionnaire: Development and evaluation. *Nurse Education Today* 39(Supp C): 122–127.

McAllister M, Oprescu F, Downer T, Lyons M, Pelly F & Barr N (2013) Evaluating STAR–A transformative learning framework: Interdisciplinary action research in health training. *Educational Action Research* 21(1): 90–106.

McAllister M, Oprescu F & Jones C (2014) N2E: Envisioning a process to support transition from nurse to educator. *Contemporary Nurse* 6(2): 242–250.

McAllister M, Tower M & Walker R (2007) Gentle interruptions: Transformative approaches to clinical teaching. *Journal of Nursing Education* 46(7): 304–312.

McAllister M, Williams LM, Gamble T, Malko-Nyhan K & Jones CM (2011) Steps towards empowerment: An examination of colleges, health services and universities. *Contemporary Nurse* 38(1/2): 6–17.

McAllister M, Wynaden D, Happell B, Flynn T, Walters V, Duggan R … Gaskin C (2015) Staff experiences of providing support to students who are managing mental health challenges: A qualitative study from two Australian universities. *Advances in Mental Health* 12(3): 192–201.

McDermott-Levy R (2013) Female Arab-Muslim nursing students' reentry transitions. *International Journal of Nursing Education Scholarship* 10(1): 163–170.

Napolitano N & Duhamel K (2017) Reflections on an innovative approach to studying abroad in nursing. *Creative Nursing* 23(1): 53–57.

Nathaniel AK (2006) Moral reckoning in nursing. *Western Journal of Nursing Research* 28(4): 419–438.

Oprescu F, McAllister M, Jones C & Duncan D (2017) Professional development needs of nurse educators. An Australian case study. *Nurse Education in Practice* 27: 165–168.

Peplau HE (1952) *Interpersonal Relations in Nursing*. New York: GP Putnam's Sons.

Perlman D, Taylor E, Moxham L, Patterson C, Brighton R, Heffernan T & Sumskis S (2017) Innovative mental health clinical placement: Developing nurses' relationship skills. *Journal of Psychosocial Nursing & Mental Health Services* 55(2): 36–43.

Roberts D & Williams A (2017) The potential of mobile technology (#MoTech) to close the theory practice gap. *Nurse Education Today* 53: 26–28.

Roy Adaptation Association (2019) Accessed at: www.msmu.edu/about-the-mount/nursing-theory/roy-adaptation-association/.

Ryan C, Heidke P, Blunt N, Williamson M & Brien D (2017) Blogging: A strategy to engage final year nursing students in reflective practice. *TEXT Special Issue 38: Illumination through narrative: Using writing to explore hidden life experience*. Accessed at: www.textjournal.com.au.

Ryan C & McAllister M (2017) Enrolled Nurses' experiences learning the nurse preceptor role: A qualitative evaluation. *Collegian* 24(3): 267–273.

Ryan C & McAllister M (2019) The experiences of clinical facilitators working with nursing students in Australia: An interpretive description. *Collegian* 26(2): 281–287.

Schlegel EFM & Selfridge NJ (2014) Fun, collaboration and formative assessment: Skinquizition, a class wide gaming competition in a medical school with a large class. *Medical Teacher* 36(5): 447–449.

Schofield L, Welfare E & Mercer S (2018) In-situ simulation. *Trauma* 20(4): 281–288.

Shulman L (2005) Signature pedagogies in the professions. *Daedalus* 134(3): 52–59.

Smith LS (2018) A nurse educator's guide to cultural competence. *Nursing Made Incredibly Easy* 16(2): 19–23.

Smith MJ & Liehr P (2005) Story theory: Advancing nursing practice scholarship. *Holistic Nursing Practice* 19(6): 272–276.

Sørensen JL, Østergaard, D, Leblanc V, Ottesen B, Konge L, Dieckmann P & Van Der Vleuten C (2017) Design of simulation-based medical education and advantages and disadvantages of in situ simulation versus off-site simulation. *BioMedCentral Medical Education* 17(20): 1–9.

Tredinnick-Rowe J (2018) The role of pedagogy in clinical education. In O Bernad Cavero & N Llevot-Calvet (Eds) *New Pedagogical Challenges in 21st century- Contributions to Research in Education* (pp. 269–285). London: IntechOpen.

Watson J (1985) *Nursing: Human Science and Human Care: A Theory of Nursing*. East Norwalk, CT: Appleton-Century-Crofts.

Woods A, Cashin A & Stockhausen L (2016) Communities of practice and the construction of the professional identities of nurse educators: A review of the literature. *Nurse Education Today* 37: 164–169.

Wynaden D, McAllister M, Happell B, Flynn T, Walter V, Duggan, R & Byrne L (2014) The silence of mental health issues within university environments: A quantitative study. *Archives of Psychiatric Nursing* 28: 339–344.

Yoder MK (2001) The bridging approach: Effective strategies for teaching ethnically diverse nursing students. *Journal of Transcultural Nursing* 12(4): 319–325.

12

SIMULATION IN NURSING EDUCATION

Leeanne Heaton, Kerry Reid-Searl and Rachelle Cole

Introduction

Simulation is an educational strategy where elements of the real world are integrated to achieve specific goals relating to learning or evaluation (Arthur, Kable & Levett-Jones, 2010). The aim of simulation is to bridge the gap between theoretical knowledge and the practical application of the knowledge (Eyikara & Baykara, 2017). In healthcare education, simulation allows for aspects of clinical practice to be reproduced in an authentic way (Jeffries, 2007). It is important to understand that simulation is a teaching strategy and is not simply the utilisation of technology in the learning environment. This chapter will present an overview of simulation, including fidelity, modalities, standards, guidelines and frameworks for simulation, phases of simulation, challenges and general tips.

Background of simulation in nursing education

Over the past 50 years, simulation has been used in many forms within nursing education. It has found its place in not only the education of learners, but also in assisting practising clinicians to refine their skills. Simulation is not just about performing a specific task; it has been used extensively to develop a range of other professional skills such as teamwork, time management, self-efficacy, self-awareness, situational awareness, effective communication and decision making (Alinier, 2011; Alinier & Platt, 2014). The modalities used within the simulated clinical setting have developed over time, reflecting the ever-changing complex needs of society (Palaganas, Epps & Raemer, 2014). Anatomically correct models have been used since ancient times and these have allowed learners to obtain a glimpse into the inner workings of the human body. As learners and clinicians often learn different skills in different ways, educators have attempted to create and apply various methods in order to accommodate these needs, such as increasing the definition and complexities of the models. As well as physical models, technology has facilitated the development of three-dimensional models (holograms) and virtual reality (VR) where learners can immerse themselves in a character or role (Foronda, Godsall & Trybulski, 2013; Cant & Cooper, 2014; Verkuyl et al., 2017).

Simulation experiences provide valuable opportunities for learners to:

- be exposed to a realistic environment within the context of a laboratory setting where they can bring together clinical skills, knowledge, communication, teamwork, situational awareness and clinical reasoning
- be exposed to critical clinical scenarios that are time-sensitive
- be actively involved in scenarios involving unpredictable patient deterioration
- make mistakes without causing harm to real patients and learn from those mistakes
- have the opportunity to repeat practice
- be involved in debriefs and then reflect on practice
- be provided with immediate feedback
- be exposed to scenarios that can address priority areas in patient safety (Arthur et al., 2010).

Fidelity in simulation

Fidelity simply means how authentic or life-like the manikin and/or the simulation is and how accurately the modality reflects a real-life situation or scenario (Arthur et al., 2010). The higher the fidelity, the higher the level of realism. Fidelity is an outcome of a collection of factors that come together in simulation to create realism and authenticity (Bussard, 2015). Using the term fidelity in relation to technology negates the contribution of other simulation modalities such as the use of simulated patients (Bussard, 2015). Fidelity can be broken down in to subcategories: low, medium and high.

Low fidelity

Low-fidelity simulation experiences include those that are often static and lack realism and/or situational context (Bogossian et al., 2018). There is a perception that low-fidelity simulation is not as valued as a teaching strategy; however, low-fidelity simulations have many positive outcomes for learners and are commonly used as a means of increasing the confidence and competence of learners (Pollard & Wild, 2014). Low-fidelity simulation can include simple items targeted at a specific task, such as a cardiopulmonary resuscitation (CPR) manikin, role playing or a model of a wound. These simple simulations allow participation in the activity in order to build confidence in a specific task or technique whilst omitting factors that may occur in real life, such as pain or emotion. For example, a wound task trainer allows the learner to practise the skill of performing wound care without elements such as patient pain or movement. The learner can focus on the skill itself and not necessarily on the management of the whole patient. In this way the learner can build confidence prior to the application of that skill in the clinical environment with other influencing factors such as patient emotions.

Medium fidelity

Medium-fidelity simulation experiences are considered to be more dynamic and realistic than low-fidelity ones (Bogossian et al., 2018). Examples include a full-body manikin with heart sounds, breath sounds and a pulse. Medium-fidelity simulations are often cost-effective and have a lower technological footprint. These elements then allow for additional use with the clinical environment. These situations are best in a higher-resourced environment such as a university clinical learning space or hospital clinical learning centre. Lapkin and Levett-Jones (2011) compared the cost and benefits of using a medium-fidelity human patient simulator compared to a more expensive and technologically advanced manikin. The result of that study indicated that, while the more expensive manikin did have some extra features, it was not necessarily beneficial to assist learners in developing knowledge acquisition or clinical reasoning skills.

High fidelity

High-fidelity simulation experiences are highly realistic and interactive (Bogossian et al., 2018). High-fidelity simulations reflect the conditions and circumstances of real life as accurately as possible. They are often utilised in circumstances where there may be high risk to learners and/or patients in a real setting, such as during a cardiac arrest, rapid deterioration or a difficult birth. Examples include a full-body patient simulator or manikin programmed for multidimensional use (Bogossian et al., 2018). These types of manikins may mimic drug effects and distribution within the body and bodily functions such as bladder control or breath sounds. High-fidelity simulation can also include simulated/standardised patients/Mask-Ed (see later) or VR stations where learners are able to place themselves in a moment that feels realistic with the sights and sounds that may occur in the real clinical environment. One distinct disadvantage of high-fidelity simulations that it exposes learners to situations that may evoke an emotional response and ultimately trigger an emotional impact within the learner, that if not dealt with during debriefing, may carry over to further simulations and ultimately clinical practice. High fidelity is often utilised with experienced clinicians who are more readily capable of making high-impact decisions in an extremely short amount of time.

Different modalities of simulation

There are a variety of different modalities in simulation. In order to determine which modality is appropriate for the simulation, the educator needs to consider:

- the learning outcomes
- the features of the particular strategy/modality/activity that make it best for learning
- the level of the learner
- the level of fidelity required.

Various modalities of simulation are summarised in Table 12.1.

Simulated patient

Simulated patients, sometimes called standardised patients, are usually volunteer members of the community or paid actors who support the education of healthcare professionals. They are provided with a background history of a patient that they will play during a scenario (Keiser & Turkelson, 2017). The use of simulated patients allows for learning on multiple levels. Learners can perform skills such as safe medication administration and procedures. They can learn to improve communication skills, particularly in relation to information gathering and challenging conversations. The benefits of simulated patients are that they are able to respond when asked a question (Slater, Bryant & Ng, 2016). A simulated patient who may be agitated and distressed creates a level of emotion that the learner must work through in order to understand the clinical indicators necessary to assist a person with his or her needs. The use of simulated patients allows for refinement of skill on multiple levels for the learner and decreases the gap between theory and practice.

Table 12.1 Modalities of simulation

Modalities	Key points
Role play	• Easy to organise; participants can take on the role of a patient • Learners can learn from each other
Simulated patients	• Actors or volunteer community members who support the education of healthcare professional learners • Effective for communication and interacting with a patient in a realistic manner
Part task trainers	• Replicate human body parts • Easy to practise skill development
Manikin (human patient simulator: HPS)	• Manikin replicating human body • Easy to practise skill development • Some interactive features such as pulse, respiration, blood pressure, bowel sounds • Able to program for scenario • Can be challenging to suspend disbelief
Hybrid	• Combination of two or more modalities to evoke sense of reality
Virtual reality (VR)/augmented reality (AR), mixed reality (MR) and serious gaming (SG)	• Realistic, exciting, engaging and interactive way of feeling like you are there
Mask-Ed (KRS simulation)	• Educator is there to direct topic
Tag team simulation	• Large number of participants able to engage in learning experience

KRS, knowledgeable, realistic and spontaneous.

Manikin

In many clinical learning spaces around the world, manikins (also referred to as human patient simulators), can be found. Manikins not only vary in price, but also range in capability. Manikins can be utilised to teach a variety of skills, including patient assessment and clinical psychomotor skills, as well as communication and work within the clinical setting (Lapkin & Levett-Jones, 2011).

Part task trainers

Part task trainers are replications of body parts that provide key elements relative to performing a procedure or learning a task. Learners can practise on these replica body parts without causing harm to a real patient. This method is often cheap with the purchase of a piece of equipment that fulfils the need of the completion of a specific task such as CPR or injections. This opportunity allows participants to build confidence and competence in a specific task. This provides a solid foundation for learners to build upon this task by eventually adding in other elements such as an emotional patient who is fearful of needles or a family member nearby watching a loved one undergoing resuscitation. The addition of these elements would lead to a higher-fidelity simulation or hybrid simulation.

Hybrid simulations

Hybrid simulations are simulations that involve more than one type of modality. For example, the learner may commence a scenario with a simulated patient and, as the simulation progresses, the addition of a task trainer may be involved for the application of intramuscular injections. This combination allows the learner to witness the emotion and communication of a live patient, along with the application of a skill within the same scenario. Hence the learner can practise multiple skills within the one setting.

An example of hybrid simulation is the utilisation of a simulated patient playing the role of a patient, and part task trainers (for example, manikin limbs) to address technical needs such as pathology and allow invasive procedures to be performed without risk (Slater et al., 2016). Here the level of technology does not dictate the realism; rather, the interaction provides the enhanced reality (Rutherford-Hemming, Simko, Dusaj & Kelsey, 2015).

One approach that has been taken in hybrid simulation is for simulated patients to wear a tracheostomy overlay system (TOS) to assist in learning how to care for a patient with a tracheostomy. Cowperthwait et al. (2015) described their study where their simulated patients wore the TOS that sits over the simulated patient's torso. Learners were required to provide full airway care and suctioning where the simulated patients were able to respond accordingly if suctioning was performed at too deep a level. The TOS has also been used on manikins, with learners reporting effective learning from the experience (Benito, Martinez & Maestre, 2015).

While hybrid simulation has normally recognised the combination of simulated patient and part task trainer, Vaughn, Lister and Shaw (2016) described how they developed a unique hybrid simulation where learners cared for a manikin while wearing augmented-reality (AR) glasses. Prior to this scenario, the learners watched a brief video of a simulated patient suffering from an exacerbation of asthma symptoms. The AR glasses projected video into the learners' field of vision to provide them with an augmented view of the manikin, assisting learners to think that the manikin was a real person (Vaughn et al., 2016). Another example of AR is the Pokemon smartphone app, where users are able to interact with the small fictional character Pikachu from their phone (Niantic, 2018).

Virtual reality, augmented reality, mixed reality and serious gaming

In recent times, the use of virtual worlds and visualisation technologies has extended the scope of high-fidelity modalities (Chia, 2013; Forneris & Scroggs, 2014;Liaw, Chan, Chen, Hooi & Siau, 2014; Hall, 2015). While technology may provide opportunities to replicate pathology that cannot readily be simulated in healthy individuals acting as patients, technology itself does not equate to authenticity or realism of the encounter. VR uses digitisation to allow users to feel like they are immersed in a situation, as if they are there in presence (Fertleman et al., 2018). AR overlays virtual things into the real world (Zhu, Hadadgar, Masiello & Zary, 2014). Vaughn et al. (2016) described the development of a unique hybrid simulation where learners cared for a manikin while wearing AR glasses. Prior to this scenario, the learners watched a brief video of a simulated patient suffering from an exacerbation of asthma symptoms. The AR glasses projected video into the learner's field of vision to provide an augmented view of the manikin, assisting the learner to think that the manikin was a real person (Vaughn et al., 2016).

Mixed reality (MR) provides the opportunity for the real and virtual world to combine where the user exists in the virtual world (Jadhav & Gonsalves, 2018).

Serious gaming (SG) or digital simulation gives the user an opportunity to provide positive health outcomes in a gaming environment (Wang, DeMaria, Goldberg & Katz, 2016; Fossum, Vivekananda-Schmidt, Fruhling & Slettebö, 2018; Johnsen, Fossum, Vivekananda-Schmidt, Fruhling & Slettebö, 2018). Avatars, or characters that take on human shape, can be used to provide healthcare in a virtual three-dimensional world (Hansen, 2008). SG allows for learning at all times of the day and can often fit around the needs of the learner; however this type of learning also presents challenges. This type of simulation can cause the learner to focus more on the physical needs of a patient as the raw emotion of the patient is less obvious to a learner. Whilst this option is often lower in cost and available to learners simultaneously in a variety of locations, it may not impact on learners as much as when they have a patient physically beside them.

Mask-Ed (KRS simulation)

Mask-Ed (knowledgeable, realistic and spontaneous (KRS) simulation) is a simulation modality that was designed by Professor Kerry Reid-Searl in 2011. Mask-Ed represents masking of the educator and the education process. It involves the educator donning realistic silicone props, including masks, hands and torsos, including functioning genitalia (Reid-Searl, Happell, Vieth & Eaton, 2011). The educator transforms into a carefully designed character who serves as the platform for learning, teaching and coaching. The character is friendly, gentle, vulnerable and wise. The character becomes the coach and direct the learner during the simulation experience through his or her knowledge and wisdom (Reid-Searl et al., 2011).

The KRS component of Mask-Ed (KRS simulation) stands for knowledgeable, realistic and spontaneous simulation:

- Knowledgeable: the educator has a deep understanding of the content being imparted through different learning styles in order to develop strategies to engage the learners (Reid-Searl et al., 2011).
- Realistic: the simulation experience mimics a real situation. The reality comes from the experience of the educator who should have a deep understanding of his or her discipline and the simulation experience (Reid-Searl et al., 2011).
- Spontaneous: the reaction of the character is unprompted (Reid-Searl et al., 2011). However, the character is directed by the educator who is in turn influenced by the learner response. Because scripts are not set, the reactions can be immediate in response to learners. The character spreads the learning through narrative and in-the-moment experiences. The technique is about constructing realities for learners and providing them with practical experiences relevant to their discipline (Reid- Searl, Happell, Vieth & Eaton, 2012; McAllister, Reid-Searl & Davis, 2013).

T= Theatrical, embracing the dramatic contribution of acting to education

A= Applied and directly relevant to clinical practice

G= Guided by a "director" who facilitates the learning experience

T= Tactical, and strategically designed to achieve predefined learning outcomes

E= Engaging through immersions of participants and observers in authentic learning experiences

A= Active involvement in dynamic and unfolding simulation experiences

M= Meaningful, memorable and designed to empower learners to become agents of change

Figure 12.1 Tag team simulation (Levett-Jones et al., 2015).

Tag team simulation

The tag team simulation approach uses applied theatre to engage large groups of participants to engage in a simulation by rotating through a scenario. As one person completes an action, he or she can tag the next person to take up where the scenario ended and continue. The approach is not dependent on specialised simulation spaces or technology (Levett-Jones et al., 2015). Tag team simulation is based upon the tenets of applied theatre (Figure 12.1) (Gervais, 2006), experience-based learning (Boud, 2010), situated learning (Lave & Wenger, 1991) and situated cognition (Brown & Duguid, 1996) as theories that bridge the learning contexts of university classroom and workplace.

Learning theories

Many learning theories are purported to be effective and commonly used when teaching nursing, particularly for assessments; however, learning theories are not necessarily related back to simulation-based education where the majority of studies concentrate more on skill transfer to the clinical setting, patient safety or outcomes (Cantrell, Franklin, Leighton & Carlson, 2017).

In nursing simulation-based education, educators often consider teaching paradigms rather than considering learning perspectives (Kaakinen & Arwood, 2009). Kolb's experiential learning theory has been identified as the theoretical positioning that underpins the pedagogy for simulation in many studies about the use of high-fidelity simulators (Rourke, Schmidt & Garga, 2010; De Oliveira et al., 2015; Bailey & Mixer, 2018; Lavoie et al., 2018; Norman, 2018). Rutherford-Hemming (2012) assessed how the cognitive (Piaget, 1972; Vygotsky & Vygotsky, 1980), social (Bandura, 1977) and constructivist (Papert & Harel, 1991) learning theories fit in simulation.

Lavoie et al. (2018) provided a theoretical review of studies that had proposed theories to explain learning in simulation. The most common theories identified between 1999 and 2015 were the National League for Nursing (NLN)/Jeffries simulation framework (Jeffries & Rogers, 2012), Kolb's experiential learning theory (Kolb & Kolb, 2005, 2009) and Bandura's social cognitive theory of self-efficacy (1977, 1986). The findings of Lavoie et al. (2018) were that there were no validated existing learning theories in the context of simulation.

Standards/frameworks and guidelines for simulation

The expansion of simulation in healthcare education necessitates that individuals who are preparing simulation experiences are educated to do so and follow quality frameworks, guidelines and or practice standards. Educators need to recognise the importance of not only what particular strategy they are choosing, but why they are choosing, it in their teaching. Whilst many publications are in existence, there are some invaluable resources that should be considered in preparing, implementing and evaluating simulations.

The International Nursing Association for Clinical Simulation and Learning (INACSL) has developed *Standards of Best Practice: Simulation*. These provide a process for not only improving the operation and delivery of simulations but also evaluation. These standards include information relating to pedagogy, simulation design, simulation format, needs assessment, objectives, pre-briefing, debriefing, fidelity and facilitation (INACSL Standards Committee, 2016). The *INACSL Standards of Best Practice: Simulation* are considered a living document because additions and revisions are ongoing. To access the standards refer to the following website:

www.inacsl.org/inacsl-standards-of-best-practice-simulation/

In 2005, Jeffries developed a simulation framework that has undergone a number of iterations to now be referred to as the NLN Jeffries simulation theory (Jeffries, 2005, 2007; Jeffries & Rogers, 2012). The concepts behind this theory relate to context, background, design, simulation experience, facilitator and educational strategies, participant and outcomes. More about this theory can be found in Jeffries and Rogers (2012).

In 2010 a team of researchers from the University of Newcastle in Australia developed quality indicators for the design and implementation of simulation experiences (Arthur et al., 2010). The quality indicators are structured under the headings of *pedagogical principles, fidelity, student preparation and orientation, staff preparation and training* and *debriefing* (Arthur et al., 2010). The resource provides quality indicator statements with supporting rationales, as well as guidelines for further reading. The resource is beneficial for educators investing in simulation. The resource can be accessed at the following website: www.newcastle.edu.au/__data/assets/pdf_file/0008/107486/quality-indicators.pdf

A further resource worthy of consideration to support high-quality simulation is the Quality Framework for Simulation Programs in Australian Health Care Settings (QualSim) (Huysmans Raven Consulting Group, 2015). This framework identified eight standards that should be met. These include:

1. a structured program
2. educationally sound
3. clear learning objectives and outcomes
4. appropriate resources, infrastructure and governance
5. qualified personnel
6. based in reality
7. safe
8. evaluated (Huysmans Raven Consulting Group, 2015).

The resource can be accessed at the following website:
https://simnet.org.au/QualSim_Framework_2016.pdf

Phases of simulation

Simulation provides an excellent way for learners to learn; however, there is a need for more than just a simulated experience. There are several phases that need to be moved through in order for the entire simulation to be successful. The Australian National Health Education and Training in Simulation (NHET-Sim) program (Monash University, 2019) refers to six phases (Figure 12.2).

Preparation and briefing

These are the planning phases and help ensure the simulation runs as the educator intends it to (Monash University, 2019). Adequate preparation, including preparatory activities, is essential for successful learner learning and to reduce the risk of cognitive overload (Page-Cutrara, 2015). In preparation, the educator needs to consider the learning outcomes, the type of modality, the level of the learner, the environment and equipment. The creation of realism is important in the preparation. A realistic environment adds to psychological realism as participants gain a sense of the authentic complexities of the situation (Waxman, 2010; Sadideen, Hamaoui, Saadeddin & Kneebone, 2012). Participants should be provided with the opportunity to feel the same perceptions and sensations as they would in a real environment.

Learners need to be provided with adequate preparation to go into a simulated experience, including a briefing about what to expect. They need to be adequately prepared with an orientation to the task, equipment, environment and expectations. Familiarity of the environment, equipment and resources to participants is beneficial to positive patient outcomes (Villemure, Tanoubi, Georgescu, Dubé & Houle, 2016). Briefing sets the scene and provides an

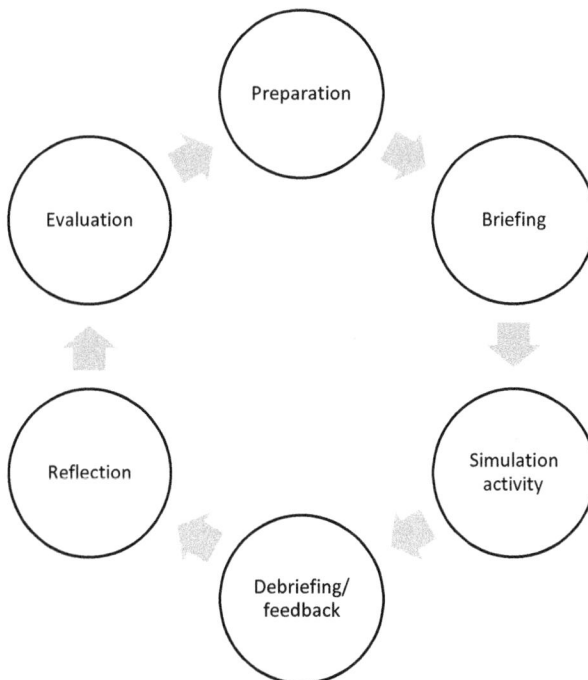

Figure 12.2 Phases of simulation (Monash University, 2019).

opportunity for learners to ask questions they might have, therefore reducing the level of anxiety of the participants. Briefing also provides an opportunity for the educator to guide learners to focus on certain aspects of a scenario that are relevant to the learning objectives.

Simulation activity

This is the do phase, where much of the knowledge is exchanged between participants and the simulation educator (Monash University, 2019).

Debriefing/feedback, reflection and evaluation

These are the review phases. For learners, debriefing/feedback is important for establishing the lessons learnt and reflection helps internalise these messages. For facilitators, evaluation is about identifying what improvements could be made and may involve self-reflection as well as feedback from peers or participants (Monash University, 2019).

> Debriefing after a simulation is a vital element for learning within the simulated session. This is a reflective experience where participants are asked to reflect on the experience they have had during the session. There are multiple debriefing models used including, for example, Pendelton's. Whatever the model chosen, it is imperative that the safety of the individuals concerned is paramount during this process.

Challenges of simulation

Simulation is not without challenges.

Mimicking reality is a challenge

Taking the time to set up and create reality is important in order for the participant to feel an emotional connection in a scenario, with the environment being seen as realistic, because this provides the opportunity for the participant to believe or suspend disbelief (Hamstra, Brydges, Hatala, Zendejas & Cook, 2014; Powers, Navathe & Jain, 2014; Bullock, Lockey & Mackway-Jones, 2015).

Maintaining simulation equipment to be in working order is a challenge

Individuals with technical skills should be employed to manage and regularly service and update the simulation equipment. If simulation equipment is not managed effectively, the equipment will not be used to its full potential, may no longer work due to poor cleaning after an event or may sit on shelves and gather dust. Spaces can become cluttered and disorganised, thus further prohibiting effective and efficient learning within the space.

Anxiety for learners is a challenge

Performance anxiety is well documented in simulation literature (Mills, Carter, Rudd, Claxton & O'Brien, 2016; Al-Ghareeb, Cooper & McKenna, 2017; Mainey, Dwyer, Reid-Searl & Bassett,

2018; Turner & Harder, 2018). Performing in front of peers in a simulated scenario has the potential to put learners in a situation where they feel that they are being judged by their peers (Hemmingway & Fitzgerald, 2016). The fear of being chastised in front of peers, clinicians or other teachers can have an overwhelming effect on performance and emotional factors in novice leaners (Mills et al., 2016). The environment should also be safe for the learner and the facilitator. Educators need to consider that structured preparation is essential for scenarios that may test participant emotions. Roussin, Larraz, Jamieson and Maestre (2018) advocate that, if participants feel safe, they will gain confidence, be prepared to take risks during their learning experience and are much more inclined to actively participate in simulation-based education.

Large cohorts of learners can be a challenge

If simulations are held with large cohorts there may only be a few participants who actually participate from a hands-on perspective and others may become the passive observers of the simulation. Learning may then be lost.

Lack of educator experience is a challenge

If educators do not have experience in preparation, do not consider learning outcomes or choose not to follow guidelines, then the simulation may not be successful as a learning opportunity. If the debriefing is not structured by an experienced facilitator, participants may leave the experience with learning opportunities lost. The participants may also carry this negative experience into their next simulation.

Educator tips

- The learning outcomes for the simulation must be clear.
- The environment must be carefully prepared.
- The modality or combination of modalities selected for a simulated experience must be able to assist the participant in meeting the planned learning outcomes of the activity.
- The financial outlay and maintenance of technological equipment should be taken into account so that equipment is used effectively (Lapkin & Levett-Jones, 2011).
- Educators should maintain training and remain contemporary with the knowledge and skills needed to work in simulation-based education, particularly when it relates to modalities such asVR, AR, MR and SG (Johnsen et al., 2018).

Box 12.1 Important note for educators involved in nursing programmes

Simulated experiences must be scaffolded throughout a curriculum. This may be achieved by embedding simulation within the course units and choosing the most appropriate modality for the year level of the learner to ensure the best learning outcomes. There is little point introducing learners to human patient simulators (manikins) when they may not have learnt a basic psychomotor skill, when a part task trainer could have been used to assist in learning the skill. The learner can concentrate on the required skill, without having to worry about other distractors such as the emotion that can also be experienced if a modality such as a simulated patient is used.

Considerations within the simulation environment

Regardless of fidelity and modality, it is essential that the learning is planned and the environment is resourced sufficiently to ensure that the sessions meet the needs of the learners. In order to prepare the space sufficiently, there are multiple elements to consider. Tips for staffing simulation spaces include the following:

- *Simulation technicians* – Having a simulation technician who understands the value of the session is vital to its success. Simulation technicians should liaise with the facilitator prior to the commencement of the session to ensure that all resources required are adequately prepared. This may include the preparation of manikins, moulage and briefing of simulated patients. The simulation technician provides valuable support to not only the host of the session, but also to learners and the simulated patients.
- *Consideration of skill requirements* – Planning is the key to success within the simulated session. Resources should reflect the desired skills that are being taught within the session to ensure that the learning objectives are met.
- *Professional development* – To ensure that the clinical learning spaces continue to move with the times, it is imperative that staff participating and planning the simulated session continue to develop and refine their understanding and skills associated with simulation. Adequate professional development should be undertaken to deliver the most appropriate education session reflective of the needs of the learners.
- *Portfolio for role* – Simulation technicians and staff who work within the simulated space may have allocated portfolios. This simple allocation ensures continued engagement within the space and allows for staff to develop a particular interest surrounding a simulation element and to share this knowledge with others within this field.
- *Simulation site* (e.g. website, learning management system (LMS)) – These sites allow for resources such as documentation, scenario templates and recipes for moulage to be maintained in one area. This allows staff to explore the various elements and have access to the same information, therefore reducing the risk of a widely varying simulated experience for the learner.

Conclusion

Simulation is an effective and efficient teaching strategy that, when utilised appropriately, enables learners to link theory to practice. Simulation, whilst common within the clinical teaching environment, is an evolving tool that, in order to maintain its effectiveness, must remain contemporary to ensure that learners obtain all the benefits of this positive teaching technique. The creation of a safe learning environment allows participants to make mistakes and the knowledgeable facilitator is able to reinforce the lessons learnt within the simulated space. This reinforcement after debriefing allows learners to take away a lesson from experience rather than from a textbook, and as a result create learning for life.

References

Al-Ghareeb A Z, Cooper S J, & McKenna L G (2017) Anxiety and clinical performance in simulated setting in undergraduate health professionals education: an integrative review. *Clinical Simulation in Nursing* 13(10): 478–491.

Alinier G (2011) Developing high-fidelity health care simulation scenarios: a guide for educators and professionals. *Simulation Gaming* 42(1): 9–26.

Alinier G & Platt A (2014) International overview of high-level simulation education initiatives in relation to critical care. *British Association of Critical Care Nurses* 19(1): 42–49.

Arthur C, Kable A, & Levett-Jones T (2010) Human patient simulation manikins and information communication technology use in Australian schools of nursing: a cross sectional survey. *Clinical Simulation in Nursing* 7(6): e219–e227.

Bailey C A, & Mixer S J (2018) Clinical simulation experiences of newly licensed registered nurses. *Clinical Simulation in Nursing* 15: 65–72.

Bandura A (1977) Self-efficacy: toward a unifying theory of behavioral change. *Psychological Review* 84(2): 191–215.

Bandura A (1986) *Social foundations of thought and action: a social cognitive theory.* Englewood Cliffs, NJ: Prentice-Hall.

Benito A, Martinez A, & Maestre J M (2015) Enhancing participants engagement during teamwork training using hybrid simulators. *Clinical Simulation in Nursing* 11(9): 433.

Bogossian F, Cooper S, Kelly M, Levett-Jones T, McKenna L, Slark J, & Seaton P (2018) Best practice in clinical simulation education – are we there yet? A cross-sectional survey of simulation in Australian and New Zealand pre-registration nursing education. *Collegian* 25(3): 327–334.

Boud D (2010) Locating immersive experience in experiential learning. In N Jackson (Ed.), *Learning to be professional through a higher education e-book.* Accessed at: http://learningtobeprofessional.pbworks.com/w/page/15914981/Learning%20to%20be%20Professional%20through%20a%20Higher%20Education%20e-Book.

Brown JS & Duguid P (1996) Stolen knowledge. In H McLellan (Ed.), *Situated learning perspectives* (pp. 47–56). New Jersey: Educational Technology Publications.

Bullock I, Lockey A, & Mackway-Jones K (Eds.) (2015) *Pocket guide to teaching for clinical instructors* (3rd ed.). Hoboken, NJ: John Wiley & Sons Inc.

Bussard M E (2015) High-fidelity simulation to teach accountability to prelicensure nursing learners. *Clinical Simulation in Nursing* 11(9): 425–430.

Cant R P & Cooper S J (2014) Simulation in the internet age: the place of web-based nursing education. An integrative review. *Nurse Education Today* 34(12): 1435–1442.

Cantrell M A, Franklin A, Leighton K & Carlson A (2017) The evidence in simulation based learning experiences in nursing education and practice: an umbrella review. *Clinical Simulation in Nursing* 13(12): 634–667.

Chia P (2013) Using a virtual game to enhance simulation based learning in nursing education. *Singapore Nursing Journal* 40(3): 21–26.

Cowperthwait A L, Campagnola B S, Doll EJ, Downs RG, Hott N E, Kelly S C, & Buckley J M (2015) Tracheostomy overlay system: an effective learning device using standardized patients. *Clinical Simulation in Nursing* 11(5): 253–258.

De Oliveira S N, Do Prado M L, Kempfer S S, Martini J G, Caravaca-Morera J A, & Bernardi M C (2015) Experiential learning in nursing consultation education via clinical simulation with actors: action research. *Nurse Education Today* 35(2): e50–e54.

Eyikara E & Baykara G Z (2017) The importance of simulation in nursing education. *World Journal on Educational Technology: Current Issues* 9(1): 02–07. Accessed at: https://files.eric.ed.gov/fulltext/EJ1141174.pdf.

Fertleman C, Aubugeau-Williams P, Sher C, Lim A N, Lumley S, Delacroix S, & Pan X (2018) A discussion of virtual reality as a new tool for training healthcare professionals. *Frontiers in Public Health* 6: 44.

Forneris S G & Scroggs N (2014) NLN scholars in residence conduct research on virtual simulation and the clinical faculty role. *Nursing Education Perspectives* 35(5): 348–349. Accessed at: https://search.proquest.com/docview/1609505362?accountid=10016.

Foronda C, Godsall L, & Trybulski J (2013) Virtual clinical simulation: the state of the science. *Clinical Simulation in Nursing* 9(8): e279–e286.

Gervais M (2006) Exploring moral values with young adolescents through process drama. *International Journal of Education & the Arts* 7(2): 1–34.

Hall SW (2015) High-fidelity simulation for senior maternity nursing learners. *Nursing Education Perspectives* 36(2): 124–126.

Hamstra S J, Brydges R, Hatala R, Zendejas B, & Cook D A (2014) Reconsidering fidelity in simulation based training. *Academic Medicine* 89(3): 387–392.

Hansen M M (2008) Versatile, immersive, creative and dynamic virtual 3-D healthcare learning environments: a review of the literature. *Journal of Medical Internet Research* 10(3): e26.

Hemmingway M & Fitzgerald B (2016) Designing effective simulation programs. *AORN Journal* 104(6): 13–14.

Huysmans Raven Consulting Group (2015) *Quality framework for simulation programs in Australian health care settings.* Accessed at: https://simnet.org.au/QualSim_Framework_2016.pdf

INACSL Standards Committee (2016) INACSL standards of best practice: simulation SM simulation design. *Clinical Simulation in Nursing* 12(S): S5–S12.

Jadhav N & Gonsalves F (2018) Mixed reality in healthcare education. *International Research Journal of Engineering and Technology* 5(6): 76–84.

Jeffries P (2007) *Simulation in nursing education.* New York, NY: National League for Nursing.

Jeffries P R (2005) A framework for designing, implementing, and evaluating simulations used as teaching strategies in nursing. *Nurse Education Perspectives* 26: 22–26.

Jeffries P R & Rogers K J (2012) Theoretical framework for simulation design. In P R Jeffries (Ed.), *Simulation in nursing education: from conceptualization to evaluation* (2nd ed., pp. 25–41). New York, NY: National League for Nursing.

Johnsen J M, Fossum M, Vivekananda-Schmidt P, Fruhling A, & Slettebö A (2018) Developing a serious game for nurse education. *Journal of Gerontological Nursing* 44(1): 15–19.

Kaakinen J & Arwood E (2009) Systematic review of nursing simulation literature for use of learning theory. *International Journal of Nursing Education and Scholarship* 6(1): 1–20.

Keiser M & Turkelson C (2017) Using students as standardized patients: development, implementation, and evaluation of a standardized patient training program. *Clinical Simulation in Nursing* 13(7): 321–330.

Kolb A Y & Kolb D A (2005) Learning styles and learning spaces: enhancing experiential learning in higher education. *Academy of Management Learning & Education* 4(2): 193–212.

Kolb A Y & Kolb D A (2009) Experiential learning theory: a dynamic approach to management learning, education and development. In S J Armstrong & C V Fukami (Eds.), *The SAGE handbook of management learning, education, and development* (pp. 42–68). Thousand Oaks, CA: SAGE.

Lapkin S & Levett-Jones T (2011) A cost-utility analysis of medium vs. high-fidelity human patient simulation manikins in nursing education. *Journal of Clinical Nursing* 20(23–24): 3543–3552.

Lave J & Wenger E (1991) *Situated learning: legitimate peripheral participation.* New York, NY: Cambridge University Press.

Lavoie P, Michaud C, Beisle M, Boyer L, Gosselin E, Grondin M, Larue C, Lavoie S & Pepin J (2018) Learning theories and tools for the assessment of core nursing competencies in simulation: a theoretical review. *Journal of Advanced Nursing* 74(2): 239–250.

Levett-Jones T, Andersen P, Reid-Searl K, Guinea S, McAllister M, Lapkin S, & Niddrie M (2015) Tag team simulation: an innovative approach for promoting active engagement of participants and observers during group simulations. *Nurse Education in Practice* 15(5): 345–352.

Liaw S Y, Chan S W, Chen F G, Hooi S C, & Siau C (2014) Comparison of virtual patient simulation with mannequin-based simulation for improving clinical performances in assessing and managing clinical deterioration: randomized controlled trial. *Journal of Medical Internet Research* 16(9): e214.

Mainey L, Dwyer T, Reid-Searl K, & Bassett J (2018) High-level realism in simulation: a catalyst for providing intimate care. *Clinical Simulation in Nursing* 17: 47–57.

McAllister M, Reid-Searl K, & Davis K (2013) Who is that masked educator? Deconstructing the teaching and learning processes of an innovative humanistic simulation technique. *Nurse Education Today* 33 (12): 1453–1458.

Mills B, Carter O, Rudd C, Claxton L, & O'Brien R (2016) An experimental investigation into the extent social evaluation anxiety impairs performance in simulation based learning environments amongst final-year undergraduate nursing learners. *Nurse Education Today* 45: 9–15.

Monash University (2019) *NHET-Sim.* Accessed at: www.nhetsim.edu.au/

Niantic (2018, October 1) *Codename: Niantic occlusion—real world AR occlusion featuring Pikachu and Eevee.* [Video file]. Accessed at: www.youtube.com/watch?v=7ZrmPTPgY3I

Norman J (2018) Differences in learning outcomes in simulation: the observer role. *Nurse Education in Practice* 28: 242–247.

Page-Cutrara K (2015) Pre briefing in nursing simulation: a concept analysis. *Clinical Simulation in Nursing* 11(7): 335–340.

Palaganas J C, Epps C, & Raemer D B (2014) A history of simulation-enhanced interprofessional education. *Journal of Interprofessional Care* 28(2): 110–115.

Papert S & Harel I (1991) *Constructionism*. Norwood, NJ: Ablex Publishing Corporation.

Piaget J (1972) *The psychology of the child*. New York, NY: Basic Books.

Pollard C L & Wild C (2014) Nursing leadership competencies: low-fidelity simulation as a teaching strategy. *Nurse Education in Practice* 14(6): 620–626.

Powers B W, Navathe A S, & Jain S H (2014) Medical education's authenticity problem. *British Medical Journal* 348: 2651.

Reid-Searl K, Happell B, Vieth L, & Eaton A (2011) The educator inside the patient: learners insights into high fidelity silicone simulation. *Journal of Clinical Nursing* 20(19–20): 2752–2760.

Reid-Searl K, Happell B, Vieth L & Eaton A (2012) High fidelity patient silicone simulation: a qualitative evaluation of nursing learners experiences. *Collegian: Journal of the Royal College of Nursing Australia* 9(2): 77–83.

Rourke L, Schmidt M, & Garga N (2010) Theory-based research of high fidelity simulation use in nursing education: a review of the literature. *International Journal of Nursing Education Scholarship* 7(1): 1–14.

Roussin C J, Larraz E, Jamieson K, & Maestre J M (2018) Psychological safety, self-efficacy, and speaking up in interprofessional health care simulation. *Clinical Simulation in Nursing* 17: 38–46.

Rutherford-Hemming T (2012) Simulation methodology in nursing education and adult learning theory. *Adult Learning* 23(3): 129–137.

Rutherford-Hemming T, Simko L, Dusaj T K, & Kelsey N C (2015) What moves simulation? *Clinical Simulation in Nursing* 11(6): 390–391.

Sadideen H, Hamaoui K, Saadeddin M, & Kneebone R (2012) Simulators and the simulation environment: getting the balance right in simulation based surgical education. *International Journal of Surgery* 10: 458–462.

Slater L Z, Bryant K D, & Ng V (2016) Nursing learner perceptions of standardized patient use in health assessment. *Clinical Simulation in Nursing* 12(9): 368–376.

Turner S & Harder N (2018) Psychological safe environment: a concept analysis. *Clinical Simulation in Nursing* 18: 47–55.

Vaughn J J, Lister M J, & Shaw R J (2016) Piloting augmented reality technology to enhance realism in clinical simulation. *Computers, Informatics, Nursing* 34(9): 402–405.

Verkuyl M, Hughes M, Tsui J, Betts L, St-Amant O, & Lapum J L (2017) Virtual gaming simulation in nursing education: a focus group study. *Journal of Nursing Education* 56(5): 274–280.

Villemure C, Tanoubi I, Georgescu M, Dubé J N, & Houle J (2016) An integrative review of in situ simulation training: implications for critical care nurses. *Canadian Journal of Critical Care Nursing* 27(1): 23–31.

Vygotsky L & Vygotsky S (1980) *Mind in society: the development of higher psychological process*. Cambridge, MA: Harvard University Press.

Wang R, DeMaria S Jr, Goldberg A, & Katz D (2016) A systematic review of serious games in training health care professionals. *Simulation in Healthcare* 11(1): 41–51.

Waxman K T (2010) The development of evidence-based clinical simulation scenarios: guidelines for nurse educators. *The Journal of Nursing Education* 49(1): 29–35.

Zhu E, Hadadgar A, Masiello I, & Zary N (2014) Augmented reality in healthcare education. *Peer Journal* 2: e469.

13

EXPLORING ARTS-BASED PEDAGOGIES IN NURSE EDUCATION

The ARTE framework

Trish Hafford-Letchfield, Kate Leonard, and Wendy Couchman

Introduction

The shift towards interest in the arts in healthcare has been concurrent with what we know about the social determinants of health (Marmot, 2010; WHO, 2013). There are many different ways in which this work is described (arts in health, arts for health, arts and health). Active engagement in the arts is not just restricted to benefits for patients and service users but has also been shown to improve care environments with benefits for staff retention and continuing professional development (Hafford-Letchfield & Huss, 2018; Huss and Hafford-Letchfield, 2018). Eisner (2004), an educationalist, asserts that the arts have the power to stimulate creative and intuitive thinking beyond text and talk given how we experience the environment through our sensory system during the lifecourse. This helps individuals to articulate their experiences, to reflect on ambiguities and uncertainties in life and often to challenge and transform long-held feelings and attitudes. In this chapter we refer to the term arts-based pedagogies (ABP), defined as "when a student learns about a subject through arts processes including creating, responding or performing" (Rieger et al., 2016: p. 142). ABP facilitates the integrative and social model of health, and has opened the space for creative arts activities in healthcare education (Couchman et al., 2014). We consider and discuss the potential for introducing and engaging with the ABP in nurse education.

We write from the perspective of our own knowledge and experiences as educators from the UK where we have been utilising novel approaches to education for nursing and social work. This has led us to experiment with the arts as a means of enriching and achieving more critical and activist pedagogies that impact on professional practice (Hafford-Letchfield et al., 2012; Leonard et al., 2016, 2018). Having conducted and evaluated a number of approaches, we will share our own learning and offer the ARTE (activate, research, teach, evaluate) framework. This framework has emerged from our enquiries and helps to conceptualise learning methods which address affective and cognitive domains within holistic approaches. We have found ABP useful for managing the increasing complexity and uncertainty of practice alongside the acquisition of technical knowledge and skills in social work and nursing.

We start by looking at some of the arguments put forward as to why the arts are considered to be helpful to the caring professions, followed by a brief review of some of the key empirical evidence in relation to ABP. We then introduce the ARTE framework and illustrate this through an example from our own practice (Leonard et al., 2013). This chapter will conclude with key points for consideration in developing your own ABP in practice.

Background to arts-based pedagogies

Other chapters in this book have already discussed the impact of unprecedented political and socio-economic challenges on professional education as a result of globalisation, dramatic demographic and cultural transformation, combined with rapid technological advances (Reisch, 2013). In some developed regions of the world, an increasingly austere, market- and individually focused context has influenced the way in which professional education, including nursing, prepares students for their role in delivering quality care (Hafford-Letchfield et al., 2016). Some have observed how these have impacted on the autonomy and creativity of the academy (Giroux, 2011), the nature of nursing scholarship and the educational process itself (McAllister, 2010).

The delivery of a nurse education curriculum has to respond to constantly changing requirements. These emphasise nursing values, attitudes, knowledge and skills prescribed by those responsible for nursing governance. The foregrounding of evidence-based practice, for example, encourages a scientific approach to nursing care. Carper's (1978) classic analysis of patterns of knowing, however, also includes essentials such as "esthetics and the art of nursing", "personal knowledge" and ethics (p. 13). How curricula are interpreted, designed and taught is often left to the discretion of members of the team in the academy.

A key role of the educator is to engage with stakeholders such as patients, service users, carers and educators from practice. Teaching and learning are also not neutral processes. The design, delivery and evaluation of any curriculum tends to reflect the values held by its stakeholders. So whilst curriculum philosophies are rarely made explicit, they may integrate a range of epistemologies (Iwasiw & Goldenberg, 2015). Ironside (2004) and McKie (2012) recognise that, with the increasing amount and complexity of knowledge needed to become a nurse, it is assumed that, if all content is covered, the requisite competent nurse will automatically emerge with the right thinking and behaviour.

Warne and McAndrew (2010) highlight how teaching methods based on these traditionally espoused knowledges have tended towards the didactic and are likely to suppress critical reflection. In order to move away from more didactic approaches (such as traditional long lectures) we need to have a range of pedagogical approaches at our fingertips. This steers away from learners "banking" knowledge which can quickly become out of date in the current context. We need to place more emphasis on developing independent creative practitioners who are capable of problem solving, critical analysis and reflection to manage the "lowlands" of practice and develop professional expertise (Schon, 1991, p. 42). This attention to holistic and flexible learning requires curriculum philosophies that support concepts such as social constructivism which give emphasis to the social, cultural and collaborative nature of learning.

Learning theorists such as Freire (1990) emphasise the political and activist role of the educator in recognising the role of power and social justice in disrupting the taken-for-granted status quo to empower learners in education and to enhance practice. ABP is one method that can be integrated into curriculum models to develop learning across affective and cognitive domains and offer creative opportunities to address the nuanced and complex nature of professional practice (McKie, 2012; Rieger et al., 2016). We now turn to the evidence of ABP as a method to understand and address these issues further.

Evidence for ABP: a short review

Arts-based approaches in education have already been embraced by disciplines such as medicine, the allied professions and social work. Some scholars have attempted to document and capture their impact (Hafford-Letchfield et al., 2012; Lake et al., 2015; Ousager and Johannessen, 2010; Perry et al., 2011). Here we examine the current evidence base for their use in nursing and draw on two significant systematic reviews for a summative review of key messages (Leonard et al., 2018; Rieger et al., 2016).

Measuring the impact of the arts on learning and practice has proved to be varied and complex. Evaluative methodologies suited to understanding subtle and contextually diverse educational interventions have not really lent themselves to scientific and technical measures (Lake et al., 2015). In this real-world research environment, the researcher is often the educator and therefore ethical and epistemological considerations are determined by their role and potential for in situ reflexivity. The value of systematic reviews is to offer some clarity in the definition of "the arts" within professional education; to capture any empirical evidence on its specific impact on nursing and other related professional education; and to consider, identify and evaluate the different approaches to measuring impact on learners. These have addressed, for example, the process of engaging with art; their acquisition of learning, knowledge and skills; and the impact on educators in their delivery of learning and teaching in education.

Rieger et al. (2016) completed a systematic review of the use of ABP with undergraduate nursing students. The objectives of their review were to find out the learners' experience of ABP. The review drew on Bloom's taxonomy (1956) to identify the affective, psychomotor and cognitive domains of learning, and review the impact of learning on competency compared to other forms of pedagogy. Rieger et al. (2016) found a total of 41 studies that met the Joanna Briggs Institute credibility levels, defined as "unequivocal" or "credible". Twenty-one studies used qualitative and 20 studies quantitative methods. The types of ABP illustrated by the studies were: reading, including poetry, writing, theatre, creating and viewing art, "creative bonding" (p. 167) interventions, films, psychodrama, music and song making, story telling and digital story making and photography. Qualitative methodologies used by educators consisted of ethnography, phenomenology, action research, descriptive, text-based or narrative approaches. The quantitative studies included three random controlled trials, quasi-experimental, pre- and post-test or descriptive designs.

The synthesised findings across the studies in Rieger et al.'s review found that ABP had potential for providing cognitive and particularly affective learning opportunities for student nurses. These illustrated a deviation from the transfer of knowledge to independent critical thinking by students which could be transformational. Areas of nursing practice where ABP were used included theoretical and clinical courses covering surgery, pharmacology, concepts of illness, professionalism, communication skills, across hospital and community and adult and child nursing practice. ABP encourages clinical knowledge, personal learning and self-awareness, "relational and reflective capacities" (p. 156) such as empathy and attitudes towards patients, collaboration and ethical and cultural competence for holistic patient-centred practice and creativity and uses experience to develop different ways of knowing, reflecting Carper's conceptual structure of nursing knowledge.

In summary, Rieger et al. (2016) concluded that there were "encouraging preliminary findings about the effectiveness of ABP that can inform educational practice and future research in nursing education" (p. 176).

In the second systematic review, Leonard et al. (2018) included nine studies on the arts in social work education which had an explicit evaluation design from which to draw some reliable conclusions. Thomas and Harden's (2008) thematic synthesis was used to report on the three analytical themes reported in the review: firstly, the exploration and development of links between social work practice at the micro level such as psychological, individualistic and familial perspectives with macro level practice perspectives. These consisted of the understanding of social structures, power, oppression, social justice and social issues and implications for the practitioner's well-being. The included studies involved community action initiatives, peer theatre, drawings, co-productive intergenerational drama and a virtual online literature group using narrative to promote professional growth. These studies also examined social workers' coping mechanisms in circumstances involving political conflict and discourses on inequalities, for example, by including auto-ethnography and cultural theory. These examples illustrated how engagement with the arts facilitated a paradigm shift in knowledge and attitudes and skills which could be applied to social work practice. Each example provided an environment where an arts focus facilitated sustained activities that required the learner to engage in active learning both individually and as part of a group, either face to face or virtually. ABP can facilitate a process of disruption (see Savin-Baden and Wimpenny, 2014: p. 198) which involves "getting it out". This theme suggests that one way in which art works is through the provision of a political vehicle for transforming troubles by healing, solving, reframing, politicising, advocating and mobilising.

The second theme (Leonard et al., 2018) addressed the role of the arts in aspects of partnership working and co-creation of learning. Engagement with the arts enabled transgression beyond verbal reasoning or rationality in participants' learning styles. ABP talked to issues of power, discrimination and equality in learning and identified the value of co-production and leadership by and with service users. Those studies that involved service users reviewed and identified aspects of "recovery" and surprise in being able to tolerate uncertainty in the face of a new experience. Teachers also took risks through sharing power in their own direct participation and being open to the unknown/unexpected. This in turn created a climate in which the feelings and attitudes of the learners were valued. These senses of levelling and participatory styles of leadership were seen to alleviate institutional dependency, a feature of managerialist discourse which is difficult to transcend.

The third theme analysed the specific processes underpinning the designs of the studies in Leonard et al.'s (2018) review to stress the importance of positioning arts-related research philosophically to establish its rigour. The theme spoke to useful typologies from "arts-enquiring pedagogy" to "arts-related evaluation" (see Savin-Baden and Wimpenny, 2014) and described a range in which arts are used. Examples are using ABP as the method or intervention and the use of arts to represent findings.

Leonard et al.'s review contributed to the debate about what constitutes effective evidence on the impact of the arts in social work education. It concluded that the application of research findings in applied contexts such as professional education needs to be supported with evaluation of quality, fitness for purpose and relevance in answering empirical questions about what works in learning and teaching. The studies reviewed drew on a range of disciplines and contributed to some theoretical perspectives on what the arts have to offer in our understanding of social structures, relationships and other cognitive and emotive aspects of our selves. What is more certain is that professionals need creative methods to find creative solutions as well as globalisation of methods to adapt to local circumstances.

In bringing the findings of these two systematic reviews together, a key point to note when developing ABP was the importance of good evaluative design from the outset. Rieger et al. found a need to explicitly address the epistemological and methodological approaches which were absent for over half of the qualitative studies, as was any discussion of the reflexivity of the researcher. This was also evident in quantitative studies where there were concerns about bias; the lack of consistency of the control group led to difficulties in managing variables that impacted on causation arguments for the effect of ABP. Leonard et al. similarly found that the epistemological bases informing the evaluations of specific arts-based methods used were not always attended to and outcomes were hard to establish from some studies. The main differences in the reviews were the attention given in social work education to the wider context for care and the integration of macro and micro perspectives. Secondly, social work educators used ABP to explore potential for collaboration, co-production, with a focus on learner and service users. They also offered insights into the benefits of interprofessional and leadership development and managing personal impacts of practice such as stress and well-being.

Introducing the activate, research, teach, evaluate (ARTE) framework

The ARTE framework is a tool to assist in going forward with ARP in nurse education. The framework has emerged from our own experience of theorising, planning and delivering ABP interprofessionally and uniprofessionally with both nurses and social workers. A summary of the framework is given in Table 13.1, following which we elaborate on each element of the framework and how you might use it.

Activate

This element of the framework refers to the political, activist and social constructivist philosophical approaches relevant to ABP. For example, the arts may be used as a method for learning, such as interacting with the visual arts or digital story telling, where learning results in the generation of an artefact. The arts may also be used as an intervention to impact or unsettle assumptions supporting the status quo.

In the activate stage the nurse educator will be thinking about ABP approaches that encourage active and deep learning and can impact on the affective and cognitive domains of professional practice. If the ABP includes working across disciplines with, for example, a musician or a film maker, then relationship building with an understanding of roles and philosophical, theoretical approaches is important for co-production. Aims and outcomes need to be aligned to any prescribed assessment of the learner (Biggs and Tang, 2011).

Consideration will need to be given to any additional costs that ABP brings. This includes people's time and payment, accessible and suitable venues that fit into everyone's timetable, resources including props, computers, cameras and recording equipment. For example, when Leonard et al. (2016) collaborated together across colleges and social work and applied drama departments a large drama space was needed and drama-gained work experience facilitating learning in the small-group work. We advise that one person leads the project management with timelines for planning delivery and evaluation. These need to be explicit and agreed by everyone.

Table 13.1 Activate, research, teach, evaluate (ARTE) framework for arts-based pedagogy (ABP)

Activate	Research	Teach	Evaluate
Articulate your philosophical approach for professional education and align with expected aims and outcomes for ABP and required assessment. Take up activist role	Ensuring you research the topic sufficiently, to engage stakeholders and collaborative partners. Ensure your ABP is underpinned by theories, pedagogies, methods and a plan for evaluation	Pay detailed attention to managing the process of engaging everybody towards your defined outcomes for ABP	Plan your evaluation from point of activation. Ensure your evaluation is aligned with the expected aims and outcomes of ABP. Consider arts-based method for your evaluation
• Identify stakeholders and partnerships • Resources required • Design with collaboration • Ensure project management timeline	• Locate and disseminate relevant literature • Begin to identify and design your evaluation framework • Put resources in place • Deal with ethical issues and any risk assessments • Obtain stakeholder sign-off	• Conduct learning agreement • Prepare learners with skills to engage in ABR • Foster positive climate for participation • Model risk taking as an educator • Formative review and adapt as required • Anticipate and respond to impact on learners' affect • Give attention to endings	• Consider models of evaluation that address cognitive and affective domains of learning • Include learners and wider stakeholders • Identify target audience for your evaluation findings • Use art as a means of dissemination

Research

Given that ABP can often be open to challenge as an approach to achieve professional nursing outcomes it is important to feel confident about introducing creative methods that may be seen as outside conventional teaching practices. Encouraging independent and critical thinkers who are reflective practitioners is a key argument for ABP. The examples from the review of the evidence in this chapter may provide some evidence to use. However, researching further the ABP the nurse educator wishes to pursue is an important element in presenting a scholarly argument of the pros and cons for the chosen method, intervention, assessment of the learner and style of evaluation. This will contribute to arguments for different types of resources, up-skilling of educators, new collaborations and consideration of timetable variations and is more likely to lead to a successful sign-off by stakeholders. Risk assessments need to be considered, especially for events away from the usual work or academic venues, to ensure accessibility and risk of adverse events. Designing the evaluation using a specified framework also adds to the growing but still limited evidence of what works with ABP in nursing and social work. Ethical considerations include agreement by the organisation and participants to contribute to an evaluation that respects confidentiality and allows dissemination through publication and networking events to share good practice.

Teach

Preparation is essential in designing, planning and evaluating an ABP activity. Having activated and researched these, they can now be embedded into the ABP teaching plan. If all stakeholders are engaged and the project is supported, then the teaching plan for the episode(s) will be designed well beforehand with resources in place and facilitators prepared. If co-production across disciplines is a feature of the ABP, then a specific teaching plan will provide clear roles for each facilitator with timings and purpose. A negotiated learning agreement to provide a conducive inclusive culture is essential and should be agreed beforehand. Information about students with particular learning needs should be integral to the design of the session. For example, how may a student with a hearing impairment interact fully in a drama session or a student who uses a wheelchair access the venue? Formative review of ABP during implementation with co-facilitators and learners will provide opportunities to negotiate and adapt the episode as required. Facilitators can model risk taking in their role and recognise the associated anxieties for students taking a risk to learn a new skill or have a new experience, especially if this to be assessed. These need to be anticipated by the facilitators and contained in a sensitive way. These new experiences may require learning new skills of technology. You also need to take account of the potential emotional impact of an embodied experience of drama, music or art. When the affective domain is evoked facilitators need to demonstrate awareness and empathy throughout and build into the ending of the episode opportunities for learners to reflect on the impact and draw on support from the facilitators as required. Facilitators need to reflect and debrief.

Evaluate

It is important to plan an evaluation that measures the learning outcomes from the point of activating the ABP. Ethical issues continue to need consideration with explicit agreement from the learners and stakeholders for use of a range of evaluation methods, including grades from an assessment, artefacts produced, classroom evaluations, attendance and purposeful focus groups as examples.

One model is Pawson and Tilley's (2000) conceptual model of "realistic evaluation". It can measure affective and cognitive domains as it takes the traditional causal model of inputs and outputs but emphasises the importance of the "real" world to find "ideas which work for certain subjects in certain situations" (p. 215). Designs tend to be formative rather than summative, characterised by greater focus on the underpinning mechanisms leading to, and the context that supports, outcomes. It therefore recognises the political dimensions of evaluation, including the reflexivity of the evaluator who may also be a member of the project team. Kirkpatrick's model (1998) is another potential measure of affective and cognitive domains. Kirkpatrick's model offers a continuum of learning, from learner responses through to changed attitude and behaviours, and impact on the service and service users. This conceptual model assists in the design of tools such as questionnaires, interviews and validated instruments to measure change before, during and after the ABP episode. Both models provide opportunities for consulting a wide range of stakeholders using creative evaluation, such as poetry, presentation of visual arts and artefacts. These products can be useful to gain funding to extend and further evaluate innovative ABP projects. Finally consider how you might use your findings to critique or promote ABP in nurse education.

Using the ARTE framework: a practice example

We now share one of our own case studies to illustrate the ARTE framework (Leonard et al., 2013). As you read through the following details of the case study, you may find it useful to try and identify the different elements of the ARTE framework.

As professionals working in interprofessional education, we introduced music and percussive activities into our curriculum for nurses and social workers engaged in leadership roles and practice/field education. This involved students, service users and academics learning to play a complex traditional piece of Balinese gamelan music led by an external facilitator. The aim was to provide opportunities for more innovative and creative co-produced learning experiences using ABP. The learning outcomes related to students' acquisition of skills and knowledge about critical reflection, collaborative teamwork and participatory leadership which could then be transferred to different settings in health and social care. Gamelan is an ideal medium for music education, providing access to a large number of students with a range of musical ability. A gamelan is a set of percussion instruments traditionally performed in Indonesian ceremonies, the playing of which constitutes a participatory and sociable activity and power relationships involved in the process.

Activate

The gamelan project sought to address the growing body of theory about what constitutes "leadership" in the sector (Hafford-Letchfield et al., 2016) and to highlight the importance of managers and practice educators being able to address these shifts through the development of more distributed or participatory leadership styles. By reflecting co-production in the design and delivery of the curriculum and learning activities, students were given an opportunity to experience teamwork that was truly participative. The literature of distributed and participatory leadership styles cites empowerment as a real substitute for leadership (Boehm and Yoels, 2008). We were focused on the *process* of participation that enables steps to be taken towards achieving stronger relationships of mutual trust with other stakeholders when working towards the same goals.

In UK health and social care, we have experienced numerous examples of public enquiries and media criticism which have promoted blame cultures, thus inhibiting openness, positive risk taking and the ongoing reflection necessary for learning and communicating more honestly. For participation to be enhanced, we placed emphasis on the process of leadership by those responsible for developing others within their practice environments. Potential leaders need to pay attention to how they actually lead, facilitate and promote more effective engagement of those with a direct stake in quality services. Learning about participatory or distributive leadership styles can also build on knowledge of how to promote learning effectively in organisations and within the different partnerships involved. Further, the notion of co-production emphasises the role that service users play in both the consumption and production of public services by highlighting the interdependence of consumer–producer relationships.

Our stakeholders were therefore leaders, educators and service users. As educators, one of our team members was a musician. We capitalised on a small grant from a national workforce development organisation aimed at demonstrating methods for involving service users in professional learning. These resources enabled us to reach out to a local arts-based practitioner to facilitate our gamelan workshops, and to fund the fee for two sessions and travel costs for participants. We had to engage more sceptical colleagues and students with enthusiasm with well-rehearsed arguments about their validity for practice.

Research

The experience of playing gamelan provided a potential metaphorical frame of reference with which to address some of the above learning needs and depart from more habitual schemas for describing and thinking about the different attributes of leading change and leading teams. Our research into the topic showed that, as an art-based method, music provides a particular metaphor within teaching with potential to offer richer insights. Its use had already been evaluated within different educational settings (Fairfield and London, 2003; Moore and Ryan, 2006). These two studies referred to the significance of generating emotional depth within individuals through such musical learning experiences and informed our own ideas of introducing gamelan into the curriculum. Participants did not need to be a musician (in the narrow Western sense) to take part. Music could be learned by ear and parts were simple and easy to memorise, leaving players free to listen to what is going on around them. Basic instructions (when to start, stop, speed up, slow down) are given by musical cues so players know how their part fits with the whole. Complete beginners can quickly learn a basic piece and play in an ensemble for perhaps the first time. With expert guidance, any member of a group could take turns in using all the instruments and lead the rhythm.

We therefore established that the accessible nature of gamelan had the potential to encourage teamwork, through listening and rhythmic skills based on its four basic structural elements (described as the branches, trunk, roots and flowers of the music). Its participatory and collaborative nature offered us great potential for active learning experiences. We were also aware of provoking anxiety associated with a new experience in a pre-mediated and safe teaching and learning environment. Prior to the session, workshop participants were given an information leaflet about gamelan and we encouraged them to ask questions and research its background. All participants gave written consent for us to undertake an evaluation, including filming of the sessions.

Teach

Our teaching plan for the gamelan sessions drew on kinaesthetic (learning by doing), aural and visual methods, as demonstrated in the VARK (visual, aural, read/write, kinaesthetic) learning styles inventory often referred to in pedagogy (Fleming, 2009). It also drew on models of critical reflection and experiential learning (Knowles, 1984), relevant to working in complex change environments common to health and social care. There was a degree of risk taking (as it may not have worked) as well as the extra time and commitment to set up a new initiative and evaluating its effectiveness. We worked through some challenges such as supporting service user and carer involvement and asking students to travel to a different venue for these specific activities. Within the design of the gamelan activity was a structure for identifying and recording any insights and perceptions gained by the students about the relevance of the gamelan experience to their day-to-day learning in the practice environment. This enabled us to evaluate the impact of the activity from a pedagogical standpoint and to help process any significant feelings and emotions that might be released during the activity. As an experiential session, some initial structure was provided through the pre-identification of learning outcomes. These focused on consideration of concepts involved in learning a new skill, such as teamwork, collaboration and creativity and the importance of group dynamics and participation in learning around power, inclusion and involvement. The significance of developing skills that enhanced both distributed and participatory leadership styles underpinned the activity throughout.

Before the sessions, learners were encouraged to recap on some of the topics already covered in their professional programme, such as on experiential learning theories, and the impact of emotions on learning with a view to developing strategies to manage these. The principles of distributed leadership theory and leading teams were also revised. Two gamelan sessions took place. Prior to each was a facilitated "group share" on expectations. Similarly, a full debriefing took place afterwards. Music making was facilitated by an experienced gamelan musician and each session lasted approximately two hours. The participant groups were relatively small due to the size and uniprofessional nature of the two cohorts. As educators, we were naturally apprehensive but modelled our own receptivity to music making by joining in and we drew on encouragement and coaching techniques to ensure that all learners participated.

Evaluate

The whole process, including briefings, debriefing and the music making, was visually recorded by a digital camcorder (we didn't report on analysis of video data). Verbal and informed written consent was obtained in advance and on the day. Participants were asked to complete a questionnaire after seven days and then four to nine months after the event. The questionnaire focused on three key areas: (1) Has any aspect of your experience of making gamelan had a lasting effect? (2) Did the experience of making gamelan contribute anything towards your own development? and (3) What would you say making gamelan has to offer the learning and development of others in health and social care?

Overall, there were 31 completed evaluations. Analysis of these data sources drew on Pawson and Tilley's (2000) "realistic evaluation", as described earlier. Formative processes during the two sessions provided feedback to participants on the progress of the initiative, from people internal to the study in order to make decisions about future action. This suited the qualitative, collaborative and ongoing nature of the gamelan project. This model also allowed the interests of different stakeholders such as service users to be addressed. Thematic analysis was used, given that our data were derived from narrative texts. Thematic narrative analysis offered potential for exploring individual accounts within the social and political context of service delivery and the role of service users. This also related to the background literature and relevant theoretical frameworks. Analysis aimed to keep the feedback from group members intact and in context. Data analysis drew on the content of the facilitated group share that explored expectations, the written evaluations and the focus group discussion at the end of each session. In addition, we observed the video of the session.

When reporting the full evaluation of this ABP (Leonard et al., 2013), we acknowledged our own insider researcher roles. This included the impact the broader social context had for different members of the group and their multiple personal and professional roles outside and within the group, such as student, service user trainer, service user, professional, teacher, and how they made sense of their experiences. Four emerging themes were identified: first, learners' experiences; second, learners' insights; third, reflective learning that engages with emotions; and, fourth, the importance of equality and co-production in learning a new skill. Using ABP proved to be a "great leveller" in achieving more satisfying and effective learning relationships whilst acknowledging the dynamics and power relationships involved in the process.

Conclusion

In this chapter we have endeavoured to convey our own enthusiasm and experience for ABP. As you will see from our ARTE framework, there is much to think about, plan for and review if you use ABP. We have brought together selected evidence from nursing and social work education which does support an argument that using the arts has many positive outcomes. The synthesis of evidence across these two professions also highlights the benefits of interdisciplinary learning for all involved.

We have offered a framework developed from the evidence so far, which can be used to develop the nurse educator's ABP. Having elaborated on what is needed to develop as an arts-based educator, including an example from our own portfolio, we hope that this generates an enthusiasm to innovate in nurse education.

References

Biggs J & Tang C (2011) *Teaching for Quality Learning at University: What the Student Does.* 4th ed. Maidenhead: McGraw.

Bloom, B.S. (Ed.). Engelhart, M.D., Furst, E.J., Hill, W.H., Krathwohl, D.R. (1956). *Taxonomy of Educational Objectives, Handbook I: The Cognitive Domain.* New York: David McKay Co Inc.

Boehm A & Yoels N (2008) Effectiveness of welfare organisations: the contribution of leadership styles, staff cohesion, and worker empowerment. *British Journal of Social Work* 39(7): 1360–1380.

Carper B A (1978) Fundamental ways of knowing in nursing. *Advances in Nursing Science* 1(1): 13–24.

Couchman W, Hafford-Letchfield T & Leonard K (2014) The practice educator as museum guide, art therapist or exhibition curator: a cross-disciplinary analysis of arts-based learning. *Journal of Practice Teaching & Learning* 12(3): 48–61.

Eisner E W (2004) *The Arts and the Creation of Mind.* London: Yale University Press.

Fairfield K D & London M B (2003) Tuning into the music of groups: a metaphor for team-based learning in management education. *Journal of Management Education* 27(6): 654–672.

Fleming N (2009) VARK: a guide to learning styles. Accessed at: www.vark-learn.com/english/index.asp.

Freire P (1990) *Pedagogy of the Oppressed.* London: Penguin.

Giroux H A (2011) *On Critical Pedagogy.* London: Continuum International Publishing Group.

Hafford-Letchfield T, Hirst K & Lane R (2016) *Tetley's Adventures: A Multigenerational Arts Project for People Living with Dementia and Early Years Children: Evaluation Report.* Sussex: Bright Shadow.

Hafford-Letchfield T & Huss E (2018) Putting you in the picture: the use of visual imagery in social work supervision. *European Journal of Social Work* 21(3): 441–453.

Hafford-Letchfield T, Lambley S, Spolander G, Cocker C & Daly N (2014) *Inclusive Leadership in Social Work and Social Care.* Bristol: Policy Press.

Hafford-Letchfield T, Leonard K & Couchman W (2012) Edited special edition 'arts and extremely dangerous', critical commentary on the arts in social work education. Social work education. *The International Journal* 31(6): 683–690.

Hafford-Letchfield T, Leonard K & Couchman W (2018) Arts-based pedagogies in social work education: does it measure up? *Social Dialogue* ISSUE 19 published by The International Association of Schools of Social Work (IASSW). Accessed at: www.academia.edu/36768819/PDF_of_Special_Issue_of _arts_in_social_work_Social_dialogue_magazine_.pdf

Huss E & Hafford-Letchfield T (2018) Using art to illuminate social workers' stress. *Journal of Social Work*. http://journals.sagepub.com/doi/10.1177/1468017318792954

Ironside P M (2004) "Covering content" and teaching thinking: deconstructing the additive curriculum. *Journal of Nursing Education* 43(1): 5–12.

Iwasiw C & Goldenberg D (2015) *Curriculum Development in Nursing Education*. 3rd ed. Boston, USA: Jones & Bartlett.

Kirkpatrick D L (1998) *Another Look at Evaluating Training Programs*. Alexandria, VA: American Society for Training & Development.

Knowles M S (1984) *Androgogy in Action: Applying Modern Principles of Adult Learning*. San Francisco: Jossey-Bass.

Lake J, Jackson L & Hardman C (2015) A fresh perspective on medical education: The lens of the arts. *Medical Education* 49(8): 759–772.

Leonard K, Gupta A, Stuart Fisher A & Low K (2016) From the mouths of mothers: can drama facilitate reflective learning for social workers? *Social Work Education* 35(4): 430–443.

Leonard, K, Hafford-Letchfield T & Couchman W (2013) "We're all going Bali" – utilising Gamelan as an educational resource for leadership and team work in Post Qualifying Education in Health and Social Care. *British Journal of Social Work* 43(1): 173–190.

Leonard K, Hafford-Letchfield T & Couchman W (2018) The impact of the arts on social work education: a systematic review. *Qualitative Social Work* 17(2): 286–304.

Marmot M (2010) Fair society, healthy lives: the Marmot Review: strategic review of health inequalities in England post-2010. Accessed at: www.instituteofhealthequity.org/resources-reports/fair-society-healthy-lives-the-marmot-review

McAllister M (2010) Awake and aware: thinking constructively about the world through transformative learning. In *Creative Approaches to Health and Social Care Education*, T. Warne & S. McAndrew (Eds.). Basingstoke: Palgrave Macmillan, pp. 157–170.

McKie A (2012) Using the arts and humanities to promote a liberal nursing education: strengths and weaknesses. *Nurse Education Today* 32(7): 803–810.

Moore S & Ryan A (2006) Learning to play the drum: an experiential exercise for management students. *Innovations in Education and Teaching International* 43(4): 435–444.

Ousager J & Johannessen H (2010) Humanities in undergraduate medical education: a literature review. *Academic Medicine* 85(6): 988–998.

Pawson R & Tilley N (2000) *Realistic Evaluation*. London: Sage.

Perry M, Maffulli N, Willson S & Morrissey D (2011) The effectiveness of arts-based interventions in medical education: A literature review. *Medical Education* 45(2): 141–148.

Reisch M (2013) Social work education and the neo-liberal challenge: The US response to increasing global inequality. *Social Work Education: The International Journal* 32(6): 715–733.

Rieger K L, Chernomas W M, McMillan D E, Morin F L & Demczuk L (2016) Effectiveness and experience of arts-based pedagogy among undergraduate nursing students: a mixed methods systematic review. *JBI Database of Systematic Reviews and Implementation Reports* 14(11): 139–239.

Savin-Baden M & Wimpenny K (2014) *A Practical Guide to Arts-Related Research*. Rotterdam: Sense Publishers.

Schon D (1991) *The Reflective Practitioner: How Professionals Think in Action*. Aldershot: Ashgate.

Thomas J & Harden A (2008) Methods for the thematic synthesis of qualitative research in systematic reviews. *BMC Medical Research Methodology* 8(45). doi: 10.1186/1471-2288-8-45.

Warne T & McAndrew S (2010) *Creative Approaches to Health and Social Care Education*, T Warne & S McAndrew (Eds.). Basingstoke: Palgrave Macmillan.

World Health Organization (2013) Transforming and scaling up health professionals' education and training: World Health Organization guidelines 2013. Accessed at: www.who.int/hrh/resources/transf_scaling_hpet/en/

SECTION 3

Contemporary issues in nurse education

Foreword: Margaret McAllister

Nursing is a career that can take you all over the world. As such, nurse educators need to understand that students must develop a global, rather than parochial, mindset if they are to deliver care that is empathic, person-centred and effective. WHO (2019) identified the top 10 health issues demanding world attention. All nursing curricula, regardless of country of offer, need to explore them because contemporary nurses are global citizens who can travel, work and make a positive contribution on the world stage. A major issue is to explore climate change, and specifically air pollution because it brings with it the risk of respiratory and heart disease as well as cancer. Another major issue is the rising prevalence of lifestyle-related non-communicable diseases, such as diabetes, cancer and heart disease, which kill 41 million people, at a young age. Cigarette smoking, poor diet and reliance on fast food, lack of exercise and living in polluted environments are practices that have reached all parts of the world. Pandemics, such as influenza and Ebola, which have devastating impacts in countries where vaccines are unavailable, are another vital inclusion in the curriculum for they require nurses to be safe early responders as effective health educators. Issues such as unstable and vulnerable living conditions, antimicrobial resistance, lack of primary healthcare and vaccine avoidance are population health issues about which nursing students need to become key advocates for change. Thus contemporary nursing issues highlight the need for nurses to be equipped with technical and psychosocial as well as social and political engagement skills.

In this section Mzwandile A. Mabhala explains the imperative for the development of the nurse's role in public health. Another contemporary issue, outlined by Helen Allan and team, is the challenges of transition to professional practice that all graduating nursing students face. It is at this time that they are most vulnerable – both to the effects of stress overload and to perceptions of inadequacy. This chapter reports on studies that interpret practices educators can make to support graduate success in their early years of qualified practice.

Helen Allan goes on in the following chapter to detail how these graduates can extend their learning to make a contribution to the knowledge and practice of nursing through doctoral studies. Likewise, Renee Kumpula discusses the facilitators of lifelong learning in graduates, for this key cognitive skill is what will enhance longevity and competence in a nurse's career.

In the twenty-first century, healthcare is assumed to involve biological, psychological, social and cultural interventions to treat illness and promote well-being. Thus, medicine no longer operates in a unidisciplinary way and neither do nurses. Instead, nurses need to learn how to work with health professionals from many disciplines, to understand the different worldviews and to appreciate that complex healthcare challenges require collaboration and communication. Forman and colleagues provide a snapshot of different approaches being undertaken across the world to enhance understanding of interdisciplinary ways of working.

In addition to diverse teams in healthcare, the student population is becoming more diverse. There are many reasons for this, as Rachael Major discusses in the penultimate chapter in this section. She explores the economic and social imperatives driving higher-education changes that are widening access to education, but also constraining ability to respond to specific learning challenges students may have. Rachael focuses particularly on the problem of dyslexia in nursing students. Finally, Gemma Ryan explores the requirements for nurses to practise effectively in the online environment, heralding the reality that nursing practice is becoming borderless.

Reference

WHO (2019) *Ten threats to global health in 2019.* Accessed at: www.who.int/emergencies/ten-threats-to-global-health-in-2019

14

PUBLIC HEALTH IN NURSE EDUCATION

Mzwandile A. Mabhala

Introduction

Making a Difference: Strengthening the Nursing, Midwifery and Health Visiting Contribution to Health and Healthcare (Department of Heath [DH], 1999) expressed the then UK Government's commitment to develop nurses, health visitors and midwives' public health role. It stated:

> Their [nurses, health visitors and midwives] contribution is crucial to high quality care and treatment in the NHS, to the success of health promotion and illness prevention and to tackling inequalities and social exclusion. We want to ensure that nurses know that the value and service they give is appreciated – by the Government, and by the people. We value the contribution of nurses, midwives and health visitors. We want to improve their education, their working conditions and their prospects for satisfying and rewarding careers. We want to expand and develop their roles.
>
> *(DH, 1999, pp. 4–5)*

In 2001 *Shifting the Balance of Power Within the NHS* (DH, 2001b) explicitly recognised nurses, health visitors and midwives as key contributors in public health strategies to reduce the health inequalities. In the same year (2001b), the Chief Medical Officer's annual report identified three major categories in the public health workforce: specialists (people who work at senior strategic and policy level, e.g. public health directors and public health consultants), practitioners (people who conduct operational, face-to-face public health work, e.g. public health nurses and public health managers) and wider workforce (who have or are developing a public health remit as part of their role) (DH, 2001a). It placed the majority of nurses within the practitioner category. In response to this policy shift, there have been attempts to integrate public health concepts within nursing education curricula (Council of Deans of Heath, 2016; Nursing and Midwifery Council, 2018).

Currently, all the UK Nursing Education Curricula claim to be either integrating or using public health principles as their core foundation. The current Nursing and Midwifery Council standards, *Future Nurse: Standards of Proficiency for Registered Nurses* (Nursing and Midwifery Council, 2018: p. 3), state:

Registered nurses make an important contribution to the promotion of health, health protection and the prevention of ill health. They do this by empowering people, communities and populations to exercise choice, take control of their own health decisions and behaviours, and by supporting people to manage their own care where possible.

These key policy documents signify the political commitment in developing nurses' public health role. However, there are limited pedagogical frameworks that provide theoretical explanation on teaching to the discourse on teaching public health within nursing curriculum. Shulman (1986) drew a distinction between curriculum content knowledge, content knowledge and pedagogical content knowledge, arguing that teaching is not just about the knowledge of what to teach (content) or how to teach (pedagogy), but a combination of both what to teach and how to teach it.

This chapter examines pedagogical approaches to teaching public health within the UK pre-registration nursing curriculum. It provides an overview of the policy context that drives the integration of public health principles within the pre-registration nursing curriculum.

Professional knowledge

While there is evidence of high priority being given to what Shulman would call "curriculum content knowledge", which is integrating public health into the nursing curriculum, there is limited evidence of priority being given to developing nurse educators' public health-specific knowledge and the pedagogical approaches to teach it.

Shulman (1986) defines *content knowledge* as the nature and organisation of knowledge in the mind of the teacher, asserting that without good understanding of discipline-specific content, even the most experienced educators lack the capacity to provide additional challenges in the exercises provided to the learners.

In making this proposition Shulman (1986) was influenced by the work of Joseph Schwab, who proposed that content knowledge requires going beyond knowledge of the facts or concepts of a subject. According to Schwab (1964), subject knowledge includes both substantive and syntactic knowledge structures.

Schwab (1964) described substantive structures as the variety of ways in which the basic concepts and principles of a discipline are organised to incorporate its facts (Schwab, 1964; Shulman, 1986, 1987). Schwab and Freeman proposed that the important features of substantive structures are the networks of meaning composed of concepts and the systematic relationships among those concepts (Freeman, 1991; Schwab, 1964). They propose that in these networks of meanings, concepts and the specific relationships among them are components of the different propositions used to describe, explain and predict phenomena (Freeman, 1991; Schwab, 1964).

In contrast, syntactic knowledge structures are the procedures of inquiry for determining the warrant of assertions offered (Freeman, 1991; Schwab, 1964). Shulman (1986) describes the syntactic structure of a discipline as the set of ways in which truth or falsehood, validity or invalidity are established. Schwab (1964) posits that when there are competing claims regarding a given phenomenon, the syntax of a discipline provides the rules for determining which claim has greater warrant. It is the set of rules for determining what is legitimate to say in a disciplinary domain, and what "breaks" the rules. Freeman (1991) posits that educators must not only be capable of defining for students the accepted truths in a domain; they must also be able to explain why a particular proposition is deemed warranted, why it is worth knowing and how it relates to other propositions, both within the discipline and without, both in theory and in practice. To illustrate this point, Freeman (1991) offers the contrast between the literary critic, who must know how to recognise "good" poetry, and the literature teacher, who must know that and in addition how to get students to recognise and understand its "goodness". Following many years of studying groups of educators, Shulman (1986) found that most educators depend on substantive structure of knowledge and never develop a syntactic one.

Pedagogical content knowledge

In recent years there have been a greater recognition of the need to re-examine the approaches to teaching public health within the nursing curriculum. Consistent with Shulman's (1986) concept of "pedagogical content knowledge", educators are calling for ways of "integrating public health into nursing curriculum, which go beyond knowledge of subject matter to the dimensions of subject matter knowledge for teaching that embodies the aspects of content most germane to its teachability" (Shulman, 1986, p. 9).

There have been claims that some conventional pedagogical approaches that are being used to educate nurses for clinical practice are not necessarily compatible with delivery of public health as a strategy to reduce the inequalities in health (McAllister et al., 2006; Nagda, Gurin, & Lopez, 2003; Vickers, 2008). Some are calling for a shift in pedagogical approaches to prepare nurses of the future for their public health role from conventional pedagogies described by Diekelmann (2001) and Ironside (2001) as qualitative, action-oriented and focused on knowledge generation to interpretive pedagogies. Diekelmann (2001) further described them as competency-based and problem-based frameworks and contrasts them with interpretive pedagogies that include narrative, critical, transformative, feminist and phenomenological pedagogies. Diekelmann (2001) asserts that such pedagogies are rooted in a philosophy of teaching and learning where learning is seen as active, reflective and socially constructed.

Several writers attempted to point out subtle differences between conventional and interpretive pedagogical approaches, and identified the following features that distinguished them. First, educators who use conventional pedagogies often worked hard to use learning strategies (e.g. active learning approaches) to make their course interesting for students (Diekelmann & Mendias, 2005). Second, these pedagogical approaches save time and resources and are easy to evaluate (Ironside, 2006). Third, they assume that learning is a rational, orderly and sequential process that leads to gaining of specific skills (Diekelmann, 2001; Ironside, 2001). These features of conventional pedagogies have been criticised for being inadequate in addressing the challenges facing the nursing profession (Allan & Smith, 2009; Brown, Kirkpatrick, Mangum, & Avery, 2008). These authors argued that, for nurses to fulfil their role as public health advocates, they need a complete empirical, ethical and humanitarian commitment to addressing the social justice issues of health inequalities (McAllister et al., 2006; Vickers, 2008).

Several researchers believed that interpretive pedagogies, particularly narrative, critical and transformative pedagogies, contained features that are consistent with the requirement for social justice learning as foundation for public health (McAllister et al., 2006; Nagda et al., 2003; Vickers, 2008). They all suggested that students and educators participating in courses in which interpretive pedagogies are being used tend to shift their attention from focusing on strategies aimed at covering content to engendering a community of learning, whereby educators and students worked collaboratively to transform practice (Brown et al., 2008; Diekelmann, 2001; Ironside, 2001). It was suggested that they tended to make interpretation of the context for learning a central focus.

Ironside (2006) posited that interpretive pedagogies proponents' concerns are how educators and students "read" or interpret what was taught and learned, and with the nature of knowledge and thinking in the context of education. Diekelmann (2001) explained that interpretative pedagogy considered presenting multiple epistemologies (knowledge) and interpretations as central to understanding the nature of experiences. She asserted that within interpretive pedagogies, the focus was on critiquing, examining, exploring and deconstructing the experiences of students for their meanings and learning.

Narrative pedagogy

Diekelmann (2001) describes narrative pedagogy as research-based interpretive phenomenological pedagogy that gathers educators and students into a converging conversation wherein new possibilities for practice and education can be envisioned. In her interpretive phenomenology research Diekelmann (2001) hermeneutically analysed the lived experiences of students, educators and clinicians in nursing education. She found that narrative pedagogy provided the context and processes for the students, educators, and clinicians to explore, critique and deconstruct issues that were pertinent to students' lives. For example, rather than focusing on delivery of content, they considered how the content connected to the personal lives of students. The focus was on addressing the challenges facing contemporary nursing education arising from increasing diversity amongst educators and students (Allan & Smith, 2009; Ironside, 2006); for example, it allowed time for discussing students' personal issues such as students who were living in poverty (Diekelmann, 2001). Major studies found that these issues were a central focus of interpretive pedagogies such as narrative pedagogy, and that they pointed toward the efficacy of creating communities of fairness and respect with limits and boundaries (Brown et al., 2008; Diekelmann, 2001; Greenhalgh-Spencer, 2018; Kirkpatrick & Brown, 2004).

Since Diekelmann's (2001) study was published, narrative pedagogy has been used by several researchers as an adjunct to course content, focusing on processes such as teaching, interpreting, critical thinking and analysing concepts, ideas and situations (Chang, Wu, An, & Zhang, 2018; Fitzpatrick, 2017; Greenhalgh-Spencer, 2018).

Ironside (2003) investigated the extent of narrative pedagogy in classrooms and clinical courses, and found this reflected a shift from thinking as problem solving or an activity to produce a certain product, to thinking as a practice geared toward an engaged understanding of both the context of care and clients' experience of health and illness. Ironside's (2003) work revealed that, because narrative pedagogy attended to students' and educators' sharing and interpreting their lived experiences of learning and practising nursing, it reflected current practice as it was experienced. Ironside (2003) observed that where narrative pedagogies were used, the emphasis shifted from students acquiring an expert's perspective (e.g. the educator's or preceptor's) to the educators, clinicians and students collectively exploring the perspective.

The latest of Ironside's (2006) studies examined the students' experiences in courses in which educators used narrative pedagogy. Ironside's (2006) research found that narrative pedagogies allowed students and educators to collectively engage in dialogue, interpreting the meaning and significance of their experiences in ways that cultivated interpretive thinking (Ironside,

2006). The participants in Ironside's (2006) project explained that, through sharing their collective interpretations, educators and students co-created, negotiated and transformed knowledge, all the while challenging the assumptions underlying nursing pedagogical practices.

The most recent research by Chang Xuejiao et al. (2018) showed that students who participated in narrative pedagogy demonstrated improvement in humanistic aspects of nursing. These include sympathy, respect, protection and care based on the perception of the value of life and nobleness of humanity. Studies found that students develop a sense of responsibility to meet the needs of care receivers, and the rational knowledge of humanitarian belief and value (Chang et al., 2018; Greenhalgh-Spencer, 2018).

A variety of modalities for infusing narrative pedagogy into nursing curricula as a humanistic educational approach have been used. Brown et al. (2008) reviewed the effect of using art, film, music, storytelling and journalling as narrative pedagogical approaches to expand the pedagogical literacy of nurse educators. This review found that the use of film helps to improve learning and effective problem solving, as well as serving as a socialisation tool, helping to establish trust and promoting bonding and fostering personal growth (Brown et al., 2008; Kirkpatrick & Brown, 2004). It was also reported that storytelling as a narrative pedagogical approach created the capacity for developing ethical knowledge in nursing, as well as an understanding of caring and culture (Brown et al., 2008). These findings were resonant with several other studies: for example, Evans and Bendel (2004) conducted an experimental study examining the effect of narrative pedagogy in nursing education on students' ability to move towards cognitive and ethical maturity. Their findings demonstrated that students taught using narrative pedagogy showed slightly more improvement in both cognitive and ethical maturity, compared to those taught using conventional pedagogies (Evans & Bendel, 2004). Narrative pedagogy's ability to move students towards cognitive and ethical maturity made it suited to teaching public health issues of social justice.

Critical pedagogy

Several studies found critical pedagogy to be amongst those that closely suit the requirements of teaching public health as a strategy to reduce the inequalities in health (Mabhala, 2012; Nagda et al., 2003; Zimmerman, McQueen, & Guy, 2007). Critical pedagogy is defined as pedagogy based on critical theory – a movement which seeks to analyse oppressive practices that lead to social inequalities experienced by members of society, especially those who are marginalised (Zimmerman et al., 2007). It keeps at its centre the need to expose and challenge both the overt and covert exercise of domination-subordination in social structures and processes, as part of exploring points of differences and commonality among various social groups (Nagda et al., 2003). Nagda et al. (2003) reported that the focus of critical pedagogy is to analyse social life through a lens of diversity and social justice, and to prepare students to be transformative democratic agents. A premise of critical theoretical perspectives is that power operates across and through all social relationships and organisations (Lynam et al., 2008). The emphasis is therefore on the importance of recognising and taking into account the broader societal context and its impact on local problems as strategies for education and social change are articulated (Lynam, 2009).

In the last 20 years critical pedagogy has begun to make an inroad into nursing curricula (Harden, 1996; Hartrick, 1998; Lynam, 2009; Lynam et al., 2008). It is particularly popular with nurse educators who are interested in promoting social justice through formal education (Harden, 1996; Jackson, 2008). The increased interest in critical pedagogy is believed to be born out of the long history of nurses' – and other clinicians' positioned at the front line of health service delivery – commitment to actively engage in addressing inequalities in health (McAllister et al., 2006). It is believed that critical pedagogy possesses useful strategies for introducing alternative viewpoints on the causes and consequences of health inequalities (Harden, 1996; Hartrick, 1998; Lynam, 2009).

Furthermore, it has been argued that nurses' interest in critical pedagogy reflects the increase in their involvement in the social justice agenda (Lynam, 2009; Lynam et al., 2008). For example, critical pedagogy proposes the need to convey the understanding that the prevalence and incidence of health and social problems are features of societal processes and practices, rather than solely products of biology and personal choice (Lynam, 2009). Such understanding requires health professionals to move beyond downstream patient/client education and behaviour change to upstream interventions that seek to address the social processes and practices that contribute to poorer health profiles (Darbyshire & Fleming, 2008; Lynam, 2009). It also requires nurse educators to assist students to develop the capacity to raise their voices for change, by helping them to ask questions about the assumptions that underpin practice, with a view to engaging with others in processes of reflection on practice (Darbyshire & Fleming, 2008). Critical pedagogy was found to encompass a number of strategies that sought to achieve social transformation at individual and social organisational levels, while also enabling learners to recognise their capacity to effect change (Darbyshire & Fleming, 2008; Lynam, 2009; Nagda et al., 2003).

Critical pedagogy uses Freire's (1972) three strategies to gain access to different points of view, namely, dialogue, conscientisation and questioning. Freire's *dialogical pedagogy*, has been hailed as a key avenue to emancipatory education and creation of a just society (Harden, 1996; Jackson, 2008). Freire (1972) attached enormous weight to the possibilities of education for transforming unjust social relations. Consistent with Freire (1972), nurse educators whose strategies are informed by critical pedagogy seek to instil the belief in students that they are social actors who have the ability, the desire and the opportunity to participate in social and political life. In his own words, Freire stated:

> Men are not built in silence, but in word, in work, in action-reflection. But while saying the true word – which is work, which is praxis – is to transform the world, saying that word is not the privilege of some few men, but the right of every man. Consequently no one can say a true word alone – nor can he say it for another, in the prescriptive act which robs others of their words.
>
> *(Freire, 1972, p. 61)*

Freire's (1972) dialogical pedagogy honours the knowledge, perspectives and experiences of students and educators as central to the education process (Nagda et al., 2003). Freirean dialogical pedagogy is directed toward the empowerment of the silenced and marginalised voices, and examining why these voices have been suppressed (Freire, 1972). Freire's (1972) pedagogy promotes multiple voices whereby students and educators examine their experiences and perspectives in light of those of other people, and in relation to larger public issues and processes of domination and liberation (Nagda et al., 2003). It is believed that such a multiplicity of perspectives under meaningful inquiry can illuminate students' understanding of why privileges and disadvantages are not evenly distributed throughout society, and identify the social orders responsible for social inequalities (Lynam, 2009; Nagda et al., 2003). In this democratic and emancipatory process, students and educators engaged in dialogical pedagogy can become active citizens, challenging injustices both within and among themselves, and in the social world around them (Nagda et al., 2003).

Nagda et al. (2003) indicated that *conscientisation* is foundational to being able to promote a critical perspective. Conscientisation is a strategy that contributes to transformation at the individual level, which they contended is evidenced in an enhanced awareness of the self in relation to others (Nagda et al., 2003: p. 168). It has been proposed that conscientisation creates opportunities for individuals to develop understanding of the experiences of persons in a range of social, usually disadvantaged, positions, in order to foster awareness of the consequences of privilege (Nagda et al., 2003). According to Freire, reflection – self and social – coupled with dialogue can foster a critical consciousness by which students and educators see their experiences situated in historical, cultural and social contexts, and recognise possibilities for changing oppressive structures (Freire, 1972). It has been argued that critical consciousness is not the result of intellectual effort alone; it results through praxis, or the authentic union of action and reflection (Freire, 1972). In Freire's words, "to speak a true word is to transform the world" (p. 60). In *Pedagogy of the Oppressed*, he recommends that students explore interdisciplinary themes of personal and social significance before engaging, ideally, in collaborative, student-led projects to better their lives (Freire, 1972). Viewing society as socially constructed by those with more power, at times against the will of those with less, it seems clear that widening the circle of political deliberation is crucial for constructing a fairer and more just society (Jackson, 2008).

The use of questioning has been recognised amongst the key strategies for nurse educators who employ critical pedagogy (Freire, 1972; Harden, 1996; Hartrick, 1998; Lynam, 2009). In the context of public health nurse education, the questioning relates to ways in which it may extend learners' understandings of inequities in health (McAllister et al., 2006). Questioning is used to prompt them to reflect on assumptions they may hold about persons who are disadvantaged, and to draw attention to both intended and unintended ways such assumptions shape their approaches to the provision of care (Harden, 1996; Lynam, 2009). It has been argued that, when using questioning to foster reflective dialogue, nurse educators can draw attention to conditions that underpin interpersonal struggle or confrontation and begin to make visible learners' points of view and the assumptions that inform them (Lynam, 2009). Arguably, such questioning may also assist learners to become aware of the discourses operating, and to recognise ways particular viewpoints are masked or countered by the dominant discourses and related practices (Lynam, 2009).

Transformative pedagogy

Similar to critical pedagogy, the popularity of transformative pedagogy amongst public health nurse educators relates to increasing acknowledgement that the fundamental causes of inequalities in health are a patriarchal and hegemonic society (Scott-Samuel, 2009; Scott-Samuel & Springett, 2007; Stanistreet, Bambra, & Scott-Samuel, 2005; UK Health Watch, 2005). It is believed that transformative pedagogy in the context of public health is primarily concerned with sensitising students to injustice, oppression, inequality and domination, issues relevant to all health contexts (McAllister et al., 2006). It helps to transform the scientific evidence that society remains unequal and divided along many lines, to make students more open, reflective and emotionally able to change (McAllister et al., 2006; Mezirow, 2003).

Many studies have shown that, for people who are vulnerable by virtue of poverty, social circumstance, ethnicity, gender or illness, it is not just extreme events that oppress them (Krieger & Bassett, 1993; Krieger & Birn, 1998; McAllister et al., 2006). Arguably, for them, inequality is experienced in everyday activities, experiences that are seemingly so mundane that they have become taken for granted and overlooked (Krieger & Bassett, 1993; Krieger & Birn, 1998; McAllister et al., 2006). A transformative pedagogical approach to public health teaching is a commitment to transformation of these taken-for-granted frames of reference, such as political power, orientation, racism, cultural bias and ideology, towards a more just, free and equal society (Fenwick, 2003; Krieger & Bassett, 1993; Mezirow, 2003). Transformative pedagogy uses the same strategies as critical pedagogy – that is, dialogue and conscientisation – to enable learners to recognise their capacity to effect change (McAllister et al., 2006; Mezirow, 2003; Nagda et al., 2003).

Though transformative pedagogy draws on Freire's (1972) concept of conscientisation, McAllister et al. (2006) contend that transformative pedagogy does not simply transmit values, beliefs and solutions to students; it seeks to build critical consciousness, collective identity and strategies for change (McAllister et al., 2006; Vickers, 2008). It is believed that, in order for student nurses to develop critical consciousness of the socially determined inequalities in health, they need to develop knowledge of what Scott-Samuel and Springett (2007) call hegemony; that is, knowledge of how nursing is shaped, constrained or silenced by dominating models of traditional science, medicine, big business, the media and even organisations within nursing itself (McAllister et al., 2006). The goal is for students to develop thinking and communication skills to challenge the tendency of some health professionals to dominate, exclude or disempower clients (McAllister et al., 2006; Vickers, 2008).

This view of conscientisation is supported by other researchers. For example, Vickers (2008) asserts that transformative pedagogy seeks to alter the discourses responsible for repressive and oppressive institutions, by empowering the individual through the process of conscientisation. Belknap (2008) contends that only when students understand and accept responsibility for either maintaining social institutions or causing them to change can there be any hope for social transformation. Furthermore, there is growing evidence that transformative pedagogy creates a learning environment that challenges students and educators to recognise, engage and transform existing health inequities and the systems that produce and sustain the oppression that leads to them (Belknap, 2008; Bountain, 2005; Fahrenwald, 2003). This pedagogical approach is said to respond to the current challenge facing nursing education, particularly in the developed world, where nurses practise within a policy context that emphasises individual responsibility as a basis for the distribution of burdens and benefits, and minimises collective obligations (Belknap, 2008). Nagda et al. (2003) assert that transformative approaches engage students as critical thinkers, participatory and active learners and envisioners of alternative possibilities.

Freirean dialogical education in the context of transformative pedagogy is believed to facilitate reflection-action dynamics (Fahrenwald, 2003). Fahrenwald, Taylor, Kneipp and Canale (2007) describe a set of ground rules for a transformative dialogue classroom as: (1) a commitment to a shared common good that binds the group; (2) a desire to learn, to receive actively knowledge that enhances intellectual ability and the capacity to live more fully in the world; (3) a recognition of the value of each individual's voice; and (4) the classroom is treated as a community where faculty members and students build mutual participation.

Evidence for the effectiveness of transformative pedagogy in facilitating social justice education has been demonstrated in several studies (Bountain, 2005, 2008; Fahrenwald, 2003; Fahrenwald et al., 2007). For example, Nagda et al. (2003) examined the impact of transformative pedagogy on raising students' participation in social justice activities, and found that it increased students' structural attributions for racial/ethnic inequality and socio-historical causation. The course also increased students' action orientation away from individual blaming, to individual action toward institutional targets and societal change (Nagda et al., 2003). Several researchers (Belknap, 2008; Bountain, 2008; Fahrenwald et al., 2007; Vickers, 2008) applied transformative pedagogy to undergraduate nursing programmes, and found that it allowed students to connect with the determinants and consequences of particular disparities, such as differences in chronic disease prevalence that parallel race and ethnic differences, and that it took the student beyond the reflective learning stage to the stage of scientific understanding. They found that principles of transformative pedagogy in the classroom establish a dialogue-based and mutually respectful learning environment that allows free exchange of ideas.

Conclusion

It emerged in this review that teaching public health within the nursing curriculum requires an understanding of the relationship between pedagogy and social justice principles of public health. This created a need to examine professional knowledge frameworks to provide a theoretical explanation of the relationship between content knowledge, curriculum content, pedagogy and professional knowledge.

A review of the literature on pedagogical approaches revealed that conventional pedagogies are not consistent with the requirements for preparing future nurses for their role as advocates for public health as a strategy to reduce inequalities in health. It identified interpretive pedagogies, particularly critical and transformative pedagogies, as more consistent with the requirement for teaching public health. Critical pedagogy was seen as the most appropriate pedagogy to achieve the social justice principles of public health.

References

Allan H T & Smith P (2009) Are pedagogies in nurse education research evident in practice? *Nurse Education Today* 30(5): 476–479.

Belknap R A (2008) Teaching social justice using pedagogy of engagement. *Nurse Educator* 33(1): 9–12.

Bountain D M (2005) Social justice as a framework for nursing profession. *Journal of Nursing Education* 44(9): 404–408.

Bountain D M (2008) Social Justice as a framework for undergraduate community health clinical experience in the United States. *International Journal of Nursing Education Scholarship* 5(1): 1–12.

Brown S T, Kirkpatrick M K, Mangum D & Avery J (2008) A review of narrative pedagogy strategies to transform traditional nursing education. *Journal of Nursing Education* 47(6): 283–286.

Chang X, Wu J, An X & Zhang X (2018) The influence of narrative education on the humanistic caring quality of undergraduate nursing students. *American Journal of Nursing* Science 7(5): 165–168.

Council of Deans of Health (2016) *Educating the future nurse – a paper for discussion our initial views on the key outcomes of future registered nurse education, across all four fields.* Retrieved from London: https://councilofdeans.org.uk/wp-content/uploads/2017/11/Educating-the-Future-Midwife-FINAL-Nov-17.pdf

Darbyshire C & Fleming V E (2008) Governmentality, student autonomy and nursing education. *Journal of Advanced Nursing* 62: 172–179.

Department of Health (2001b) *Shifting the balance of power within the NHS: securing delivery.* London: The stationery Office.

Department of Health (1999) *Making a difference: strengthening the nursing, midwifery and health visiting contribution to health and healthcare.* Retrieved from webarchive.nationalarchives.gov.uk/20120524072447/www.dh.gov.uk/prod_consum_dh/groups/dh_digitalassets/@dh/@en/documents/digitalasset/dh_4074704.pdf

Department of Health (2001a) *Annual report of the Chief Medical Officer 2001.* Retrieved from www.dh.gov.uk/en/Publicationsandstatistics/Publications/AnnualReports/DH_4005607

Diekelmann N (2001) Narrative pedagogy: Heideggerian hermeneutical analyses of lived experiences of students, teachers, and clinicians. *Advances in Nursing Science* 23(3): 53–71.

Diekelmann N & Mendias E P (2005) Being a supportive presence in online course: knowing and connecting with students through writing. *Journal of Nursing Education* 44(8): 344–345.

Evans B C & Bendel R (2004) Cognitive and ethical maturity in baccalaureate nursing students. *Nursing Education Perspectives* 25(4): 188–195.

Fahrenwald N L (2003) Teaching social justice. *Nurse Educator* 28(5): 222–226.

Fahrenwald N L, Taylor J Y, Kneipp S M & Canale M K (2007) Academic freedom and academic duty to teach social justice: A perspective and pedagogy for public health nursing faculty. *Public Health Nursing* 24(2): 190–197.

Fenwick T (2003) Ethical dilemmas Of transformative pedagogy in critical management education: stream 20: activism and teaching. Retrieved from Alberta:

Fitzpatrick J J (2017) Narrative nursing: applications in practice, education, and research. *Applied Nursing Research* 37: 67.

Freeman D (1991) Mistaken constructs: re-examining the nature and assumptions of language teacher education. In J. E. Alatis (Ed.), *Linguistics and language pedagogy: the state of the art*, pp. 25–39. Washington DC: Georgetown University Press.

Freire P (1972) *Pedagogy of the oppressed*. London: A Penguin Book.

Greenhalgh-Spencer H (2018) Teaching with stories: ecology, haraway, and pedagogical practice. *Studies in Philosophy and Education* 38(1): 43–56.

Harden J (1996) Enlightenment, empowerment and emancipation: the case for critical pedagogy in nurse education. *Nurse Education Today* 16(1): 32–37.

Hartrick G (1998) A critical pedagogy for family nursing. *Journal of Nursing Education* 37(2): 80–84.

Ironside P M (2001) Creating a research base for nursing education: an interpretive review of conventional, critical, feminist, postmodern, and phenomenologic pedagogies. *Advances in Nursing Science* 23(3): 72–87.

Ironside P M (2003) New pedagogies for teaching thinking: the lived experiences of students and teachers enacting narrative pedagogy. *Journal of Nursing Education* 42(11): 509–516.

Ironside P M (2006) Using narrative pedagogy: learning and practising interpretive thinking. *Journal of Advanced Nursing* 55(4): 478–486.

Jackson L (2008) Dialogic pedagogy for social justice: a critical examination. *Studies in Philosophy & Education* 27: 137–148.

Kirkpatrick M K & Brown S (2004) Narrative pedagogy: teaching geriatric content with stories and the "Make a Difference" Project (MADP). *Nursing Education Perspectives* 25(4): 183–187.

Krieger N & Bassett M (1993) *The health of black folk: disease, class and ideology in science*. Indiana: Indiana University Press.

Krieger N & Birn A E (1998) A vision of social justice as the foundation of public health: commemorating 150 years of the Spirit of 1848. *Am J Public Health* Retrieved from www.ncbi.nlm.nih.gov/pmc/articles/PMC1508556/pdf/amjph00023-0009.pdf

Lynam MJ (2009) Reflecting on issues of enacting a critical pedagogy in nursing. *Journal Of Transformative Education* 7(1): 44–64.

Lynam M J, Loock C, Scott L & Khan K B (2008) Culture, health, and inequalities: new paradigms, new practice imperatives. *Journal of Research in Nursing* 13(2): 138–148.

Mabhala M (2012) Embodying knowledge of teaching public health. Doctorate thesis. Faculty of education. University of Brighton. Brighton: UK.

McAllister M, Rowe J, Venturato L, Tower M, Johnston A & Moyle W (2006) Solution focused teaching: a transformative approach to teaching nursing. *International Journal of Nursing Education Scholarship* 3(1): 1–13.

Mezirow J (2003) Transformative Learning as Discourse. *Journal of Transformative Education* 1(1): 58–63.

Nagda B. N, Gurin P & Lopez G E (2003) Transfortive pedagogy for democracy and social justice. *Race Ethnicity and Education* 6(2): 165–191.

Nursing and Midwifery Council (2018) *Future nurse: Standards of proficiency for registered nurses*. Retrieved from www.nmc.org.uk/globalassets/sitedocuments/education-standards/future-nurse-proficiencies.pdf

Schwab J J (1964) The structure of the disciplines: meanings and significances. In G.W. Ford & L. Pugno (Eds.), *The structure of knowledge and the curriculum*, pp. 6–30. Chicago: Rand McNally.

Scott-Samuel A (2009) Patriarchy, masculinities and health inequalities. *Gaceta Sanitaria* 23(2): 159–160.

Scott-Samuel A & Springett J (2007) Hegemony or health promotion? prospects for reviving England's lost discipline. *Journal of the Royal Society of Promotion of Health* 127(5): 211–214.

Shulman L S (1986) Those Who Understand: knowledge growth in teaching. *Educational Researcher* 15(4): 4–14.

Shulman L S (1987) Knowledge and teaching: foundations of the new reforms. *Harvard Educational Review* 57(1): 1–21.

Stanistreet D, Bambra C & Scott-Samuel A (2005) Is patriarchy the source of men's higher mortality? *Journal Epidemiology Community Health* 59: 873–876.

UK Health Watch (2005) The experience of health in an unequal Society. Retrieved from www.pohg.org.uk/support/publications.html

Vickers D A (2008) Social justice: a concept for undergraduate nursing curricula? *Southern Online Journal of Nursing Research* 8(1): 1–19.

Zimmerman L W, McQueen L & Guy G (2007) Connections, interconnections, and disconnections: the impact of race, class and gender in the university classroom. *Journal of Theory Construction & Testing* 11(1): 16–21.

15

LEARNING TO KEEP PATIENTS SAFE

Helen Allan, Carin Magnusson and Alison Steven

Introduction

The focus in this chapter is on the experiences of student nurses and newly qualified nurses (NQNs) as they transition into independent practice and their learning from and in practice. In an investigation into NQNs' ability to re-contextualise knowledge to allow them to deliver, organise and supervise care (Allan et al. 2016), Allan et al. (2017) found that NQNs progressively put knowledge learnt in university to work by drawing on interconnected domains of learning, including embodied and emotional knowledge. These projects found that attaining competence during the transition period to confident professional is underpinned by knowledge re-contextualisation (Evans et al., 2010).

Findings from the project which investigated the effects of academic award on registered nurses' ability to re-contextualise knowledge to allow them to deliver, organise and supervise care (Allan et al. 2016), referred to hereafter as Study 1 are drawn on to illustrate arguments in this chapter

Pearson et al. (2010) investigated formal and informal ways pre-registration students, from a range of healthcare professions, learn about patient safety in order to become safe practitioners. This project sought to identify, describe and understand issues which impact upon teaching, learning and practising patient safety in the academic, organisational and practice "knowledge" contexts. The project concluded that a number of tensions and paradoxes exist across the academic, organisational and practice contexts which influence practice learning about patient safety and impact upon students' "emotional safety" for learning (ESFL). This study is referred to hereafter in this chapter as Study 2.

In this chapter, extracts from Studies 1 and 2 are used to illustrate that students and NQNs need emotional safety in order to re-contextualise or learn across knowledge contexts (KCs) – learning is the production of new knowledge, which allows students and NQNs to develop in their journey to independent and competent practice as a registered nurse. The chapter concludes by showing how safe challenge in the clinical learning environment can contribute to the development of a skilled reflective professional.

Workforce changes in increasingly complex nursing teams

The demand for nurses able to manage complex clinical nursing teams is predicted to increase due to an ageing population with more people suffering from long-term, manageable conditions (Shin et al., 2006; Worrell, 2007). Caring for patients with long-term conditions will become as important to the health service as delivering new technological advances (Dawoud & Maben, 2008). However, there are acute nurse shortages globally and, as a result, nurses are increasingly delegating tasks to unregistered healthcare staff due to rising healthcare costs, the need to maximise resources, skill mixes and the general expansion of health workers' roles (Gillen & Graffin, 2010; Weydt, 2010).

To prepare for the rising demand for nursing, the UK Government has said that nurses, equipped with critical thinking skills, will increasingly take up leadership positions to meet these challenges in future healthcare and delegate care to the unregistered nursing assistant workforce. In the UK, this expanded care workforce will comprise the existing healthcare support workers (HCSWs) at different bands of competency, including nursing associates and nursing apprentices. This ambitious nursing leadership agenda will be achieved through a number of policy changes:

- a career framework to retain highly skilled nurses in the workforce (Department of Health [DH], 2007);
- the introduction of all undergraduate pre-registration programmes (Nursing and Midwifery Council [NMC], 2010) which was itself shaped by *Lord Willis' Review of the Future Education and Training of Registered Nurses and Care Assistants* (Health Education England, 2014);
- the latest proficiency and education standards: *Future Nurse: Standards of Proficiency for Registered Nurses* (NMC, 2018a), *Standards Framework for Nursing and Midwifery* (2018b) and *Standards for Preregistration Nursing Programmes* (2018c).

At the heart of these policy strands is the aspiration for nurses who are prepared prior to registration to manage care and lead changes within health services through appropriate delegation and teamwork. Delegation is closely related to other concepts, such as responsibility, accountability and authority (Weydt, 2010). Cipriano (2010) maintains that delegation is an underdeveloped skill among nurses which is difficult to assess as it relies on personality, communication style and mutual respect between the registered nurse and the care assistant.

Theoretical framework: re-contextualisation, emotions and learning and knowledge contexts

In this chapter three theoretical frameworks are synthesised: (1) re-contextualisation (Evans et al., 2009); (2) emotions and learning (Allan, 2011); and (3) KCs (Steven, 2009), to discuss how student nurses and NQNs learn to keep patients safe while feeling safe themselves in their own learning.

Re-contextualisation

The knowledge re-contextualisation perspective introduces fresh thinking about the theory–practice relation by recognising that all the forms of knowledge that come together at the point of registration have been re-contextualised, that is, changed in the move from one context to another (e.g. university, clinical placements) to serve a new purpose. The approach of Evans et al. (2010) concentrates on different forms of knowledge that students learn from and the ways in which these are contextualised and "re-contextualised" in movements between different sites of learning in colleges and workplaces. In Study 2, it was recognised that NQNs continue re-contextualising knowledge during the early days as a registered nurse.

Emotions and learning in nursing practice

Drawing on a psychodynamic theory where emotions are fundamental to all human interaction and contact (Menzies-Lyth, 1970; Fabricius, 1995), Allan (2011) has proposed using a psychodynamic approach to emotional learning in nursing curricula or learning to work with feelings. She suggests that feelings shape learning both consciously and unconsciously in interactions with patients, their families and colleagues. She shows how supervision can assist students to integrate theory and practice through guided reflection on feelings arising from their learning in placements in small-group work with a skilled teacher and/or tutor who works psychodynamically (Allan & Parr, 2010; Allan, 2011).

Learning to work with feelings means that the nurse is aware that, as well as the clinical dimension of delivering care, there are social and emotional processes at work in interactions with patients (and, one could argue, other practitioners) which affect how we feel (Fabricius, 1991a). Sometimes nurses are aware of these feelings and can reflect in action – this means nurses are able to recognise the patient's feelings and their own responses and act appropriately. A concept with some similarities to *reflection-in-action* is "reflexivity" (Iedema, 2011). Unlike reflection-in-action, which is personal, in relation to patient safety Iedema (2011) describes reflexivity as more collaborative in nature, and the "capacity to monitor and affect events, conducts and contexts in situ".

However sometimes nurses can only reflect on action, i.e. after the event, and learn from that reflection to work differently in similar situations in the future. These feelings are frequently buried and, although they shape action, are not processed or learnt from. More worryingly, emotions are frequently buried as there is no one with whom students can easily process them (Fabricius, 1991a, 1991b; Röndahl et al., 2004; Allan & Parr, 2010).

Several studies have highlighted the need for emotions to be managed by students if they wish to "fit" into a clinical placement or ward culture during their often short placements (Levett-Jones et al., 2008, 2009a, 2009b; Pearson et al., 2009; Steven, 2009; Allan, 2011; Steven et al., 2014; Bickhoff et al., 2016; Borrott et al., 2016; Allanet al., 2017). Students become reluctant to rock the boat and learn to manage themselves to fit in; Steven et al. (2014) argue that this arises from a lack of ESFL. Drawing on data from Study 1, a large patient safety education research project (Pearson et al., 2009), Steven expanded her analysis of emotions and identified situations which lacked ESFL (Steven et al., 2014). In later research regarding qualified nurses undertaking continuing professional development Steven identified some core elements of ESFL (Steven et al., 2018).

Knowledge contexts

Steven's work is a further development of these ideas around the interplay between context, here referred to as *KCs*, emotions and learning, where she develops a framework for understanding student nurses' learning in practice as ESFL. Students traverse a series of KCs during their education and, while contexts are sometimes viewed as purely geographical locations, Steven et al. (2014) conceptualise KCs as much more. Drawing on the work of

Eraut (1994), KCs can be identified as pertaining to: *organisational* (health care organisations such as NHS trusts), *academic* (universities or colleges) and *practice* (ward or team level of day-to-day practice) (Pearson et al., 2009; Steven et al., 2014). Although these KCs sometimes share physical locations, they hold different perceptions of what is valuable in terms of knowledge types and ways of working. For example, a healthcare organisational KC encompasses managerial, human resource, work flow processes, policies and so on. This KC could be defined as bureaucratic and concerned with systems, targets and procedures. Thus the organisational KC values knowledge which may partially draw on empirical evidence, but which is legitimised and "verified" through stakeholder support, agreement and consensuses (for example, policies and strategies).

The academic KC is predominantly based in, or informed by, research and higher education and privileges scientific "evidence" and theory based on empirical work (often traditional science) and validated by "experts". The academic KC is underpinned to a large extent by technical rationality (Schön, 1991; Usher et al., 1997; Steven, 2009) and is concerned with imparting "evidence-based" knowledge, theory and techniques. This KC aims to have students reach certain thresholds on qualification – knowledge, theory and technique levels as measured by tests and examinations, and underpinned by "robust" evidence. The practice KC is characterised by traditions, routines and accepted ways of working and values mainly experiential knowledge developed through everyday "doing" and transmitted through working together (Eraut, 1994; Steven, 2009). While the practice KC (and organisational KC, to a certain extent) espouses "evidence-based" practice, the everyday concern within both is "getting the work done" and drawing on what appears to "work". Thus, value is placed on qualitative, narrative "craft" knowledge from both individual and shared practitioner experience (Usher et al., 1997; Steven, 2009). Such knowledge is "validated" by personal and/or group judgement (Steven et al., 2014).

These are of course simplified caricatures of KCs which are highly complex and overlap to some degree in their espousing of the inclusion of differing types of knowledge. KCs can be viewed as socially constructed, perpetuated via language and social practices (Gergen, 2015) and potentially serving multiple agendas. Thus students not only navigate between physical settings (classroom to ward) and social environments (student cohort to ward team), but also between diverse KCs – with their inherent discourses of what is useful or valuable knowledge and consequentially diverse approaches to "practice".

Study 1: re-contextualising knowledge as a newly qualified nurse

In Study 1, into NQNs' experiences of their transition from senior student nurse to registered nurse (Allan et al. 2016), only a few NQNs were able to describe an awareness of their learning. Thirty-three NQNs working in three different acute hospitals in England participated in the study. The nurses were based in general medical, surgical and accident and emergency inpatient wards.

Mostly NQNs described the early months of their registered practice as a "muddle" and a "struggle". NQNs described an almost textbook case of re-contextualisation, for example, knowing the knowledge was there and being able to pull things together from wherever it was stored, while at the same time not necessarily knowing what it is to be a nurse.

Many NQNs found it difficult to identify and access the knowledge that they needed in the early days of practice to organise and delegate care. However, NQNs were able to articulate a perception of things fitting into place, usually after some six months of practice – in other words, a re-contextualising moment, which suggests some resolution to a difficult learning period, which implies new knowledge.

While the re-contextualisation of knowledge may occur over time NQNs identified the stress related to being newly qualified. Furthermore, finishing one's workload on time is contingent upon adequate staffing, which suggests that more learning remains in order for NQNs to feel like an independent and competent practitioner.

This finding conveys how difficult learning is as an NQN. It seems the muddle described by the NQNs is caused by strong emotions arising from the struggle to organise themselves, prioritise care and supervise HCSWs. NQNs learn through the fear of mistakes or the observation of others' mistakes.

Learning through mistakes

The fear of making a mistake is quite striking. Findings from Study 1 illustrate NQNs often perceive fears regarding what could go wrong. However, facing these fears allows NQNs to reflect, and to "step back". Yet this doesn't seem to be an example of re-contextualisation in that reflecting on feelings of fear didn't appear to result in an awareness that such fears are manageable, which would suggest new knowledge. It would appear from these data from Study 1 that re-contextualisation may not always result from reflection as the emotions may not be processed. Somehow the emotions interfere with re-contextualisation. This may be because learning through mistakes evokes emotions which are powerfully uncomfortable and stressful and NQNs may not have any support to process them (Johnson et al., 2015).

The fears observed during fieldwork in clinical areas, followed by informal conversations with NQNs in practice, illustrate how NQNs are often "nervous" of the responsibility embedded within the new role, for example fears that patients will die. Moreover, when NQNs supposedly "learn" through others' experiences this does not necessarily equate with less anxiety. Furthermore, there is no evidence of reflection or re-contextualisation. The NQN in Study 1 who reported feeling unsafe (nervous) had an overwhelming feeling of responsibility, which needed to be borne alone, especially in circumstances where patients had died unexpectedly, with no explanation or context. When knowledge is not re-contextualised and the student and NQN lack the emotional safety to learn (argued here to happen much of the time), the consequences for the learner are potentially further mistakes, further muddling through and huge amounts of anxiety and fear. This, in turn, blocks developing authority, being accountable, finding one's voice as a delegator, developing confidence and competence.

Unsafe learning

Data from Study 1 suggest that NQNs had to learn from negative experiences, trial and error, as well as using untested strategies. Although most of the mistakes recounted by NQNs were minor, there were some examples of more serious mishaps. For example, one event was described by a nurse who had trusted a healthcare assistant to check that the patient going to theatre had the correct name on the wristband, and therefore just signed off the paperwork. While NQNs' learning is invisible, it is generally unprocessed or unreflected upon (Allan et al., 2015, 2016a). However, there is evidence of at least an awareness among mentors and ward managers that NQNs should be supported to learn as they settle into their new roles.

Emotional safety and support

NQNs also described learning through watching how more senior staff performed, explicitly learning in a supportive nursing team. For example, one NQN in Study 1 described a sense of awareness that support is available from nursing team members, both registered and unregistered care staff. When reflection on fear of making mistakes occurs a new awareness based on new knowledge follows.

NQNs also described learning through watching how more senior staff performed, explicitly learning in a supportive nursing team. An awareness of support was not always present in the interview data but, where it was described, it indicates an awareness of emotions in learning on the part of the NQN and shows an ability to re-contextualise learning – as Steven et al. (2014) suggest, an ESFL.

Study 2: emotional safety for learning

ESFL can be described as a "milieu" or ambience in which the learner (student, NQN or nurse undertaking continuing professional development) feels able to question, comment, seek clarification, sensitively challenge and be challenged in a supported, facilitated way without fear of repercussions or penalties (Steven et al., 2014, 2018). Such an ambience of ESFL would also lend itself to the surfacing, discussion and processing of emotions – those of the students and perhaps of others (patients, relatives and other staff). Core elements or mechanisms in the development of ESFL appear to include reciprocity, relevance and inter-activity, which encourage feeling relaxed and safe to discuss concerns, experiences and areas of uncertainty (Steven et al., 2018). We contend that the presence of ESFL may enhance knowledge re-contextualisation (see following sections for illustrations).

Although ESFL may be experienced by pre- and post-registration nurse students (Steven et al., 2014, 2018), it is arguable that pre-registration students feel this much more acutely. Unlike qualified nurses engaged in continuing professional development (who are already professionally socialised), pre-registration students face the complexity of learning to traverse unfamiliar settings, cultures and KCs; working with complex nursing teams; while also learning to work with feelings, undertake critical self-reflection and re-contextualise knowledge. In addition, a series of issues, tensions and paradoxes in nurse education appear to further influence a learner feeling ESFL (Figure 15.1).

Tensions and dilemmas influencing ESFL

Steven (2009) has suggested that students need to believe in the education type or practice they are involved in to maintain motivation. In the academic context, such motivation may be exhibited in a general desire to achieve good grades or do well. Indeed, Dornyei's (2000) student motivation model describes an "actional" phase (e.g. during the course or task) which includes a process of "ongoing appraisal" in which students evaluate a multitude of environmental stimuli as a means of judging and monitoring their progress towards their goal. Likewise in the practice context the student may instinctively wish to "fit in" or "belong". In relation to the organisational context (and dependent on exposure and permissions), students may feel that if they do engage with organisational systems (such as incident reporting) they need to adhere closely to them to follow procedure. These desires to fit in, do well and adhere may be present in and across all KCs to differing degrees and may influence the dilemmas and tensions felt with a knock-on

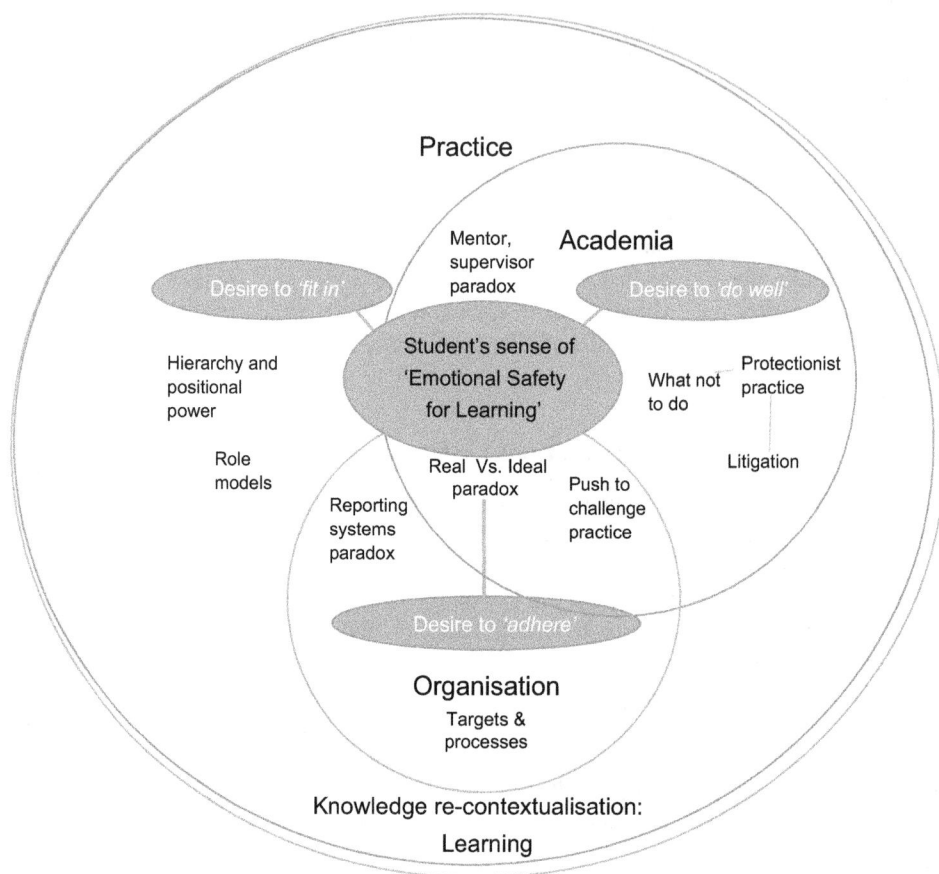

Figure 15.1 Knowledge contexts, emotional safety for learning and knowledge re-contextualisation.

effect for their sense of ESFL. Some of these dilemmas and tensions will now be illustrated using data from Study 2.

Protectionist practice

It was evident from Study 2 that in the academic setting students were taught "protectionist" practice. Curriculum documents and academic staff emphasised the importance of professional registration and the code of conduct. For example, academic staff reported teaching about professional standards, professionalism and clinical governance from the beginning of the programme as being driven by the requirements of the professional code.

However, students in Study 2 also noticed implicit messages from the hidden curriculum about what not to do, with an underlying sense of the risk and fear of losing registration signified by the NMC pin number.

Such caution may be seen as implicitly and insidiously portraying patient safety as predominantly related to the risks of practice – independent of the type of practice involved – and may have a detrimental effect upon students' self-confidence, encouraging fear and tentative "protectionist" practice. This tension may then influence students' sense of ESFL when in practice. Indeed, students in Study 2 and NQNs in Study 1 struggled emotionally with the wish to put their academic context learning into practice (re-contextualisation) whilst facing the messy reality of clinical practice and the pressures of protectionist practice, compounded by their positional power (or lack of) in the nursing hierarchy.

Hierarchy and power

Hierarchy was also evident, with both NQNs and students in Study 2 perceiving it impossible to question or challenge someone more senior. Thus the issue of questioning or challenging practice was a dilemma and major tension for the students, and indeed such challenge was in some ways encouraged and reinforced by the university, which espoused principles of evidence-based best practice. This created dissonance for the student: a potential burden of guilt for not using correct techniques and further feelings of not "belonging" which conflict with their desire to fit in. A sense of struggle and dissonance was evident in the reported discourses of students and NQNs. This burden and hierarchical position were compounded when students and NQNs perceived a need to be accepted into their new roles.

Role models

The issue of questioning, querying or challenging was never more present than in relation to role models, and while there were many good role models, those who were perceived as "poor" by students and NQNs in Study 2 seem to have been highly influential. For example, the perceived issue of a gap between theory and practice was justified by qualified nurses, in other words more senior staff, whereby "corners were cut" in the name of expediency.

Witnessing this practice and feeling unable to challenge may heighten the emotional burden for students (thus negatively impacting on their ESFL) who are fearful of challenging, want to fit in and perceive their position as being at the bottom of the hierarchy. In response to the perceived difficulties in questioning, exploring or challenging practice an alternative approach is that of a need for assertiveness education. However, it could be argued that such assertiveness education or training may have the tendency to "individualise" the issue, making it the problem of the student or NQN. Such an approach (as often present in discourses of resilience) removes the focus from wider systems, culture, community of practice and so on, and fails to also consider the need for students to learn to re-contextualise knowledge and develop understandings of practice as enacted.

Mentor/supervisor paradox

A further important tension which can be viewed as heavily influencing ESFL regards the relationship between a student and the person assigned as "practice mentor" or educational supervisor. An ideal educational relationship could perhaps be viewed as a relaxed relationship where it feels safe to disclose and discuss concerns, experiences and areas of uncertainty and to question and challenge. In essence such a relationship would ideally engender trust and facilitate interactivity and reciprocity (Steven et al., 2018). However, while qualified nurses in Study 1 acknowledged the need for such a trusting relationship, students were cognisant of the variation which existed, reporting practice learning to be variable depending on the practice placement, on whether or not the mentor is motivated to teach. Moreover, the students often would not know in advance the nature of the mentor–student relationship.

The desire for an effective educational relationship was compounded by the need to fit in and do well and the student's place in the hierarchy, and conditioned by the awareness that practice mentors were reported in Study 2 to be solely responsible for assessing place- ment learning and "signing off" competencies. A paradoxical situation seemed to exist where the mentor had a dual role: facilitating learning and also assessing or grading practice- based elements of the pre-registration course. Students often felt conflicted and were there- fore reticent about raising and discussing any issues that may potentially influence their grades, be they emotional issues or questions about practice.

Reporting systems paradox

A further paradox existed regarding the organisational reporting systems, which were espoused as promoting an open culture, encouraging reporting and learning from errors and mistakes. However such systems also served (and it could be argued, still serve) as a mechanism for identi- fying underperformance. Thus, the systems embody what has been called the "dual imperatives of accountability and organizational learning" (Dodds & Kodate (2011, 328). Although the stu- dents may not have engaged directly with these systems they may have been aware of staff scep- ticism and mistrust of the systems through throw-away comments and remarks. This feeling of organisational mistrust, whether conscious or not, could again impinge on decisions to chal- lenge, question or report aspects of practice they may have perceived as unsafe.

Discussion

In 1964, in a national study in the UK, Revans (1964) was able to demonstrate a clear asso- ciation between an infrastructure for care and positive staff and patient outcomes. He showed that organisations with high morale had effective communication systems where ward sisters spoke frequently with junior nurses, were able to retain a stable workforce and consequently showed better than average patient recovery times than in comparable hos- pitals. The caring organisation, therefore, is one that engenders high morale which in turn sustains and supports the delivery of front-line care (Smith et al., 2009). Any consideration of ESFL and organisations (Smith et al., 2009) needs to account for the connections between how staff are managed, how they feel about their work and the outcomes for patients (West & Dawson, 2013). The complex relationship between staff and patient safety, emotions and the impact of these two complex factors on quality of care is highlighted by quantitative and qualitative studies spanning two decades in both the UK and US (Woo- drow & Guest, 2008). Unfortunately, research shows that ESFL is not the normative experi- ence of nursing students and NQNs in the English NHS; in fact, as Melia (2005) has argued, the NHS is not a learning organisation.

We have explored how the theory of re-contextualisation could help students learn across a disintegrated learning context during their preparatory professional nursing pro- grammes. In this chapter, we have integrated work on *emotions and learning* (Smith & Allan, 2010; Allan, 2011) and *ESFL* (Steven et al., 2014) to argue that re-contextualisation may be developed as a useful theoretical framework to understand student nurses' and NQNs' requirement for emotional safety in order to learn. We have explored how emotional safety might support current workforce developments in increasingly complex nursing teams. Such an approach to learning (that learners need to feel emotionally safe to learn and that learning occurs across settings and is context-dependent) at this stage of a professional career (as stu- dents transition to NQN) may be a way to resolve tensions for students and NQNs which "splits" their thinking about different practice priorities. In both studies, participants (students and NQNs) reported tension between their understanding of the NMC code which is reinforced frequently in their university teaching and written work, and their observations of ward team customs and practices which do not meet the NMC code. This frequently led to "splits" in their thinking. This might be described as a split between higher-education institution and practice which is talked about as the "theory–practice" gap (Smith & Allan, 2010), but in reality is an emotional splitting which is frequently manifested as anger towards either practice colleagues or lecturers (Allan, 2011). Both Steven et al. (2014) and Allan et al. (2015, 2016a, 2017) have shown that students and NQNs learn how to bring together the reality of making decisions within local workplace custom and practice – accountability – with what they've been taught about ideal practice in higher-education institutions, although sometimes at a cost (Allan, 2011; Allan et al., 2017). An example of how this split is reproduced in students' and NQNs' talk is the way they talk about "losing their PIN [personal identification number]". In both studies, students and NQNs described tutors scaring them with "horror" stories about losing their PIN through unprofessional practice. Data from both studies suggest that this talk of losing their PIN can inhibit students and NQNs from learning. The emotions evoked by being fearful of losing their PIN are rarely acknowledged.

This lack of emotional processing has been found before in healthcare professionals' practice. Emotions are rarely referred to when talking (and writing) about the work that is done in healthcare (Taylor, 2006; Allan, 2011) and descriptions of work are often bland (Fineman, 1993). Yet emotions abound and are the crux of errors and patient safety incidents (Smith et al., 2009); learning from these and effective communication in teams are integral to becoming confident and competent as an NQN (Allan et al., 2017).

The Francis report highlighted the importance of proper support and supervision for HCSWs, to ensure they are not just "left to their own devices", potentially exposing patients to unacceptable risks (Francis, 2013). The Francis report also indicated a need for more effective delegation by nurses in relation to HCSWs. However, despite the increasing relevance of delegation and supervision skills among nurses, these do not yet form a central component of nurse training or preceptorship programmes (Allan et al., 2015, 2016a, 2017). With increasing pressures on NHS resources and the introduction of nursing associates and apprentices, there will be more reliance on streamlining tasks and roles between nurses and their support workers in nursing teams. Maximising these clinical teams' performance via effective working between them, and in particular, appropriate task allocation and completion respectively, will form a crucial component in safe and efficient patient care and outcomes. These workforce changes currently place great demands on *students* as they observe what their future roles may involve and on *NQNs* as they begin to take responsibility for new nursing teams. We argue that greater focus should be given to creating emotionally safe learning spaces for both students and NQNs in curricula.

We have argued that:

- In addition to the individual ability to critically self-reflect and re-contextualise knowledge when working in complex nursing teams, students and NQNs require a learning culture which encourages "emotional safety".
- Learning to work with feelings or "emotional learning" is enhanced by understanding how the learning takes place across such environments and contexts.
- Students and NQNs traverse and negotiate a range of physical and social environments and KCs.

Conclusion

In this chapter, we have argued that students and NQNs need emotional safety in order to re-contextualise or learn across KCs – learning is the production of new knowledge, which allows students and NQNs to develop in their journey to independent and competent practice as a registered nurse. We have illustrated our argument with extracts from two large-scale qualitative studies from the UK. We have shown how safe challenge in the clinical learning environment can contribute to the development of a skilled reflective professional.

References

Allan H T (2011) Using psycho-dynamic small group work in nurse education: Closing the theory-practice gap? *Nurse Education Today* 31(5): 521–524.

Allan H T, Magnusson C, Ball E, Evans K, Horton K, Curtis K & Johnson M (2015) People, liminal spaces and experience: Understanding re-contextualisation of knowledge for newly qualified nurses. *Nurse Education Today* 35(2): e78-e83.

Allan H T, Magnusson C, Evans K, Ball E, Westwood S, Curtis K, Horton K & Johnson M (2016) Delegation and supervision of healthcare assistants' work in the daily management of uncertainty and the unexpected in clinical practice: Invisible learning among newly qualified nurses. *Nursing Inquiry* 23(4): 377–385.

Allan H T, Magnusson C, Johnson M, Evans K, Ball E, Horton K, Curtis K & Westwood S (2017) Putting knowledge to work in clinical practice: Understanding experiences of preceptorship as outcomes of interconnected domains of learning. *Journal of Clinical Nursing* 12(1–2): 123–131.

Allan H T & Parr S (2010) "We were given a map of the hospital and told to find our own way" – student nurses' experiences of support. *Nursing Standard* 24(26): 69.

Bickhoff L, Levett-Jones T & Sinclair P M (2016) Rocking the boat — nursing students' stories of moral courage: A qualitative descriptive study. *Nurse Education Today* 42: 35–40.

Borrott N, Day G E, Sedgwick M & Levett-Jones T (2016) Nursing students' belongingness and workplace satisfaction: Quantitative findings of a mixed methods study. *Nurse Education Today* 45: 29–34.

Cipriano P (2010) Overview and summary: Delegation dilemmas: Standards and skills for practice. *The Online Journal of Issues in Nursing* 15(2): 1–11.

Dawoud D & Maben J (2008) Nurses in society: Starting the debate (report of written evidence). National Nursing Research Unit publication, King's College, London. Accessed at: www.kcl.ac.uk/content/1/c6/04/32/16/Nursesinsocietywrittenevidence.pdf.

Department of Health (2007) Towards a framework for post-registration nursing careers: A national consultation. Accessed at: webarchive.nationalarchives.gov.uk/20071104144315/www.dh.gov.uk/en/Consultations/Liveconsultations/DH_079911.

Dodds A & Kodate, N (2011) Accountability, organisational learning and risks to patient safety in England: Conflict or compromise? *Health, Risk & Society* 13(4): 327–346.

Dornyei Z (2000) Motivation in action: Towards a process orientated conceptualisation of student motivation. *British Journal of Educational Psychology* 70: 519–538.

Eraut M (1994) *Developing Professional Knowledge and Competence*. London: Falmer Press.

Evans K, Guile D, Harris J & Allan H T (2010) Putting knowledge to work: A new approach. *Nurse Education Today* 30: 245–251.

Fabricius J (1991a) The crisis in nursing: Reflections on the crisis. *Psychoanalytic Psychotherapy* 13(3): 203–206.

Fabricius J (1991b) Running on the spot or can nursing really change? *Psychoanalytic Psychotherapy* 5: 97–108.

Fabricius J (1995) Psychoanalytic understanding and nursing: A supervisory workshop with nurse tutors. *Psychoanalytic Psychotherapy* 9: 17–29.

Fineman S (editor) (1993) *Emotions in Organisations*. London: Sage, pp. 94–117.

Francis R (chair) (2013) *Report of the Mid Staffordshire NHS Foundation Trust Public Inquiry*. The Stationery Office. Accessed at: https://www.gov.uk/government/publications/report-of-the-mid-staffordshire-nhs-foundation-trust-public-inquiry.

Gergen K. (2015) *An Invitation to Social Construction*. London: Sage.

Gillen P & Graffin S (2010) Nursing delegation in the United Kingdom. *The Online Journal of Issues in Nursing* 15(2). Accessed at: http://ojin.nursingworld.org/MainMenuCategories/ANAMarketplace/ANAPeriodicals/OJIN/TableofContents/Vol152010/No2May2010/Delegation-in-the-United-Kingdom.html.

Health Education England (2014) *Lord Willis' Review of the Future Education and Training of Registered Nurses and Care Assistants*. Chair: Lord Willis. Health Education England: London. www.hee.nhs.uk/sites/default/files/documents/2348-Shape-of-caring-review-FINAL.pdf.

Iedema R (2011) Creating safety by strengthening clinicians' capacity for reflexivity. *BMJ Quality and Safety* 20(Suppl 1): i83–i86.

Johnson M, Magnusson C, Allan H T, Evans K, Ball E & Horton K (2015) Doing the writing and working in parallel: How 'distal nursing' affects delegation and supervision in the emerging role of the newly qualified nurse. *Special Edition. Nurse Education Today* 35(2): e29–33. doi: 10.1016/j.nedt.2014.11.020

Levett-Jones T & Lathlean J (2008) Belongingness: A prerequisite for nursing students' clinical learning. *Nurse Education in Practice* 8(2): 103–111.

Levett-Jones T & Lathlean J (2009a) 'Don't rock the boat': Nursing students' experiences of conformity and compliance. *Nurse Education Today* 29(3): 342–349.

Levett-Jones T, Lathlean J, Higgins I & Mcmillan M (2009b) Staff–student relationships and their impact on nursing students' belongingness and learning. *Journal of Advanced Nursing* 65: 316–324.

Melia K (2005) Nursing in the New NHS: *A Sociological Analysis of Learning and Working*. Accessed at: www.researchcatalogue.esrc.ac.uk/grants/R000271191/outputs/read/f513ae62-6f5f-403d-9796-135a576f339f

Menzies-Lyth I E P (1970) *The Functioning of Social Systems as a Defence against Anxiety: Report on a Study of the Nursing Service of a General Hospital*. London: The Tavistock Institute of Human Relations.

Nursing & Midwifery Council (2010) Standards pre-registration nursing education. Accessed at: www.nmc.org.uk/standards/standards-for-nurses/pre-2018-standards/standards-for-pre-registration-nursing-education/

Nursing & Midwifery Council (2018a) Future nurse: Standards of proficiency for registered nurses. Accessed at: www.nmc.org.uk/globalassets/sitedocuments/education-standards/future-nurse-proficiencies.pdf?utm_source=Council+of+Deans+of+Health+Policy+Bulletin&utm_campaign=2c5365ca7f-EMAIL_CAMPAIGN_2018_05_14&utm_medium=email&utm_term=0_7c5e43a9b0-2c5365ca7f-171617605

Nursing & Midwifery Council (2018b) Standards framework for nursing and midwifery education. Accessed at: www.nmc.org.uk/globalassets/sitedocuments/education-standards/education-framework.pdf?utm_source=Council+of+Deans+of+Health+Policy+Bulletin&utm_campaign=2c5365ca7f-EMAIL_CAMPAIGN_2018_05_14&utm_medium=email&utm_term=0_7c5e43a9b0-2c5365ca7f-171617605

Nursing and Midwifery Council (2018c) Standards for preregistration nursing programmes. Accessed at: www.nmc.org.uk/globalassets/sitedocuments/education-standards/programme-standards-nursing.pdf?utm_source=Council+of+Deans+of+Health+Policy+Bulletin&utm_campaign=2c5365ca7f-EMAIL_CAMPAIGN_2018_05_14&utm_medium=email&utm_term=0_7c5e43a9b0-2c5365ca7f-171617605

Pearson P, Steven A, Howe A, Smith P, Magnusson C, et al (2009) Patient safety in health care professional educational curricula: Examining the learning experience. Report to the Patient Safety Research Portfolio/Department of Health. Accessed at: www.birmingham.ac.uk/Documents/college-mds/haps/projects/cfhep/psrp/finalreports/PS030PSRPReportFINAL0609.pdf

Pearson P H, Steven A, Howe A, Sheikh A, Ashcroft D & Smith P (2010) Learning about patient safety: Organisational context and culture in the education of health care professonals. *Journal of Health Services Research & Policy* 15(supplement 1): 10.

Revans R W (1964) *Standards for Morale: Cause and Effect in Hospitals*. Oxford: Nuffield Hospital Trust.

Röndahl G, Innala S & Carlsson M (2004) Nursing staff and nursing students' emotions towards homosexual patients and their wish to refrain from nursing, if the option existed. *Scandinavian Journal of Caring Sciences* 18(1): 19–26.

Schön D (1991) *The Reflective Practitioner*. London: Basic Books.

Shin K, Jung D Y, Shin S & Kim M S (2006) Critical thinking dispositions and skills of senior nursing students in associate, baccalaureate, and RN-to-BSN programs. *Journal of Nurse Education* 45(6): 233–237.

Smith P & Allan H T (2010) We should be able to bear our patients in our teaching in some way' theoretical perspectives on how nurse teachers manage their emotions to negotiate the split between education and caring practice. *Nurse Education Today* 30(3): 218–223.

Smith P, Pearson P & Ross F (2009) Emotions at work: What is the link to patient and staff safety? Implications for nurse managers in the NHS. *Journal of Nursing Management* 17: 230–237.

Steven A (2009) *Knowledge Discourses and Student Views*. Saarbrucken: VDMVerlag.

Steven A, Larkin V, Stewart J & Bateman B (2018) The value of continuing professional development: A realistic evaluation of a multi-disciplinary workshop for Health Visitors dealing with children with complex needs. *Nurse Education Today* 67: 56–63.

Steven A, Magnusson C, Smith P & Pearson P (2014) Patient safety in nursing education: Contexts, tensions and feeling safe to learn. *Nurse Education Today* 34(2): 4(2): 277–284.

Taylor D (2006) *What immortal hand or eye has framed their fearful symmetry?* Paper presented at Governed State of Minds: thinking Psychoanalytically. Oxford: St Hugh's College, Oxford, 24–25 March 2.

Usher R, Bryant I & Johnstone R (1997) *Adult Education and the Postmodern Challenge: Learning Beyond the Limits*. London: Routledge.

West M & Dawson J (2013) NHS staff management and health service quality. Accessed at: https://assets.publishing.service.gov.uk/government/uploads/system/uploads/attachment_data/file/215454/dh_129658.pdf

Weydt A (2010) Developing delegation skills. *The Online Journal of Issues in Nursing* 15(2): http://ojin.nursingworld.org/MainMenuCategories/ANAMarketplace/ANAPeriodicals/OJIN/TableofContents/Vol152010/No2May2010/Delegation-Skills.aspx

Woodrow C & Guest D (2008) Workplace bullying, patient violence and quality of care: A review. PSSQ Working Paper.

Worrell J A & Profetto-McGrath J (2007) Critical thinking as an outcome of context-based learning among post RN students: A literature review. *Nurse Education Today* 27(5): 420–426.

16

RESEARCH IN AND "OF" NURSING PRACTICE

Doctoral education in nursing

Helen Allan

Introduction

The need for improved research literacy at registration and throughout the nurse's career is urgent (Oliver, 2017). Nursing research in practice is required to answer ongoing questions about the effectiveness of nursing procedures, the delivery of care and its impact on clients, as well as the outcomes of nurse education and learning in practice. In this chapter I will evaluate different forms of doctoral programmes offered for study in nursing globally and compare the most popular forms: the traditional PhD and the professional or clinical doctorate. I will argue that doctorally educated nurses from both programmes may lead a nursing research agenda in practice to improve patient outcomes and experience (practitioner-based research). But their skills can equally be used to lead academic research centres which offer mentorship and research training for early-career nurses as well as investigate research questions which have less direct clinical impact.

What is doctoral study in nursing?

Nursing as a discipline with a body of knowledge was well established by the mid twentieth century in some countries, notably the USA, UK and continental Europe (McKenna & Cutliffe, 2001). The purpose of doctoral degrees in any discipline is to critically generate, test, challenge and disseminate knowledge in the field (Lanara, 1994; Azusa et al., 2012). In nursing, this is for the benefit and comfort of patients and their families. There are four ways to be awarded a doctoral degree:

1. By thesis: this is the "traditional" route (PhD). These programmes of study vary globally: an American PhD generally involves accompanying coursework, European and British models have no formal taught component, although the British Research Councils

recommend a graduate personal development plan (The Roberts Review, 2002) and Australian PhDs can involve supervised project work or a combination of course and thesis work.

2. By published work: this involves the aggregation of a series of published academic articles or book chapters that pursue and build on a line of inquiry into a specific subject area.
3. By integrated PhD: this involves completion of a coursework research-oriented master's degree with an additional doctoral thesis.
4. By a taught doctoral pathway: examples include: Doctor of Business Administration (DBA), Doctorate of Clinical Psychology (DclinPsy), Doctor of Education (EdD), Doctor of Medicine (MD), Doctor of Engineering (EngD), Doctorate in Clinical Practice (DCP) and Doctorate in Professional Practice (DProf).

The history of the doctor of philosophy in nursing

Philosophy is the study of meaning and, while those awarded a doctor of philosophy in nursing are usually not philosophers, they are considered expert in finding meaning in the world and solving research questions. Jolley (2007) traces the first use of the title PhD to medieval France, and only much later in the nineteenth century in Germany and in America in 1850; the UK awarded a PhD (DPhil from Oxford) only in 1920. The first doctoral degree in nursing was awarded by Columbia University of America in 1923 (Burns & Grove, 2009). Doctoral nursing study was introduced more widely into the USA in the 1950s (Florczak et al., 2014). Only a small number of nurses studied for PhDs in nursing as a disciplinary subject; until the mid-1970s, nurses were more likely to study for PhDs in other disciplines such as sociology, psychology and physiology.

Indeed, until the 1990s, there were only a few nursing departments in the UK and it wasn't until the 1990s in the UK, as all nursing pre-registration programmes entered the university system (McKenna & Cutliffe, 2001), that nursing began to establish itself as a discipline across higher education and nurses began to study and gain PhDs in their disciplinary subject – however the numbers were and remain small. To use the UK as an example, McKenna and Cutliffe (2001) suggest there were about 300 British nurses with PhDs in 1997 and 10 Irish nurses with PhDs. They suggested that the numbers would increase with the move of nursing into universities.

While writing this chapter, I have been unable to find out the exact number of PhDs in nursing or nurses employed as nurses with PhDs in other disciplines in the UK. An educated guess can be made: in summer 2018, 1,540 PhDs are archived in the Steinberg Collection of Nursing Research at the Royal College of Nursing Library in London. These are British theses by nurses or about nursing deposited at the collection since it opened in 1974. Alternatively, one can use the Ethos database where I located 943 awarded with nursing in the title since 1990; this means there may be approximately 33 doctorates awarded per year. These numbers and timings are similar to those awarded PhDs in nursing in countries like Japan and Australia, largely driven by the expansion of undergraduate BSc nursing programmes (Azusa et al., 2012) and the need for firstly, faculty to teach the enrolling students and secondly, an evidence base for practice to improve productivity in increasingly complex healthcare systems (Rudge, 2015).

After having completed an honours degree or master's programme, nurses usually study for their PhD degrees part-time (Wilkes et al., 2015). In 2001, McKenna and Cutliffe found that the average age is relatively older for nursing PhD students – 35 years of age, compared with 21 years in the basic sciences. Perhaps worryingly in view of the recruitment of younger nurses into research careers, Wilkes et al. (2015) found in their survey of 27 doctoral students (traditional PhD and clinical/professional doctoral candidates) in Australia and the UK that the mean age had increased to 50 years old and the majority of this sample were working in academic posts. This may have changed since the introduction of Clinical Academic Careers fellowships funded by the Department of Health (see below).

In continental Europe there are also opportunities for funded PhD scholarships. UK and continental European countries hold to a "European" study pattern that culminates in a written thesis which is examined by a viva voce (oral examination after the examiners have read the thesis) where candidates are expected to "defend" their work in front of two examiners who are also PhDs and familiar with the candidate's field of knowledge. However, the European model also includes the requirement that the PhD candidate publishes four or five papers and the thesis is shorter (40,000–50,000 words) than the British version (commonly 80,000–100,000 words).

Traditionally there is minimal research training in this study pattern, although since 2002 the UK has introduced a fourth mode of doctoral study: the four-year integrated PhD, which includes an master's in research (MRes) followed by a PhD. The American PhD requires a five-chapter thesis, so it is shorter than the UK model, with four papers required to be submitted rather than published. The doctoral programmes offered in Australia approximate to the traditional European PhD and the clinical/professional doctorate offered in the UK with taught modules and a large research project (Walker et al., 2016).

Professional doctorates have a long tradition in Europe, as the medical degree, the MD, shows. The DClinPsy has likewise been the entry qualification to become a practising clinical psychologist for some time. In the latter part of the twentieth century (Watson et al., 2011), as part of a move to develop leaders in practice educated to doctoral level (Ellis, 2005), both the USA and the UK saw the introduction of clinical doctorates in nursing. These had different titles: Doctorate in Clinical Practice or Professional Doctorate in the UK and Doctorate in Nursing Science in America. In 2004, the clinical practice doctorate, the Doctor of Nursing Practice (DNP) degree, was introduced as the entry to advanced practice roles in America (Dreher, 2011; Watson et al., 2011; Ketefian & Redman, 2015) and has proved hugely popular. In 2016 773 nurses graduated as PhD in the USA, while 4,855 graduated as DNPs.

Conversely, after an initial surge in popularity from 2000 to 2005, the taught doctorates in nursing in the UK are proving less popular and programmes have stopped recruitment altogether while the traditional PhD continues to recruit largely through self-funded students. The professional doctorates offered as an interdisciplinary work-based programme in some universities still see nurses complete their doctorate, albeit as part-time students, and professional doctoral programmes continue to recruit (Ellis, 2005). There is no funding for this option and students generally self-fund.

The American DNP is not the same as the European or British professional or clinical doctorate and is criticised as research training is not part of the curriculum and it does not require a substantial component of empirical research (Dreher, 2011). The DNP programmes are poorly evaluated and their contribution to practice is under-researched (Green, 1997; Edwardson, 2001; Terhaar & Sylvia, 2015). The DNP aims to produce graduates who practise at a higher level and have "mastery of advanced speciality within nursing practice" (AACN, 2006: p. 20). However, concern is expressed that the contribution of doctoral study and its product, a contribution to knowledge in a field, is threatened by a doctoral programme that does not generate substantive new knowledge for the respective discipline (Florczak, 2010; Dreher, 2011).

In the UK, taught doctorates were introduced after the NHS Plan in 1997 as part of a drive to reinvigorate nursing leadership in the NHS; it was hoped that they would provide nurse leaders in new posts such as nurse consultants with a professionally relevant higher-education qualification (Ellis, 2005). They were hugely popular between 2000 and 2005 (Ellis, 2005; Watson et al., 2011). This is partly because it was seen as a good option for those universities wishing to develop their nurse lecturing staff through to doctoral level and, hence, through the traditional university promotional tracks, and partly because the traditional PhD has been criticised for not being relevant for a practice discipline like nursing (McKenna & Cutliffe, 2001; Walker et al., 2016). Rolfe and Davies (2009) argue that the traditional model of identifying a research question at PhD (from the literature) should be turned on its head and be derived solely from practice. As McKenna and Cutliffe (2001) suggest: "patient care should be the seedbed for substance. Knowledge is generated in practice and has to be refined and returned to inform or be tested in practice". This is certainly the philosophy behind many clinical doctorate curricula and follows other disciplines such as engineering and psychology, as well as industry as a whole. In these practice disciplines research questions around the nature of work, learning and pedagogies to underpin effective and inquiry-based learning in work are increasingly encouraged as industry strives to retain an innovative and creative workforce (Evans et al., 2006). However, these degrees have declined in popularity in nursing since 2005 (Ellis, 2005) for a number of reasons:

- wide variation leading to a lack of understanding of their value
- perception that they were irrelevant to practitioners
- little clarity, even among academics with responsibility for these programmes, of the value of taught doctorates both in respect of practice and in relation to the traditional PhD
- lack of support for these forms of doctoral award among academic staff responsible for these programmes and from students' peers both in practice and at university
- lack of post-award career structure and resistance in practice to nurses utilising both their degree and their title
- an explanation for their decline in nursing may be because the health workplace is a barrier rather than a facilitator for learning (Melia, 2005).

Since the Bologna agreement (1999) there is synergy across Europe for doctoral-level study. The Bologna agreement was reached after a series of meetings between higher-education leaders internationally, to ensure comparability in the standards and quality of higher-education qualifications. The taught element of the clinical doctorate and the relationship between practice and the topic area for study are influenced by other work-based learning innovations at doctoral level (Fink, 2006), such as the need for advanced practice (McKenna, 1997).

In the UK, since 2009, the Department of Health has invested in funding clinical academic careers for nurses and midwives (UK Clinical Research Collaboration, 2009). This initial funding programme has now merged into one programme funded by Health Education England (HEE): HEE/National Institute Health Research (NIHR) Integrated Clinical Academic (ICA) programme. However data on the funded fellowships for nurses and midwives from pre-doctoral through doctoral to post-doctoral level are disappointing. The number of career progressions among nurses and midwives has remained relatively static compared to other allied health professionals; after initial master's/PhD funding, successful PhDs have not progressed to senior academic appointments as in other allied and medical professions (Medical Research Council [MRC] Report, 2017). The survey's conclusions are salutary in respect of access to and support for doctoral study in the UK among nurses (and midwives): the majority of the increase in the 1,660 fellowships awarded in 2017 is due to increased numbers of pre-doctoral Academic Clinical Fellowship posts supported by NIHR. The overwhelming majority of those identified were medical graduates (76%).

It is unfortunate that nursing as a discipline entered the university system throughout UK and continental Europe at a time when the nursing global workforce was shrinking (Open University, 2018). At the same time, the nursing workforce are not educated to bachelor's level globally (Ketefian & Redman, 2015) and governments are having to be creative in how they attract students into nursing who do not have the qualifications for degree level, and to alter aspirations for postgraduate and *then* doctoral-level study. And pressures on the workforce have occurred at the same time as the existing nursing faculty age and retire. While the new Nursing and Midwifery Council (NMC) standards for teaching and learning (2018) require less teaching of academic subjects such as sociology and psychology, they call for more extensive and complex skills acquisition which will further strain the academic and teaching workforce in nursing. Consequently, there is an urgent need to recruit into both teaching and research (Institute of Medicine [IoM], 2012; MRC, 2017) and to support new academic staff to develop their careers (McKenna, 2005). These factors may shape both applications and completions of doctoral studies in nursing.

Other factors which affect PhD completion across subjects at British universities and may be important in shaping the context of doctoral study in nursing include the following:

- Mode of study: part-time students are significantly more likely not to complete compared to full-time students. Few nurses study for PhDs full-time and many self-fund part-time study.
- Subject: those with large, well-established research fields with largely agreed methodologies are more likely to complete. Nursing is still a new academic discipline and, with the introduction of non-university-based programmes of studying nursing in the UK and existing non-graduate nursing qualifications remaining popular in the USA, it remains under threat from shrinkage as an academic discipline.

Ketefian and Redman (2015) argue that the American model of doctoral study for nurses needs urgent evaluation of the current DNP. They cite a lack of standardisation, a lack of research methods training (in comparison with PhDs), a lack of mapping of advanced practice standards against doctoral-level programmes and poor employment outcomes for DNPs on graduation. Importantly, as the current master's level advanced practice study continues, employers are more familiar with this and reluctant to employ DNPs, as little is known about the level of practice and their (potential and actual) contribution to patient outcomes.

Nurses' disciplinary knowledge

Despite expanding numbers of PhDs in nursing and the number of clinical doctorates, many questions remain about the purpose of doctorally prepared nurses in nursing practice and the nature of nursing as a body of disciplinary knowledge, specifically about what a PhD in nursing is and whether it is possible to hold a PhD in nursing which draws on other forms of disciplinary knowledge (psychology and sociology are common examples). The critique is that, by drawing on disciplinary knowledge from outside nursing, the coherence of nursing knowledge is threatened (Donaldson & Crowley, 1978). I believe that as a nurse with a BSc in sociology and a PhD in nursing, I draw on sociological and psychological knowledge in a unique way to answer nursing questions. Certainly when working in interdisciplinary teams, my views draw on knowledge from a number of disciplines to give a nursing point of view. And my views are usually different to those of the sociologist or the psychologist on the team!

Donaldson and Crowley (1978) argue that there are three areas of research which make up the nursing field for research:

1. concern with principles and laws which govern life processes, well-being and optimum functioning of human beings – sick or well
2. concern with patterning of human behaviour in interaction with the environment in critical life situations
3. concern with the processes by which positive changes in health status are affected.

While these may well be included in nursing concerns, I believe we can broaden our research and knowledge endeavours to include:

1. concern with the social structures which act as constraints and/or facilitators in which society lives – sick or well
2. concern with the emotional, social and psychological responses of patients, their families and healthcare staff in acute and chronic life situations
3. concern with the delivery of care.

Another debate in relation to nursing knowledge at doctoral level is whether a professional or clinical doctorate is the "equivalent" of a traditional PhD (Dreher, 2011). Rather than think of the two routes as equivalent and argue that one is more or less than the other, it might be more productive to think of them as serving different purposes. As Florczak et al. (2014) suggest, PhDs are research-focused and clinical or professional doctorates practice-focused; they may just produce a different outcome. Walker et al. (2015) cite Bourner et al. (2001) who have called nurses with professional or clinical doctorates "researching professionals" as opposed to "professional researchers" who hold a traditional PhD. Gregory (1997) calls them "scholarly professionals" and those with a PhD in nursing "professional scholars".

However, if we think of the two routes as serving different purposes, does either fulfil that purpose? PhDs in nursing can fulfil Donaldson and Crowley's (1978) three principles of nursing research and hence produce nursing knowledge, especially if we extend these to include ways in which the social and psychological affect how nurses deliver and patients experience nursing in increasingly complex nursing teams. It has been argued that it is unclear how doctorally prepared nursing leaders benefit practice and improve patient outcomes (McKenna & Cutliffe, 2001; Brown-Benedict, 2008; Florczak et al., 2014) and whether the purpose of clinical doctorates is to translate evidence into practice and improve practice expertise (Brown & Crabtree, 2013; Wilkes et al., 2013). Given that research critique and review have been part of undergraduate nurse education for some years now in the UK, doctorates with this purpose may have already become superfluous. Or, as Rolfe and Davies (2009) argue, clinical doctorates may be more relevant for nursing if their purpose is practitioner-based research (Walker et al., 2016), which might have a direct impact on patient outcome and/or experience (Wilkes et al., 2013).

It is noteworthy that, in the UK, the NIHR-funded scholarships and fellowships for postgraduate study (including MRes and PhD) are called "clinical fellowships" in the medical tradition of "clinical research". Clinical research is a branch of healthcare science that determines the safety and effectiveness (efficacy) of medications, devices, diagnostic products and treatment regimens intended for human use. As such it has been traditionally a term associated with medicine rather than nursing. The choice of the term "clinical fellow" therefore seems to describe a certain type of research which isn't traditional in nursing academia or practice, but rather is more like the role of clinical research nurses in the UK, whose role is primarily to assist with medical research.

The medical "clinical" model appears to influence nursing PhDs if we look at the subjects of nursing theses retrieved from Ethos database. The majority are health and social care services research and medical care. However, the subject area of the thesis may not tell us much about the focus of the research. It is also important to understand the focus and impact of the PhD, which we can do through publication title and journal. When examining publications between 2004 and 2008, Wilkes et al., (2011) found the focus was on practice issue research with patients/family participants. In their small interview of 27 doctoral students in Australia and the UK in 2015, Wilkes et al. found that the top three research areas were paediatrics (6, 22.2%), acute care (5, 18.5%) and the role of nurses in practice (4, 14.8%) which, like the subjects in the Ethos data, fit into established subject areas. However, analysis of the titles and abstracts showed that 23 (85%) of these had a patient focus. Four (15%) were related to nursing issues of unethical conduct, resilience in the workplace and nurse/midwife roles. Wilkes et al. (2015) conclude that there seems to be an increasing emphasis on patient- and practice-focused research as nurses end the first decade of the twenty-first century. Yet Borbasi et al. (2002), using a similar methodology, found the most common topic of research was education, with a focus on nurse participants, after reviewing Australian nurse researchers' publications from 1995 to 2000. To understand this conundrum, as Wilkes et al.'s (2015) results suggest, fewer than 50% of respondents describe any impact of their research. This indicates that, while the focus of research might be more patient-focused, clinical studies in nursing may have variable impact (Borbasi & Emden, 2001). This seems to be largely because most doctoral students work in academic posts rather than clinical posts, which makes the sharing of knowledge difficult, daunting and perhaps impossible.

This trend of "clinical" research questions emerging as the *new* nursing research, shaped by the medical understanding of what constitutes clinical, is also seen in American nursing research. Broome et al. (2013a) found that the most widely reported types of publication by doctorally educated American nurses were clinical intervention studies, not Mode-2 (second-generation) knowledge production research which develops questions from practice to resolve practice problems (Rolfe & Davies, 2009). Rolfe and Davies (2009) argue that Mode-2 doctorates subvert the idea of the traditional PhD (knowledge production largely divorced from practical application) as they focus on practice issues which are embedded in a society's economy and therefore have direct practical application.

Advanced practice and doctorates in nursing

The demand for clinical or professional doctorates emerged or increased in practice disciplines where the volume of science to be applied in practice demanded careful evaluation and application to improve care (Sperhac & Clinton, 2008) at a particular time, i.e. late twentieth/early twenty-first century. At this time, national healthcare systems were undergoing challenges to become more productive (Rudge, 2015). Advanced nursing practice emerged at this time as a potential solution to the need for increasingly complex healthcare delivery (Allan & Barber, 2005); it was part of a solution in some healthcare systems to the pressure on junior doctors' time (Rudge, 2015). As Walker et al. (2016) argue, the professional/clinical doctorate emerged at a time when universities were "encouraged" to forge clearer links with industry or, as they argue, citing Lyotard (1987), to fulfil the demands of the economy and late capitalism – part of the move to increasing productivity in education and professional work (Rudge, 2015; Allan et al., 2016).

Fink also noted that "[d]octoral education in Australia is currently under pressure to become more industry focussed and advocated that professional doctorates may be able to fulfil this role by developing and sustaining closer collaboration between universities and industry" (Fink, 2006: p. 35). This is essentially what happened.

Advanced nursing practices have, of course, also brought about shifts in delineated boundaries between doctors and nurses and between nursing support staff and nurses. And this situation has all been informed by wider influences including, but not limited to, the emergence of a so-called "knowledge society"; globalisation; and other social, economic and cultural transformations internationally. These influences have exerted a number of pressures for doctoral education to change and, in the words of Scott (2006):

> the boundaries for doctoral education have become fuzzier – with master programs on the one hand and professional development and lifelong learning on the other, and even the highest levels of adult and continuing education … the whole higher education system, and also the research system, have been stretched and, at the same time, become more diffuse and permeable.
>
> *(Scott, 2006)*

As a result, the nature of disciplinary knowledge and its relationship to practice are also blurred and shifting.

Rolfe and Davies (2009: p. 1265) make two important points in respect of the development of the professional doctorate in nursing: "Professional doctorates have arisen out of dissatisfaction with the traditional PhD which is perceived as too distant from practice; study at doctoral level is now increasingly relevant to those working outside academe". Rolfe and Davies (2009) argue that a response to this situation is to develop Mode-2 or second-generation doctorates where the focus becomes practice problems rather than doctoral projects centred on problems identified by academics in academic practice.

The purpose of doctoral education

It might be assumed that there is agreement in nursing that nurses educated to the doctoral level will enhance the health of people through discovery and dissemination of new knowledge (Kim et al., 2006). Even here there is debate about what outcomes might be expected of doctorally prepared nurses and what their career pathways might look like in order to promote and capture potential doctoral nurses at the start of their career and benefit from their potential. Given the debates over the nature of disciplinary knowledge in nursing, it is not surprising that there are different views about the purpose of doctoral study in nursing. This is reflected in the provision and popularity of doctoral programmes in nursing. We have already seen that the DNP in America is very popular while registrations to professional or clinical doctoral programmes have declined in the UK. And we have noted that the PhD in nursing in the UK remains popular for students on a self-funded part-time basis while, in America, the traditional PhD route (with some taught elements, as described above) is less popular.

Why is this important? Ultimately doctoral education in nursing is important for three reasons and, if entrants to doctoral programmes decline, then nursing as a discipline with an identifiable disciplinary knowledge will be affected. Doctorates in nursing aim:

1. to undertake research to challenge accepted practices, develop clinical knowledge and provide an evidence base for nursing practice
2. to provide a future supply of nurse teachers who will teach nursing students, design curricula and assess them in practice
3. to practise at advanced level in a complex, changing and challenging health environment.

It is clear that the current global nursing shortage raises particular problems in terms of nursing faculty (American Association of Colleges of Nursing [AACN], 2010). Both American and British authorities argue that highly qualified nursing faculty are needed to teach future nurses (IoM, 2012; NMC Standards, 2018). Having doctorally prepared teachers who are research-active will not only enhance the level of curricula and teaching, but they will act as role models for those students to develop their own career in education and research. However, even where nurse teachers are doctorates, their age on graduating is 46 (AACN, 2010) and therefore the number of years for their full participation in research and teaching is less than 20 years compared to most disciplines where the average age on completion of a doctorate is 35 years old. In the USA, baccalaureate-to-PhD and accelerated programmes have been introduced and evaluated (Squires et al., 2014; Nehls et al., 2016; Smith et al., 2016). To date evaluation data from these programmes are equivocal. A key predictor of success for graduation is the presence of an academic mentor, access to funding and preparation for teaching. Graduates without clinical experience unsurprisingly feel they lack clinical skills (Squires et al., 2014; Nehls et al., 2016). This issue is also recognised by the NIHR in the UK and is one of the reasons for funding schemes to attract good honours graduates in nursing who have some clinical experience into MRes programmes prior to doctoral programmes (UK Clinical Research Council [UKCRC], 2009).

The global nursing shortage is caused by several intersecting factors:

- increasing acuity and complexity of patients in both acute care hospitals and community settings (Aiken et al., 2003; Walker et al., 2016)
- an ageing nursing workforce retiring at the same time as younger nurses who hold different satisfactions from their working life (Heidemeier & Staudinger, 2015)
- funding and economic constraints on government budgets globally at the same time as expensive technologies and treatments (Baal et al., 2014)
- the need for new ways of thinking about how we deliver healthcare which will utilise the new technologies effectively yet retain a caring and interpersonal ethos (Elf et al., 2015).

These challenges call for competent, but above all critical, thinkers who are able to problem solve, manage teams and take on additional responsibility and who also have highly attuned interpersonal skills (AACN, 2006; NMC, 2018). Internationally, it was hoped within nursing that master's-prepared nurses in acute care settings would educate both student nurses and experienced nurses in caring for a changing patient population with increased acuity

(Abraham et al., 2015). However, even if nurses qualify with the knowledge and skills to care for this level of acuity and experienced nurses continue with professional development in both academic and skills-based programmes, implementation of changes in practice is often difficult. This may be because, once in practice, lead nurses and their teams lack knowledge in using evidence-based practice and research methods as a problem-solving approach to achieve positive patient outcomes on an everyday basis (Fineout-Overholt et al., 2005). In the USA, when all formal education is taken into account, 51.2% of the current registered nurse (RN) workforce has less than a four-year college degree. Of those prepared at the associate degree level, 20.7% returned to school and 30.2% of those prepared in diploma programmes obtained post-RN nursing or nursing-related degrees (Health Resources and Services Administration, 2004). The introduction of the DNP in America was a strategy to introduce *more* highly educated and technically competent nurses, practising at advanced level, to lead teams in place of the master's-prepared nurses. and above all to evaluate care and implement change using their enhanced research skills acquired during doctoral education. The DNP's purpose is to conduct evidence-based practice change projects and translate research/evidence into practice (Brown & Crabtree, 2013); to "reduce time-lag between discovery of knowledge and its implementation" (p. 331). The DNP is not considered to have addressed this need for a research-informed practice developmental approach with a doctorate who synthesises evidence and produces new local knowledge. A lack of research training in the existing DNP programmes and a lack of mapping of doctoral-level competencies against advanced practice make it difficult to see what difference a DNP makes to patient care against existing master's-prepared advanced nurses (Green, 1997; Edwardson, 2001; Ellis, 2005).

In the UK, the workforce figures are compiled slightly differently as there is (currently) only one level of RN; healthcare assistants are not registered. Nursing associates will be registered from 2019 with the NMC after a two-year educational programme. The NMC only holds information on the nursing qualifications for each person on the register. The approved programmes that can be undertaken to earn nursing qualifications can be offered at different academic levels depending on the institution running the course. For example, a Community Practitioner Nurse Prescribing V100 course may be offered at either BSc or MSc level. Employers (private or the NHS) only keep records of academic qualifications if they are required for the role.

In the UK, nursing leadership is part of a strategy to address low morale in nursing, poor recruitment and retention (Department of Health, 1997; National Health Service Executive [NHSE], 1999). A cadre of newly appointed specialist, advanced and consultant nurses spearheaded the popularity for master's in advanced practice and professional or clinical doctorates in the early 2000s. In the USA too, policy changes under the Obama administration were part of the driver for the expansion and call for better-educated nurses in advanced clinical roles – the DNP (Murphy et al., 2015).

However clear I might think the need for doctorally educated nurses to be, as outlined above, repeated studies into nurses' perceptions of the purpose of doctoral education in nursing show that there is a large amount of ambiguity (Ellis, 2005; Kot & Hendel, 2012; Uldis & Mancuso, 2015). Uldis and Mancuso (2015) found that nurses sampled at two large nursing conferences in America clearly supported the DNP degree. They believed the DNP-educated nurse's goal was to improve healthcare outcomes as a leader in health organisations, through influencing policy, working interprofessionally and translating evidence into practice. However, even in this sample, who were generally supportive and informed about the DNP, there were many areas of confusion concerning the role of DNP-prepared nurses. Uldis and Mancuso (2015) argue that, to reduce role ambiguity, the distinctive contributions of the DNP-prepared nurse must be embraced, valued and operationalised. Otherwise, the role of the DNP-prepared nurse will continue to be discussed, debated and challenged.

Clarifying the purpose of doctoral study in nursing is an urgent one. Currently the DNP is undervalued and the PhD seen by some as less relevant for a practice discipline (Walker et al., 2016). In their discussion paper on this topic, Walker et al. (2016) adapt ideas around "signature pedagogies" used in educational studies in calling for new thinking about the purpose of doctorally prepared nurses. Shulman (2005) describes signature pedagogies as "the characteristic forms of teaching and learning … that organize the fundamental ways in which future practitioners are educated for their new professions" (p. 52). Walker et al. (2016) cite Golde (2007) in calling for a doctoral signature pedagogy which would not follow the traditional PhD programme. It would instead:

> socialis[e] doctoral students into the discourse community of the profession, providing practice in articulating a summary and critique of research literature, helping faculty and students keep up with the latest literature and with active controversies in their fields, making connections around disciplinary boundaries and helping doctoral students discover and claim a topic and direction for their dissertation projects.
>
> *(Golde, 2007: p. 349)*

Wilkes et al. (2015) argue that the fundamental problem with doctorates in nursing is the failure to disseminate new knowledge into practice where it could have an effect on patient care and care delivery. They adopt the Canadian Institute of Health Research's view on this (2012: p. 1), namely that dissemination of research as a form of knowledge translation is "the exchange, synthesis and ethically sound application of knowledge … within a complex system of interactions among researchers and users … to accelerate the capture of the benefits of research". However, this implies that knowledge is static and unchanged as it is used across settings; it is the interactions in the system which will change the knowledge and produce new knowledge which is localised but valid for practice. This is what Rolfe and Davies (2009) argue should be the purpose and focus of doctoral clinical nurses: the production of local knowledge for practice – known as second-generation doctorates. As we have seen in previous chapters, nurses continually re-work knowledge to meet their own needs. We are still left with the question: how do we evaluate the value of doctorally prepared nurses?

Outcomes/evaluation of nursing doctorates

Golde and Walker (2006: p. 5) argue that a doctorate "prepare[s] future leaders of the discipline, who will creatively generate new knowledge, critically conserve valuable and useful ideas and responsibly transform those understandings through writing, teaching and applications". The question about whether their actions and leadership improve patient care and/or outcomes remains unanswered (Watson et al., 2011; Wilkes et al., 2015). Indeed, Borbasi and Emden (2001) concluded that most nursing doctoral students pursued their doctorate for personal goals rather than professional or patient-centred ones.

Unfortunately the evidence base to support master's-level education in nursing, namely that nurses educated to master's level will improve patient care, directly does not exist. We know that master's-educated nurse report development in personal and professional qualities such as confidence, which may have an indirect benefit on patient care. Cotterill-Walker (2012) concludes from her systematic review of the literature on the outcomes of master's-level nurse education that direct benefits need to be measured along with understanding what hinders and what facilitates a nurse's ability to apply knowledge and skills acquired at this level of study. We also know that, indirectly, well-educated nursing workforces (to graduate level or higher) produce patient benefit in terms of reduced surgical patient mortality (Aiken et al., 2003).

Terhaar and Sylvia (2015) argue that outcomes of the DNP (in America) are implicit in the aim of the professional or clinical doctorate concerned. So some programmes will require a "translational project" (as Terhaar and Sylvia describe it), while others will require a standard doctoral thesis which is familiar to the traditional PhD programme. Others will require an account of learning or a full reflexive explanation of what impact the work has had on practice. Some final projects will be required to address a "problem" in practice; others will emerge from an examination of the literature over the programme itself. Terhaar and Sylvia describe one programme which required students to undertake a scholarly project where the problem arises in practice and which encompasses four phases of planning, initiation, monitoring and controlling and closing a practice project. In this model, they argue, the outcomes of the DNP are clear and patient-focused.

In their small survey of doctoral students, Wilkes et al. (2015: pp. 9–10) explicitly asked respondents whether they felt their doctoral thesis (either a traditional PhD thesis or a shorter clinical/professional thesis) had produced changes in nursing practice in any of the listed areas: education and training, management, practice, politics, workplace issues and other. Most of the respondents believed their doctoral research had led to changes in nursing. Fourteen (51.9%) respondents thought their research had made an impact in at least one of the areas listed. There was a fairly even spread across the two countries with six of the 14 (42.9%) respondents from the UK highlighting impacts. Two respondents noted their research had an impact in five of the areas listed. Four respondents stated their research had an impact in two areas. Three (11.1%) respondents did not provide an answer to this section of the survey. Three (11.1%) respondents noted personal change related to career development and development of research partnerships. Another 10 respondents (37.0%) stated their doctoral research had not changed nursing.

The reasons given for this lack of change were:

- recent completion of doctoral thesis
- limited dissemination
- change of field or redundancy
- type of research
- perceived lack of interest in research by senior managers.

A direct quote from this study illustrates the lack of career structures in clinical practice for doctoral nurses:

> My disappointment from the lack of interest by key nursing managers … resulted in my choice to cease working as a nurse in any capacity.
>
> *(R3)*

The following quotation shows what a barrier a perceived split between practice and academia might be to disseminating at the very least a doctoral study's results:

> I am not working in the environment, so difficult to influence practice personally.
>
> *(R20)*

One respondent suggested it was difficult to gauge impact, although s/he suggested his/her publication and conference presentations may have had some impact. This suggests a lack of guidance or perhaps even awareness in his/her supervisory team about the purpose of the doctorate and the best way to influence practice.

Little is known nationally or globally about the impact or outcomes of doctorally or even master's-level educated nurses (Bombard et al., 2010; Sorbello, 2010; Stanton et al., 2011; Hicks & Rosenberg, 2016); in the UK, RNs' educational qualifications beyond their bachelor's (BSc) degree are not recorded by their employer and are largely immaterial to the role descriptions for nurses in direct patient care roles. Nurses who complete master's-level study are often confused about what their academic achievement brings to their practice (Bombard et al., 2010) and their employer is a key figure in supporting them to build on their studies and develop skills in practice (Stanton et al., 2011; Bender, 2014; Hicks & Rosenberg, 2016); clarifying their academic development or contribution to practice becomes less and less important. However, some universities are offering master's in nursing as part of a retention programme with local NHS trusts for their qualifying BSc graduates (Birmingham, Northumbria, York). Doctoral study is not required in academic/teaching roles at all universities in the UK. Nor is it required in clinical research nurse (CRN) posts in NHS trusts, although, increasingly, CRNs are attaining their higher-level degrees.

In a survey study in the USA by Abraham et al. (2015), in one acute care hospital, 54% of doctorally educated nurses reported that their motivations for doctoral study were personal and professional growth, and that they aspired to remain in direct patient care. Incentives for their educational development were unrelated to their pay and conditions as there was no role descriptor which included education beyond bachelor (BS) degree. Abraham et al. (2015) go on to say that there are few job descriptions for doctorally educated nurses who remain in direct patient care. Hicks and Rosenberg (2016) argue that providing the evidence for such roles in terms of impact on patient outcomes and/or experience is vital to start designing innovative curricula to prepare RNs to work at doctoral level in direct patient care roles. They argue that such evidence will only emerge as academia and practice become more aligned in promoting the discipline of nursing.

Warren and Mills (2009) give an example of a practice-based project in one American hospital to attract, recruit and retain nurses who aspire to master's-level study and practice – these nurses are called clinical nurse leaders in the USA (Hicks & Rosenberg, 2016). They conclude that the employer needs to offer incentives to successfully motivate RNs to return for advanced degrees (Box 16.1). Professional commitment at the same time as lower career satisfaction are predictors of nurses' willingness to enrol on an advanced nursing degree programme.

Box 16.1 Motivating incentives to encourage registered nurses to return for advanced degrees

- The knowledge that an advanced degree will provide greater job and promotional opportunities
- Innovative partnership models and the sharing of resources between healthcare agencies and schools of nursing to recruit and train clinical instructors
- Successful completion of advanced degrees by nurses working full-time can be facilitated by mentors, tutoring, tuition support and academic support and guidance

---

Abraham et al. (2015) report an evaluation of DNPs in one state in America. The aim of the study was to identify any impact on patient care delivery that nurses with advanced education might have, and to understand how DNPs contribute to the overall culture of hospital teams. The evaluation was particularly interested in identifying how master's- and doctoral-prepared nurses were employed/involved in direct patient care, and whether there were specific job responsibilities necessary to fulfil the role. The work is ongoing but a supplementary project has begun to assist nurse managers to provide support and incentives to retain DNPs in the hospital's workforce by identifying competencies, rewriting job descriptions, identifying work-based projects which utilise DNPs' skills to the full and adjusting pay to reflect higher educational achievement.

Examples of local practice change through doctoral work

Despite there being little research evidence of the impact of doctorally educated nurses, there is plenty of published evidence reporting local, small-scale contributions to knowledge and practice. In America, Murphy et al. (2015) give an example of work by DNP and PhD-prepared faculty members in one university hospital to highlight collaborative efforts to prepare students with skills to participate as full partners in the redesign of healthcare models to improve quality, access and cost. The expertise, knowledge and skill set of each faculty member contributed to the success of this innovative effort that restructured seven medical practice sites as patient-centred medical homes (Swartout et al., 2014). As a result, advanced-practice nursing students were placed in the sites over the two-year patient-centred medical home restructuring and were integral to the efforts with the interprofessional teams. This collaborative effort prepared students for leadership roles, particularly interprofessional team-based practice, and the use of technology to increase access, improve outcomes and reduce cost (Swartout et al., 2014).

In my own practice, as a PhD and clinical doctorate supervisor, I have supervised doctoral students who remain in clinical practice and those who are academics; both of these types of work inform practice.

Examples include those given in Table 16.1.

Even where the topics are educational (Callwood et al., 2012, 2015, 2016), the effects of the research have a direct effect on recruitment of midwives to the professional programme and therefore in the care they deliver to women and their families. Callwood's thesis is that, by recruiting using multiple mini-interviews (MMIs), universities are able to craft MMIs which select for compassionate and caring values as well as for academic grades on leaving school.

Table 16.1 Comparison between thesis subjects of clinical doctorate and traditional PhD students

Clinical doctorate	*Traditional PhD*
An ethnographic exploration of blood transfusion practice (Bishop et al., 2011)	The sexual experiences of women following radical cancer therapy (White et al., 2011)
The experiences of women in choosing keyhole surgery for cancer of the endometrium (Hughes et al., 2010)	The use of multiple mini-interviews in midwifery selection (Callwood et al., 2012, Callwood et al., 2015, Callwood et al., 2016)
Community nurses' learning of physical assessment skills (Raleigh et al., 2016)	Guyanese women's experiences of diabetes and transition (Mitchell et al., 2017)

Conclusions: research in and "of" practice

Wilkes et al. (2013) argue that clinical scholarship needs defining and reinvigorating so that it becomes much more prolific, more widely known and understood as a product. They propose a re-visioning of nursing clinical scholarship and draw on Boyer's (1990) framework to help us understand scholarship in a practice discipline such as nursing.

Box 16.2 Four dimensions of scholarship in practice disciplines

1. Scholarship of discovery investigative work: research
2. Scholarship of integration: giving fuller meaning to isolated facts fitting one's own research to others into larger intellectual patterns – making connections across disciplines
3. Scholarship of teaching: creating teaching in a planned and evaluated form
4. Scholarship of application: how the knowledge can be helpful to society

Source: Wilkes et al. (2013), citing Boyer (1990).

Boyer's work focused on teaching and university teaching. After empirical work with nurses in practice and education, Wilkes et al. (2013) suggest two of the essential elements of clinical scholarship in nursing are vision and passion. And components of clinical scholarship in nursing are:

1. building and disseminating nursing knowledge
2. sharing knowledge
3. linking academic research to practice
4. doing practice-based research.

They conclude, like others (Florczak et al., 2014), that nurse academics and clinical scholars (both doctorally educated) need to work together to encourage researching in practice as well as translating research into nursing practice. To do this, however, nursing leaders in both academia and practice should focus on increasing research literacy in practice at the registration and immediately post-registration points in nurses' careers as well as developing doctorally prepared nurse leaders. These leaders may lead a nursing research agenda in practice to improve patient outcomes and experience (practitioner-based research) or they may lead academic research centres, which offer mentorship and research training for early-career nurses. Nursing research in practice includes clinical research questions as well as questions about the delivery of care, nurse education and learning in practice.

References

Abraham P J, Gohan La Donna D M & Pfrimmer D M (2015) Retaining master and DNP registered nurses in direct patient care: utilizing nurses to the fullest extent of their education. *Nurse Leader* 13(1): 70–74.

Aiken L H, Clarke S P, Cheung R B, Sloane D M & Silber J H (2003) Educational levels of hospital nurses and surgical patient mortality. *JAMA* 290: 1617–1623.

Allan H T & Barber D (2005) Emotion boundary work in advanced fertility nursing roles. *Nursing Ethics* 12(4): 391–400.

Allan H T, Tapson C, O'Driscoll M, Savage J, Lee G & Dixon R (2016) A critical integrative literature review of governing body nurses on Clinical Commissioning Groups in the UK. *Nursing Inquiry* 23(2): 178–187.

American Association of Colleges of Nursing (2006) *The essentials of doctoral education for advanced nursing practice*. Washington, DC: American Association of Colleges of Nursing. Retrieved from www.aacn. nche.edu/DNP/pdf/Essentials.pdf.

American Association of Colleges of Nursing (2010) The research-focused doctoral program in nursing: Pathways to excellence. Retrieved from www.aacn.nche.edu/education-resources/PhDTaskForceReport.pdf Accessed: 31st March 2018.

Azusa A, Misuzu F G, Satoko N, Yuko M, Sachiyo M (2012) Evaluation of doctoral nursing programs in Japan by faculty members and their educational and research activities. *Nurse Education Today* 32: e1–e7.

Baal P, Meltzer D & Brouwer W (2014) Future costs, fixed healthcare budgets, and the decision rules of cost-effectiveness analysis. *Health Economics* 25(2): 237–248.

Bender M (2014) The current evidence base for clinical nurse leader: a narrative review of the literature. *Journal of Professional Nursing* 30: 110–123.

Bishop E, Faithfull S & Allan H T (2011) An exploration of the influences on clinical decision making and the culture of blood transfusion practice in cancer related anaemia using an ethnographic methodology. *Supportive Care in Cancer* 19: 203–210.

Bombard E, Chapman K, Doyle M, Wright D K, Shippee-Rice R & Kasik D (2010) Answering the question 'what is a clinical nurse leader?' Translation experience of four direct-entry masters students. *Journal of Professional Nursing* 26: 332–340.

Borbasi S & Emden C C (2001) Is a PhD the best career choice? Nursing employers' views. *Contemporary Nurse: A Journal for the Australian Nursing Profession* 10(3–4): 187–194.

Borbasi S, Hawes C, Wilkes L, Stewart M & May D (2002) Measuring the outputs of Australian nursing research published 1995–2000. *Journal of Advanced Nursing* 38(5): 489–497.

Bourner T, Bowden R & Lang S (2001) Professional doctorates in England. *Studies in Higher Education* 24(2): 75–93.

Boyer E (1990) *Scholarship reconsidered: priorities of the professoriate*. Princeton, NJ: Carnegie Foundation.

Broome M E, Riner M E & Allam E S (2013a) Scholarly publication practices of doctor of nursing practice-prepared nurses. *Journal of Nursing Education* 52(8): 1.

Broome M E, Riner M E & Allam E S (2013b) Scholarly publication practices of doctor of nursing practice-prepared nurses. *Journal of Nursing Education* 52(8): 429–434.

Brown M A & Crabtree K (2013) The development of practice scholarship in DNP programs: a paradigm shift. *Journal of Professional Nursing: Official Journal of the American Association of Colleges of Nursing* 29(6): 330.

Brown-Benedict D (2008) The doctor of nursing practice degree: lessons from the history of the professional doctorate in other health disciplines. *Journal of Nursing Education* 47(10): 448–457.

Burns N & Grove S K (2009) *The practice of nursing research: appraisal, synthesis, and generation of evidence* (6th ed.). St. Louis, MO: Saunders Elsevier.

Callwood A, Allan H & Courtenay M (2012) Are current strategies for pre-registration student nurse and student midwife selection 'fit for purpose' from a UK perspective?: introducing the multiple mini interview'. *Nurse Education Today* 32(8): 835–837.

Callwood A, Allan H T & Cooke D (2015) Developing a robust tool: advancing the multiple mini interview in pre-registration student midwife selection in a UK setting. *Nurse Education Today* 34(12): 1450–1454.

Callwood A, Cooke D & Allan H T (2016) Values based recruitment in midwifery: do the values align with what women say is important to them? *Journal of Advanced Nursing* 72(10): 2358–2368. doi: 10.1111/jan.13038. Epub 2016 Jul 4.

Canadian Institute of Health Research (2012) Canadian Institute of Health Research annual report. Retrieved from www.cihr-irsc.gc.ca/e/47320.html

Cotterill-Walker S M (2012) Where is the evidence that master's level nursing education makes a difference to patient care? A literature review. *Nurse Education Today* 32(1): 57–64.

Department of Health (1997) *The new NHS: modern, dependable*. London: HMSO, Department of Health.

Donaldson & Crowley (1978) The discipline of nursing. *Nursing Outlook* 26(2): 113–120.

Dreher H M (2011) global perspectives on the professional doctorate. *International Journal Nursing Studies* 48: 403–408.

Edwardson (2001) Nursing education and doctoral study in the United States. In *Doctoral education and professional practice: the next generation*. Green B, Maxwell T W & Shanahan P (Eds.). Sydney, NSW: Kardoorair Press 5: 85–106.

European Commission (1999) The Bologna Process and the European Higher Education Area. https://ec.europa.eu/education/policies/higher-education/bologna-process-and-european-higher-education-area_en. Accessed: 20th September 2019.

Elf M, Fröst P, Lindahl G & Wijk H (2015) Shared decision making in designing new healthcare environments—time to begin improving quality. *BMC Health Services Research* 15(114): 1–7.

Ellis L B (2005) Professional doctorates for nurses: mapping provision and perceptions. *Journal of Advanced Nursing* 50(4): 440–448.

Evans K, Hodkinson P, Rainbird H & Unwin L (2006) *Improving workplace learning*. Abingdon: Routledge.

Fineout-Overholt E, Melnyk B M& Schultz A (2005) Transforming health care from the inside out: advancing evidence-based practice in the 21st century. *Journal of Professional Nursing* 21: 335–344.

Fink D (2006) The professional doctorate: its relativity to the PhD and relevance for the knowledge economy. *International Journal of Doctoral Studies* 1(1): 35–44.

Florczak K L (2010) Research and the doctor of nursing practice: a cause for consternation. *Nursing Science Quarterly* 23(1): 13–17.

Florczak K L, Poradzisz M & Kostovich C (2014) Traditional or translational research for nursing: more PhDs please. *Nursing Science Quarterly* 27(3): 195–200.

Golde C (2007) Signature pedagogies in doctoral education: are they adaptable for the preparation of education researchers? *Educational Researcher* 36(6): 344–351.

Golde, C M & Walker, G E (Eds.) (2006). *Envisioning the future of doctoral education: preparing stewards of the discipline. Carnegie essays on the doctorate*. San Francisco, CA: Jossey-Bass.

Green B (1997) *Theorising the professional doctorate: representation, practice and the curriculum problem in post graduate education*. Symposium paper 'Professional doctorates in new times in the Australian University' presented at AARE Annual National Conference Brisbane 3 December.

Gregory M (1997) Professional scholars and scholarly professionals. *The New Academic* Summer: 19–22.

Health Resources and Services Administration (2004) *The registered nurse population: findings from the 2004 national sample survey of registered nurses*. Retrieved July 24, 2018 from http://bhpr.hrsa.gov/healthworkforce/rnsurvey04

Heidemeier H & Staudinger U M (2015) Age differences in achievement goals and motivational characteristics of work in an ageing workforce. *Ageing and Society* 35(04): 809–836.

Hicks F D & Rosenberg L (2016) Enacting a vision for a master's entry clinical nurse leader program: rethinking nursing education. *Journal of Professional Nursing* 32(1) (January/February): 41–47.

Hughes C, Knibb W & Allan H T (2010) Laparoscopic surgery for endometrial cancer: a phenomenological study. *Journal of Advanced Nursing* 66(11): 2500–2509.

Institute of Medicine (2012) *The future of nursing: leading change, advancing health*. Washington, DC: National Academies Press. Retrieved from www.thefutureofnursing.org/recommendation Accessed: December 27.

Jolley J (2007) Choose your doctorate. *Journal of Clinical Nursing* 16: 225–233.

Ketefian S & Redman W (2015) A critical examination of developments in nursing doctoral education in the United States. *Revista latino-americana de enfermagem* 23(3): 363–371.

Kim M J, McKenna H P & Ketefian S (2006) Global quality criteria, standards, and indicators for doctoral programs in nursing; literature review and guideline development. *International Journal of Nursing Studies* 43(4): 477.

Kot F C & Hendel D D (2012) Emergence and growth of professional doctorates in the in the United States, United Kingdom, Canada and Australia: a comparative analysis. *Studies in Higher Education* 37(3): 345–364.

Lanara V A (1994) *The contribution of nursing research to the development of the discipline of Nursing in Europe*. Proceedings from the 7th Biennial Conference (pp. 33–46) Oslo: European Workgroup of Nurse Researchers.

Lyotard J-F (1987) *The postmodern condition: a report on knowledge*. (Bennington, G. and Massumi, B. Trans.). Manchester: Manchester University Press. (Originally published in 1979).

McKenna H (2005) Doctoral education: some treasonable thoughts. *International Journal of Nursing Studies* 42(3): 245–246.

McKenna H P (1997) *Nursing models and theories*. London: Routledge.

McKenna H & Cutliffe J (2001) Nursing doctoral education in the United Kingdom and Ireland. *Online Journal Issues in Nursing* 6(2). Retrieved from http://ojin.nursingworld.org/MainMenuCategories/ANAMarketplace/ANAPeriodicals/OJIN/TableofContents/Volume62001/No2May01/ArticlePreviousTopic/UKandIrelandDoctoralEducation.html.

Medical Research Council (2017) UK-wide survey of clinical and health research fellowships. Retrieved from https://mrc.ukri.org/publications/browse/clinical-and-health-research-fellowships-survey-2017/ Accessed: 29th June 2018.

Melia K (2005) Nursing in the new NHS: a sociological analysis of learning and working. Retrieved from www.researchcatalogue.esrc.ac.uk/grants/R000271191/outputs/read/f513ae62-6f5f-403d-9796-135a576f339f

Mitchell A, Koch T & Allan H T (2017) 'It's a *touch of sugar*': Guyanese women's beliefs about diabetes'. *Action Research Journal*. doi: 10.1177/1476750317721303,

Murphy M P, Staffileno B A & Carlsson E (2015) Collaboration among DNP and PhD prepared nurses: opportunity to drive positive change. *Journal of Professional Nursing* 31: 388–394.

National Health Service Executive (1999) Nurse, midwife and health visitor consultants: establishing posts and making appointments. Health Service Circular 217. Retrieved from webarchive.nationalarchives.gov.uk/+/www.dh.gov.uk/en/Publicationsandstatistics/Lettersandcirculars/Healthservicecirculars/DH_4003972

Nehls N, Barber G & Rice E (2016) Pathways to the PhD in nursing: an analysis of similarities and differences. *Journal of Professional Nursing* 32(3): 163–172.

Nursing and Midwifery Council (2018) Standards for preregistration nursing programmes. Retrieved from www.nmc.org.uk/globalassets/sitedocuments/education-standards/programme-standards-nursing.pdf?utm_source=Council+of+Deans+of+Health+Policy+Bulletin&utm_campaign=2c5365ca7f-EMAIL_CAMPAIGN_2018_05_14&utm_medium=email&utm_term=0_7c5e43a9b0-2c5365ca7f-171617605 Accessed: 22nd May 2018.

Oliver D (2017) Why shouldn't nurses be graduates? *British Medical Journal* 356: j863. doi: 10.1136/bmj.j863.

Open University (2018) *Tackling the nursing shortage*. Milton Keynes: Open University.

Raleigh M, Knibb W & Allan H T (2016) A qualitative study of nurses' use of physical assessment skills in primary and community care: shifting skills across professional boundaries. *Journal of Clinical Nursing* 26(13–14): 2025–2035. doi: 10.1111/jocn.13613.

Rolfe G & Davies R (2009) Second generation professional doctorates in nursing. *International Journal of Nursing Studies* 46(9): 1265–1273.

Rudge T (2015) Managerialism, govermentality and the evolving regulatory climate. *Nursing Inquiry* 22(1): 1–2.

Scott P (2006) *The global context of doctoral education. EUA Bologna Handbook: making Bologna work*. European University Association.

SET for Success (2002) *The supply of people with science, technology, engineering and mathematics skills. The report of Sir Gareth Roberts' Review*. London: Universities and Research Councils UK.

Shulman L S (2005) Signature pedagogies in the professions. *Daedalus* 134(3): 52–59.

Smith C R, Martsolf D S, Draucker C B, Shambley-Ebron D Z, Pritchard T J & Maler J (2016) Stimulating research interest and ambitions in undergraduate nursing students: the research-doctorate pipeline initiative. *Journal of Nursing Education* 55(3): 133.

Sorbello B (2010) *Clinical nurse leaders stories: a phenomenological study about the meaning of leadership at the bedside*. PhD Dissertation Florida Atlantic University. (Publication number AAT 3407171).

Sperhac A M & Clinton P (2008) Doctorate of nursing practice: blueprint for excellence. *Journal of Pediatric Health Care* 22(3): 146–151.

Squires A, Kovner C, Faridaben F & Chyun D (2014) Assessing student intent for PhD study. *Nurse Education Today* 34: 1405–1410.

Stanton M P, Barnett Lammon, C A & Williams E S (2011) The clinical nurse leader: a comparative study of the American Colleges of Nursing vision to role implementation. *Journal of Professional Nursing* 27: 78–83.

Swartout K, Murphy M, Dreher M & Bahal R (2014) Advanced practice nursing students in the patient-centred medical home: preparing for a new reality. *Journal of Professional Nursing* 30: 139–148.

Terhaar M F & Sylvia M (2015) Scholarly work products of the doctor of nursing practice: one approach to evaluating scholarship, rigour, impact and quality. *Journal of Clinical Nursing* 25: 163–174.

UK Clinical Research Collaboration (2009) *Clinical academic careers for nurses, midwives and allied health professionals.* Retrieved from www.ukcrc.org/workforce-training/clinical-academic-careers-for-nurses-midwives-and-allied-health-professionals/ Accessed: 29th June 2018.

Uldis K A & Mancuso J M (2015) Perceptions of the role of the doctor of nursing practice-prepared nurse: clarity or confusion? *Professional Nurse* 31: 274–283.

Walker K, Campbell S, Duff J & Cummings E (2016) Doctoral education for nurses today: the PhD or professional doctorate? *The, Australian Journal of Advanced Nursing* 34(1): 60–69.

Warren J I & Mills M E (2009) Motivating registered nurses to return for an advanced degree. *The Journal of Continuing Education in Nursing* 40(5): 200–207.

Watson R, Thompson D R & Amella E (2011) Doctorates and nurses. *Contemporary Nurse* 38(1–2): 151–159.

White I, Allan H T & Faithfull S (2011) Assessment of treatment-induced female sexual morbidity in oncology: is this part of routine medical follow-up after pelvic radiotherapy? *British Journal Cancer* 105: 903–910.

Wilkes L, Cummings J, Ratanapongleka M & Carter B (2015) Doctoral theses in nursing and midwifery: challenging their contribution to nursing scholarship and the profession. *The Australian Journal of Advanced Nursing* 32(4): 6–14.

Wilkes L & Jackson D (2011) Trends in publication of research papers by Australian-based nurse authors. *Collegian* 18(3): 125–130.

Wilkes L, Mannix J & Jackson D (2013) Practicing nurses perspectives of clinical scholarship: a qualitative study. *BMC Nursing* 12(1): 21.

17

EXPANDING LIFELONG LEARNING OPPORTUNITIES

Finding interprofessional models
to forge change

Renee S. Kumpula

Introduction

Nurses and leaders face rising expectations and new realities with the complexity of health-care and the consumer-driven quest for quality and options for optimal care. Not only are nurse educators striving to stay ahead of the challenges, but the public expects healthcare teams to solve tomorrow's problems in the here and now. The nature of current advances and global connectedness have created a sense of urgency in isolating the best treatments and solutions for symptoms or conditions that are not yet fully understood or defined. Amid the expectations and accompanying pressures of time in resolving crises, nurses can discover new intersections and possibility for cultivating transformation within the interpersonal, community, and societal structures that surround healthcare.

Changing the way nurses and healthcare teams are educated becomes more important when considering the timely care of vulnerable populations such as infants and children, the disabled, the mentally ill, the frail, the chronically ill, the elderly, and those at the end of life. Currently, healthcare systems are overwhelmed with issues and initiatives to over-come the problems of those who struggle. In a world that esteems health and vitality, nurses consistently advocate for those who fall between the cracks in systems and experience inequity. With compassion and grace, nurses attend to vulnerable individuals as they come into and go out of the lifespan with dignity. Moreover, nurses continue this cycle throughout the career.

Critical changes in healthcare delivery come at a time when it may be difficult for nurses throughout the globe to accrue hours or credits for continuing education and continuing professional development, the very programs that update them on the latest standards of care and newer evidence-based practices. The Royal College of Nursing (RCN) (2017, 2018a, 2018b) in the UK reported an increase in problems with continuing nursing education. Nurse scholars in the UK, US, and other countries have identified difficulty for nurses to access and complete contact hours or credits, have staffing coverage that allowed training, obtain reimbursement or support, and travel distances to large centers with educational offerings (Glasper, 2018; Lee, Tiwari, Hui Choi, Yuen, & Wong, 2005; McCafferty, Ball, & Cuddigan, 2017). In addition, constructs of continuing education, continuing professional development, and lifelong learning have continued to evolve over time (Jarvis, 2005; Qaleh-sari, Khaghanizadeh, & Ebadi, 2017). These problems persist when the previous emphasis on improving individual performance as a practice standard has shifted to include individual team member performance and the quality improvement for an entire team in all practice settings.

In this chapter, interprofessional education (IPE) and interprofessional continuing education (IPCE) to ensure the best team-based care for vulnerable individuals in academic programs and professional practice will be described. The constructs of continuing education, continuing professional development, and lifelong learning will be discussed. The importance of accreditation of programs for professional training and interprofessional teams will be described. These perspectives can provide the nursing profession in general, and nurse educators and faculty in particular, an unprecedented opportunity to enhance and expand best practices beyond the medical and disease model of the past to a person-centered wellness and wholeness model for the future.

Moving from multidisciplinary to interprofessional team-based care

There has been renewed focus on the importance of interprofessional team-based care in all practice settings since the 1960s, especially as its importance has been continually repeated and reinforced. In national initiatives in the US, UK, Canada, Australia, and other countries, the necessity of healthcare professions providing integrated care to promote quality and safety has been established (Croenewett et al., 2007; Disch, 2013). Moreover, there have been recent calls for making substantive advances and closing the gap in continuing education for preparing teams with membership among the various healthcare professions.

The emphasis on interprofessional collaborative practice and team performance has come by way of lessons learned from the past on how professional identities are constructed and how particular disciplines socialized their future members in academic programs. Social identity theory and social theory provide understanding for how the structure of various professions may limit the effectiveness of interprofessional practice. Traditional training models were constructed to inculcate uniprofessional ideals and identity in future practitioners. Because professions perpetuated a narrative that supported the preservation of the particular discipline and professional identity, the long-held safeguards that legitimated the profession may conflict with newer social constructions needed for building interprofessional teams (Bourdieu & Passeron, 1990; McNeil, Mitchell, & Parker, 2013. Social identity threats can produce withdrawal from team activities or sharing information during interprofessional collaboration; such a threat would indicate tension with both the current circumstances and the historical tensions that affect the various disciplines (McNeil et al., 2013). Due to a need to share knowledge and decision making in collaborative practice, barriers to team behaviors include factors such as medical dominance, lack of respect toward other professions, and tendencies for stereotyping among the disciplines (McNeil et al., 2013).

Traditional power structures situated nursing and other professions in subordination to medicine where there was a history of domination (Blue & Fitzgerald, 2002). Physicians were socialized through educational, legal, organizational, social, and cultural structures in a particular identity and understood their role was to be the key decision maker and lead "over" rather than "with" nurses and other members of the healthcare team (Bourdieu & Passeron, 1990; Foucault, 1980; Nugus, Greenfield, Travaglia, Westbrook, & Braithwaite,

2010). Eisler and Potter (2014) proposed medicine and nursing were historically situated in a domination paradigm that prevented collaboration. A newer partnership paradigm has been proposed that focuses on equal respect and validation of professional roles and structures that support equitable partnerships in practice. The partnership paradigm sets as primary tenets the respect for and honoring of patient-centered care, mutual priorities in sharing information, and joint decision making among multiple health professions (Bleich, 2016b; Eisler & Potter, 2014).

With a definition of an interdisciplinary team being two or more disciplines working together, Boon, Verhoef, O'Hara, and Findlay (2004) characterized team functioning in seven levels: independent teams, consultative teams, collaborative teams, coordinated teams, multidisciplinary teams, interdisciplinary teams, and fully integrated teams. These types of teams can be observed in many organizations since improving patient outcomes became a renewed focus. However, the interprofessional teams that are being proposed globally reference the last two types of interdisciplinary and fully integrated teams. Bleich (2016a) qualified that the goal for interprofessional teams should not result in a team being homogeneous in function, but rather that teams would consider and gauge different perspectives from each discipline and position integrated teams to utilize differing perspectives and thus ensure positive outcomes.

Moving from uniprofessional silos to interprofessional models

In creating partnerships on interprofessional teams, team members must develop a capacity to exchange information and consider other viewpoints without being restricted by existing social identities and hierarchies (Meleis, 2016). In order to negotiate collaborative practices, team members must acknowledge the reality of both "competitive" and "collaborative" power existing in practice structures (Nugus et al., 2010). One of the difficulties in forging collaboration is each profession's perception of autonomy over the scope of practice in the particular discipline. Several factors affect negotiating collaboration across professions, including managing patient care, understanding where both competitive and collaborative powers already exist, decision making for quality care, the acuity of the care setting, and the actual quantity of interprofessional contributions included in case conference discussions (Nugus et al., 2010). One challenge is to transform historical uniprofessionalism into a new type of interprofessional identity for collaborative practice similar to developing a new ethnic identity in accordance with social theory (Pecukonis, 2014). Building the Robert Woods Johnson Foundation's (RWJF) (2015) culture of health may be one mechanism for developing such an identity of authentic interprofessional collaboration.

Earlier efforts to establish continuing education for each profession resulted in the formation of the Alliance for Continuing Medical Education in 1974 to increase the efficiency and effectiveness of continuing education across the disciplines (Balmer, 2014). The organization expanded to the Alliance for Continuing Education in the Health Professions (AACEhp) that purposed to move even further toward interdisciplinary collaboration (Balmer, 2014). The Josiah Macy Jr. Foundation (2014) convened a conference with an imperative: a call for partnership across the professions. In response to the conference report, DeSilets (2014) posited the importance of nurse educators leading in continuing education and continuing professional development efforts. She proposed nurse leaders be involved in forming and sustaining partnerships by demonstrating the following principles: create role model partnership values and behaviors; create new mission, vision, and value statements emphasizing partnership; establish expectations and incentives for partnerships; and promote leadership, governance, structures, and alliances with like-minded professional organizations that understand and support partnership. DeSilets (2014) quoted a Macy conference participant, "What we [are] really talking about is turning it [the American healthcare system] right side up and placing the focus on where it should have been all along: on the patients" (Josiah Macy, Jr., Foundation, 2014, p. 1).

The RWJF (2015) set a national priority for its vision for building a culture of health across all of the health professions. For the nursing profession, Balmer (2014) posited that nurses have always advocated for the health of individuals, families, and communities, and therefore, should move this vision of a health culture to action. One component particularly relevant to nurses is to foster collaboration across all sectors to improve the well-being of everyone in society (RWJF, 2016). Nurses demonstrate ability to actively build a culture of health, which is inherent in promoting IPCE, continuing professional development, and lifelong learning (Balmer, 2014; Billings, 2016; RWJF, 2016).

Cultivating interprofessionality among the healthcare professions

Moving from multidisciplinary teams to interprofessional practice has been a goal for several decades. Since the World Health Organization (WHO) (1988) position on *Learning Together to Work Together*, recent efforts are producing results (Hammick, Freeth, Koppel, Reeves, & Barr, 2007). In Canada, the move from uniprofessional to interprofessional approaches met with resistance (Borduas et al., 2006). The resistance in healthcare systems was coupled with barriers in integrating IPE in higher education due to lack of: government and professional funding, institutional funding, programs for faculty development in IPE, supportive organizational structures to support IPE, and buy-in and commitment across all professions involved in IPE programming (Lawlis, Anson, & Greenfield, 2014).

The Joint Commission accredits healthcare facilities and services in the US. Indicators for reimbursement are tied to improving patient outcomes and reducing medical errors. Initiatives such as the TeamSTEPPS master's training program through the Agency for Healthcare Research and Quality (AHRQ) (2018), a quality improvement program in the US, is changing how healthcare teams learn to communicate and function through continuing education (Roman, Abraham, & Dever, 2016).

TeamSTEPPS has been implemented in healthcare systems in the US where medical errors have occurred. The traditional remediation for cardinal errors had been continuing education. With the move to team measures as an indicator of quality outcomes linked to reimbursement, the training of all professions on standardized methods for team communications became paramount (Sexton & Baessler, 2016). With the development of the TeamSTEPPS standardized language, strategies for conveying critical information with a common coded language allowed professionals to communicate critical data in patient situations that required prompt action to prevent or minimize harm (AHRQ, 2018). One example with the TeamSTEPPS program is teaching teams to use the SBAR (situation, background, assessment, recommendation) pneumonic in care transitions or critical situations, by using a standard format to provide instant context for critical data in patient transfers. Another example is using the CUS pneumonic (for expressing *concern*, being *uncomfortable*, and citing *safety*) in stating key words to convey urgency, such as: "I have a concern," "I am uncomfortable with this situation," and "I have a concern with safety" in an emergency, critical care, or surgical environment (AHRQ, 2018).

In response to the WHO (2010) framework for action, the Interprofessional Education Collaborative (IPEC) (2011) formed with the following members: American Association of

Colleges of Nursing, Association of American Medical Colleges, American Associations of Colleges of Osteopathic Medicine, American Association of Colleges of Pharmacy, American Dental Education Association, and Association of Schools of Public Health. The WHO (2010) goal to prepare all students in healthcare professions to be "collaborative practice ready" for team-based care now necessitated the integration of IPE in higher education (Kuper & Whitehead, 2012).

Interprofessional education

Perhaps more effective than the training or re-training of interprofessional teams already in practice, academia has been instituting IPE in pre-professional programs. The purpose of IPE is to intentionally foster an open mindset and initiate conversations among students in multiple health professions during their programs of study. IPE programs in academia focus on students gaining awareness and appreciation for the roles of other professions.

With this inclusive approach, students can begin to understand the similarities and differences among the roles and responsibilities of other disciplines before their professional identities are fully developed or integrated. This awareness is essential prior to licensure and professional practice. The net gain of IPE in academic programs is the likelihood that professionals will respect and seek opinions from other professions on teams. IPE draws from education, sociology, and psychology theory for both its rationale and design of delivery, often drawing from social constructions involving interaction with others (Thistlethwaite, 2012).

The case for IPE and the involvement of the nursing profession has grown in the literature and in the consciousness of healthcare professionals. With the Institute of Medicine (IOM) (2003) *Health Professions Education: A Bridge to Quality*, core competencies were to "cooperate, collaborate, communicate, and integrate care in teams to ensure that care is continuous and reliable" (p. 4). Whether in pre- or post-licensure educational programs, students and professionals are cognizant of the expectations for quality interprofessional care from healthcare teams.

With a rising increase in healthcare specialties, it is becoming more important for pre-professional students and professionals to have experiences that cultivate positive behaviors for teamwork (IPEC, 2011; Smith, 2014). The Centre for the Advancement of Interprofessional Education (2002) in the UK defined IPE as activities when two or more professions learn with, from, and about each other to enhance collaboration and the quality of care. The case for interprofessional teams grew with the Canadian Interprofessional Health Collaborative (CIHC) work on a National Interprofessional Competency Framework for Canada (CIHC, 2010; Hammick et al., 2007).

Nurse faculty can create IPE experiences that utilize innovation and interprofessionality at its best. Barnsteiner, Disch, Hall, Mayer, and Moore (2007) described six characteristics of integrated IPE: an explicit IPE philosophy in the organization; evidence of faculty from different professions co-creating curricula; experiential student learning with collaboration with others in other disciplines; having IPE experiences embedded in nursing curricula; providing students opportunity to demonstrate core competencies; and having structures that foster interprofessional experiences in the organization. Ironside and Valiga (2006) posited the import of nurse faculty teaching content reflective of their passion and expertise; challenging students with hard questions by acknowledging even those that cannot be answered; creating environments that encourage a "lively exchange of ideas" and introducing discussion of critical issues where all contributions are valued (p. 120). In addition, scholars reported the importance of faculty development for all IPE activities and especially for advanced and graduate students with preceptors in clinical settings (Berman, 2013; Bleich, 2016b; Chen, Rivera, Rotter, Green, & Kools, 2016). Because of nurse ability to provide leadership for teams, they have opportunity for central roles in planning effective IPE to shape nursing practices.

The call for interprofessional competencies

More recently, the World Health Organization (WHO (2010) established evidence and support for IPE and collaborative practice in its framework for action. With the IOM (2011) report, *The Future of Nursing: Leading Change, Advancing Health*, the interdisciplinary panel identified the importance of nursing taking a primary role in transforming healthcare and improving outcomes. Kowalski (2012a) reported the importance of nurse-led initiatives for collaborative improvements, especially in nurse-led clinics and joint practices, along with the need for action coalitions to assemble at the state level to support national level efforts (2012b). Sigma Theta Tau International's global advisory panel convened to determine how nurses could develop global relationships and inform policy (Yoder-Wise, 2015).

The IPEC (2011) expert panel's *Core Competencies for Interprofessional Collaborative Practice* report recommended that nursing education would foster a culture for lifelong learning (Gaberson & Langston, 2017). IPEC developed core competency domains for healthcare teams that include interprofessional communication, values and ethics for IPE practice, roles and responsibilities, and teams and teamwork (Pardue, 2015). The American Association of Colleges of Nursing has established integrated interprofessional competencies for every essential pertaining to nursing education at all levels from bachelor to doctoral programs (Disch, 2013).

The effectiveness of interprofessional education

Hammick et al. (2007) found in a systematic review that students had positive perceptions of IPE and that it enabled their knowledge and skills for future practice. The researchers reported the importance of using adult learning principles in designing IPE and customizing content for specific groups of students. Reeves et al. (2009) cited examples in a systematic review, yet stated there was difficulty in drawing direct inferences due to the heterogeneity among the compiled results. Thistlethwaite and Moran (2010) reported that early IPE programming can promote positive attitudes toward IPE in practice. Mitchell, Groves, Mitchell and Batkin (2010) found that students reported an appreciation of the importance of effective communications in practice due to IPE. However, another study found IPE did not produce a sustaining effect on students' eventual practices on healthcare teams (Curran, Sharpe, Flynn, & Button, 2010). Rosenfield, Oandasan, and Reeves (2011) reported concerns that poorly designed IPE activities actually diminished medical student interest in interprofessional collaboration. Hudson, Sanders, and Pepper (2013) described the need for longitudinal studies to determine IPE effectiveness and the actual transfer of student learning to eventual practice. Some studies found that, although students reported the positive attitudes acquired in early IPE programming, they were affected by exposure to negative attitudes and stereotypes later in their professional training (Smith, 2014). Hart (2015) reported that, despite nurse commitment to interprofessional practice, the embedded messages of power and status that exist in some organizational cultures rendered nurses unable to overcome barriers for collaborating in interprofessional practice. With these results in mind,

Bleich (2016b) proposed that the mantle of IPE has now shifted to healthcare systems that employ the very professionals who were educated with IPE programming in their pre-licensure studies.

The continuum of lifelong learning

There are different standards around the globe for continuing education and continuing professional development that apply to lifelong learning in the nursing profession. Generally, pre-professional education (becoming a nurse or healthcare professional) prepares one for licensure to practice a chosen profession. The continuing education model of the past, where professionals collected attendance hours to acquire knowledge and skills for practice, has evolved to one of continuing professional development and lifelong learning. Continuing education is understood to be further education for professionals to stay on the forefront of best practices and the latest standards for quality patient care, which is applied to maintain a license for practice or to obtain additional credentials for a nursing specialty, advanced practice, or nursing leadership. Whereas before, nurses and other professionals primarily measured improvement in their individual knowledge and skills as continuing education, they now engage in interactive strategies and activities that allow them to explore or exercise new skills in concert with other professionals as continuing professional development.

Early proponents proposed that continuing professional development included continuing education, professional development, staff development, continuing professional development, and lifelong learning (James & Francis, 2011). Today, continuing professional development has come to mean a blending of traditional components of knowledge, skills, and attitudes along with applications of clinical reasoning and reflection about clinical practice. These aspects add a personal dimension for professional practice and developing competence. Continuing professional development is now understood as an individualized plan for cultivating both personal and professional growth and improvement in the career, rather than being dependent upon the workplace or system for mandated training and to keep training records. Lawton and Wimpenny (2003) proposed that the broad nature of continuing professional development includes not only personal and professional development, but also differentiation in structured and unstructured activities.

Lifelong learning is a principle value upheld by the professional commitment to a profession, implying personal responsibility and accountability for one's own competence and performance. The meaning of lifelong learning continues to evolve and has various meanings throughout the world, yet nurses understand the importance of improving their performance and quality improvement in their profession (Jarvis, 2005; Qalehsari et al., 2017). Although varied requirements exist for licensure and credentialing even within countries such as the US, the importance of lifelong learning as a value and necessary goal for nursing practice is upheld globally.

The evolution from continuing education to continuing professional development

In the US, national accreditation bodies provide the standards and oversight for continuing education and continuing professional development. Nursing has its own American Nurses Credentialing Center (ANCC) that accredits schools of nursing, professional organizations, and other entities to become providers or approvers of contact hours for nurses who are practicing in clinical settings. Medicine has the Accreditation Council for Continuing

Medical Education (ACCME) and pharmacy has the Accreditation Council for Pharmacy Education (ACPE) as counterparts to ANCC. In addition, other national accrediting bodies and state boards exist for approving continuing education and continuing professional development hours or credits for other professions on healthcare teams.

Accreditation and the advent of joint accreditation

With the similarities and differences for accreditation among the disciplines, some scholars have posited that providing educational programming for multiple professions has promoted uniprofessionalism and redundancy. With the advent of joint accreditation in the US, the Joint Accreditation Commission (JAC) consolidated ANCC, ACCME, and APCE standards for continuing education and continuing professional development in nursing, medicine, and pharmacy while consolidating multiple providers into one accreditation body (JAC, 2018). The WHO (2010) defined interprofessional collaborative practice as "when multiple health workers from different professional backgrounds work together with patients, families, careers, and communities to deliver the highest level of care." The new definition for IPCE with the JAC (2016) is: "when members from two or more professions learn with, from, and about each other to enable effective collaboration and improve health outcomes." Thistlethwaite (2012) had stipulated that the prepositions "with, from, and about" were essential and fundamental for learning to be interprofessional, therefore all three must be applied together in educational practice where interactive learning occurs (p. 59).

According to Dickerson and Bernard (2018), the goal of all IPCE is to improve team outcomes by addressing team-focused gaps in practice and collaboratively planning activities to improve or influence individual skills, team performance, and patient outcomes. What sets apart an IPCE activity from a multidisciplinary activity is that two or more professions plan the activity collaboratively and participants learn and interact with other disciplines during the activity itself (Dickerson & Bernard, 2018). Collaboration has led to benefits such as ensuring consistent content and improving the care team partnership along with enriching the education. This can result in gaining learning approaches for developing common content while respecting the divergent needs among various disciplines (Glossenger, Bennett, Ferren, & Sageser, 2016). Therefore, the hallmark of team-based education is that IPCE is planned "by" the healthcare team "for" the healthcare team (JAC, 2016).

The nursing profession's role in shaping the future and forging change

It has become clear that emerging leaders in healthcare teams may well come from professions that have not traditionally served as principle leaders. Rather, future leaders have likely been serving in the background as the foundation and bedrock for the medical profession, as physicians have traditionally been at the forefront. In the past, physicians depended on nurses to conduct accurate assessments, provide critical data, make patient-centered recommendations, and articulate the best choices to solve patient problems. At this juncture in time, the fluidity and flexibility of teams to respond to rapidly changing crises are taxed and tested. This has led to new calls for collaborative team leadership and decision making to ensure critical information is shared. Today, there are major initiatives to reduce medical errors, improve quality and safety, and improve patient outcomes.

If change is needed and afoot, nurse leaders may be best suited to provide leadership in establishing connection, building synergy, and shaping innovative interprofessional models for the care of vulnerable groups in the decades ahead. It is imperative that futuristic models are person-centered. It is imperative for models to be created that generate and increase resilience, not only among individuals who require customized care, but also among those individuals who deliver quality care.

In developing interprofessional collaboration, there are a number of assets that nurses can contribute. Nurses have the most patient contact during assessments, diagnoses, and treatments, and can therefore articulate how holistic team-based care can be delivered. Nurses are advocates and core healthcare team members who have the public trust and can accurately communicate the needs of vulnerable individuals, groups, and populations. Nurses can translate evidence-based knowledge into practice for improving patient outcomes. Nurses can forge change in creating interprofessional models that promote holistic, team-based practices and secure a real impact on the future of healthcare.

References

Agency for Healthcare Research and Quality (AHRQ). (2018). TeamSTEPPS© strategies and tools to enhance performance and patient safety. Accessed at www.ahrq.gov/teamstepps/index.html

Balmer, J. T. (2014). The alliance for continuing education in the health professions: A brief overview of health care CE professionals. *The Journal of Continuing Education in Nursing* 45(4): 153–154.

Barnsteiner, J., Disch, J., Hall, J., Mayer, D., & Moore, S. M. (2007). Promoting interprofessional education. *Nursing Outlook* 55(3): 144–150.

Berman, R. O. (2013). Moving out of one's comfort zone: Developing and teaching an interprofessional research course. *The Journal of Continuing Education in Nursing* 44(7): 303–308.

Billings, D. M. (2016). Building a culture of health: Implications for nurse educators. *The Journal of Continuing Education in Nursing* 47(5): 210–211.

Bleich, M. (2016a). Interprofessional education: Background and purpose, Part 1. *The Journal of Continuing Education in Nursing* 47(2): 55–57.

Bleich, M. (2016b). Interprofessional education: Selecting faculty and course design, Part 2. *The Journal of Continuing Education in Nursing* 47(3): 106–108.

Blue, I., & Fitzgerald, M. (2002). Interprofessional relations: Case studies of working relationships between registered nurses and general practitioners in rural Australia. *Journal of Clinical Nursing* 11(3): 314–321.

Boon, H., Verhoef, M., O'Hara, D., & Findlay, B. (2004). From parallel practice to integrative health care: A conceptual framework. *BMC Health Services Research* 4(15). doi: 10.1186/1472-6963-4-15

Borduas, F., Frank, B., Hall, P., Handfield-Jones, R., Hardwick, D., Ho, K., Jarvis-Selinger, S., Lockyear, J., Lauscher, H. N., MacLeod, A., Robitaille, M.-A., Rouleau, M., Sinclair, D., & Wright, B. (2006). *Facilitating the integration of into quality health care: Strategic roles of academic institutions.* Canada: Ottowa Health.

Bourdieu, P., & Passeron, J. C. (1990). *Reproduction in education, society, and culture.* (2nd ed). Thousand Oaks, CA: Sage.

Canadian Interprofessional Health Collaborative: A national interprofessional competency framework. (2010). Accessed at www.cihc.ca/files/CIHC_IPCompetencies_Feb1210.pdf

Centre for the Advancement of Interprofessional Education. (2002). Defining IPE. Accessed at www.caipe.org.uk/resources/defining-ipe/

Chen, A. K., Rivera, J., Rotter, N., Green, E., & Kools, S. (2016). Interprofessional education in the clinical setting: A qualitative look at the preceptor's perspective in training advanced practice nursing students. *Nurse Education in Practice* 21: 29–36.

Croenewett, L., Sherwood, G., Barnsteiner, J., Disch, J., Johnson, J., Mitchell, P., Warren, J. (2007). Quality and safety education for nurses. *Nursing Outlook* 55(3): 122–131.

Curran, V. R., Sharpe, D., Flynn, K., & Button P. (2010). A longitudinal study of the effect of an interprofessional education curriculum on student satisfaction and attitudes towards interprofessional teamwork and education. *Journal of Interprofessional Care* 24(1): 41–52. doi: 10.3109/13561820903011927

DeSilets, L. D. (2014). Turning the health care system right side up. *The Journal of Continuing Education in Nursing* 45(9): 375–376.

Dickerson, P. S., & Bernard, A. (2018). What's in a word? Understanding terms in continuing nursing education and professional development. *The Journal of Continuing Education in Nursing* 49(1): 19–25.

Disch, J. (2013). Interprofessional education and collaborative practice. *Nursing Outlook* 61: 3–4.

Eisler, R., & Potter, T. M. (2014). *Transforming interprofessional partnerships: A new framework for nursing and partnership based health care.* Indianapolis, IN: Sigma Theta Tau International.

Foucault, M. (1980). *Power/Knowledge.* New York, NY: Pantheon.

Gaberson, K. B., & Langston, N. F. (2017). Nursing as knowledge work: The imperative for lifelong learning. *AORN Journal.* 10.1016/J.aorn.2017.06.009

Glasper, A. (2018). Problems affecting the continuing professional development of nurses. *British Journal of Nursing* 27(12): 714–715.

Glossenger, A., Bennett, D., Ferren, M., & Sageser, P. E. (2016). Breaking down silos: An interprofessional approach to education. *The Journal of Continuing Nursing Education* 47(1): 5–7.

Hammick, M., Freeth, D., Koppel, I., Reeves, S., & Barr, H. (2007). A best evidence systematic review of : BEME guide no. 9. *Medical Teacher* 29: 735–751.

Hart, C. (2015). The elephant in the room: Nursing and nursing power on an interprofessional team. *The Journal of Continuing Education in Nursing* 46(8): 349–355.

Hudson, C. E., Sanders, M. K., & Pepper, C. (2013). Interprofessional education and prelicensure baccalaureate nursing students: an integrative review. *Nurse Education in Practice* 38(2): 76–80. doi: 10.1097/NNE.0b013e318282996d

IOM (Institute of Medicine). (2003). *Health Professions Education: A Bridge to Quality.* Washington, DC. The National Academies Press.

IOM (Institute of Medicine). (2011). *The Future of Nursing: Leading Change, Advancing Health.* Washington, DC: The National Academies Press. doi: 10.17226/12956

IOM (Institute of Medicine). (2012). *Redesigning continuing education in the health professions.* Washington, DC: National Academies Press.

Institute of Medicine (U.S.). (2012). *Interprofessional education for collaboration: Learning how to improve health from interprofessional models across the continuum of education to practice.* Washington, DC: National Academy Press.

Interprofessional Education Collaborative. (2011). Core competencies for interprofessional collaborative practice: Report of an expert panel. Washington, DC: Interprofessional Education Collaborative. Accessed at https://nebula.wsimg.com/2f68a39520b03336b41038c370497473?AccessKeyId=DC06780E69ED19E2B3A5&disposition=0&alloworigin=1

Ironside, P. M., & Valiga, T. M. (2006). Creating a vision for the future of nursing education: Moving toward excellence through innovation. *Nursing Education Perspectives* 27(3): 120–121.

James, A., & Francis, K. (2011). Mandatory continuing professional education: What is the prognosis? *Collegian* 18: 131–136.

Jarvis, P. (2005). Lifelong education and its relevance in nursing. *Nurse Education Today* 25: 655–660.

Joint Accreditation Commission. (2016) Joint accreditation for interprofessional continuing education. By the team for the team: Evolving interprofessional continuing education for optimal patient care— Report from the 2016. Accessed at www.jointaccreditation.org/

Joint Accreditation Commission. (2018). Joint accreditation for the provider of continuing education for the healthcare team. Accessed at www.jointaccreditation.org/

Josiah Macy Jr. Foundation. (2014). Conference recommendations: Partnering with patients, families, and communities: An urgent imperative for health care. Recommendations for the Macy Foundation Conference on partnering with patients, families and communities to link interprofessional practice and education. New York, NY: Author. Accessed at http://macyfoundation.org/docs/macy_pubs/JMF_ExecSummary_Final_Reference_web.pdf

Kowalski, K. (2012a). Recommendations of the future of nursing report. *The Journal of Continuing Education in Nursing* 43(2): 57–58.

Kowalski, K. (2012b). Working to implement the recommendations of the future of nursing report. *The Journal of Continuing Education in Nursing* 43(3): 104–105.

Kuper, A., & Whitehead, C. (2012). The paradox of : IPE as a mechanism of maintaining physician power? *Journal of Interprofessional Care* 2: 347–349.

Lawlis, T. R., Anson, J., & Greenfield, D. (2014). Barriers and enablers that influence sustainable : A literature review. *Journal of Interprofessional Care* 28(4): 305–310.

Lawton S., & Wimpenny P. (2003). Continuing professional development: A review. *Nursing Standard* 17(24): 41–44.

Lee, A. C. K., Tiwari, A. F. Y, Hui Choi, E. W. H., Yuen, K. H., & Wong, A. (2005). Hong Kong nurses. Perceptions of and participation in continuing nursing education. *The Journal of Continuing Education in Nursing* 36(5): 205–212.

McCafferty, K. L., Ball, S. J., & Cuddigan, J. (2017). Understanding the continuing education needs of rural Midwestern nurses. *The Journal of Continuing Education in Nursing* 48(6): 265–269.

McNeil, K. A., Mitchell, R. J., & Parker, V. (2013). Interprofessional practice and professional identity threat. *Health Sociology Review* 22: 291–307.

Meleis, A. (2016). Interprofessional education: A summary of reports and barriers to recommendations. *Journal of Nursing Scholarship* 48: 106–112.

Mitchell, M., Groves, M., Mitchell, C., & Batkin, J. (2010). Innovation in learning: An inter-professional approach to improving communication. *Nurse Education in Practice* 10(6): 379-384. doi: 10.1016/j.nephr.2010.05.008

Nugus, P., Greenfield, D., Travaglia, J., Westbrook, J., & Braithwaite, J. (2010). How and where clinicians exercise power: Interprofessional relations in health care. *Social Science & Medicine* 71: 898–909.

Pardue, K. T. (2015). A framework for the design, implementation, and evaluation of interprofessional education. *Nurse Educator* 40(1): 10–15.

Pecukonis, E. (2014). Interprofessional education: A theoretical orientation incorporating profession-centrism and social identity theory. *Journal of Law, Medicine & Ethics* 42(4): S60(5). doi: 10.1186/1472-6963-4-15

Qalehsari, M. Q., Khaghanizadeh, M., & Ebadi, A. (2017). Lifelong learning strategies in nursing: A systematic review. *Electronic Physician* 9(10): 5541–5550.

Reeves, S., Zwarenstein, M., Goldman, J., Barr, H., Freeth, D., Hamrich, M., & Koppel, I. (2009). Interprofessional education: Effects on professional practice and health care outcomes. *Cochrane Database of Systematic Reviews* 1: CD002213. doi: 10.1002/14651858.CD002213.

Robert Wood Johnson Foundation. (2015). From vision to action: Measures to mobilize a culture of health. Accessed at www.rwjf.org/content/dam/files/rwjf-web-files/Research/2015/From_Vision_to_Action_RWJF2015.pdf

Robert Wood Johnson Foundation. (2016). About a culture of health. Accessed at www.rwjf.org/content/rwjf/en/cultureofhealth/taking-action.html

Roman, T. C., Abraham, K., & Dever, K. (2016). TeamSTEPPS in long-term care: An academic partnership: Part 1. *The Journal of Continuing Education in Nursing* 47(11): 490–492.

Rosenfield, D., Oandasan, I., & Reeves, S. (2011). Perceptions versus reality: A qualitative study of students' expectations and experiences of interprofessional education. *Medical Education* 45(5): 471–477.

Royal College of Nursing. (2017). The domino effect: The RCN reveals the results of its latest employment survey. RCN Bulletin 29 November 2017. Accessed at https://tinyurl.com/yaqs4n2m

Royal College of Nursing. (2018a). Nursing staff miss out on training amid NHS cuts. Accessed at https://tinyurl.com/y9xurfdl

Royal College of Nursing. (2018b). Investing in a safe and effective workforce continuing professional development for nurses in the UK. Accessed at https://tinyurl.com/y8ue7dte

Sexton, M., & Baessler, M. (2016). Interprofessional collaborative practice. *The Journal of Continuing Education in Nursing* 47(4): 156–157.

Smith, K. A. (2014). Health care : Encouraging technology, teamwork, and team performance. *The Journal of Continuing Education in Nursing* 45(4): 181–187.

Thistlethwaite, J. (2012). Interprofessional education: A review of context, learning, and the research agenda. *Medical Education* 46: 58–70.

Thistlethwaite, J., & Moran, M. (2010). Learning outcomes for interprofessional education (IPE):Literature review and synthesis. *Journal of Interprofessional Care* 24(5): 503–513. doi: 10.3109/13561820.2010.483366

World Health Organization. (1988). Learning together to work together. Geneva: WHO.

World Health Organization, Department of Human Resources for Health. (2010). Framework for action on and collaborative practice. Geneva: WHO. Accessed at http://whqlibdoc.who.int/hq/2010/WHO_HRH_HPN_10.3_eng.pdf

Yoder-Wise, P. (2015). The future of nursing: A worldwide perspective. *The Journal of Continuing Education in Nursing* 46(4): 147.

18

GLOBAL APPROACHES TO INTERPROFESSIONAL EDUCATION

Dawn Forman, Roger Dunston, Simeon Mining, Sue Fyfe, Keryn Bolte, Marion Jones, Tagrid Yassin and Alistair Turvill

Introduction

It is clear that healthcare policies internationally recognise the need to ensure graduates entering the health and social care professions apply and practise knowledge and skills beyond theoretical knowledge learned at university, and implement newly acquired competencies (Higgs, Andresen & Fish, 2004). The development of these competencies differs in accordance with local cultural and environmental demands as this learning is context-based in the community of practice (Dahlgren, Richardson & Sjostrom, 2004). Peers, role models, mentors and supervisors can significantly influence the quality of learning (Goldenberg & Iwasiw, 1993; Ajjawi & Higgs, 2008; Johnsson & Hager, 2008).

It has been said that successful adaptation relies on social learning and active participation in reflection, and feedback from reliable others to judge actions and decisions (Regehr & Eva, 2007). Self-directed learning, critical thinking, reflective practice, adaptability and flexibility are highlighted as skills for lifelong learning (Barr, 2002; Smith & Pilling, 2007), and development of these skills in the practice environment during this critical transition time facilitates graduates' successful progression to the workforce (Smith & Pilling, 2007; Johnsson & Hager, 2008).

Research into best practice in interprofessional education (IPE) and its sustainability is ongoing (Reeves, Zwarenstein, Goldman, Barr, Freeth, Hammick & Koppel, 2009; Forman, Jones & Thistlethwaite, 2016). As nurses are described as healthcare leaders who "spearhead organisational change and systems improvements and teachers and mentors who prepare the next generation of direct care providers, educators, and nurse scientists" (Institute of Medicine, 2009, p. 5), it is vital that nurses both participate in and lead interprofessional collaboration in all aspects of their roles.

This chapter will therefore outline the differing approaches being taken internationally. Four case studies from different countries will be described, which collectively provide examples of how interprofessional collaboration fits with the country's health education priorities and cultural perspectives, the research which is being undertaken and how interprofessional curriculum is being developed and delivered.

Case study 1 – Australia

A number of government grants focused on the development of Australian educational practice have made it possible to track and learn from an 11-year programme of research in the area of IPE. This case study tracks major developments in this journey.

The context

This national development case study provides an account of how a group of individuals, universities, peak bodies and funders have come together over a period of 11 years to contribute to the further development of Australian IPE. The development programme we refer to is named the Curriculum Renewal Studies (CRS). The CRS consists of seven distinct development and research studies conducted between 2008 and 2019. Studies making up the CRS programme are:

1. *Interprofessional Health Education in Australia: The Way Forward* (Dunston, Lee, Matthews, Nisbet, Pockett, Thistlethwaite & White, 2009)
2. *Interprofessional Health Education: A Literature Review* (Nesbit, Lee, Kumar, Thistlethwaite & Dunston, 2011)
3. *Interprofessional Education for Health Professionals in Western Australia: Perspectives and Activity* (Nicol, 2011)
4. *Curriculum Renewal for Interprofessional Education in Health* (Interprofessional Curriculum Renewal Consortium, 2014)
5. *Work Based Assessment of Teamwork* (The iTOFT Consortium, 2015)
6. *Curriculum Renewal in Interprofessional Education in Health: Establishing Leadership and Capacity* (Dunston, Forman, Moran, Rogers, Thistlethwaite & Steketee, 2016)
7. *Securing an Interprofessional Future [SIF]: Establishing an Australian Interprofessional Education Governance and Development Framework* (Dunston, Fisher, Canny, Steketee, Forman, Rodgers, O'Keefe, Oates, Moran & Yassine, 2018) (This is an interim report; the final report will be available in 2019.)

Human research ethics approval was obtained for each of the studies. Details of the above studies can be found at: https://sifproject.com/projects/

As we initiated our first study three things stood out. Firstly, we knew almost nothing about Australian IPE in general – how it was understood and defined across universities and, more specifically, how IPE was configured in individual universities, faculties and schools. We would need to learn. Secondly, from everything we knew about working with and benefiting from cultural diversity, we recognised the need to find ways to invite, enable and sustain individuals, groups and academic communities who operated in different uniprofessional spaces to come together, stay together and inquire together. Thirdly, although the idea was little developed at the time, it seemed to us that any significant change in how Australian IPE was designed and delivered would need to be inclusive, collaborative, developed at the national level and consensus-based – this has proved to be the case.

What follows is a summary of how the CRS programme developed, our theoretical and methodological framework, what we learned and how we responded. As an indication of how this work developed we will discuss how the "we" – initially a small grouping – expanded to become a national cross-sector mobilisation including nursing and midwifery, medicine, allied health, consumers, the registration and accreditation system, health policy and, more broadly, government. Whilst these developments occurred as a response to Australian circumstances, we believe there is much that will resonate with those involved with IPE in a wide range of jurisdictions.

Aims, theorisation, methodology and methods

In this section, we look at the aims, theorisations, methodology and methods of the CRS. We identified five broad aims:

1. to identify how Australian IPE existed across the periods of our studies – 2007–2019
2. to understand the various ways in which IPE was experienced by those involved – the stakeholder experience
3. to understand the institutional dynamics and the factors that were constraining and/or enabling IPE at local and national levels
4. to work closely with CRS participants to identify what would be required to improve the sustainability and outcomes of Australian IPE
5. to use what we were learning to design and facilitate positive change for interprofessional programmes.

To assist with the design and collective development of the studies, we drew extensively on a group of theories that are particularly suited to understanding and working with cultural diversity and cultural change, in particular socio-cultural, socio-material and practice theories (Hager, Reich & Lee, 2012). As distinguished from individually focused, cognitive and behavioural theories of learning – theories that tend to be dominant in the area of health professional education – socio-cultural theories draw attention to the complex social, cultural and environmental elements and negotiations that constitute and shape health practice, the process of education and learning and the management of change. These ideas shaped our design and methods; in particular they underlined the importance of working inclusively, iteratively, respectfully and collectively. What would be required was an ongoing conversation in which all parties felt included, respected, valued and heard. In terms of methods, the CRS was developed utilising a mixed methods approach. In particular:

*   Surveys that focused on categorisation, frequency and description were used to build activity profiles that related to curriculum and educational practice – what was occurring, where, how, and so on.
*   Documentary sources – the IPE research literature and university curriculum and performance documents were utilised.
*   Interviews, focus groups, fora and collective narrative development activities were used to elicit the experience of participants.
*   Wherever possible and meaningful, comparative analyses were developed using Australian and overseas examples of curriculum, education practice, evaluation data, and so forth.
*   A particular emphasis on futures thinking (Hager, Reich & Lee, 2012) was also developed. Participants in all studies were asked to pay particular attention to what would be required to create and sustain a significant and positive change in Australian IPE. (We return to this issue in studies 6 and 7.)

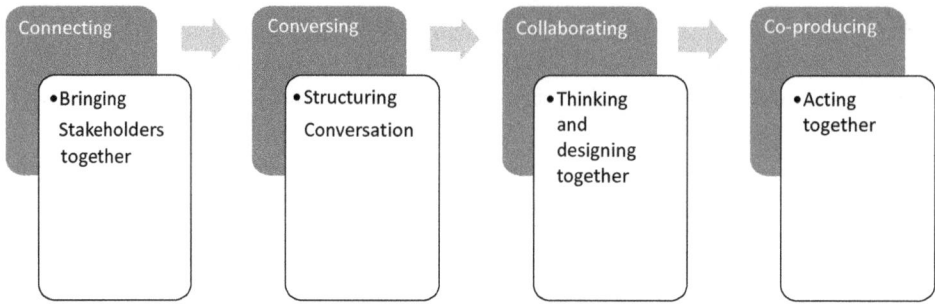

Figure 18.1 Sequencing the studies.

The curriculum renewal studies – connecting, conversing, collaborating and co-producing

In this section, we look at the sequencing and focus of each of the seven studies.

From the commencement of our first study, *The Way Forward*, we saw each study as, firstly, an opportunity to elicit information – addressing the descriptive and information-gathering aims of the CRS; and, secondly, as an opportunity to develop trust and identity building work which would support the development aims of the CRS.

Whilst Figure 18.1 presents a simple view of what was a complex process developed across time, it pictorially represents the process logic we designed into the studies.

Study 1: mapping the territory

Study 1, a national scoping and development study, was a summary description of the Australian IPE landscape. We developed and utilised a broadly scoped national survey. Study 1 was descriptive rather than analytic. Critically, study 1 also focused on "connecting" – bringing stakeholders together – and on trust and relationship building. Its publications, including an Australian-focused IPE literature review (Nesbit, Lee, Kumar, Thistlethwaite and Dunston (2011) were, we believe, the first time that an "Australian" IPE focus was foregrounded and studied.

Methodologically, our stakeholders – all our stakeholders – were the "experts". We sought to develop a series of narratives as to how Australian IPE was experienced. What was identified was provisional, open to elaboration; meanings were checked. What was clear was immense diversity in every area. We identified "diversity" and "locality" as the two defining characteristics of Australian IPE. This initial work was also about engaging with the subjective experience of those involved. Our intent was to begin the cultural move away from existing as competing tribes with closed boundaries toward the recognition that we were all health professionals and that we were all struggling with complexity, uncertainty, the wish to add value and change.

Studies 2, 3 and 4: description, analysis and national resource development

Studies 2, 3 and 4 were strongly focused on more in-depth description, detailed analysis and the identification of Australian resources and exemplars that could be used by all universities. Study 3 (Nicol, 2011) was particularly important, with its ethnographic approach used to develop in-depth understandings of the complex dynamics at play as universities in one Australian state sought to develop their interprofessional curriculum and educational practices.

Returning to the idea of relationship and identity building, studies 2 and 4 moved beyond engagement and conversation to opening boundaries and sharing experiences and resources – the intellectual property of universities and professions. What was noticeable was the degree of generosity and openness to sharing and working together that occurred. Importantly, the work that was occurring, and the resources that were being developed, began to be located on university and government websites. The CRS programme began to be discussed in terms of national leadership and the resources identified as "national" resources. A small but important degree of interprofessional identity development and national mobilisation was occurring (Dunston, Forman, Thistlethwaite, Rogers, Steketee & Moran (2018).

Study 5

Study 5 was far more particular in its aims. It addressed an issue that is, both nationally and globally, a major focus of IPE discussion and scholarship, that is, how to "assess" individual students participating in IPE teamwork activities.

The study reviewed and evaluated existing pre-qualification work-based assessment across the health professions with a focus on assessment for collaborative teamwork competencies. As part of this review, the study also explored the conceptual underpinnings and the definitions of teamwork competencies, considering teamwork as both a set of linked attributes and a global construct. The outcome of this work was the development of a framework for the work-based assessment of teamwork. Exemplary instruments are being piloted to explore the application of this framework in a range of different contexts. The instrument, individual Observation and Feedback Tool (iTOFT) (The iTOFT Consortium, Australia, 2015), focuses on formative assessment, with an educational impact arising from its usefulness as a means of giving timely and constructive feedback.

Study 6

Returning to the focus on IPE futures, studies 6 and 7 were developed as transition and action or co-production studies. By the time we were part-way through study 5, it seemed to us that we had reached a national consensus on what was required to make a major shift in how Australian IPE was being conceptualised, designed and implemented. Study 6, *Establishing Leadership and Capacity* (Dunston, Forman, Moran, Rogers, Thistlethwaite & Steketee, 2016), was designed with the intent of testing these ideas. Did we have a national consensus and what would it require to shift this consensus from ideas to practice?

Study 6 was developed as a series of deliberative fora – a national event, a state-based event and a series of focus groups and individual events/interviews. There were differences in emphasis. Not surprisingly, the state-based forum focused on state-based issues and development, whereas the national forum focused on the development of national issues and national developments. However, what was common across all fora and consultations was the need not just for the development of individual areas, but for something that would exist and work as an integrated system of national IPE governance and development. This was a major step and a new way of thinking about what would be required to shift Australian IPE from the margins to the centre of education practice.

What emerged from the fora can be described as the design for a "national IPE architecture". This architecture is to build an inclusive, collegial and participatory national approach to understanding, communicating, learning about and developing IPE/interprofessional practice in Australia. This is about the development of an interprofessional approach involving the widest possible participation of all groups involved with or impacted by IPE/interprofessional practice (Dunston, Forman, Moran, Rogers, Thistlethwaite & Steketee, 2016).

Study 7

Study 7 took its point of departure from the system development focus of study 6. Funding was sought and granted for the SIF project to focus on the implementation of an Australian IPE governance and development framework and system. This would target:

1. national IPE leadership – bringing all professions and all sectors together, to establish an enduring interprofessional national body. This mechanism will be a point of inclusive coordination and will give direction and support to the further development of Australian IPE
2. embedding and supporting an IPE and interprofessional collaborative focus as part of the Australian health accreditation scheme. A partnership with bodies in the existing accreditation system
3. the further development of IPE capacity and capability across all relevant universities and regulatory bodies to further cement a partnership between the higher-education and health sectors
4. establishing an Australasian IPE/interprofessional collaborative practice (IPCP) knowledge and information hub. This work will also include the development of Australian IPE-focused research and knowledge development agenda
5. the development of an "Australian IPE work plan" for all healthcare professionals.

Methodologically and practically, success in developing and sustaining national IPE governance would require not only the normative agreement of other already established bodies, but also their ownership and active participation in working for the further development of Australian IPE. We have referred to this work and to this stage of the CRS programme as developing a co-productive approach.

Close to the end of study 7 (December 2018), we can report that the co-productive work is progressing well. The focus of the SIF study has been working with over 13 national peak bodies with an interest in or involvement with IPE to operationalise the national governance and development framework and system discussed above. An update in our last newsletter captures this well:

> One of the most significant outcomes from the day [a national IPE round table convened by SIF] was regarding the next stages of design and implementation work being undertaken by a "Collaboration" comprised of a small number of key cross-sector peak bodies [establishing the Collaboration was a recommendation made by the participant peak bodies]. It was agreed that the Collaboration would auspice the development of a more broadly based "National IPE Advisory Group" – a group whose membership would include representatives of key bodies and individuals with high levels of IPE and IPCP expertise. To date, five peak bodies are working with the SIF project to finalise

the design and implementation details of the National IPE Advisory Group and the Collaboration.

(Dunston, Fisher, Canny, Steketee, Forman, Rogers, O'Keefe,
Oates, Moran & Yassine, 2018a)

"Terms of reference" of the National Advisory Group were agreed. The Advisory Group will:

1. provide vision and leadership for the development of IPE and collaborative practice across all areas of Australian health professional education and health service delivery
2. make recommendations and provide policy advice based on a strategic knowledge of the field of IPE, the priorities and development of Australian health services and health professional education
3. advocate for IPE to be adopted and developed across all health profession education and health services
4. support initiatives that enable interaction, learning and shared decision making across uniprofessional and interprofessional educators and practitioners
5. demonstrate an interactive and participatory approach to engaging with the international interprofessional community (National SIF Project IPE Round-Table 21 September 2017) https://sifproject.files.wordpress.com/2018/02/sif-project-round-table-21-sep-17_out comes-report.pdf

The curriculum renewal studies – a critical review

One of the most striking features of the decade-long CRS cycle has been the positive response from the many organisations we approached. Our experience challenges the widely held view that what primarily constrains the development of IPE and, as a consequence, interprofessional and collaborative practice, is the resistance of key stakeholders, in particular the professions. On the contrary, many professions have a long-standing commitment to recognising the importance of a need for interprofessional collaborative practice and there-fore IPE. For example, the Australian nursing and midwifery professions make the following statement:

> Registered Nurse Accreditation Standards (2012) require that workplace experience opportunities are provided for interprofessional and interprofessional learning and development of knowledge, skills and behaviours for collaborative practice.

(Woods, 2017: p. 23)

Our experience requires a different explanation. We suggest that what has been missing is the existence of any enduring mechanisms to bring professions and other key stakeholders together over time to work through what will be required to establish and sustain a shared approach to the further development of IPE. Whilst the larger and more powerful profes-sions, such as nursing, midwifery and medicine, have traditionally been the leaders in initiat-ing IPE-focused activity, it is not surprising, given the already well-developed focus of and demands on these professions, that many of these initiatives have failed to move from intent to action.

The most important learnings we draw from the CRS experience are as follows.

Firstly, good intent, regardless of how powerful and influential the professions involved are, whilst necessary, will not be sufficient to progress IPE as a national and system-wide outcome. Secondly, what will be required is the establishment of an enabling framework and system dedicated to the governance and development of IPE as its primary aim. The SIF project is an Australian attempt to design and implement such a system. Thirdly, given the need for an IPE system that is coherent and sustainable, its development must be an ongoing and collectively owned activity.

Case study 2 – New Zealand

As with Australia, IPE and collaborative practice in New Zealand have been themes in nursing curricula for many years. This case study provides an overview of the background and current developments in New Zealand.

The context

New Zealand (Aotearoa) is a three-island country in the South Pacific and did not have a public health system until the 1860s (Gage & Hornblower, 2007). However, with a developing population, nursing changed rapidly from the 1880s onwards with the Nurse Registration Act of 1901 being passed at the same time as hospital-trained nurses became evident. Over the next 50 years there was discussion on how nursing and nurse education would develop, with university education being considered in multiple years over this period. The major shift in nurse education came in the early 1970s with the Carpenter report of 1971 (Kirkman, 2019) recommending the transfer of the training of nurses to educating nurses in tertiary education institutions such as polytechnics and universities (Gage & Hornblower, 2007). The shift resulted in funding through Vote Health to the education sector to support IPE and collaborative practice. As Gage and Hornblower (2007: p. 333) stated, "New Zealand nursing has the opportunities to develop areas of independent practice to emphasise a *collaborative* rather than a subordinate relationship with medicine and to contribute nursing expertise to scientific knowledge and research".

All programmes, including those which are interprofessional, which are developed within universities are approved through Universities New Zealand Committee for Universities Approval of Programmes (CUAP) of all academic programmes in New Zealand's eight universities. The work of CUAP includes assessing that all New Zealand's universities fulfil the rules for the approval and accreditation of qualifications and programmes within those qualifications, as provided for in section 253(a) of the Education Act 1989 (Handbook of CUAP, 2018). Alongside this are programmes within the polytechnic system, and these programmes are approved through the New Zealand Qualification Authority (NZQA). NZQA's role in the education sector is to ensure that New Zealand qualifications are regarded as credible and robust, nationally and internationally, in order to help learners succeed in their chosen endeavours and to contribute to New Zealand society. For nursing, the Nursing Council of New Zealand works with NZQA in the approval process so statutory requirements are clearly evident within the programmes.

Alongside the approval processes for universities is the Academic Quality Agency for New Zealand (AQA), which is a body operationally independent of Universities New Zealand, and set up by the universities to ensure the quality of their academic activities is maintained and consistent with the CUAP processes and policy. There were several challenges for nursing in that there were now student-based comprehensive nursing programmes in 16 schools of nursing; nursing-focused knowledge was needed to be developed along with nursing research and dissemination of that knowledge. Between the 1970s and today's nursing workforce development, nursing has a degree-entry qualification to practice; it has the opportunity to complete master's and doctoral degrees, with nurses holding positions throughout the health sector, from bedside to heads of departments, with academia and government positions at their fingertips. Originally, the development of programmes concentrated on both the generic and multidisciplinary aspects of practice, along with moving to provide logical pathways for health professionals from many disciplines. Partnership in care and a philosophy of care developed, which not only reflected the patient code of rights, but altered the balance of power between the disciplines, client and health professional, and accentuated the need to strengthen interprofessional collaboration. All of the programmes developed have been approved through either CUAP or NZQA, providing consistency in standards across New Zealand.

Nursing opportunities

Under the Health Practitioners Competence Assurance Act (HPCA) 2003, the Nursing Council of New Zealand continues as the statutory body which has responsibility for nurse registration and ongoing speciality accreditation, such as prescribing, surgical assistant and multiple nurse practitioner status opportunities. This also provided the change in practice for "interprofessional working, which the World Health Organization (WHO) believes is interprofessional collaboration in education and practice as an innovative strategy that will play an important role in mitigation in the global workforce crisis" (WHO, 2010: p. 7). Collaborative practice not only indicates the health team will work together but also requires nursing and other health disciplines to change from uniprofessionalism to interprofessionalism (Jones, Jamieson & Anderson, 2015).

While interprofessional development originally occurred more as parallel practice (Boon, Verhoef, O'Hara & Findlay, 2004), solid cross-disciplinary relationships have developed over the years as academics have worked more closely together. In New Zealand this is still in development. To help this there are some postgraduate programmes that are open to all health professionals and promoting interprofessional working. The programme includes students from disciplines such as psychology, nursing, midwifery, oral health, physiotherapy, occupational therapy, podiatry, psychotherapy, applied science, sport and recreation undertaking papers (modules) together, such as health professional education, ethics, health law, leadership, health systems analysis, management, child health, emergency management, rehabilitation and occupational practice, to name a few.

The New Zealand context: biculturalism and the Treaty of Waitangi

Also unique in some respects to New Zealand is the development of cultural safety underpinned by the Treaty of Waitangi (te Tiriti o Waitangi) of 1840. Health professional education led by nursing, for example, is shaped by its commitment to biculturalism and cultural safety. Biculturalism represents "the relationship between Maori [the indigenous people of New Zealand] and others, particularly the Crown" (Ramsden, 2005: p. 5). Health professionals and health educators recognise the significance of the Treaty of Waitangi because of the interconnections between the health status of Maori, the Treaty of Waitangi and health service delivery in New Zealand. The three main tenets of the treaty are partnership, participation and protection. These principles have raised cultural awareness and cultural sensitivity through to cultural safety as being paramount within education and practice and "challenge many health care professionals and health providers [who] are required to be culturally sensitive to alternative ways of looking at the world" (Wareham, McCallin &

Diesfeld, 2005: p. 350). While many countries are very familiar with multicultural concerns, the distinctive bicultural emphasis in New Zealand raises significant issues. "It is not so much the presence of differing beliefs and ideals that makes bicultural issues unique, but rather the progressive integration of the principles right across every part of New Zealand society" (Main, McCallin & Smith, 2006: p. 145). The implications of the Treaty of Waitangi and bicultural issues are considered as core to all educational programmes. This includes a commitment to partnership in identifying and meeting health needs of Maori along with integrating the principles of partnership, protection and participation, as mentioned above (Moss, 2005). The Nursing Council's (2011, p. 7) definition of cultural safety is the effective nursing practice of a person or family from another culture, and is determined by that person or family. Culture includes, but is not restricted to, age or generation; gender; sexual orientation; occupation and socioeconomic status; ethnic origin or migrant experience; religious or spiritual belief; and disability. The nurses delivering the nursing service will have undertaken a process of reflection on their own cultural identity and will recognise the impact that their personal culture has on their professional practice. Unsafe cultural practice comprises any action which diminishes, demeans or disempowers the cultural identity and well-being of an individual.

Nursing in New Zealand today is continuing its development in all levels of education and practice with a strong focus on interprofessional learning and working. Cultural safety in practice encourages collaboration which in turn promotes the ongoing development needs for interprofessional practice being a reality.

Case study 3 – Malaysia

Dr Wendy Shoesmith, Dr Loo Jiann Lin, Ms Waidah Sawatan

In this case study we look at how interprofessional collaboration has been implemented in the community setting in Sabah, Malaysia.

The context

Malaysia is a middle-income country in Asia with a relatively well-developed health system that has focused on acute and infectious diseases to reduce maternal and infant mortality, although non-communicable and chronic diseases are becoming more prevalent. The state of Sabah (population 3.5 million) on the island of Borneo differs from most other parts of Malaysia, both socioeconomically and culturally, with higher rates of poverty and lower levels of healthcare staff than the rest of the country. The Malaysian public sector has a hierarchical culture, with top-down decision making the norm and few decisions made collaboratively. In the healthcare system, most patient care decisions are made by doctors with little interprofessional input. The training system for staff reflects the previous focus on acute and infectious diseases, in that training is task-focused, rather than relationship-focused. In this context, collaborative practice is difficult to achieve (Shoesmith, Sawatan, Abdullah & Fyfe, 2016). Since there is minimal collaborative practice in the healthcare system, it is very difficult to establish IPE. Academic staff awareness of collaborative practice is low, there are no accreditation requirements for IPE in either nursing or medicine and there are few appropriate "communities of practice" for students to learn the skills needed.

Programmes and IPE for health students in Sabah

Universiti Malaysia Sabah (UMS) was established in 1994 and started enrolling students into medicine in 2003 and nursing in 2008. A form of IPE has been introduced into two programmes: the health promotion programme and later into the university community partnership programme (PuPUK).

In the health promotion programme, a group of around 15 students go to a rural community for two weeks, during which time they conduct a rapid rural appraisal. This appraisal involves undertaking some key informant interviews and then identifying health issues in the community. The students then develop a health promotion campaign focusing on raising awareness and changing attitudes and behaviour that could help improve that health issue. In the PuPUK programme, the students are "adopted" by a rural family for five years. They visit the family three times per year for the duration of their course and develop a relationship with the family members, learning about their culture, family dynamics, health issues, health-related behaviour and how all of these factors interact. In later years, they conduct an intervention in the family to help to improve their health. The medical students have been taking part in these two community programmes since 2004. The nursing students have been taking part in the health promotion programme since 2011 and the PuPUK programme since 2014.

These programmes were introduced with minimal training and awareness about IPE or collaborative practice in staff or students. Formal staff training on IPE was conducted in 2013 in two one-day workshops, in which approximately 40% of the staff participated. These workshops aimed to help staff understand the rationale behind IPE and collaborative practice. The nursing students were formally introduced to the ideas of IPE and collaborative practice, with a two-hour workshop-style class, but the medical students have no formal teaching on IPE or collaborative practice.

A realist evaluation of the IPE in these programmes was conducted in 2015, using focus groups of medical and nursing students (Shoesmith, Sawatan, Abdullah & Fyfe, 2016). These focus groups indicated that the programmes were having an impact on intermediate outcomes, including a reduction of stereotypes, increased contact between the professional groups and a better understanding of roles. The nursing students had some understanding of the goals of IPE and collaborative practice and both the nursing and medical role. The medical students' understanding of these things was less, which was assumed to be because they had no formal introduction to IPE and collaborative practice. The medical students who had the most contact with the nursing students were more positive about the PuPUK programme, they appeared to be more relationship-oriented (rather than task-oriented) and described learning from the nursing students in the way that they communicated with the family.

Despite the loss of many of the staff who were trained in 2014, there is now a growing awareness in the academic staff of the importance of collaborative practice and IPE. This growing awareness has partly been because some of the newer staff have spent time training abroad in healthcare systems with established collaborative practice. A new medical curriculum will be implemented in 2020 and this includes a final-year module where medical students will be attached to a "community of practice" where collaborative practice skills are used. The new curriculum will also include theoretical teaching on IPE and collaborative practice, high-fidelity interprofessional simulations and joint sessions for medical and nursing students to plan care for complex patients. The new University Hospital (currently under construction) also aims to develop systems around the principles of collaborative practice.

These programmes have brought IPE into the learning experience, without it being an explicit focus. The response from students suggests that they see benefits from learning with and about each other. The experience with the PuPUK and health promotion programme have shown that IPE can be introduced with minimal staff training and awareness and with some of the aims being met without being explicitly identified. The way IPE was introduced was far from ideal, but it does appear to be having an effect and we hope that this will lead to slow systems change.

Case study 4 – Kenya

In this case study we provide an interprofessional problem-based learning example being used in a university in Kenya. In many ways this tutorial example could be used internationally but it is particularly important in the context in Kenya where the healthcare needs of mothers and children under five are a priority.

The context

Kenya is classed as a lower-middle-income country with a complexity of healthcare needs, including an under-five mortality rate of double the global average (www.who.int/gho/countries/ken.pdf).

Moi University College of Health Sciences, Eldoret, Kenya has utilised an interprofessional curriculum since 1989 (Mining, 2014) and problem-based learning case studies (Owino, 2010), are one mechanism which is used to facilitate interprofessional learning in the basic sciences, pathology and clinical courses. For the case studies the nursing students are integrated in tutorial groups where appropriate, with students studying to be medical laboratory scientists, physiotherapists, pharmacists, medical psychologists and public health professionals. Tutorials can take place in the classroom, on wards and in the community. All students in the clinical areas have log books to document their activities and the procedures they have undertaken.

The log books are signed by the immediate supervisor in the ward and countersigned by the academic tutor responsible for the course. Table 18.1 shows how the tutorial process is conducted in Moi University.

Student case study

An eight-year-old girl has been brought by her mother to the paediatric unit of a community hospital with chief complaints of hotness of the body, chill and global headache. The mother tells the nurse that the child became unwell five days ago and the symptoms, especially the headache, have been worsening in severity over the last two days. The mother also reports that the girl has not been feeding well lately and has been vomiting each time she tries feeding her. It is also reported that the girl has had four seizures over the last day and has been unusually sleepy since the previous night. On examination, the admitting clinician observes that the girl has a stiff neck, stiff leg joints and a purpuric rash on the trunk and legs. The clinician makes a decision to refer the patient to the Moi Teaching and Referral Hospital for further investigations and proper management.

- What further investigations may be necessary?
- How will we decide which investigations are undertaken and ensure a patient-centred approach?

Table 18.1 The tutorial process

1.0 Initial encounter with the problem: problem formulation
1.1 Clarify terms and concepts
1.2 Formulate the problem and identify its components
1.3 Suggest possible explanations
1.4 Collect data
1.5 Schematise and classify the hypotheses in step 3
1.6 Formalise and select learning issues
2.0 Self-directed learning activities
2.1 Locating and consulting learning resources outside the classroom
2.2 Reading and interpreting text in the light of the problem
2.3 Questioning and verifying own understanding with relevant human resources (subject experts, patients and/or relatives, policymakers, etc.)
3.0 Subsequent encounter with the problem: synthesis and review of newly acquired information
3.1 Formulate most likely explanation
3.2 Propose what action should or would be taken
3.3 Carry out action where feasible or appropriate
3.4 Verify effectiveness of action
4.0 Attain problem closure
4.1 Formulate further study questions
4.2 Review group process and progress

- Which healthcare professions may be involved and how will they communicate between one another and with the mother of the child?
- What responsibilities do the healthcare professions have for the ongoing health and welfare of the mother and child?

Key for the tutor guide: paediatric healthcare and theory

- Have the students addressed the common microbial and viral infections of newborns?
- Have the students checked on the medical history of childhood immunisation?
- Have the students interpreted the whole blood count and specific microbial laboratory test suspected in the test?
- Have the students clarified the reasons why the clinician ordered further investigations and management in a specialised paediatric unit in a referral hospital?
- Have the students collectively identified the investigations needed?
- Have the students ensured effective communication between the professions?
- Have the students identified the ongoing health and welfare considerations of the mother and child?

There are many examples of case studies, curriculum developments and collaborative tools being used internationally. As yet, however, there is no international "go to" place where health professionals who are developing, implementing and refining IPE can access the best from around the world. It is hoped that the SIF project manages to take a leap in this direction.

Conclusion

This chapter has provided four case studies from four countries and showcased how countries with differing strategic healthcare priorities are adapting to ensure all healthcare professionals are equipped with the skills to work interprofessionally and collaboratively with a focus on the needs of the patient and the community in which they live.

It is clear that, for all healthcare professionals and the people in their care, we still need to develop a range of IPE tools for students to learn in different contexts, continue our research and publish in this area and find ways of sharing good practice and sustaining good practice across the globe. The nursing profession internationally is embracing and often leading these interprofessional developments and is key to ensuring interprofessional collaboration, and research in this area continues. In doing so it is imperative that leaders of these developments learn from the developments which have taken place in other countries. It is hoped that the case studies provided give some insight into the research and developments taking place internationally and the importance of taking into account the cultural aspects of the community in which interprofessional practice will be offered when the provision is implemented.

References

Ajjawi R & Higgs J (2008) Learning to reason: a journey of professional socialisation. *Advances in Health Sciences Education: Theory and Practice* 13(2): 133–150.

Barr H (2002) *Interprofessional education: today, yesterday and tomorrow.* Commissioned by the learning and teaching support network of the health sciences and practice from the UK Centre for the Advancement of Interprofessional Education London: CAIPE.

Boon H, Verhoef M, O'Hara D & Findlay B (2004) From parallel practice to integrative health care: a conceptual framework. *BMC Health Services Research, [Electronic]* 4: 15–20. Accessed at: www.biomed central.com/1472-6963/4/15.

Dahlgren M A, Richardson B & Sjostrom B (2004) Professions as communities of practice. In J Higgs, B Richardson & M A Dahlgren (Eds) *Developing practice knowledge for health professionals.* Edinburgh: Butterworth Heinemann, pp. 71–88.

Dunston R, Fisher A, Canny B, Steketee C, Forman D, Rogers G D, O'Keefe M, Oates M, Moran M & Yassine T (2018a) *Securing an interprofessional future. Establishing an Australian interprofessional education governance and development framework – a compelling case.* Information brochure Canberra: Australian Government Department of Education and Training.

Dunston R, Forman D, Moran M, Rogers G D, Thistlethwaite J & Steketee C (2016) *Curriculum renewal in interprofessional education in health: establishing leadership and capacity.* Canberra: Commonwealth of Australia, Office for Learning and Teaching.

Dunston R, Forman D, Thistlethwaite J, Rogers G D, Steketee C & Moran M (2018b) Repositioning interprofessional education from the margins to the centre of Australian health professional education – what is required? *Australian Health Review.* Accessed at: https://doi.org/10.1071/AH17081.

Dunston R, Lee A, Matthews L, Nisbet G, Pockett R, Thistlethwaite J & White J (2009) *Interprofessional health education in Australia: the way forward.* Sydney: University of Technology Sydney.

Forman D, Jones M & Thistlethwaite J (Eds) (2016) *Leading research and evaluation in interprofessional education and collaborative practice.* London: Palgrave Macmillan.

Gage J D & Hornblower A R (2007) Development of the New Zealand nursing workforce: historical themes and current challenges. *Nursing Inquiry* 14(4): 330–334.

Goldenberg D & Iwasiw C (1993) Professional socialsation of nursing students as an outcome of a senior clinical preceptorship experience. *Nurse Education Today* 13: 3–15.

Hager P, Reich A & Lee A (2012) *Practice, learning and change: practice-theory perspectives on professional learning.* Dordrecht: Springer.

Higgs J, Andresen L & Fish D (2004) Practice knowledge – its nature, sources and contexts. In J Higgs, B Richardson & M Dahlgren (Eds) *Developing practice knowledge for health professionals.* Edinburgh: Butterworth Heinemann, pp. 51–69.

Institute of Medicine (2009) *Roundtable on evidence-based medicine. Leadership commitments to improve value in healthcare: finding common ground: workshop summary.* Washington, DC: National Academies Press (US). Accessed at: www.ncbi.nlm.nih.gov/books/NBK52851/.

Interprofessional Curriculum Renewal Consortium, Australia (2014) *Curriculum renewal for interprofessional education in health.* Canberra: Commonwealth of Australia, Office for Learning and Teaching.

Johnsson M C & Hager P (2008) Navigating the wilderness of becoming professional. *Journal of Workplace Learning* 20(7/8): 526–536.

Jones M, Jamieson I & Anderson E (2015) Perioperative practice in the context of client-centred care. In C Orchard & L Bainbridge (Eds) *Interprofessional client-centred collaborative practice. What does it look like? How can it be achieved?* New York: Nova Science Publishers, pp. 25–36.

Kirkman A (2019) Health practitioners – Nurses and midwives. Te Ara – the Encyclopedia of New Zealand. Accessed at: www.TeAra.govt.nz/en/health-practitioners/page-3.

Main C A, McCallin A M & Smith N (2006) Cultural safety and cultural competence: what does this mean for physiotherapists? *NZ Journal of Physiotherapy* 34(3): 144–150.

Mining S (2014) Community development of interprofessional practice in Kenya. In D Forman, M Jones & J Thistlethwaite (Eds) *Leadership development for interprofessional education and collaborative practice.* London: Palgrave MacMillan, pp. 196–205.

Moss L (2005) Biculturalism and cultural diversity: how far does state policy in New Zealand and the UK seek to reflect, enable or idealise the development of minority culture? *International Journal of Cultural Policy* 11(2): 187–197.

Nesbit G, Lee A, Kumar K, Thistlethwaite J & Dunston R (2011) *Interprofessional health education: a literature review.* Canberra: Australia Learning and Teaching Council.

Nicol P (2011) *Interprofessional education for health professionals in Western Australia: perspectives and activity.* Sydney: University of Technology Sydney.

Nursing Council of New Zealand (2011) *Guidelines for cultural safety, the Treaty of Waitangi and Maori health in nursing education and practice.* Auckland: Nursing Council of NZ.

Owino C (2010) Perceptions of interns' performance: a comparison between a problem-based and a conventional curriculum journal. *East African Medical Journal* 87(7): 15–20.

Ramsden I (2005) Towards cultural safety. In D Wepa (Ed) *Cultural safety in Aotearoa New Zealand.* Auckland, New Zealand: Pearson Education, pp. 2–19.

Reeves S, Zwarenstein M, Goldman J M, Barr H, Freeth D, Hammick M & Koppel I (2009) Interprofessional education: effects on professional practice and health care outcomes (Review). *Cochrane Database System Review* 1(1): CD002213.

Regehr G & Eva K W (2007) Self-assessment, self-direction, and the self-regulating professional. *Clinical Orthopaedics and Related Research* 449: 34–38.

Registered Nurse Accreditation Standards (2012) Australian Nursing and Midwifery Accreditation Council.

Shoesmith W, Sawatan W, Abdullah A F & Fyfe S (2016) Leadership and evaluation issues in interprofessional education in Sabah Malaysia. In D Forman, M Jones & J Thistlethwaite (Eds) *Leading research and evaluation in interprofessional education and collaborative practice.* London: Palgrave, pp. 193–212.

Smith R A & Pilling S (2007) Allied health graduate program – supporting the transition from student to professional in an interdisciplinary program. *Journal of Interprofessional Care* 21(3): 265–276.

The iTOFT Consortium, Australia (2015) *Work based assessment of teamwork: an interprofessional approach.* Canberra: Australian Government, Office for Learning and Teaching.

Universities New Zealand (2018) *Handbook of Committee of Universities Approval Processes (CUAP).* Accessed at: www.universitiesnz.ac.nz/quality-assurance/

Wareham P, McCallin A M & Diesfeld K (2005) Advance directives: the New Zealand context. *Nursing Ethics: An International Journal for Health Care Professionals* 12(4): 3.

Woods M (2017) *Australia's health workforce: strengthening the education foundation.* Independent review of accreditation systems within the national registration and accreditation scheme for health profession. Accessed at: www.coaghealthcouncil.gov.au/Projects/Accreditation-Systems-Review

World Health Organization (WHO) (2010) *Framework for action on interprofessional education & collaborative practice.* Geneva: World Health Organization. (WHO/HRH/HPN/10, 349–359.

19

DYSLEXIA AND NURSE EDUCATION

Rachael Major

Introduction

Dyslexia is a specific learning difficulty or difference, which affects around 10 per cent of the population, 4 per cent severely (British Dyslexia Association, 2012). It is not known how many nurses have the condition (Sanderson-Mann, 2006). However, research has shown that people with dyslexia might be drawn to people-orientated careers, such as nursing, which exhibit a higher practical component and less structure than an office-based profession (Taylor and Walter, 2003). This way of working appears to suit individuals with dyslexia (Bartlett et al., 2010), therefore the number of nurses with dyslexia might be higher than in the general population. In this context it is important to note that nursing practice is changing, with a requirement for a more flexible workforce and higher academic qualifications to meet the increasing demands of an ageing population and more complex health problems (Willis, 2015). These increasingly complex care requirements require the nursing student to continue to engage in lifelong learning after registration on the professional register. With a shortage of nurses (NHS Improvement, 2016) and a potential for more than the average 4–10 per cent of the nursing population having dyslexia (Taylor and Walter, 2003), the needs of this group of nurses cannot be ignored, either legally due to equality legislation (Equality Act, 2010), or practically.

This chapter explores the concept of dyslexia within the context of nurse education in higher-education settings. The chapter concentrates on professional concerns for nurse educators of managing the needs of nursing students with dyslexia and the prerequisite to prepare nurses to practise safely. While it is recognised that mentorship and attrition from nurse education are important, these issues are discussed elsewhere in this book. However, it is important to note that mentorship is an important consideration for students with dyslexia. Furthermore, a lack of or poor mentorship for students with dyslexia may disproportionately impact attrition from nursing programmes.

The chapter begins by considering the potential benefits to nursing students and nurses of having dyslexia, which are often not well recognised. The chapter then moves to consider dyslexia within the higher-education setting, attitudes of teaching staff towards students with dyslexia and issues of safety within the nursing profession, which may or may not be impacted by nurses having dyslexia. Throughout the chapter recent narrative research undertaken by the author as part of doctoral studies into the experiences of registered nurses with dyslexia and nurse lecturers who have supported nurses with dyslexia (hereafter called the doctoral study) is contrasted with existing literature.

Dyslexia and potential benefits to nursing student and nurses

Although there are many definitions of dyslexia (McLoughlin and Leather, 2012), it is generally accepted that it primarily affects skills in accurate and fluent word reading and spelling, causes difficulties in phonological awareness, verbal memory and verbal processing speed and occurs across the range of intellectual abilities (Rose, 2009). The condition is lifelong, but compensatory strategies can be developed over time, with dyslexia in adults manifesting signs of "poor spelling, slow reading, poor time management, difficulty with tasks that require sequencing, difficulty working in noisy environments, low self-esteem, anxiety and frustration" (Brunswick, 2012: p. 4). It has been argued that those adults who have made it as far as university have managed to overcome some of these barriers (Brunswick, 2012). However, there is also evidence of a significant number of students only being identified as having dyslexia once at university (Singleton et al., 2009), which could be due to the increasing academic requirements.

It is important to recognise the potential benefits that individuals with dyslexia can bring to healthcare and teaching professions. Individuals with dyslexia are often insightful and intuitive (Davis, 2010), have good problem-solving skills (Reid, 2009) and increased spatial awareness (Roberts, 2009), are caring and empathetic (Francis-Wright, 2007; Glazzard and Dale, 2013) and have good long-term memory (Doyle, 2014). While individuals with dyslexia may have difficulty with working memory (Bartlett et al., 2010), they are likely to be creative and lateral thinkers (Leather et al., 2011). In several studies students and practitioners identified positive benefits from having dyslexia (Price and Gale, 2006; Francis-Wright, 2007; Roberts, 2009; Child and Langford, 2011; Griffiths, 2012; Glazzard and Dale, 2013; Evans, 2014a). Student teachers with dyslexia used their experiences to shape themselves into the type of teacher that they would have wanted as a child and were able to identify children with difficulties more quickly (Burns and Bell, 2011; Glazzard and Dale, 2013). Student healthcare practitioners in have also identified greater potential for empathy due to the difficulties experienced due to disabilities, which subsequently enhanced patient care (Hargreaves et al., 2013) .

In getting to university many of the students will have overcome difficulties and developed compensatory strategies (Pollak, 2005). Several studies identified dyslexic students needed to be more organised (Francis-Wright, 2007; Harriss and Ricketts, 2009; Jelfs and Richardson, 2010; Griffiths, 2012; Glazzard and Dale, 2013; Evans, 2014a) and had developed strategies such as using assistive technology (Murphy, 2011), notes and prompts (Burns et al., 2013) and over-checking (White, 2007). However, many of these strategies take time and can be tiring for learners (Murphy, 2011).

Dyslexia and higher education

An increasing body of research on professional students with disabilities identifies students are experiencing difficulties and barriers within higher education (Baron et al., 1996; Holloway, 2001; Kolanko, 2003; Fuller et al., 2004; Carroll and Iles, 2006; Prowse, 2009; Collinson and Penketh, 2010; Ricketts et al., 2010; Rickinson, 2010; Brandt, 2011; Bevan, 2013; Evans, 2014b). This literature demonstrates continuing barriers to learning despite a UK report into dyslexia in higher education making 101 recommendations to improve higher-education policy, practice and provision (National Working Party on Dyslexia in Higher

Education, 1999). Students in the UK are not alone in experiencing difficulties attributed to dyslexia. Pre-registration nursing students in the US with learning disabilities (the term used in the US for specific learning difficulties) are reported as having to work harder than their peers for less positive outcomes (Kolanko, 2003). A similar situation is reported from research undertaken with students in Ireland (Evans, 2014a). It is worth noting the attitudes of teaching staff towards students with dyslexia, as this may explain reported student experience.

Attitudes of teaching staff

Attitudes of teaching staff have been found to be key in the support of students with dyslexia (Storr et al., 2011; Cameron and Nunkoosing, 2012; Ashcroft and Lutfiyya, 2013). For example, when lecturers have personal experience of dyslexia, whether through colleagues or relatives, or through increasing contact with students with dyslexia, they are more likely to show an interest in and understanding of the condition and be proactive in tailoring appropriate support (Cameron and Nunkoosing, 2012). The longer lecturers had been in service and the more knowledge they had about the disability, the more positive they were about students being able to meet the professional requirements and to make adjustments (Ashcroft and Lutfiyya, 2013). Storr et al. (2011) produced an interesting literature review which identified that negative attitudes to students with a disability and a lack of understanding of the condition were barriers to student progression. Furthermore, lack of awareness and lack of support resulted in adverse student experiences. There is increasing evidence of the need to support the education of both lecturers (Sowers and Smith, 2004; Kong, 2012; Evans, 2014b) and practice colleagues (Hargreaves and Walker, 2014; Howlin et al., 2014), as means to recognise the implications and thus support the needs of students with dyslexia. A wider debate should include how healthcare professionals view students with a disability, especially as many are situated within a medical model as part of professional role (often subordinated to medicine), which frames disability as a deficit or impairment (Bevan, 2013). The notion of professional risk avoidance is important here as it has the potential to influence the views of the academic staff in relation to patient safety.

Maintaining safety

Nurses are required to meet professional standards to maintain patient safety and the trust of the public, as well as the integrity of the profession (Nursing and Midwifery Council, 2015). Research conducted with several professional groups, including teachers, nurses, occupational therapists and radiographers, has identified that there is still an on-going concern about the inclusion of disabled professionals and in particular those with dyslexia from both lecturers and practice providers (Sowers and Smith, 2004; Murphy, 2009; Rankin et al., 2009; Carey, 2012; Ashcroft and Lutfiyya, 2013; Evans, 2014b; McPheat, 2014; Nolan et al., 2015). In the research by Carey (2012), the 15 nurse lecturers identified a disparity between the notion of inclusivity required by the Equality Act and the regulatory requirements of the professional body (Nursing and Midwifery Council, 2010a). They felt that there was a risk of undermining clinical standards with the use of reasonable adjustments (Carey, 2012). This is supported by research by Walker et al. (2013) and Nolan et al. (2015) where participants shared similar concerns about the risks posed to the nursing and allied health professions by disabled students.

Research by Sanderson-Mann et al. (2012) however identified that students with and without dyslexia both identified drug calculations as an area of practice that they found difficult (Sanderson-Mann et al., 2012). This is of interest, as in the non-comparative studies, the nursing students with dyslexia were very aware of the importance of drug administration and their perceived difficulties and therefore took longer over this skill to ensure that they did not make mistakes (Morris and Turnbull, 2006, 2007a; White, 2007; Ridley, 2011).

This increased awareness of safety issues in relation to drug administration by students mirrors the concerns of the 12 nurse lecturers interviewed in the discourse analysis study by Evans (2014b). Evans (2014b) found that there was still a significant debate amongst nurse lecturers regarding the inclusion of individuals with disabilities in nursing and, in particular, those with dyslexia. Safety concerns were seen to legitimise students not progressing rather than identifying problems that could be resolved. Students who required extra support were viewed negatively and the duty of care to the student was not greater than the duty of care to the patients. In research carried out as part of doctoral studies lecturers and the nurses identified that there was a professional requirement to maintain service user safety. For the nurses, this was demonstrated through the narratives with explanations of taking extra time and care with drug administration and documentation, mirroring the research results from student nurses (Morris and Turnbull, 2006, 2007a; White, 2007; Ridley, 2011). It is of interest that most of the nurses in the doctoral study were identified as having dyslexia before or during their nurse training, although two of the participants had been qualified for many years when they were diagnosed and both were very aware of taking extra care with both drug administration and documentation. This was taken further by one of those participants who refused to administer drugs unsupervised, which adhered to the participant's current job description but limited promotion prospects. As in previous studies, some lecturers in the doctoral study continued to be concerned about the safety of drug administration (Evans, 2014b). However, the majority of lecturers felt that there were misconceptions with regard to the risk and there was little evidence of risk in the literature.

Compensatory learning strategies

The nurses taking part in the doctoral study identified that they had to be organised and spent a great deal of time in preparation for activities, although organisational skills have been identified as a problem for those with dyslexia (Moody, 2009; Brunswick, 2012) and were identified as an issue by the lecturers. A study by Leather et al. (2011) identified that adults with dyslexia who had developed higher-level executive functioning reported higher levels of job satisfaction, self-efficacy and perceived personal success, although they did not achieve higher levels of pay or promotion.

Disguise and avoidance were another set of strategies that were identified by the nurses, and this was also identified in a study of teenagers with dyslexia by Alexander-Passe (2006). In the doctoral study, many of the nurses interviewed identified that they would avoid reading out loud and would either use alternative words if they could not spell or write in an untidy manner to disguise the spelling. There could be many reasons for this behaviour, not least the stigma associated with dyslexia (Evans, 2015) and other psychological and emotional effects (Armstrong and Humphrey, 2009; Macdonald, 2010). While the strategies could have a personal protective effect (Armstrong and Humphrey, 2009), they also could have professional consequences.

Many of the nurses in the doctoral study also discussed how they used memory to compensate for difficulties that they encountered, for example, spending hours memorising written work so that it did not have to be read in public. For many people with dyslexia, whilst their long-term memory is often good (Kibby and Cohen, 2008), working memory has been identified as a potential deficit (Beneventi et al., 2010; Callens et al., 2012). However, visual memory has been identified as a potential compensatory mechanism (Callens et al., 2012; Bacon and Handley, 2014). Working memory is the process by which information is stored in the short term to enable it to enter the long-term memory, as well as retrieving information from the long-term memory (McLoughlin and Leather, 2012). Working memory has been found to be impaired by stress (Qin et al., 2009) and most of the nurses identified that their dyslexia symptoms were worse when they were tired. The nurses in the doctoral study attempted to compensate for this as much as possible by seeking additional support or, in the case of one participant, changing working patterns. The extra effort required both in theory and practice was recognised by the nurses and lecturers. It took extra time to complete documentation and to learn new skills, words and templates by which to structure their work. The ability to recognise how and when to use strategies for learning (metacognition) is often not automatic for those with dyslexia (McLoughlin and Leather, 2012) and therefore it will take time and extra effort to engage in activities that others may not have to think about. This will increase the level of tiredness and stress that nurses with dyslexia may experience, which has been shown in my study to increase the difficulties experienced from dyslexia and will reduce the ability to engage in learning activities.

Preferred ways of learning

Many of the participants were drawn to nursing because of the practical nature of the career, some before nursing became a graduate profession. The nurses in my study identified that they were very practical and enjoyed learning in this way. Many also discussed how they preferred more visual methods of learning. It can be argued that, over time, people will identify ways of learning that are effective and they will continue to use these strategies, forming a preferred learning style (Mortimore, 2008). Several studies have sought to identify the preferred learning styles of nursing students (Rassool and Rawaf, 2008; Fleming et al., 2011; Ponto et al., 2014) as well as students with dyslexia (Exley, 2003), although the methodology and findings of this study have been criticised (Mortimore, 2005). It has been argued that the use of learning styles is controversial as the tools used are in the main not valid or reliable (Coffield et al., 2004a, 2004b). However, the process of self-reflection and interest in the students' learning can be beneficial (Mortimore, 2008). What appears to be important is identifying what methods work best for the learner (Reid and Strnadova, 2008). It must also be recognised that the use of the term learning styles is very much common practice in nursing literature (Rassool and Rawaf, 2008; Fleming et al., 2011; Ponto et al., 2014; Gopee, 2015) and was used extensively by the participants within their narratives. The term learning styles is, therefore, used to describe the participants' preferred approach to learning.

The nurses within my study identified that they learnt best when they were engaged in the learning either at a practical level or when it was applied to their area of practice, and this is supported by the literature (Kirby et al., 2008). Post-registration continuing professional development is often very applied to the nurse's area of interest and practice, and this will encourage nurses to invest the time and effort required for deep learning (Roberts, 2010). A comparative study of dyslexic and non-dyslexic students at universities in Canada demonstrated that the dyslexic students were more likely to use deep approaches to learning

(Kirby et al., 2008). This was also seen in my study, with the nurses preferring to actively engage with the learning process, which helped them to learn more effectively and reduce the challenges that dyslexia posed for them.

There were, however, conflicts and challenges in how participants demonstrated their learning and personal compensatory strategies. The nurses within my study identified that they had developed their verbal skills but these did not match their ability to write. Two participants described how they were able to talk through complex issues and would rather do this than write an email or letter. This was also identified by the lecturers and is commonly one of the earliest signs of dyslexia (Mather and Wendling, 2012). Verbal skills are important in nursing, and all of the nurses sought to use these skills to teach others. The teaching of others could be viewed as a way of enhancing self-esteem (Heinz, 2015), as nurses feel valued for their knowledge and experience (Alexander-Passe, 2015). The nurses also felt that they had developed particular skills in teaching, as they had different ways of approaching learning that they had developed over the years. This is mirrored in studies of teachers with dyslexia (Burns and Bell, 2010; Burns et al., 2013). They felt that they had higher levels of empathy and caring, which may be related to their previous experiences and is a positive trait cited by other authors (McLoughlin and Leather, 2012; Glazzard and Dale, 2013).

Transitions in learning for dyslexic students

The nurse participants in the doctoral study identified that they found changes to the style of academic assessments, as well as changes in the academic level of study, challenging and often their compensatory strategies were initially insufficient to meet these demands. It took students time to learn how to structure an assignment in a certain way and once students had done this they used this as a template for future work. This is in contrast to current educational thinking where a variety of assignment types are used to cater for different student preferences and to enhance student engagement (Fry et al., 2014). This may, in fact, be detrimental to learners with dyslexia, as the structure is often a problem in academic writing (Tops et al., 2013). Students could actually spend more time trying to navigate how to structure the assignment than on the actual content required. Qualified nurses who engage in continuing professional development may find that universities, other than the one first engaged with, have a variety of requirements, for example, the structure of an assignment and assessment protocols, which magnifies the difficulties some students with dyslexia face in transitions in learning.

The use of templates in the form of exemplars or main headings was also a key theme in practice, with nurses developing an individual approach to structuring documentation. However, successfully managing this way of working was identified as requiring a degree of stability and the nurses in the doctoral study moved to areas that were more supportive, where the documentation was perceived as more manageable. This could be in the form of electronic healthcare records or areas such as intensive care where the documentation is set out in a structured manner. A change in role or job is likely to cause difficulties initially and therefore support may be required in the first instance for nurses new to the area/role to adapt individual compensatory strategies to the new situation (Reid et al., 2008). This is a further consideration for student nurses who are required to change placements regularly to meet course requirements (Nursing and Midwifery Council, 2018). Weedon and Riddell (2010) recognised that students with a disability may find transitions more difficult due to complex psychological issues and past educational experiences. However, Alheit (2012) suggests that transitions are an opportunity for learning depending on how important the change is seen to be and how the learner is able to reflect on it. Compensatory strategies are likely to be developed as part of the lifelong learning process along with other skills.

Support and disclosure

Many people are involved in the professional development of a nurse, but for nurses with dyslexia, professional and educational support is particularly important in areas where these students experience greatest difficulty. To be able to access additional resources and obtain reasonable adjustments, dyslexia needs to be recognised and disclosure has to occur. The lecturers in the doctoral study identified that, whilst some nurses were aware that they had dyslexia, support was sometimes only requested when the student was failing. Unsurprisingly, Goldberg et al. (2003) found that students with dyslexia are more successful when they actively seek support and accept it when it is offered.

Disclosure is well recognised in dyslexia literature and within the doctoral study referred to here. Disclosure of dyslexia in practice is also an issue in that the majority of the research studies found student nurses with dyslexia had raised it as such. While the pre-registration student nurses generally disclosed their dyslexia in the classroom, some, but not all, chose to do so in practice (Morris and Turnbull, 2006, 2007a; Sanderson-Mann, 2006; Ridley, 2011; Evans, 2014a). There is very little literature regarding disclosure of dyslexia by qualified nurses in practice; the results of both studies mirrored that of the research with dyslexic student nurses, showing that not all qualified nurses disclosed their dyslexia (Illingworth, 2005; Morris and Turnbull, 2007b). Furthermore, the decision to disclose appears to be dependent on the culture of the area and perceived benefits to the nurse or student nurse (Morris and Turnbull, 2006, 2007a, 2007b; Ridley, 2011). Students on professional courses will have had previous educational experiences, which may have a detrimental effect on individual emotional well-being and learning (Price and Gale, 2006; Collinson and Penketh, 2010; Gwernan-Jones and Burden, 2010; Griffiths, 2012). The pervasive discourse of either feeling stupid or being called stupid is evident in dyslexic students in all professional groups (Dale and Taylor, 2001; Wright and Eathorne, 2003; Sanderson-Mann, 2006; Morris and Turnbull, 2007b; Murphy, 2009, 2011; Griffiths, 2012; Kong, 2012; Evans, 2014a). Students with a disability are entitled to have reasonable adjustments that will enable them to reach their full potential (Riddell and Weedon, 2006; Equality Act, 2010; Ricketts et al., 2010). However, there is also evidence that students do not want to be treated differently (Walker et al., 2013; Evans, 2014a), with adjustments potentially causing social embarrassment (Riddell and Weedon, 2009). Some students would not disclose that they had dyslexia or access services so that they were not treated differently (Miller et al., 2009; Kong, 2012), identifying that adjustments could be seen by themselves and others as gaining an advantage (Kolanko, 2003; Miller et al., 2009; Hargreaves and Walker, 2014). Some students wanted to prove that they could achieve on their own merit (Kong, 2012).

One reason that nurses may be reluctant to disclose dyslexia is the stigma attached to the condition (Riddick, 2000; Morris and Turnbull, 2007a), with students feeling that they will be labelled as stupid (Roberts, 2009; Evans, 2014a) or even dangerous (Morris and Turnbull, 2007a; Sanderson-Mann et al., 2012). Without disclosure, nurses are unable to access the support that they are entitled to under the Equality Act (2010). One of the main reasons identified for disclosure in both student and qualified nurses was to maintain patient safety (Illingworth, 2005, Morris and Turnbull, 2007a). This was also evident in research focused on the placement experiences of both student and qualified healthcare professionals, including nurses (Hargreaves et al., 2013; Walker et al., 2013; Hargreaves and Walker, 2014), healthcare professionals and student teachers (Nolan et al., 2015). Students in the study by White (2006) wanted control of who to disclose to and when to disclose, with the decision influenced by previous experience and attitudes of staff.

Nurses in the doctoral study had a variety of reasons for choosing whether to disclose, including a need to know and a supportive work environment. The nurses who had developed compensatory strategies, self-confidence and achieved successfully in their nursing career were more likely to disclose. McLoughlin and Leather (2012) suggest that success at work depends on many factors, including individuals being aware of their skills, feeling supported and being valued for their skills and knowledge. Dyslexia can be seen as a hidden disability (Nalavany et al., 2015) and therefore it is possible for nurses not to disclose. My study identified that nurses can achieve very successful careers without either being aware of or disclosing their dyslexia. Disclosure poses the risk of a change in social identity (Riddell and Weedon, 2014; Evans, 2015) and, for most of the nurses in the study, this was not something that they were willing to chance until they had established themselves within the nursing team. This was also something that was identified by the lecturers who found that disclosure was much more likely to occur once they had developed a relationship with the student. Both nurses and lecturers were aware that there still is a stigma attached to the label of dyslexia (Riddick, 2000; Evans, 2015).

As qualified nurses, all of the participants had developed compensatory strategies that had enabled them to achieve their qualification and to progress their careers. The nurses in the study valued the support to enable them to use these strategies. This support could come from colleagues, managers or lecturers. It is recognised that each person with dyslexia is an individual (Day, 2013) and that a uniform approach to dyslexia support is not going to be effective (Busgeet, 2008).

Assessment

Access to assessment for dyslexia was identified as a potential problem by both nurses and lecturers. For students to be identified as requiring assessment for dyslexia, lecturers have to recognise the signs. This requires the lecturer to have knowledge about the signs of dyslexia and access to written work. In my study, lecturers identified that early formative assessment of written work enabled earlier identification. Provision of assessment for dyslexia was particularly difficult at the beginning of the academic year. For qualified nurses accessing continuing professional development units, they may have finished their course of study before assessments can be completed. A more inclusive approach to teaching and assessment may help these students until their diagnosis is confirmed and specialist support can be arranged (Mortimore, 2013). From the results of my study, this will rely on the universities increasing the level of training of all lecturing staff so that they are aware of the needs of students with dyslexia so that they can adopt inclusive practices as well as early identification of students with possible dyslexia. This will include the use of assistive technologies, although students with dyslexia need to be trained and supported to use these, otherwise the technology will not be effective or valued (Stewart, 2002), as demonstrated by the findings of my study where one participant described not having taken the software that he or she had been given out of the box as he or she did not know how to use it.

Specialist support

In a survey commissioned by the *Times Higher Education*, this inequality in provision was also highlighted (Speed, 2014). The British Dyslexia Association has developed a quality mark for higher education with the aim of improving the provision of support and under-standing of dyslexia (van Daal and Tomlin, 2016). However, at the time of writing only one university faculty had achieved this award (Speed, 2014). The level of provision and specialist support available to students with dyslexia at universities was reported as variable in the doctoral study reported here, and was dependent on the personnel available and the uni-versity policies and philosophy. Relatively few lecturers reported having a specific role in supporting nurses with disabilities. However, those lecturers were experienced in ensuring that students were able to access specialist services. A significant number of lecturers dis-cussed how their university was moving to a more inclusive way of working. Changes to government funding of the Disabled Students' Allowance that came into effect from Sep-tember 2016 will affect students with dyslexia attending English universities. Universities will be expected to take responsibility for funding non-medical support staff such as scribes, readers and proof readers and there will be reduced funding for computers and peripheral devices (Johnson, 2015). This is in keeping with the notion of a more inclusive approach to teaching in higher education and the obligation to meet the Equality Act (2010), although there have been arguments that this will increase the financial pressure on universities and students, as well as possibly reducing the quality of specialist student support, as the market for this is opened up (Cameron, 2015). For many nurses on continuing professional devel-opment courses, funding could come from the Access to Work scheme, as reasonable adjust-ments would also be needed within the workplace (GOV.UK, 2016). Students on courses less than a year long are also not eligible for Disabled Students' Allowance (GOV.UK, 2016). None of the nurses interviewed for the doctoral study had accessed the Access to Work scheme, which may well impact practice learning as well as everyday work.

Inclusive teaching and learning in higher education

The basic premise of inclusive learning and teaching is to remove barriers to participation in higher education so that all students are able to fully participate in learning and achieve their potential (Hockings, 2010). Whilst this has been debated for a number of years, it could be argued that it has been slow to become established within the higher-education sector (Gibson, 2015). Inclusive teaching and learning promote the concept that all learners have different strengths and weaknesses which should be considered in "curriculum design, cur-riculum delivery, assessment and institutional commitment to and management of inclusive learning and teaching" (Thomas and May, 2010: p. 9). Diversity can be seen as a benefit in education, enriching society as a whole (Moriña, 2017), with Healey et al. (2006) suggesting that we should start from the assumption that everyone is impaired in some way and all would benefit from inclusive approaches. Inclusive approaches to assessment have been shown to increase student satisfaction and grades, although took more of the lecturer's time to implement (Waterfield and West, 2008). This was a case study in a single UK university; however, it is one of the few evaluative studies on inclusive approaches to teaching and learning. Students in a qualitative study in Northern Ireland identified that they preferred methods of assessment that did not require reasonable adjustments that could be disclosed to other students (Redpath et al., 2013).

Inclusive learning and teaching are based on the social model of disability but disability legislation could be argued to come from a medical model, with the Equality Act (2010) focusing on a deficit model requiring reasonable adjustments to be implemented to enable those with disabilities to fit into the curriculum (Pleasance, 2016). Many studies have emphasised difficulties that students have found in accessing reasonable adjustments at university (Fuller et al., 2004; Dalun et al., 2010; Equality Challenge Unit, 2010; Zhang et al., 2010). However, an inclusive approach does not mean that students should not have reasonable adjustments, rather a shift to meeting the needs of the majority so that few adjustments would be required (Halligan and Howlin, 2016; Disabled Students Sector Leadership Group, 2017). This would be particularly beneficial to students who have not disclosed a disability or have not been assessed to meet Disabled Students' Allowance requirements (Wray et al., 2012a). In a case study of a London university, Masterton (2010) suggested that there was a focus on individual adjustments and an awareness of the legislation, although staff had not embraced inclusive education. It has been argued that inclusive education benefits all through effective teaching and learning methods (Moriña, 2017), as well as being ethically right (Bolt, 2004; Bleich et al., 2015; Reindal, 2016). Inclusive approaches may also be more cost-effective as the number of individual accommodations required for students is reduced (Disabled Students Sector Leadership Group, 2017). It has also been argued that these approaches enable students to become more independent lifelong learners, especially with the use of technology (Tonge and Treanor, 2017).

A model of inclusive education which was devised in the US is Universal Design for Learning (UDL), although it is also termed Universal Design for Instruction (UDI) and Universal Instructional Design (UID) (CAST, 2011). The principle of UDL is to address variability between learners by developing a flexible curriculum using three principles: "provide multiple means of representation, provide multiple means of action and expression, and provide multiple means of engagement" (CAST, 2011: p. 5). In this way UDL allows students to engage in learning and demonstrate their understanding in a way that suits them, reducing the need for individual accommodations (Halligan and Howlin, 2016). There is an increasing body of literature about the implementation of UDL, especially in the US (Scott et al., 2003; Orr and Hammig, 2009; Lombardi and Murray, 2011; Lombardi et al., 2011; Smith, 2012; Mole, 2013) and Ireland (Heelan et al., 2015; Tonge and Treanor, 2017), with evidence that it is emerging in Australia (Hitch et al., 2015) and at least one university in the UK (Disabled Students Sector Leadership Group, 2017). However, as the studies are mainly descriptive, there is very little evidence to demonstrate how effective UDL is (Pliner and Johnson, 2004; Atkinson, 2012; Mole, 2013; Rao et al., 2014). This could be because UDL is relatively new and still being defined (Rao et al., 2014) and not fully embedded in practice (Fovet, 2017).

Hitch et al. (2015) conducted a review of policies along with a survey of Australian universities regarding inclusivity. They found that one-third of universities included inclusive teaching and learning in their policies, with one referring to UDL. However, there was a wide range of training for staff on inclusivity, with online training and one-off workshops at staff induction being most common (Hitch et al., 2015).

Despite the increasing prominence of inclusive education as a philosophy, a Spanish study by López Gavira and Moriña (2015) demonstrated that policies were not always implemented in practice and that attitudes of lecturers were a common barrier. This was supported by many other studies from the US and Europe (Hanafin et al., 2007; Zhang et al., 2010; Black et al., 2014; Strnadová et al., 2015; Morgado et al., 2016), with students finding lecturers reluctant to use inclusive technology (Moriña et al., 2015; van Jaarsveldt and Ndeya-Ndereya, 2015). One mixed methodology case study of a UK university even identified a discourse that inclusive practices may compromise academic standards (Mortimore, 2013). Inclusive approaches were also seen to interfere with the competitive nature of assessment with reasonable adjustments seen to give an unfair advantage to some students (Hanafin et al., 2007). Students with a disability were seen as the responsibility of disability services (van Jaarsveldt and Ndeya-Ndereya, 2015), with students with more visible disabilities being more accepted and accommodations agreed (Hanafin et al., 2007; Zhang et al., 2010; Magnus and Tøssebro, 2014; Strnadová et al., 2015). It has been argued that inclusive approaches that reduce the need for common individual accommodations may be more beneficial for these students, which would include students with dyslexia.

Conclusion

Whilst dyslexia could be seen to impact nursing students and registered nurses personally and professionally, it is evident that students and practitioners with dyslexia are able to develop compensatory mechanisms to enable effective practice and engagement in learning. However, these strategies come at a cost in both effort and in some cases career progression. The strategies developed were not always effective and were dependent on the personality traits and resilience of the individual. Childhood and early-career experiences of supportive relationships impacted on how individuals were able to engage in learning and how they viewed capabilities as learners. Early identification of dyslexia also had a positive effect, with difficulties attributed to dyslexia, rather than lack of intellectual ability and accessing support earlier. There is clearly a persistent lack of understanding of dyslexia and a fear that nurses with dyslexia are a risk to patient safety or the profession. This is not the case, as demonstrated in the literature and the narratives of the nurses within the doctoral study recounted here. However, myths regarding the capacity of nurses and by implication nursing students to practise safely perpetuate the stigma associated with dyslexia in nursing, Inclusive approaches to teaching and learning would help mitigate this problem, premised on wider education and understanding of dyslexia.

References

Alexander-Passe N (2006) How dyslexic teenagers cope: an investigation of self-esteem, coping and depression. *Dyslexia*, 12(4): 256–275.

Alexander-Passe N (2015) *Dyslexia and Mental Health*. London: Jessica Kingsley Publishers.

Alheit P (2012) The Biographical Approach to Lifelong Learning. In Jarvis P & Watts M (eds.) *The Routledge International Handbook of Learning*. London: Routledge, pp. 168–175.

Armstrong D and Humphrey N (2009) Reactions to a diagnosis of dyslexia among students entering further education: development of the "resistance-accommodation" model. *British Journal of Special Education*, 36(2): 95–102.

Ashcroft T J and Lutfiyya Z M (2013) Nursing educators' perspectives of students with disabilities: a grounded theory study. *Nurse Education Today*, 33(11): 1316–1321.

Atkinson R (2012) The Life Story Interview as a Mutually Equitable Relationship. In Gubrium J F, Holstein J A, Marvasti A B & McKinney K D (eds.) *The SAGE Handbook of Interview Research: The Complexity of the Craft*. Thousand Oaks, CA: SAGE, pp. 115–129.

Bacon A M and Handley S J (2014) Reasoning and dyslexia: is visual memory a compensatory resource? *Dyslexia: An International Journal of Research and Practice*, 20(4): 330–345.

Baron S, Phillips R and Stalker K (1996) Barriers to training for disabled social work students. *Disability & Society*, 11(3): 361–378.

Bartlett D, Moody S and Kindersley K (2010) *Dyslexia in the Workplace*. Chichester: Wiley-Blackwell.

Beneventi H, Finn Egil T, Ersland L and Hugdahl K (2010) Working memory deficit in dyslexia: behavioral and fMRI evidence. *International Journal of Neuroscience*, 120(1): 51–59.

Bevan J (2013) Disabled occupational therapists – asset, liability … or 'watering down' the profession? *Disability & Society*, 29(4): 583–596.

Black D R, Weinberg L A and Brodwin M G (2014) Universal design for instruction and learning: a pilot study of faculty instructional methods and attitudes related to students with disabilities in higher education. *Exceptionality Education International*, 24(1): 48–64.

Bleich M R, MacWilliams B R and Schmidt B J (2015) Advancing diversity through inclusive excellence in nursing education. *Journal of Professional Nursing*, 31(2): 89–94.

Bolt D (2004) Disability and the rhetoric of inclusive higher education. *Journal of Further and Higher Education*, 28(4): 353–358.

Brandt S (2011) From policy to practice in higher education: the experiences of disabled students in Norway. *International Journal of Disability, Development & Education*, 58(2): 107–120.

British Dyslexia Association (2012) *What are Specific Learning Difficulties?* Available at: www.bdadyslexia. org.uk/about-dyslexia/schools-colleges-and-universities/what-are-specific-learning-difficulties.html

Brunswick N (2012) Dyslexia in UK Higher Education and Employment. In Brunswick N (ed.) *Supporting Dyslexic Adults in Higher Education and the Workplace*. Chichester: Wiley-Blackwell, pp. 33–42.

Burns E and Bell S (2010) Voices of teachers with dyslexia in Finnish and English further and higher educational settings. *Teachers and Teaching: Theory and Practice*, 16(5): 529–543.

Burns E and Bell S (2011) Narrative construction of professional teacher identity of teachers with dyslexia. *Teaching & Teacher Education*, 27(5): 952–960.

Burns E, Poikkeus A M and Aro M (2013) Resilience strategies employed by teachers with dyslexia working at tertiary education. *Teaching and Teacher Education*, 34: 77–85.

Busgeet T (2008) *Dyslexia in higher education: exploring lecturers' perspectives of dyslexia, dyslexic students and support strategies*. Doctor in Philosophy, University of Liverpool, Liverpool.

Callens M, Tops W and Brysbaert M (2012) Cognitive profile of students who enter higher education with an indication of dyslexia. *Plos One*, 7(6): e38081-e38081.

Cameron H (2015) The narrow way. *Times Higher Education*, 17th December. Available at: www. timeshighereducation.com/comment/the-market-will-drive-out-dyslexic-students

Cameron H and Nunkoosing K (2012) Lecturer perspectives on dyslexia and dyslexic students within one faculty at one university in England. *Teaching in Higher Education*, 17(3): 341–352.

Carey P (2012) Exploring variation in nurse educators' perceptions of the inclusive curriculum. *International Journal of Inclusive Education*, 16(7): 741–755.

Carroll J M and Iles J E (2006) An assessment of anxiety levels in dyslexic students in higher education. *British Journal of Educational Psychology*, 76(3): 651–662.

CAST (2011) *Universal Design for Learning Guidelines version 2.0*. Wakefield, MA: CAST. Available at: www.udlcenter.org/aboutudl/udlguidelines/downloads

Child, J. and Langford, E. (2011) Exploring the learning experiences of nursing students with dyslexia. *Nursing Standard*, 25(40): 39–46.

Coffield F, Moseley D, Hall E and Ecclestone K (2004a) *Learning Styles and Pedagogy in Post-16 Learning*. London: Learning and Skills Research Centre. Available at: http://sxills.nl/lerenlerennu/bronnen/ Learning%20styles%20by%20Coffield%20e.a.pdf (Accessed: 25th February 2016).

Coffield F, Moseley D, Hall E and Ecclestone K (2004b) *Should We Be Using Learning Styles? What Research Has to Say to Practice*. London: Learning and Skills Research Centre. Available at: www.itslifejimbutnotasweknowit.org.uk/files/LSRC_LearningStyles.pdf

Collinson C and Penketh C (2010) 'Sit in the corner and don't eat the crayons': postgraduates with dyslexia and the dominant 'lexic' discourse. *Disability & Society*, 25(1): 7–19.

Dale M and Taylor B (2001) How adult learners make sense of their dyslexia. *Disability & Society*, 16(7): 997–1008.

Dalun Z, Landmark L, Reber A, Hsien Yuan H, Oi-man K and Benz M (2010) University faculty knowledge, beliefs, and practices in providing reasonable accommodations to students with disabilities. *Remedial & Special Education*, 31(4): 276–286.

Davis R (2010) *The Gift of Dyslexia*. 3rd edn. London: Souvenir Press.

Day K (2013) Coping with dyslexia. *Nursing Standard*, 28(4): 74.

Disabled Students Sector Leadership Group (2017) Inclusive teaching and learning in higher education as a route to excellence. Available: Department for Education. Available at: www.gov.uk/govern ment/uploads/system/uploads/attachment_data/file/587221/Inclusive_Teaching_and_Learnin g_in_Higher_Education_as_a_route_to-excellence.pdf

Doyle N (2014) Supporting stressed staff. *Occupational Health*, 66(5): 14–16.

Equality Act (2010) *(c.15)*. London: HMSO.

Equality Challenge Unit (2010) *Managing Reasonable Adjustments in Higher Education*. London: Equality Challenge Unit. Available at: www.ecu.ac.uk/publications/managing-reasonable-adjustments-in-higher-education/

Evans W (2014a) 'I am not a dyslexic person I'm a person with dyslexia': identity constructions of dyslexia among students in nurse education. *Journal of Advanced Nursing*, 70(2): 360–372.

Evans W (2014b) "If they can't tell the difference between duphalac and digoxin you've got patient safety issues". Nurse Lecturers' constructions of students' dyslexic identities in nurse education. *Nurse Education Today*, 34(6): e41-6.

Evans W (2015) Disclosing a dyslexic identity. *British Journal of Nursing*, 24(7): 383–385.

Exley S (2003) The effectiveness of teaching strategies for students with dyslexia based on their preferred learning styles. *British Journal of Special Education*, 30(4): 213–220.

Fleming S, McKee G and Huntley-Moore S (2011) Undergraduate nursing students' learning styles: a longitudinal study. *Nurse Education Today*, 31(5): 444–449.

Fovet F (2017) Doing what we preach: examining the contradictions of the UDL discourse in faculties of education. *Presentation at AHEAD 2017 Conference*, Dublin. Available at: www.youtube.com/watch?v=LxTvtcQHAyg

Francis-Wright M J (2007) *Living with dyslexia: a phenomenological study of in-service part-time undergraduate occupational therapy students' experiences*. Doctorate of Education, University of East Anglia, Norwich.

Fry H, Ketteridge S and Marshall S (2014) *A Handbook for Teaching and Learning in Higher Education: Enhancing Academic Practice*. London: Routledge.

Fuller M, Healey M, Bradley A and Hall T (2004) Barriers to learning: a systematic study of the experience of disabled students in one university. *Studies in Higher Education*, 29(3): 303–318.

Gibson S (2015) When rights are not enough: what is? Moving towards new pedagogy for inclusive education within UK universities. *International Journal of Inclusive Education*, 19(8): 875–886.

Glazzard J and Dale K (2013) Trainee teachers with dyslexia: personal narratives of resilience. *Journal of Research in Special Educational Needs*, 13(1): 26–37.

Goldberg R J, Higgins E L, Raskind M H and Herman K L (2003) 'Predictors of success in individuals with learning disabilities: a qualitative analysis of a 20-year longitudinal study. *Learning Disabilities Research & Practice*, 18(4): 222–236.

Gopee N (2015) *Mentoring and Supervision in Healthcare*. London: SAGE Publications.

GOV.UK (2016) *Access to Work*. Available at: www.gov.uk/access-to-work

Griffiths S (2012) 'Being dyslexic doesn't make me less of a teacher'. School placement experiences of student teachers with dyslexia: strengths, challenges and a model for support. *Journal of Research in Special Educational Needs*, 12(2): 54–65.

Gwernan-Jones R and Burden R L (2010) Are they just lazy? Student teachers' attitudes about dyslexia. *Dyslexia (Chichester, England)*, 16(1): 66–86.

Halligan P and Howlin F (2016) *Supporting Nursing and Midwifery Students with a Disability in Clinical Practice: A Resource Guide*. Dublin: University College Dublin.

Hanafin J, Shevlin M, Kenny M and Mc Neela E (2007) Including young people with disabilities: assessment challenges in higher education. *Higher Education: The International Journal of Higher Education and Educational Planning*, 54(3): 435–448.

Hargreaves J, Dearnley C, Walker S and Walker L (2013) The preparation and practice of disabled health care practitioners: exploring the issues. *Innovations in Education and Teaching International*, 51(3): 303–314.

Hargreaves J and Walker L (2014) Preparing disabled students for professional practice: managing risk through a principles-based approach. *Journal of Advanced Nursing*, 70(8): 1748–1757.

Harriss A and Ricketts K (2009) Dealing with dyslexia. *Occupational Health*, 61(11): 18–20.

Healey M, Fuller M, Bradley A and Hall T (2006) Listening to Students: The Experience of Disabled Students of Learning at University. In Adams M & Brown S (eds.) *Towards Inclusive Learning in Higher Education: Developing Curricula for Disabled Students*. London: Routledge Falmer, pp. 32–43.

Heelan A, Halligan P and Quirke M (2015) Universal design for learning and its application to clinical placements in health science courses (practice brief). *Journal of Postsecondary Education & Disability*, 28(4): 469–479.

Heinz M (2015) Why choose teaching? An international review of empirical studies exploring student teachers' career motivations and levels of commitment to teaching. *Educational Research and Evaluation*, 21(3): 258–297.

Hitch D, Macfarlane S and Nihill C (2015) Inclusive pedagogy in Australian universities: a review of current policies and professional development activities. *The International Journal of the First Year in Higher Education*, 6(1).

Hockings C (2010) Inclusive learning and teaching in higher education: a synthesis of research. *Evidence Net*, Available: Higher Education Academy. Available at: www.heacademy.ac.uk/resources/detail/resources/detail/evidencenet/Inclusive_learning_and_teaching_in_higher_education

Holloway S (2001) The experience of higher education from the perspective of disabled students. *Disability & Society*, 16(4): 597–615.

Howlin F, Halligan P and O'Toole S (2014) Evaluation of a clinical needs assessment and exploration of the associated supports for students with a disability in clinical practice: part 2. *Nurse Education in Practice*, 14(5): 565–572.

Illingworth, K. (2005) The effects of dyslexia on the work of nurses and healthcare assistants. *Nursing Standard (Royal College Of Nursing (Great Britain)*, 19(38): 41–48.

Jelfs A and Richardson J T E (2010) Perceptions of academic quality and approaches to studying among disabled and nondisabled students in distance education. *Studies in Higher Education*, 35(5): 593–607.

Johnson J (2015) *House of Commons Written Statements 2nd December 2015*. London: Parliament.uk. Available at: www.publications.parliament.uk/pa/cm201516/cmhansrd/cm151202/wmsindx/151202-x.htm

Kibby M Y and Cohen M J (2008) Memory functioning in children with reading disabilities and/or attention deficit/hyperactivity disorder: a clinical investigation of their working memory and long-term memory functioning. *Child Neuropsychology*, 14(6): 525–546.

Kirby J R, Silvestri R, Allingham B H, Parrila R and La Fave C B (2008) Learning strategies and study approaches of postsecondary students with dyslexia. *Journal of Learning Disabilities*, 41(1): 85–96.

Kolanko K M (2003) A collective case study of nursing students with learning disabilities. *Nursing Education Perspectives*, 24(5): 251–256.

Kong S Y (2012) The emotional impact of being recently diagnosed with dyslexia from the perspective of chiropractic students. *Journal of Further & Higher Education*, 36(1): 127–146.

Leather C, Hogh H, Seiss E and Everatt J (2011) Cognitive functioning and work success in adults with dyslexia. *Dyslexia (10769242)*, 17(4): 327–338.

Lombardi A R and Murray C (2011) Measuring university faculty attitudes toward disability: willingness to accommodate and adopt universal design principles. *Journal of Vocational Rehabilitation*, 34(1): 43–56.

Lombardi A R, Murray C and Gerdes H (2011) College faculty and inclusive instruction: self-reported attitudes and actions pertaining to Universal Design. *Journal of Diversity in Higher Education*, 4(4): 250–261.

López Gavira R and Moriña A (2015) Hidden voices in higher education: inclusive policies and practices in social science and law classrooms. *International Journal of Inclusive Education*, 19(4): 365–378.

Macdonald S J (2010) Towards a social reality of dyslexia. *British Journal of Learning Disabilities*, 38(4): 271–279.

Magnus E and Tøssebro J (2014) Negotiating individual accommodation in higher education. *Scandinavian Journal of Disability Research*, 16(4): 316–332.

Masterton H (2010) The SENDA agenda: the vision for inclusive higher education. *At the Interface/Probing the Boundaries*, 60: 211–225.

Mather N and Wendling B (2012) *Essentials of Dyslexia Assessment and Intervention*. Hoboken: John Wiley and Sons.

McLoughlin D and Leather C (2012) *The Dyslexic Adult: Interventions and Outcomes - An Evidence-based Approach*. 2nd edn. Oxford: John Wiley & Sons.

McPheat C (2014) Experience of nursing students with dyslexia on clinical placement. *Nursing Standard*, 28(41): 44–49.

Miller S, Ross S and Cleland J (2009) Medical students' attitudes towards disability and support for disability in medicine. *Medical Teacher*, 31(6): 556–561.

Mole H (2013) A US model for inclusion of disabled students in higher education settings: The social model of disability and Universal Design. *Widening Participation and Lifelong Learning*, 14(3): 62–86.

Moody S (2009) *Dyslexia and Employment: A Guide for Assessors, Trainers and Managers*. Malden, MA: Wiley-Blackwell.

Morgado B, Cortés-Vega M D, López-Gavira R, Álvarez E and Moriña A (2016) Inclusive education in higher education? *Journal of Research in Special Educational Needs*, 16: 639–642.

Moriña A (2017) Inclusive education in higher education: challenges and opportunities. *European Journal of Special Needs Education*, 32(1): 3–17.

Moriña A, Cortés-Vega M D and Molina V M (2015) Faculty training: an unavoidable requirement for approaching more inclusive university classrooms. *Teaching in Higher Education*, 20(8): 795–806.

Morris D and Turnbull P (2006) Clinical experiences of students with dyslexia. *Journal of Advanced Nursing*, 54(2): 238–247.

Morris D and Turnbull P (2007a) The disclosure of dyslexia in clinical practice: experiences of student nurses in the United Kingdom. *Nurse Education Today*, 27(1): 35–42.

Morris D and Turnbull P (2007b) A survey-based exploration of the impact of dyslexia on career progression of UK registered nurses. *Journal Of Nursing Management*, 15(1): 97–106.

Mortimore T (2005) Dyslexia and learning style – a note of caution. *British Journal of Special Education*, 32(3): 145–148.

Mortimore T (2008) *Dyslexia and Learning Style: A Practitioner's Handbook*. 2nd edn. Chichester: John Wiley and Sons.

Mortimore T (2013) Dyslexia in higher education: creating a fully inclusive institution. *Journal of Research in Special Educational Needs*, 13(1): 38–47.

Murphy F (2009) The clinical experiences of dyslexic healthcare students. *Radiography*, 15(4): 341–344.

Murphy F (2011) On being dyslexic: student radiographers' perspectives. *Radiography*, 17(2): 132–138.

Nalavany B A, Carawan L W and Sauber S (2015) Adults with dyslexia, an invisible disability: the mediational role of concealment on perceived family support and self-esteem. *British Journal of Social Work*, 45(2): 568–586.

National Working Party on Dyslexia in Higher Education (1999) *Dyslexia in Higher Education: Policy, Provision and Practice*. Hull: National Working Party on Dyslexia in Higher Education.

NHS Improvement (2016) *Evidence from NHS Improvement on Clinical Staff Shortages: A Workforce Analysis*. London: NHS Improvement.

Nolan C, Gleeson C, Treanor D and Madigan S (2015) Higher education students registered with disability services and practice educators: issues and concerns for professional placements. *International Journal of Inclusive Education*, 19(5): 1–16.

Nursing and Midwifery Council (2010a) *Reasonable adjustments*. Available at: www.nmc-uk.org/Students/Good-Health-and-Good-Character-for-students-nurses-and-midwives/Reasonable-adjustments/ (Accessed: 1st January 2015 2015).

Nursing and Midwifery Council (2015) *The Code: Professional Standards of Practice and Behaviour for Nurses and Midwives*. London: Nursing and Midwifery Council.

Nursing and Midwifery Council (2018) *Future nurse: Standards of proficiency for registered nurses* London: Nursing and Midwifery Council. Available at: https://www.nmc.org.uk/globalassets/sitedocuments/education-standards/future-nurse-proficiencies.pdf (Accessed: 1st June 2018).

Orr A C and Hammig S B (2009) Inclusive postsecondary strategies for teaching students with learning disabilities: a review of the literature. *Learning Disability Quarterly*, 32(3): 181–196.

Pleasance S (2016) *Wider Professional Practice in Education and Training*. London: SAGE.

Pliner S M and Johnson J R (2004) Historical, theoretical, and foundational principles of universal instructional design in higher education. *Equity & Excellence in Education*, 37(2): 105–113.

Pollak D (2005) *Dyslexia, the Self and Higher Education*. Stoke on Trent: Trentham Books.

Ponto M, Ooms A and Cowieson F (2014) Learning styles and Locus of control in undergraduate medical, nursing and physiotherapy students: a comparative study. *Progress in Health Sciences*, 4(1): 172–178.

Price G A and Gale A (2006) How do dyslexic nursing students cope with clinical practice placements? the impact of the dyslexic profile on the clinical practice of dyslexic nursing students: pedagogical issues and considerations. *Learning Disabilities – A Contemporary Journal*, 4(1): 19–36.

Prowse S (2009) Institutional construction of disabled students. *Journal of Higher Education Policy & Management*, 31(1): 89–96.

Qin S, Hermans E J, van Marle H J F, Luo J and Fernández G (2009) Acute psychological stress reduces working memory-related activity in the dorsolateral prefrontal cortex. *Biological Psychiatry*, 66(1): 25–32.

Rankin E R, Nayda R, Cocks S and Smith M (2009) Students with disabilities and clinical placement: understanding the perspective of healthcare organisations. *International Journal of Inclusive Education*, 14(5): 533–542.

Rao K, Ok M W and Bryant B R (2014) A review of research on universal design educational models. *Remedial and Special Education*, 35(3): 153–166.

Rassool G H and Rawaf S (2008) The influence of learning styles preference of undergraduate nursing students on educational outcomes in substance use education. *Nurse Education in Practice*, 8(5): 306–314.

Redpath J, Kearney P, Nicholl P, Mulvenna M, Wallace J and Martin S (2013) A qualitative study of the lived experiences of disabled post-transition students in higher education institutions in Northern Ireland. *Studies in Higher Education*, 38(9): 1334–1350.

Reid G (2009) *Dyslexia: A Practitioners Handbook*. 4th edn. Chichester: Wiley-Blackwell.

Reid G, Came F and Price L (2008) Dyslexia: Workplace Issues. In Reid G, Fawcett A J, Manis F & Siegel L (eds.) *The SAGE Handbook of Dyslexia*. London: SAGE, pp. 474–487.

Reid G and Strnadova I (2008) Dyslexia and Learning Styles: Overcoming the Barriers to Learning. In Reid G, Fawcett A J, Manis F & Siegel L (eds.) *The SAGE Handbook of Dyslexia*. London: SAGE, pp. 369–381.

Reindal S M (2016) Discussing inclusive education: an inquiry into different interpretations and a search for ethical aspects of inclusion using the capabilities approach. *European Journal of Special Needs Education*, 31(1): 1–12.

Ricketts C, Brice J and Coombes L (2010) Are multiple choice tests fair to medical students with specific learning disabilities? *Advances in Health Sciences Education*, 15(2): 265–275.

Rickinson M (2010) *Disability Equality in Higher Education: A Synthesis of Research*. York: Higher Education Academy Action on Access. Available at: www.heacademy.ac.uk/assets/EvidenceNet/Syntheses/disability_equality_in_he_synthesis.pdf

Riddell, S. and Weedon, E. (2006) What counts as a reasonable adjustment? dyslexic students and the concept of fair assessment. *International Studies in Sociology of Education*, 16(1): 57–73.

Riddell S and Weedon E (2009) The Idea of Fitness to Practise. In Fuller M, Georgeson J, Healey M, Hurst A, Kelly K, Riddell S, Roberts H and Weedon E (eds.) *Improving Disabled Students' Learning*. Abingdon: Routledge, pp. 57–73.

Riddell S and Weedon E (2014) Disabled students in higher education: discourses of disability and the negotiation of identity. *International Journal of Educational Research*, 63: 38–46.

Riddick B (2000) An examination of the relationship between labelling and stigmatisation with special reference to dyslexia. *Disability & Society*, 15(4): 653–667.

Ridley C (2011) The experiences of nursing students with dyslexia. *Nursing Standard*, 25(24): 35–42.

Roberts H (2009) Listening to Disabled Students on Teaching, Learning and Assessment. In Fuller M, Georgeson J, Healey M, Hurst A, Kelly K, Riddell S, Roberts H & Weedon E (eds.) *Improving Disabled Students' Learning: Experiences and Outcomes*. Abingdon: Routledge, pp. 38–59.

Rose, J. (2009) *Understanding and Teaching Children and Young People with Dyslexia and Literacy Difficulties* Annesley: DCSF Publications. Available at: http://webarchive.nationalarchives.gov.uk/20130401151715/https://www.education.gov.uk/publications/eOrderingDownload/00659-2009DOM-EN.pdf

Roberts S (2010) Reflection on life experience as an aid to deeper learning. *Nursing Older People*, 22(10): 33–37.

Sanderson-Mann J (2006) Understanding dyslexia and nurse education in the clinical setting. *Nurse Education in Practice*, 6(3): 127–133.

Sanderson-Mann J J, Wharrad H and McCandless F (2012) An empirical exploration of the impact of dyslexia on placement-based learning, and a comparison with non-dyslexic students. *Diversity & Equality in Health & Care*, 9(2): 89–99.

Scott S S, McGuire J M and Shaw S F (2003) Universal design for instruction. *Remedial & Special Education*, 24(6): 369–379.

Singleton, C., Horne, J. and Simmons, F. (2009) Computerised screening for dyslexia in adults. *Journal of Research in Reading*, 32(1): 137-152.

Smith F G (2012) Analyzing a college course that adheres to the Universal Design for Learning (UDL) framework. *Journal of the Scholarship of Teaching & Learning*, 12(3): 31–61.

Sowers J-A and Smith M R (2004) Nursing faculty members' perceptions, knowledge, and concerns about students with disabilities. *Journal of Nursing Education*, 43(5): 213–218.

Speed B (2014) No standard offering of aid for dyslexia. *Times Higher Education*, 2146: 20–21.

Stewart W (2002) Electronic assistive technology for the gifted and learning disabled student. *Australian Journal of Learning Disabilities*, 7(4): 4–12.

Storr H, Wray J and Draper P (2011) Supporting disabled student nurses from registration to qualification: a review of the United Kingdom (UK) literature. *Nurse Education Today*, 31(8): e29-e33.

Strnadová I, Hájková V and Květoňová L (2015) Voices of university students with disabilities: inclusive education on the tertiary level – a reality or a distant dream? *International Journal of Inclusive Education*, 19(10): 1080–1095.

Taylor K E and Walter J (2003) Dyslexia and occupation. *Dyslexia*, 9(3): 177–185.

Thomas L and May H (2010) *Inclusive Learning and Teaching in Higher Education.* York: Higher Education Academy. Available at: www.heacademy.ac.uk/resource/inclusive-learning-and-teaching-higher-education

Tonge J and Treanor D (2017) UDL and reasonable accommodations – the systemic changes required in higher education in Ireland. *Presentation at AHEAD Conference 2017*, Dublin. Available at: www.youtube.com/watch?v=Si5zL0hxz1Q&feature=youtu.be

Tops W, Callens C, Cauwenberghe E, Adriaens J and Brysbaert M (2013) Beyond spelling: the writing skills of students with dyslexia in higher education. *Reading & Writing*, 26(5): 705–720.

van Daal V and Tomlin P (2016) *The Dyslexia Handbook 2016.* Bracknell: British Dyslexia Association.

van Jaarsveldt D E and Ndeya-Ndereya C N (2015) It's not my problem': exploring lecturers' distancing behaviour towards students with disabilities. *Disability & Society*, 30(2): 199–212.

Walker S, Dearnley C, Hargreaves J and Walker E A (2013) Risk, fitness to practice, and disabled health care students. *Journal of Psychological Issues in Organizational Culture*, 3(S1): 50–63.

Waterfield J and West B (2008) Towards inclusive assessments in higher education: case study. *Learning and Teaching in Higher Education*, 3: 97–102.

Weedon E and Riddell S (2010) Disabled Students and Transitions in Higher Education. In Ecclestone K, Biesta G & Hughes M (eds.) *Transitions and Learning through the Lifecourse.* Abingdon: Routledge, pp. 103–117.

White, J. (2006) *Dyslexia in pre-registration nursing students: strategies for developing clinical competencies.* Doctor of Philosophy, Cardiff University, Cardiff.

White J (2007) Supporting nursing students with dyslexia in clinical practice. *Nursing Standard*, 21(19): 35–42.

Willis G P (2015) *Shape of Caring Review: Raising the Bar.* London: Health Education England.

Wray J, Aspland J, Taghzouit J and Pace K (2012a) Making the nursing curriculum more inclusive for students with specific learning difficulties (SpLD): Embedding specialist study skills into a core module. *Nurse Education Today*, 33(6): 602–607.

Wright D J and Eathorne V (2003) Supporting students with disabilities. *Nursing Standard*, 18(11): 37–42.

Zhang D, Landmark L, Reber A, Hsien Yuan H, Oi-man K and Benz M (2010) University faculty knowledge, beliefs, and practices in providing reasonable accommodations to students with disabilities. *Remedial & Special Education*, 31(4): 276–286.

20

E-PROFESSIONALISM AND NURSE EDUCATION

The Awareness to Action (A2A) educational framework

Gemma Sinead Ryan

Introduction

In the UK, all professionally registered nurses are required to operate within the scope of the Nursing and Midwifery Council (NMC) Code of Conduct (2018). Internationally, there are a range of different regulators of the nursing profession. For example, American Nurses Association, Nursing and Midwifery Board of Ireland, National Council of State Boards of Nursing, British Columbia College of Nursing Professionals and Australian Nursing and Midwifery Federation. Professional codes published by regulators outline the conduct that patients, the public and professional bodies expect of registered professionals and students and thus underpin the values of the nursing profession. Operating within the scope of the NMC (2018) requires awareness and understanding of how the professional and personal context may impact on the individual ability to uphold the values of the profession.

Registered nurses and pre-registration nurses are held accountable to their professional regulator. Therefore, their employer/university must act ethically and within legal frameworks (Caulfield, 2005). This means professionals need to be able to justify their actions, decisions and omissions whether in practice, outside of the workplace or in the online environment. Consequently, the concept of e-professionalism (also used interchangeably with e-accountability), defined as "the attitudes and behaviours reflecting traditional professional paradigms that are manifested through digital media" (Cain & Romanelli, 2009: p. 1) has posed emerging issues for nursing (Thompson et al., 2008; Cain et al., 2009).

This chapter discusses the concept of e-professionalism (or e-accountability) and the socialisation of student nurses into the nursing profession. The argument is made for active and reflective educational interventions and tools to raise awareness of and facilitate the behaviours that reflect e-professionalism. Student nurses (and nurses) need to become unconsciously competent in the management of their digital footprint (i.e. the information and data trail that exist about individuals every time they engage with the internet in some way).

The chapter offers strategies for nurse education, including learning from a series of research projects: (1) 42-month realist ethnography; (2) development of an educational intervention for student nurses (and nurses) (Ryan, 2017); and (3) validation and evaluation of a decision-making tool to facilitate consistent decisions about online behaviours, collectively known as the Awareness to Action (A2A) framework.

Background to e-professionalism and student nurses

Several recent studies have emphasised the issue of unprofessional behaviours in the online social networks (OSNs) such as Facebook, with many students expressing confusion about what is acceptable (Ginory et al., 2012; Henry & Molnar, 2013; Mamocha et al., 2015). Twenty-one per cent of students are reported to have shared clinical images without obtaining permission (O'Sullivan et al., 2017), while 25% of profiles presented "unprofessional" content (Nason et al., 2018). Nursing students are generally thought to "use social media irresponsibly" and to "lack accountability" (Nyangeni et al., 2015). Thirty-eight NMC competency hearings have been linked to unprofessional behaviours on Facebook: boundary violation (communication with or "friending" patients); information sharing (details about the workplace); breach of confidentiality; and failure to uphold the reputation of the profession (Ryan, 2017a, 2017b). More recently, in several legal cases student nurses have been investigated for breaches of confidentiality and inappropriate photographs posted on OSN (Westrick, 2016).

Professional guidance warns nurses of the implications of OSN presence due to the wide range of individuals who may be able to view and "[mis-]interpret" profiles and posts (Ryan, 2016). Guidance documents present advice in a range of ways, and while there are clear "violations" (such as those above), a grey area still exists where unprofessional versus unacceptable behaviours occur, for example, photos of drinking alcohol during a social occasion (Ryan, 2016). Conversely, such behaviour does not reflect poorly on an individual, with patients and members of the public stating that "nurses are entitled to a life outside of work" (Ryan et al., in press). Members of the public stress the need for student nurses and nurses to be more "aware" of what they share publicly for their own safety but also in the interests of patient confidentiality.

In terms of healthcare student awareness and understanding of online professionalism, most students expressed that professional–personal–social domains should be separate. However, comments such as "we should be held accountable, but I have a right to a personal life" suggest the presence of conflicting values (White et al., 2013; Maloney et al., 2014; Usher et al., 2014). While (online) self-efficacy is shown to improve as they approach the end of their training (Ness, 2013; Alber et al., 2016), it has already been argued that "self-efficacy" does not necessarily equate to "actual behaviours" (Ryan, 2017). There are clearly issues of boundary management, with confidence not necessarily meaning competence. The lack of definition of "physical boundaries" in OSNs (e.g. leaving the workplace or university) exacerbates these concerns. Discrepancies between what "should" be shared, "could" be shared, and what should be challenged and/reported in student nurse, clinical and academic nurse groups further complicate matters (Ryan, 2017). Conversely, such evidence suggests the need for educational interventions to promote "unconscious competence" in the way the profession operates online. Students agree that they should be held accountable for online behaviours (Cain et al., 2009; Finn et al., 2010; Hall et al., 2013) (Kumar, 2014). However, large numbers of students and organisations report observing unprofessional behaviours; some even report doing this themselves (Langenfeld et al., 2016; Levati, 2014; Wang et al., 2019).

The conflict between self-awareness/efficacy and actual behaviour is reflected in perceived awareness of professionalism, self-awareness and behaviours, which did not always correspond (Ryan, 2017b; Alber et al. 2016; Wissinger & Stiegler, 2019). This disconnect is likely to impact on the way in which boundaries exist and information is shared in OSNs (Ollier-Malaterre et al., 2013). Furthermore, it is known that many student nurses use OSN more frequently than academics and are considered "digital natives" (i.e. having been born post-1995 and having been "socialised" into a world that is "online") (Prensky, 2001; Frazier et al., 2014; Duke et al., 2017). Thus, a lack of knowledge, confidence and competence of those in educational roles, many of whom are digital immigrants (i.e. they were socialised into the online environment in later life, born "post-1995"; Prensky, 2001), along with lack of consensus, compound this problem (Lahti & Salminen, 2017; Ryan, 2016, 2017).

More recently, the concept of "patient-targeted Googling" (PTG) and "healthcare-professional targeted Googling" (HCPTG) has become a topic for debate. PTG is defined as "clinicians' practice of searching the internet for information about their patients" (Gershengoren, 2019: p. 134). Research literature suggests that, in psychiatry, counselling and medicine, up to 53% of students and professionals engage in PTG (Ben-Yakov et al., 2015; Eichenberg et al., 2016; Omaggio et al., 2018; Thabrew et al., 2018).

There are clear ethical dilemmas associated with such activity. Many students and professionals engage in PTG, while others consider it unethical (Thabrew et al., 2018; Weijs et al., 2019). Professionals have also been reported to conduct PTG without informing patients or asking for consent (Harris & Kurpius, 2014; Kuhnel, 2018; Gershengoren, 2019). Arguably, the information obtained via PTG is publicly available, but the question remains whether, without clear rationale of the benefit to the patient, or patient consent, this is an invasion of privacy. If there is an ongoing therapeutic relationship, in this case with adolescent patients, there may be justification for obtaining information via PTG (Jent et al., 2011). However, this behaviour risks damaging patient–professional trust (Harris & Kurpius, 2014).

Other concerns include the use of potential "misinformation" in decisions about patient care (Jent et al., 2011), the currency, lack of clarity, context and confirmability of information found on the internet and how people might misrepresent themselves on social media sites (Jent et al., 2011; Ryan, 2017a). Currently, there is significant debate about the nature of PTG and, in the absence of education, training and guidance, many professionals are conflicted about how this should be managed, when and if it should be employed (i.e. before, during or after monitoring patient care) (Chester et al., 2017; Omaggio et al., 2018).

Less documented in literature, doctor-targeted Googling or HCPTG) refers to the practice of patients or members of the public searching for information about their healthcare professional(s) on the internet (Chester et al., 2017; Omaggio et al., 2018; Thabrew et al., 2018). "Information" in the literature most commonly refers to that shared publicly on social media profiles such as Facebook or LinkedIn. However, it could also be information contained in online reviews of organisations or organisation staff profile pages.

HCPTG is less commonly referenced (Chester et al., 2017); however, Bosslet et al. (2011) identified 43% of US physicians and student physicians have received friend requests on social media from patients and Wang et al. (2019) suggest that in nursing this figure is closer to 50%. Ryan (2017) identified several student nurses who had been searched for and/or contacted by patients or relatives on Facebook, which suggests a need for effective nurse education interventions relating to privacy settings, information sharing, appropriate use of OSN platforms for personal and professional purposes and actions they should take in such circumstances.

Registered nurses are accountable to their employer; student nurses are further accountable to their training provider. This type of accountability refers to the need to abide by university and placement policy, procedure and corporate values. Many universities and organisations now have policy and/or guidance relating to the internet and the use of social media (NMC, 2016; Ryan, 2016; Open University, 2019). However, there is evidence to suggest that just having these in place and telling students that they exist is simply not enough to embed e-professionalism in a curriculum (Duke et al., 2017; Mariano et al., 2018). The need for reflective and active interventions that facilitate awareness, acknowledgement of "risk" and navigate the complex nature of OSN is identified widely in research literature (Ramage & Moorley, 2019; Wissinger & Stiegler, 2019). DeGagne et al. (2019) further discuss the need for "cyber-civility", promoting socially acceptable values that might or might not be unprofessional; for example, sexually suggestive material posted publicly. Hence, there is a wider need for promoting "ethical" behaviour that reflects social and professional values and culture.

Pre-registration student nurses are undertaking an educational programme aimed at facilitating their professional socialisation into nursing. As part of this, they are required to develop their professional accountability in order to demonstrate and uphold the values of the profession. However, the values of the professional are (in part) subjectively applied and may conflict with the values of the person. It is argued that prior to Facebook these were more easily managed as there were clear "physical presence" boundaries and changes in behaviours to comply with the "norms" or "values" of life modes. It is also known that, despite the existence of professional codes of conduct, nurses and pre-registration nurses are being held to account for unprofessional behaviours in the OSNs. Correspondingly, they are also held to account for actions and omissions in the physical environment. Is this due to the subjective nature of acceptability, "accountability" or "professional values"? Or is there more clarity needed based on the "values" of the profession? Is it OSN/online social media (OSM) that is the "problem" or are there deeper mechanisms influencing professional behaviours?

In educating nursing students, it is not only of interest to the professional body and education institutions but also to those in the profession to be able to understand and explain the impact and nature of the relationship that OSN/OSM has had.

To summarise, despite professional guidance and organisational policy being in place for several years, there is evidence to suggest that: (1) students need further guidance and input from educators; and (2) the nursing profession has not reached explicit consensus about what accounts for "unprofessional" behaviour.

E-professionalism and professional accountability

Internationally, guidance documents for the professional use of OSNs do exist; for example, those produced by NMC (2016), Nursing and Midwifery Board of Ireland (2013) and Nursing and Midwifery Board Australia (2014). However, the type of advice, structure and level of detail varies, with much of the content reflecting what professional codes of conduct already state (Ryan, 2016). Where nurses and nursing students are aware of the guidance available there are some behaviours and actions that achieve consensus as being unprofessional, such as a breach of confidentiality. However, there are other behaviours where this is less clear, for example, photos of drinking alcohol and being intoxicated (Ford, 2011; Levati, 2014; Barnable et al., 2018).

There is also evidence to suggest that self-assessed online behaviour does not reflect in "actual" online behaviours. For example, awareness of privacy settings does not mean that they are used effectively (Ross et al., 2013; Alber et al., 2016; Ryan, 2017). This suggests that there are still grey areas of understanding relating to what constitutes e-professionalism in nursing. As part of their educational journey, pre-registration student nurses should be learning or "socialising" themselves into the professional values associated with being "registered".

Professional socialisation and the learning journey

Socialisation is "the process by which the objective world of reality is internalised and becomes subjectively meaningful" (Jarvis, 1983: p. 88). Individuals learn, interact, develop and adapt to accepted "social norms and values" as they grow into and throughout adulthood. Socialisation is a fluid, unique and individual process depending on the environment and people someone is exposed to and how the person responds to these. Social trust is enhanced by operating within accepted social norms, acceptable behaviours and values. In the virtual network, these may be more complex, but widely different from those typically found in the physical environments, due to the enhancement across three levels of social capital and because boundaries between personal, public and professional spheres are less defined in OSNs than is the case in the physical world.

Professional socialisation is the process by which individuals acquire knowledge, skills and values relating to their profession (Mackintosh, 2006). For nursing students, this includes understanding the concept and demonstration of professional accountability and how personal and professional identity in which behaviours and values reflect those of the profession is developed. The outcome of professional socialisation is that:

> newcomers ... make sense of their surroundings and ... acquire the kinds of knowledge which would enable them to produce conduct which allowed ... that group [professional body, qualified practitioners] to recognise them as competent.
> *(Howkins & Ewens, 1999: p. 1)*

Professional socialisation begins upon entry to pre-registration nurse education and the journey is influenced by prior life experiences, individual motivations and external factors and continues throughout the professional career (Weidman et al., 2001; Lai & Lim, 2012). Educational establishments are therefore required to facilitate the development of knowledge and skills for reflection, on-going professional development and accountability, to enable the desired outcomes of professional socialisation: development of professional identity, ability to practise within a professional role and demonstration of professional and organisational commitment (Dinmohammadi et al., 2013). Nurse educators are responsible for providing learning activities which improve the knowledge, skills and attitudes explicitly related to professional accountability and the core values of the nursing profession, providing an understanding that actions and professional standards are inextricably linked (Fahrenwald et al., 2005; Krautscheid, 2014).

Online social networks

OSN refers to people connecting online through a range of platforms, enabling users to share personal or professional information on a profile, their online presence and the "platform" for this. OSM places emphasis on social relationships but is better used to describe the "media" by which those relationships exist, such as videos, photos and blogs. Hence, OSNs represent the platform for the online presence and the relationships associated with them, while OSM is a facilitator and method of communication that links the online presence. Globally, the most used OSNs are Facebook, YouTube, WhatsApp, Facebook Messenger, WeChat and Instagram (Statista, 2019).

Ryan (2017a) introduces the concept of "online socialisation" and argues that socialisation, professional socialisation and becoming socialised "online" are interdependent with the relationship between them being individual, complex and evolving (ICE):

- individual: becoming socialised is influenced by values, experiences and culture
- complex: as a result of OSNs and the interaction between the online and offline world
- evolving: continuously exposed to learning and experiencing the online and offline world, they are also *becoming* socialised as a professional.

Rejon and Watts (2014) and Rejon (2013) have previously suggested that OSNs may have a role to play in professional socialisation and more recent research indicates that students are using OSNs such as Facebook and WhatsApp messaging groups to stay in contact with each other about their academic programme and practice placements (Ryan, 2017). This suggests that OSNs do have an impact on the professionally accepted values, behaviours and skills, particularly for pre-registration nursing students on their journey of professional socialisation.

The role of nurse education

Pre-registration student nurses are in the early stages of their professional career, still developing their own understanding and practice around professional accountability, and on their own journey of professional socialisation. Understanding the values and accepted norms of the nursing profession is not always easy and yet is "required" for an individual to be accountable. Conversely, *being* accountable is an inherent component.

As individuals registered on professionally recognised programmes of education, students are accountable, and are thus required to uphold the values of the profession outlined by the regulator, enshrined within the four pillars of accountability (Caulfield, 2005). Professional guidance and codes of conduct often provide examples of professional and unprofessional behaviours and attributes for professional accountability, including the values of the profession through academic conduct and personal behaviour. Codes of conduct emphasise the importance of personal behaviour and conduct outside of the workplace (including OSNs) and in maintaining a positive reputation of the nursing profession, which confirms registered professionals are accountable for opinions, behaviours and actions in OSN/OSM.

While individuals may believe their privacy settings limit what is shared widely, in reality it is difficult to know how far a post will reach, and who it may be visible to. Furthermore, the complex nature of OSNs does not guarantee information will not be shared with patients or the public. Personal opinions and data shared to OSN timelines may potentially be shared much more widely than if discussed verbally in the "family/personal" domain.

If nurses can be held accountable for their actions then, in theory, their behaviours should reflect those values of the profession. Conversely, these values may conflict with their personal values, personal values which, prior to OSN/OSM, would only have been shared within the family/personal domain. This poses a dilemma: the right to a personal "life" versus the requirements of the profession. It also raises further questions: what is acceptable? and what is unprofessional?, when? and in what circumstances? And, what are the online social norms accepted by the nursing profession?

Introducing the Awareness to Action framework

As discussed, there are some clear boundaries about what is professional and unprofessional, such as breaches in confidentiality. Professional guidance often makes further reference to political, religious and moral opinions not being shared inappropriately. However, such a stipulation is subjective: what one person (based on his or her own experiences, thoughts and values) believes to be acceptable may not be acceptable to another. Conversely, OSNs such as Facebook are often viewed as a personal domain where individuals feel they should be able to have their own opinions and beliefs; they are more than a nurse. Arguably this means that the boundary between unprofessional and unacceptable is opaque, leading to confusion and inconsistency when making decisions about what, how, when and in what context an individual can be held to account. This section discusses the A2A framework; the two tools in the A2A framework can be used as the basis for reflective discussion and "'active" learning on the topic of e-professionalism.

Being reactive: Awareness to Action decision-making tool

One component of the A2A framework is the A2A 3Cs decision-making tool. As part of current research evidence and the programme of research previously discussed, it is known that there are four pillars of accountability (Caulfield, 2005) and that there are three components or "Cs" to be considered as part of online actions, incidents or events (Ryan & Cornock, 2018): clarity, context and confirmability. The A2A tool (Ryan, 2017; Ryan et al., in press) enables nurses and nursing students to assess particular behaviours and incidents on OSNs under each of the 3Cs and asks them to consider whether there is evidence of a breach under one or more of the four pillars of accountability: professional, legal, employer and/or ethical (Caulfield, 2005). In the ethical component, this is assessed by the principles of Beauchamp and Childress (2004): justice, autonomy, beneficence and non-maleficence. By evidence, this means that there has to be an explicit guideline or policy that can be applied; the scenarios later in this chapter provide examples of this. A recent project to validate this tool showed excellent reliability, consistency and internal validity (Ryan & Cornock, 2018a, in press). Each of the 3Cs needs to be met for a person to be "held to account" and indicates what, if any, consequence should be pursued; they should be considered in sequence, with the latter dependent on the former (i.e. if the first (clarity) does not evidence a breach, then the final two do not need to be assessed).

Clarity asks the assessor, "Does the behaviour explicitly breach policy and/or guidelines?"

1. *Professional*: is there any evidence of a professional breach? For example, a breach of patient confidentiality or professional code?
2. *Legal*: is there explicit evidence of criminal activity or civil violations, such as fraud, theft or breach of government legislature?
3. *Employer*: is there evidence that the behaviour is a breach of contractual obligation or employer policy and procedure? For example, being on a leave of sickness absence and showing photos of being on holiday or bullying against staff members?
4. *Ethical*: consider the behaviour in the context of justice, autonomy, beneficence and non-maleficence.

Context asks the assessor: "Can you explain/describe the context of the situation, when and where it occurred?"

1. *Professional*: was the offender in a professional capacity at the time and place? What would be expected of another professional of this standing in this circumstance?
2. *Legal*: is the action legal in time and place? Is this explicit and not implied?
3. *Employer*: can the action or behaviour be associated directly with the workplace? For example, does the person name his or her employer or place of work?
4. *Ethical*: are the consequences acceptable given the context of the situation? What was the intent? Who was it accessible to and what would the consequences be? Were there exceptional circumstances?

Confirmability asks the assessor: "Can you be sure that it was the professional who committed this activity while that person was in a professional capacity? Can you confirm the consequences and the outcome?"

1. *Professional*: is the person clearly identifiable as a professional from the online information? Can you confirm that the person shared the content him- or herself or whether it was someone else?
2. *Legal*: was the action legal at the time it occurred? Has the illegal activity already been punished?
3. *Employer*: can you be sure that the individual was working for that employer at the time? Could the information be dated but just shared recently?
4. *Ethical*: can you confirm when, how and what the impact of the consequences were? Did harm come to anyone? If so, what level of harm and what was the intent?

A2A 3Cs: example scenario A

A scenario where a nurse shared images of a patient's leg with a chronic leg ulcer in a closed professional group was met with debate; there are clearly identifiable ethical, legal, professional and employer issues and the post was eventually removed by group moderators. However, the scenario failed to evidence a clear professional breach at the first stage, when considering clarity; as such it would perhaps recommend "no intervention or a reflective activity" for the individual in question. Interestingly, the public participants in Ryan et al. (in press) felt that, as long as the nurse was acting within the "best interests" of the patient, consent was obtained from the patient and this was documented (as was care), the patient remained anonymous and all other options for treatment had been explored, this was innovative, efficient and acceptable use of OSN/OSM. This does suggest that there is a lack of *consensus* within and outside of the profession about what actions nurses should be held to account for.

Consider clarity

Professional: outcome – no breach

There was no evidence that the nurse breached confidentiality. She had documented consent from the patient. The picture did not show the patient's face or identifiable information.

All discussions and activity related to such decisions need to be documented as per professional guidance, including guidance on the use of social media/internet where this is available.

Legal: outcome – no breach

There was no evidence of criminal or civil law being broken as consent was obtained and documented according to General Data Protection Regulations (GDPR) (Information Commissioners Office, ICO, 2018) and Data Protection Act (UK Government, 2018).

All discussions and activity related to such decisions need to be documented as per legal frameworks in the practising country and within the parameters of the usage policy of the OSN platform being used.

Employer: outcome – no breach

This was a closed professional group. The nurse identified with the profession, but the employer was not identifiable from the image shown so there is no way of identifying if it breached any organisational policy on use of the internet.

However, employer policy should be consulted before pursuing such activity to ensure that it is not in breach. If there was a policy in place that was explicit about this then it would suggest that stage 2, context, would need to be considered.

- *Ethical*: outcome – no breach. However, there are some points for reflection, noted above.
- *Justice* – the use of a professional OSN group may be efficient and successful in reaching a wide range of other nurses and their associated experience.
- *Autonomy* – assuming the situation was explained to the patient and patient consent was documented then there is no evidence of a breach in this scenario.
- *Beneficence* – all treatment options had been exhausted; the nurse had consulted with colleagues on a face-to-face basis with no success or improvement. The patient wanted to 'get better'.
- *Non-maleficence* – the nurse needs to consider the potential "harm". Can the nurse confirm the information or suggestions received are from reliable sources? If not, then these need to be discussed with senior staff or peers before implementation.

There is also the component of "unintended consequence". For example, could someone copy, edit and share the image more widely?

Here there is a potential "risk" but considering the other "pillars of accountability" and that there is no evidence that harm came to the patient, then this is limited.

A2A 3Cs: example scenario B

Example scenario B considers the concept of PTG. A woman in her 20s with low mood presents to a mental health nurse who has been a qualified practitioner for 10 years and explains that she had separated from her boyfriend 3 months ago and requested some medication to help with her anxiety, During the discussion the patient talks about her living situation and financial circumstances; she explains that she does not drink alcohol or take any illegal substances. Once the patient leaves, the nurse, out of curiosity and because she feels suspicious of the information provided, searches for the patient using an internet search engine. She finds the patient's Facebook page and it states that she is still in a relationship; there are recent photos and there are also pictures from the previous weekend that show her drinking (what looks like) a glass of wine. At their next meeting, the nurse questions the patient about what she found, and the patient becomes very upset, storms out and makes a complaint. The nurse's defence was that the information was public, and she wanted to find out whether the patient was lying.

Consider clarity – possible breach

Professional

The nurse did not necessarily breach any confidentiality of the patient. However, professionally it is not considered "good practice" to use a patient's personal information or access a patient's personal details unless there is a clinical, safety-related or justifiable need to do so.

From the perspective of professional guidance and the need to employ an evidence-based approach to decisions. However, research evidence to date generally considers it unjustifiable to search for a patient out of "curiosity" or because a patient might be lying (Clinton et al., 2010; Harris & Kurpius, 2014; Eichenberg et al., 2016; Kuhnel, 2018; Omaggio et al., 2018). This literature on the topic of PTG also recommends that, wherever possible, patient consent is obtained and documented for such activity.

Conversely, many professional guidance documents state that nurses should maintain a therapeutic relationship; the actions of the nurse damaged this.

The nurse did not document this as part of the patient's care and is not able to strongly justify how this was for the benefit of the patient.

Legal

There is some legal debate surrounding PTG. However, in using the internet to search for information that is publicly available it is not likely that any criminal or civil laws have been broken.

However, it might be that a disciplinary review panel and professional body review considers that the use of personal information obtained through a professional capacity and would not have been available otherwise (such as a patient's name) is a possible breach of the Data Protection Act (UK Government, 2018) or similar.

Employer

This would depend on whether there was any employer policy in place on the topic of internet use and/or PTG. Employers typically have a policy that reflects the requirements for confidentiality, GDPR (ICO, 2018) and data protection (UK Government, 2018).

Ethical

- *Justice* – it is difficult to determine a clinical or patient need other than the nurse's curiosity. Her intent was not necessarily in the "best interests" of the patient.
- *Autonomy* – the patient was not consulted and did not provide consent. Her reaction and complaint imply that she was not pleased with the actions of the nurse.

- *Beneficence* – it is difficult for the nurse to justify how this has been of benefit to the patient or her care. She explains that she was curious and felt that the patient was lying but the internet should not have been the first route of action here.
- *Non-maleficence* – the patient did become upset and submitted a complaint. Also, she had visited the clinic for "low mood" and this might have a negative impact on this. The nurse might not have intended to cause harm, but this could be considered an unintended consequence of her actions.

Consider context – possible breach

Professional

The nurse was acting in a professional capacity but only through "curiosity" and "because the patient might be lying".

Legal

This is less easy to define. However, as the nurse conducted this on the employer's premises it might be possible to identify when and what search was conducted. This would also help to identify how the patient's personal information was used. It would be useful to consider what another nurse of the same level of training would do in the same circumstances.

Employer

This is directly related to the nurse's employment as she conducted the activity on the premises and in her capacity as an employee.

Ethical

The patient is upset and has made a complaint so, ethically, the nurse has potentially caused harm with little justification. The actions in the circumstances are not supported by research evidence in this context. There was no evident risk of harm to the patient, for example.

However, we do need to consider that the information the patient shared online (however naively) was publicly accessible information. Conversely, there needs to be some consideration that the information she presented online might not be "accurate" or timely. Regardless of this, it did not serve any benefit towards her care.

Consider confirmability – possible breach

Therefore, this scenario could lead to disciplinary, performance management and/or referral to the professional body.

Professional

The nurse conducted this search during her working hours. She also admitted her actions to the patient and the employer in her attempt to justify these.

Legal

There are emerging guidelines and frameworks on the topic of PTG but these are not (in the UK) part of a legal framework. It would be reasonable to consider case law at the time of the event to establish what the precedent is.

Employer

This could be established through the nurse's admittance and through the IT department/internet history. The employer will likely investigate this as part of the complaints process.

Ethical

This would need to be assessed through discussion with the patient and a possible clinical discussion. There would be an investigation associated with the patient's complaint.

Being proactive: Awareness to Action educational tool

From current literature, discussed earlier in this chapter, it is known that there is a need for more active and reflective educational interventions for nurse education on e-professionalism. Conversely, Olliere-Malaterre et al. (2013) describe the need to promote a "hybrid approach" to managing boundaries in the online domain. Ryan (2017) identified a model by which this reflects a student nurse's ability to become "unconsciously competent" (Kruger & Dunning, 1999) through the use of "hybrid boundary management. *Hybrid boundary management* involves the competent application of custom privacy settings so that certain types of OSM are only shared with close friends or family, using appropriate OSN platforms for their intended purpose (e.g. LinkedIn for professional purposes and Facebook for personal use), regular assessment of privacy settings and publicly accessible information and challenging behaviour where needed.

It is recognised that becoming "unconsciously-competent" is a learning process and certain events might challenge an individual's ability to comply with this, for example, when exposed to emotive images or subjects that trigger strong opinions or emotions. However, lifelong learning theory (Jarvis, 2006) and evidence discussed in this chapter suggest that repeated exposure to concepts facilitates reflection and experiential (lifelong) learning. Conversely, it is also known that sites such as Facebook change their privacy and security settings intermittently, and this tool supports individuals to consider how these changes may have affected what they share and who they share it with.

Hence, based on a review of the available evidence earlier in this chapter and that discussed in Ryan (2017), the "proactive" component of the A2A framework consists of the following parts and may be used by an individual or as small-group activity (Figure 20.1 outlines the suggested process and role of each part) to promote personal reflection and repeated exposure to the principles of *hybrid boundary management*:

- part 1: a checklist and traffic light scoring system on an individual's "awareness" and perceived self-efficacy about what he or she shares on his or her OSN profile with a checklist of questions
- part 2: a checklist and reflective process that requires review of a public and personal OSN profile to identify "actual" behaviours

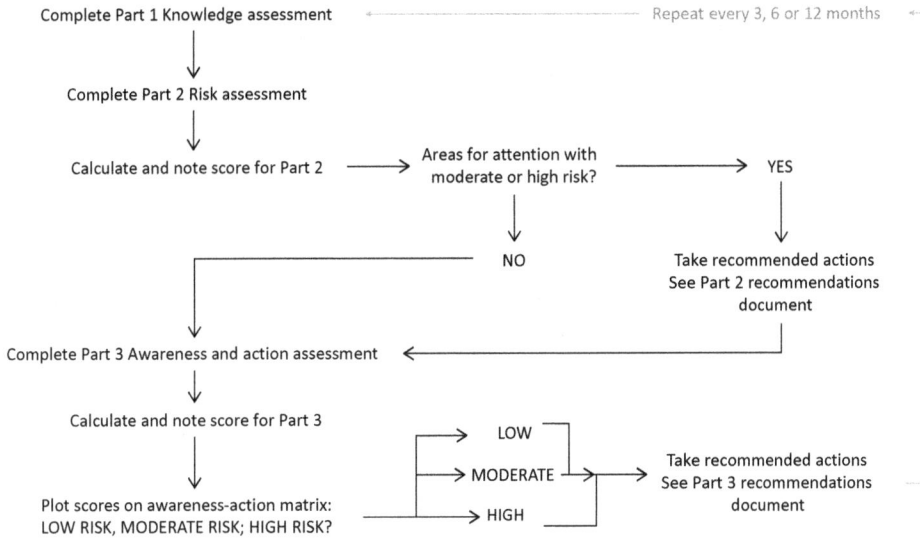

Figure 20.1 Awareness to Action (A2A) assessment process.

- part 3: a risk assessment score that combines the difference between "awareness and action"
- recommendations document: this provides actions that can be taken to reduce the "risk" of unprofessional behaviours
- action plan: this requires the individual to identify areas of moderate and high risk and note what actions can be taken to avoid this risk. This activity also requires individuals to plan when they will conduct the A2A assessment again (e.g. 3, 6 or 12 months) based on their level of assessed "risk".

The A2A awareness tool can be used for professional development, either on entry to nursing or during nurse training. For example, at the beginning of each stage and towards the end of a programme of study, for registered nursing staff or as part of the "recommended actions" in the A2A decision-making process (reactive component, discussed previously). This is an ongoing and evolving process that can be repeated at entrance to and throughout nurse training but also during the professional career.

While this assessment seeks to facilitate reflection of self-efficacy (awareness) of online behaviours versus "actual" behaviours, it also serves to prompt discussion about what *being professionally accountable* means in reality. Furthermore, group discussion as part of conducting the assessment will serve to negotiate and confirm the values of the profession in relation to online socialisation – what is simply unacceptable or what is clearly unprofessional and requires action.

The nursing profession is not well socialised into the online environment at this point and there is a clear lack of consensus about acceptable, professional and unprofessional behaviour. Rogers (2003) represents this concept as "critical mass"; innovations (or values, in this case) are unlikely to be advantageous if there are only a small number of adopters; these are not yet "the norm". Hence the benefit of a generic A2A assessment, adopted as part of nurse education more widely, could help to set these "norms" and thus, professional values, creating consensus and consistency.

Conclusion: becoming unconsciously competent

From the background research and evidence on the topic of e-professionalism discussed in this chapter, it is known that there are a range of legal, ethical, employer and professional issues associated with the use of OSN. What is also known is that there is a need for reflective and active interventions to facilitate nurses' knowledge and activity associated with e-professionalism (especially student nurses being socialised into the profession and as the "future" for promoting and establishing these values in the context of "online").

This chapter presents the A2A framework that consists of two components: a proactive: A2A assessment tool and a reactive A2A decision-making tool. The first can be used as part of individual or group educational activities for student nurses, and indeed nurses in the educational sector to raise awareness of e-professionalism but also the behaviours associated with it. The second can be used when assessing online incidents or behaviours as part of formal "review" processes or as an educational intervention to generate debate about example scenarios. It seeks to promote consensus, consistency and an evidence base for decision making when considering online behaviours.

References

Alber J M, Paige S, Stellefson M & Bernhardt J M (2016) Social media self-efficacy of health education specialists: training and organizational development implications. *Health Promotion Practice* 17(6): 915–921.

Barnable A, Cunning G & Parcon M (2018) Nursing students' perceptions of confidentiality, accountability and e-professionalism in relation to Facebook. *Nurse Educator* 43(1): 28–31.

Beauchamp T L & Childress J F (2004) *Principles of biomedical ethics*. London: Oxford University Press.

Ben-Yakov M, Kayssi A, Benardo J D, Hicks C M & Devon K (2015) Do emergency physicians and medical students find it unethical to look up their patients on Facebook or Google? *Western Journal of Emergency Medicine* XVI(20): 234–239.

Bosslet G T, Torke A M, Hickman S E, Terry C L & Helft P R (2011) The patient-doctor relationship and online social networks: results of a national survey. *Journal of General Internal Medicine* 26(10): 1168–1174.

Cain J & Romanelli F (2009) E-professionalism: a new paradigm for a digital age. *Curriculum Pharmacy Teaching & Learning* 1(2): 66–79.

Cain J, Scott D R & Akers P (2009) Pharmacy students' Facebook activity and opinions regarding accountability and e-professionalism. *American Journal of Pharmaceutical Education* 73(6): article 104.

Caulfield H (2005) *Vital notes for nurses: accountability*. Oxford, UK: Blackwell Publishing.

Chester A N, Walthert S E, Gallagher S J, Anderson L C & Stitely M L (2017) Patient-targeted Googling and social media: a cross-sectional study of senior medical students. *BMC Medical Ethics* 18(70).

DeGagne J C, Hall K, Conklin J L, Yamane S S, Roth N W, Chang J & Kim S S (2019) Uncovering cybercivility among nurses and nursing students on Twitter: a data mining study. *International Journal of Nursing Studies* 89: 24–31.

Dinmohammadi M, Hamid P & Neda M (2013) Concept analysis of professional socialization in nursing. *Nursing Forum* 48(1): 26–34.

Duke V J A, Anstey A, Carter S, Gosse N, Hutchens K M & Marsh J A (2017) Social media in nurse education: utilization and e-professionalism. *Nurse Education Today* 57: 8–13.

Eichenberg C, Nabil P, Herzberg P Y & Habil D (2016) Do therapists google their patients? A survey among psychotherapists. *Journal of Medical Internet Research* 18(1): e3.

Fahrenwald N L, Bassett S D, Tschetter L, Carson P P, White L & Winterboer V J (2005) Teaching core nursing values. *Journal of Professional Nursing* 21(1): 46–51.

Finn G, Garner J & Sawdon M (2010) You're judged all of the time! Students' views on professionalism: a multicentre study. *Medical Education* 44: 814–825.

Ford S (2011) Nurses breaching online rules. *Nursing Times.net*. 26th July 2011 [Available Online] www. nursingtimes.net/nursing-practice/clinical-zones/management/nurses-breaching-online-rules/5032948.article.

Frazier B, Culley J M, Hein L C, Williams A & Tavakoli A S (2014) Social networking policies in nursing education. *Computers, Informatics, Nursing* 32(3): 110–117.

Gershengoren L (2019) Patient-targeted googling and psychiatric professionals. *The International Journal of Psychiatry in Medicine* 54(2): 133–139.

Ginory A, Sabatier L M & Eth S (2012) Addressing therapeutic boundaries. *Psychiatry* 75(1): 40–48.

Hall M, Hannah L A & Huey G (2013) Use and views on social networking sites of pharmacy students in the United Kingdom. *American Journal of Pharmaceutical Education* 77(1): article 9.

Harris S E & Kurpius S E (2014) Social networking and professional ethics: client searches, informed consent and disclosure. *Professional Psychology, Research and Practice* 45(1): 11–19.

Henry R K & Molnar A L (2013) Examination of social networking professionalism among dental and dental hygiene students. *Journal of Dental Education* 77(11): 1425–1430.

Howkins E J & Ewens A (1999) How students experience professional socialisation. *Nursing Studies* 36(1): 41–49.

Information Commissioners Office (2018) *Guide to the General Data Protection Regulation (GDPR).* [Available Online] www.gov.uk/government/publications/guide-to-the-general-data-protection-regulation.

Jarvis P (1983) *Professional Education.* London: Croom Helm.

Jarvis P (2006) *Towards a comprehensive theory of learning, lifelong learning and the learning society volume 1.* London, UK: Routledge.

Jent J F, Eater C K, Merrick M T, Englebert N E, Dandes S K, Chapman A V & Hershorin E R (2011) The decision to access patient information from a social media site: what would you do? *Journal of Adolescent Health* 49: 414–420.

Krautscheid L C (2014) Defining professional nursing accountability. a literature review. *Journal of Professional Nursing* 30(1): 43–47.

Kruger J & Dunning D (1999) Unskilled and unaware of it: how difficulties in recognizing one's own incompetence lead to inflated self-assessments. *Journal of Personality and Social Psychology* 77(6): 1121–1134.

Kuhnel L (2018) TTaPP: together take a pause and ponder: a critical thinking tool for exploring the public/private lives of patients. *The Journal of Clinical Ethics* 29 Summer 2018: 102–113.

Kumar K (2014) Views of medical e-professionalism: a comparison. *The Clinical Teacher* 11: 70–73.

Lahti M & Salminen L (2017) Use of social media by nurse educator students: an exploratory study. *The Open Nursing Journal* 28(11): 26–33.

Lai P K & Lim P H (2012) Concept of professional socialization in nursing. *IeJSME* 6(1): 31–35.

Langenfeld J, Hall C J, Tran A, Sison-Martinez J, Finke D, Buzalko R & Lnagenfeld S (2016) 38 Social media and medical professionalism: an assessment of behaviour of Facebook by emergency medicine residents. *Annals of Emergency Medicine* 68(4): S17.

Levati S (2014) Professional conduct among registered nurses in the use of online social networking sites. *Journal of Advanced Nursing* 70(10): 2284–2292.

Mackintosh C (2006) Caring: the socialization of pre-registration student nurses: a longitudinal qualitative descriptive study. *International Journal of Nursing Studies* 43(8): 953–962.

Maloney S, Moss A & Ilic D (2014) Social media in health professional education: a student perspective on user levels and prospective applications. *Advances in Health Science Education* 19(5): 687–697.

Mamocha S, Mamoncha M R, Pillow T (2015) Unprofessional content posted online among nursing students. *Nurse Educator* 40: 119–123.

Mariano M C O, Maniego J C M, Manila H L M D, Mapanoo R C C, Maquiran K M A, Macindo J R B, Tejero L M S & Torres G C S (2018) Social media use profile, social skills, and nurse-patient interaction among registered nurses in tertiary hospitals: a structural equation model analysis. *International Journal of Nursing Studies* 80: 76–82.

Nason K N, Byrne H, Nason G J & O'Connell B (2018) An assessment of professionalism on students Facebook profiles. *European Journal of Dental Education* 22(1): 30–33.

Ness G L, Sheehan A H, Snyder M E, Jordan J, Cunningham J E & Gettig J P (2013) Graduating pharmacy students' perspectives on e-professionalism and social media. *American Journal of Pharmaceutical Education* 77(7). article 146.

Nursing and Midwifery Board of Australia (2014) *Social media policy.* [Available Online] www.nursingmidwiferyboard.gov.au/Codes-Guidelines-Statements/Policies/Social-media-policy.aspx.

Nursing and Midwifery Board of Ireland (2013) *Guidance to nurses and midwives on social media and social networking.* [Available Online] www.nmbi.ie/Standards-Guidance/More-Standards-Guidance/Social-Media-Social-Networking

Nursing and Midwifery Council (2016) *Guidance on using social media responsibly*. [Available Online] www.nmc.org.uk/standards/guidance/social-media-guidance/

Nursing and Midwifery Council (2018) *The code*. [Available Online] www.nmc.org.uk/standards/code/

Nyangeni T, Du Rand S & Van Rooyen D (2015) Perceptions of nursing students regarding responsible use of social media in the Eastern Cape. *Curatonis* 38(2): 1496.

O'Sullivan E, Cutts E, Kavikondala S, Salcedo A, D'Souza K, Hernandez-Torre M, Anderson C, Tiwari A, Ho K & Last J (2017) Social media in health science education: an international survey. *JMIR Medical Education* 3(1): e1.

Ollier-Malaterre A, Rothbard N P & Berg J M (2013) When worlds collide in cyberspace: how boundary work in online social networks impacts on professional relationships. *Academy of Management Review* 38(4): 645–669.

Omaggio N F, Baker M J & Conway L J (2018) Have you ever googled a patient or been friended by a patient? Social media intersects the practice of genetic counselling. *Journal of Genetic Counselling* 27: 481–491.

Open University (2019) *Student computing policy*. [Available Online] https://help.open.ac.uk/documents/policies/computing

Prensky M (2001) Digital natives, digital immigrants. *On the Horizon* 9(5): 1–6. [Available Online] www.marcprensky.com/writing/Prensky%20-%20Digital%20Natives,%20Digital%20Immigrants%20-%20Part1.pdf (Accessed 24 July 2019) .

Ramage C & Moorley C (2019) A narrative synthesis on healthcare students use and understanding of social media: implications for practice. *Nurse Education Today* 77: 40–52.

Rejon J C (2013) Appendix 2: Social learning tools: are we online? In Rejon J C & Watts C (Eds.). *Supporting professional nurse socialisation: findings from evidence reviews*. London, UK: Royal College of Nursing, p. 28.

Rejon J C & Watts C (2014) *Supporting professional nurse socialisation: findings from evidence reviews*. London, UK: Royal College of Nursing.

Rogers E (2003) *Diffusion of innovations*. 5th ed. London, UK: Free Press.

Ross S, Lai K, Walton J M, Kirwan P & White J S (2013) "I have the right to a life": medical students' views about professionalism. *Medical Teacher* 35: 826–831.

Ryan G S (2016) International perspectives on social media guidance for nurses: a content analysis. *Nursing Management* 23(8): 28–35.

Ryan G S (2017) *Online social networks and the pre-registration student nurse: a focus on professional accountability*. [Available Online] www.dora.dmu.ac.uk/handle/2086/16379.

Ryan G S (2017a) Professional socialisation, accountability and social media: what's the relationship and why should we care? *Nursing Educational and Professional Development: The Global Perspective Conference and Exhibition Hosted by the RCN Education Forum*. 21-22 March 2017. Cardiff, Wales.

Ryan G S (2017b) What do nurses do in professional Facebook groups and how can we explain their behaviours. *RCN International Research Conference 2017*. 5-7 April 2017, Oxford, UK.

Ryan G S & Cornock M (2018) Professionalism in social media: the 3Cs rule. *RCN International Research Conference*. University of Birmingham Medical School, Birmingham, UK.

Ryan G S & Cornock M (2018a) Awareness into Action (A2A): a tool for making decisions about professionalism on social media. *2nd Digital Health and Wellbeing Conference*. 1-3 May, Open University, Milton Keynes.

Ryan G S & Cornock M (in press) PRISM: Professional Regulation in Social Media: validation and evaluation of a decision making tool. *Nurse Researcher*.

Ryan G S, Cornock M & Jackson J (in press) What is the patient and public position on e-professionalism in social media. *Nursing Management*.

Statista (2019) *Most popular social networks worldwide as of July 2019, ranked by number of active users (in millions)*. [Available Online] www.statista.com/statistics/272014/global-social-networks-ranked-by-number-of-users/ (Accessed 22 July 2019).

Thabrew H, Sawyer A & Eischenberg C (2018) Patient-targeted Googling by New Zealand mental health professionals: a new field of ethical consideration in the internet age. *Telemedicine and e-Health* 24(10): 818–824.

Thompson L, Dawson K, Ferdig R, Black E, Boyer J, Coutts J & Black N (2008) The intersection of online social networking with professionalism. *Journal of General Internal Medicine* 23(7): 954–957.

UK Government (2018) *Data protection act*. [Available Online] www.gov.uk/government/collections/data-protection-act-2018 (Accessed 22 July 2019).

Usher K, Woods C, Wilson R, Mayner L, Jackson D, Brown J, Duffy E, Mather C, Cummings E & Irwin P (2014) Australian health professions use of social media. *Collegian* 21: 95–101.

Wang Z, Wang S, Zhang Y & Jiang X (2019) Social media usage and online professionalism among registered nurses: a cross sectional survey. *International Journal of Nurse Education* 98: 19–26.

Weidman J C, Twale D J & Stein E L (2001) Socialisation of graduate and professional students in higher education: a perilous passage. *ASHE-ERIC Higher Education Report* 28(3). Jossey-Bass. San Francisco: USA.

Westrick S J (2016) Nursing students' use of electronic and social media: law, ethics and e-professionalism. *National League for Nursing*. January/February 16-22.

White J, Kirwan P, Lai K, Walton J & Ross S (2013) Have you seen what is on Facebook? The use of social networking software by healthcare professions students. *British Medical Journal Open* 3: 1–8.

Weijs C, Coe J, Majowicz S & Jones-Bitton A (2019) Effects of mock Facebook workday comments on public perception of professional credibility: a field study in Canada. *Journal of Medical Internet Research* 21(4): e12024.

Wissinger C L & Stiegler Z (2019) Using the extended parallel process model to frame e-professionalism instruction in healthcare education. *Teaching and Learning in Medicine* 31(3): 335–341.

SECTION 4

Nurse education and social commentary

Foreword: Sue Dyson

This section is premised on the words of Paulo Freire, who said education either functions as an instrument which is used to facilitate integration of the younger generation into the logic of the present system and bring about conformity, or it becomes the practice of freedom, the means by which men and women deal critically and creatively with reality and discover how to participate in the transformation of their world. Nurse educators are obliged to prepare nurses to take the world of nursing forward. This section considers some of the strategies for ensuring nurses are able to engage with critical social commentary on behalf of and for patients and clients, no matter the context or community. Change is fundamental to nursing, and often the pace of change makes planning for the future challenging. However, nurse educators do have a responsibility to prepare professional nurses for all possible contingencies, and to engage in future thinking about what will and ought to be the mandate for nursing. Environmental change has seen the mass migration of people, created huge inequalities in health and has led to many more people in poverty, homeless and in crisis with mental health issues. This section considers the role nurse education has in social commentary, and the responsibility therein for nurse educators to prepare politically, environmentally and socially aware professionals.

The section opens with Michael Traynor's chapter, where he discusses the profession's aspirations, changes in regulation, neoliberal policies affecting UK higher education, national economic performance and nursing shortages, as well as contingent events such as highly publicised NHS care scandals. He argues all these shift what is seen as desirable and possible in nurse education. Michael suggests the question of the best educational preparation for nurses generally stimulates fierce and polarised debate and offers insight into how nurse educators might think through these important issues.

Priya Martin and Dawn Forman's chapter considers various leadership approaches drawing on contemporaneous literature. Using two lenses (health services leadership and clinical supervision), the authors unpack how these leadership models and strategies can be applied in day-to-day situations at the coalface, as a means of facilitating transformation in healthcare to meet emerging population needs.

Renee Kumpula focuses her chapter on the differences as well as the commonalities that hold all of humanity together. She describes various pedagogical lenses for cultivating the workforce of the future, giving specific consideration to how to work with student populations, enhance student involvement and create an equitable climate for student participation in nursing programmes.

David Robertshaw's chapter draws our attention to the use of technology in nurse education. Technology and the internet have made learning accessible to almost everyone and the benefit of knowledge sharing is felt globally. However, David points out nurse education should study carefully the impact and nature of technology, and how it affects nursing students and patients alike, considering at every stage whether technology is the right pedagogy to use or not.

In Ruta Renigere's chapter, she discusses the ecological approach in education and healthcare. Ruta refers to this as a value-oriented transformation process of students from *I-ego* to *I-eco* in their life activities and systemic thinking in social, education and healthcare environments, complementing the professional code of ethics.

Steve Parker and Sandra Egege's chapter discusses the significance of critical thinking to nursing practice. The authors introduce the basic concepts of epistemology deemed essential in understanding the broader context of critical thinking to nursing practice and discuss cultural issues related to the teaching and learning of critical thinking, so relevant for a globalised and international environment. The chapter turns its attention to what is meant by critical thinking in general and then within the nursing context.

Finally, Sue Dyson's chapter draws the section and the book to a close. Sue discusses the importance of transformational pedagogy for nurse education, wherein students are situated at the centre of learning. She argues, in the context of nursing as risky business, regulation of nurse education becomes the mainstay for nurse educators, thus taking on the role of pseudo-pedagogy. Structured volunteering within the nursing curriculum is suggested as one way students may come to know safe nursing practice (knowledge), and how to practise nursing safely (competence).

21

THE POLITICS OF NURSE EDUCATION

Michael Traynor

Introduction

We can think of the education and training of an occupational group as part of a professionalising project. The higher the level, the longer the preparation and the harder it is to enter, the more likely that occupation is to be considered to have professional standing. Over the course of the twentieth century in many developed countries those promoting nursing's professional status have generally been successful in persuading governments that nurse education belongs in the highest educational position – the university. Labelled however, in the early 1960s, a semi-profession, nursing has not, at least in the UK, achieved an unchallengeable professional status. This precarious position has at least two effects. The first is that many commentators outside the profession, along with a not inconsiderable number inside, remain unconvinced that the high-status/high-level educational model for nursing is the right one. The second is that when the policy context shifts it continually appears to undermine nursing's professional achievements. I am thinking both of health services policy, to do with the make-up of the NHS workforce for example, and higher-education policy which has promoted initiatives that threaten the unique status of the university, particularly in the preparation of public-sector professionals – nurses, social workers and teachers being the largest groups. Earlier chapters have presented this history and surrounding debates in detail. In this chapter I want to document the intersection of forces that are acting on nursing and nurse education in the UK today. Each historical and policy period has its own unique features but the forces and debates underlying them tend to have a longer timescale. In this chapter I will be discussing:

- the current and anticipated shortage of nurses in the UK – with a comparison to other countries – and responses from the NHS and Departments of Health, including the introduction of a new type of worker, the nursing associate
- changes in the character of the profession's regulator, the Nursing and Midwifery Council
- the continuing advance of neoliberal policy as it affects the university sector
- debates about the character of nursing in the light of much publicised "nursing failures" in the opening decade of the twenty-first century.

Why are there not enough nurses?

In November 2013 the World Health Organization released a report in which it claimed that the world was short of 7.2 million nurses (Global Health Workforce Alliance and World Health Organization, 2013). The report identified several key causes. They include an ageing health workforce and staff retiring or leaving for better-paid jobs without being replaced, while not enough young people were entering the profession or being adequately trained. The report also considered that increasing demands are being put on the healthcare sector as a whole from a growing world population with risks of non-communicable diseases increasing. Internal and international migration of health workers also contributes to regional imbalances. The authors of the report made a number of recommendations, including the following:

1 increased political and technical leadership in countries to support long-term human resource development efforts
2 collection of reliable data and strengthening human resource for health databases
3 maximising the role of mid-level and community health workers to make front-line health services more accessible and acceptable
4 retention of health workers in countries where the deficits are most acute and greater balancing of the distribution of health workers geographically
5 providing mechanisms for the voice, rights and responsibilities of health workers in the development and implementation of policies and strategies towards universal health coverage.

In 2014 the *Australia's Future Health Workforce* report (Health Workforce Australia, 2014) estimated that the nation would need an extra 123,000 nurses by 2030. Reasons for this predicted shortage include demographic changes and reduced recruitment of nurses from overseas. The report also noted an increase in student nurse attrition during training from an overall 21 per cent (2000–2006) to 34 per cent (2009–2012).

In the UK, a report by the King's Fund claimed that the number of nurses employed in the NHS (on a headcount or full-time equivalent basis) fell in 2017 for the first time in more than three years. It also noted that the number of nurses was failing to keep pace with population growth: the number of nurses per 100,000 population in England declined from 604 in 2009 to 576 by 2016. After a decade of rapid growth in both budgets and staff during the 2000s, the slowdown in NHS spending growth began in 2010 as the Conservative–Liberal Democrat government attempted to reduce the UK's budget deficit. For the NHS this meant a switch to low real-terms growth in spending rather than actual cuts at that point. However that still meant that increasing the number of staff was no longer affordable once other cost pressures were taken into account (Murray, 2017). In early 2017, the Royal College of Nursing (RCN) estimated that there were 40,000 unfilled nursing posts in England (Royal College of Nursing, 2017).

A report from the Health Foundation identifies one cause for this shortage – poor overall workforce planning:

> Following on from the report by Sir Robert Francis into the care failings at Mid Staffordshire NHS Foundation Trust, published in 2013, national policy focus on staffing levels in the NHS in England has not been robust or consistent. The approach has been caught between concern about staffing levels (with the aim of

assuring care is safe) and the need to contain staffing costs as part of the financial challenge.

(Buchan et al., 2017: p. 15)

As evidence of the long-term nature of this problem, in 2006 a "boom or bust" rather than a coordinated policy approach to the commissioning of nurse education places was blamed for unstable numbers in the UK nursing workforce and a repeated cycle of nurse shortages causing NHS bodies to undertake various targeted overseas recruitment drives (Buchan and Seccombe, 2006: p. 5):

> The current organisational changes in the NHS in England … the de-concentration of some workforce planning and policy responsibilities, such as international recruitment and large scale workforce change, to NHS employers means that the NHS workforce planning process in England is once again confused, with multiple stakeholders and uncertainties about future focus, responsibilities and structures. There is a danger of a fragmented system emerging, with overlap and gaps, a lack of clear lines of responsibility; an absence of effective integration and oversight at national level, and, inadequate capacity at local and regional level.

Why is this short summary of workforce issues important for a consideration of the politics of nurse education? I think because it highlights the fact that the aspirations of the profession and government policy concerning the public sector and its workforce are not necessarily aligned. While a professional group is likely to be most concerned with advancing its own interests, governments as employers are likely to focus on overall cost containment and the maximising of efficiency. Regarding this chapter, the arena where this encounter is played out is in state healthcare provision and in state-funded universities. While each party claims that the well-being of patients is its paramount concern, the fact of regular conflict between them reveals their differing interests.

So what might we consider to be the interests of a professional group? Such a question has been, for many decades, at the centre of sociology's historical fascination with professions such as medicine (Freidson, 1970; Atkinson et al., 1977), but also, more recently, nursing (Melia,1987; Walby and Greenwell, 1994; Traynor, 2009; Traynor et al., 2015). We might consider the following as core professional concerns:

- control over entry to the profession
- specialised high-level educational preparation
- autonomy of practice
- clear boundaries around their sphere of authority
- a high degree of responsibility
- a direct relationship with its clients
- an ethical code of practice to deter exploitation of those clients
- a high degree of public trust and respect
- to be financially rewarded in line with the high level of responsibility
- to have influence to shape the context of their work.

The authors of other chapters have set out the history of nurse education in a range of countries, including the UK. However an identification of the educational recommendations of the Briggs report (Committee on Nursing, 1972) and the implementation of the, more or less, resulting Project 2000 (United Kingdom Central Council for Nursing Midwifery and Health Visiting, 1986) is necessary for this chapter because it remains a landmark in the professional progress of nursing in the UK. As is well known and well repeated, the Committee on Nursing chaired by historian Asa Briggs saw a great deal of unfulfilled potential in nursing. A more highly educated workforce could make a significant contribution to ever more complex healthcare. It could attract a broader cohort of recruits into training and become a more structured and attractive career. The committee recommended both a restructuring of the profession's regulatory bodies and a radical reform of nurse education. The report concluded that existing training was spread too thinly across nearly 655 schools of nursing in England and Wales and 62 in Scotland. The committee however rejected the RCN's call for an increase in the qualifications required of recruits to nurse training. Instead it wanted to place more emphasis on motivation than on formal academic achievement. The report recommended reducing the age of entry to training from 18 to 17 and changing the structure of education involving two 18-month parts. The 1979 Nurses, Midwives and Health Visitors Act inaugurated five new statutory bodies; key perhaps was the UK Central Council for Nursing, Midwifery and Health Visiting (UKCC). The UKCC was required to establish and improve standards of professional conduct and training.

So, in the mid-1980s, the UKCC, itself a young organisation, started work on devising a major reform of nursing education in the UK. That reform became known as Project 2000. The first aim was to change the character of nurse education from a system which was largely driven by the requirement to meet the NHS workforce needs with its large contribution of student labour to one that would expose its students, as well as those who educated them, to the likely beneficial effects of mainstream higher education. Nurse training before the university was often described as "an apprenticeship model". Whatever variety of actual practices is included within that term, the association was one of how trade skills were transmitted from experienced tradesmen to their "apprentices". Alongside all the other arguments for university-based education, many in nursing felt that the association with trades did not help the overall status of the profession. Today apprenticeships have been revitalised, particularly by the recent coalition government, as a way of dealing with the country's deficit in intermediate-level skills and improving the job prospects of young people which have been deteriorating since the mid-2000s. (In the mid-1990s the Conservative government introduced "modern apprenticeships" which form the basis of today's conceptualisations.) Nevertheless, in the mid-1980s, a new identification of trainee nurses with the higher-education sector as well as their new "supernumerary" position releasing them from being used as a cheap source of labour was seen by most (but not all) as a significant professional advancement.

The implementation ran into a number of unforeseen problems, some the effect of unco-ordinated government policy across sectors (Davies, 1995; Draper, 1995). Perhaps most significantly, the government of the day considered the scheme far too costly. It is not a coincidence that the 1990s in the UK saw increased policy attention to issues of "skill mix" in the healthcare and particularly nursing workforce. A government already committed to managerialist strategies for organising and controlling the health service saw increasing the division of nursing labour as an urgent issue (Traynor, 1999; Allen, 2001). The rise of the healthcare support worker/assistant caused predictable issues on the border of the nursing profession. The profession and those who argued for the expansion (in numbers and scope) of workers in such assistant roles had to emphasise their differentiation from nursing and subordination to registered nurses. If the promoters of Project 2000 had hoped to walk away with an increase in the overall qualification level of the nursing workforce, they ended up having to convince managers and politicians that highly educated nurses bring the benefits of their education even to the apparently low-skilled work of bathing patients.

The same array of changes both to society and to healthcare delivery named in support of Project 2000 have been, 20 years later, marshalled as the impetus for further attention to the structure of nurse education and to the establishment of all-degree entry to the profession (Department of Health and CNO's Office, 2006). This degree-level entry was implemented from 2013 in England. As a mark of its professionalising significance the then general secretary of the RCN, Peter Carter, described the change as "an important and historic development" (BBC News, 2009). However, as might have been foreseen, a step forward for UK nursing is often shortly followed by two steps back, in this case by two problematic announcements from the Department of Health. The first concerned the proposal for a new "nursing" worker, the nursing associate, intended to work with a range of skills "between" (such a seductively simple spatial metaphor) a registered nurse and existing healthcare assistants (Cummings, 2016). The second concerned the removal of the Department of Health-funded bursary for student nurses (Department of Health, 2015), meaning that prospective student nurses had to consider whether they wanted to accumulate £50,000 of debt (including interest – at a shamefully high rate) for the privilege of training to be a nurse, earning a salary just above the threshold of eligibility to repay their loan (Gill, 2016).

But let's look at the nursing associate first. In a chapter about nurse education we need to focus on the implications for entry into the profession. The new nursing associate worker offers many advantages to health service managers, or at least appeared to at the time of its proposal, but it could be that its main impact will be in having created a new route into nursing for motivated recruits who do not have the qualifications for traditional entry into university courses and who are not in a position to accumulate the associated debt. In research into the implementation of the nursing associate pilot in London that I have been involved in, the majority of trainee nursing associates told me that they see the nursing associate role as a step toward becoming a registered nurse, via the various shortened courses, or newly designed apprenticeships, being offered by universities with an eye on diversifying their offerings in the face of difficulties recruiting for nursing degrees. My sense is, as one of the reports chaired by Lord Willis suggested (Willis, 2015), the new role gives many talented and motivated individuals a route into nursing, a career that they perhaps otherwise would not have considered. It might, perhaps, give the architects of Project 2000 and of the degree-entry initiative pause for thought. Is this, through unanticipated folds of politics and history, the reappearance of "the apprenticeship model" of nurse preparation? Or is it a serendipitous solution to the crisis of the nursing shortage and a key to social mobility and diversity of entry, all in one initiative?

University education: nursing education

The nursing associate and associated alternative routes into nursing are likely to be of considerable interest to a current government that seems unable to stop itself sabotaging the nursing workforce by any means possible. Since the scrapping of separate treatment for university students studying nursing, in the form of the NHS bursary, applications by students in England to nursing and midwifery courses at British universities have fallen by 23 per cent. We ought to remember in passing that undergraduate numbers across other courses fell in 2012 when UK tuition fees rose to £9,000 a year, but later recovered (Adams, 2017). Nevertheless expediency sometimes helpfully supports ideology and it could be that a government, never entirely convinced of the need for a degree-qualified nursing workforce, sees this "crisis" as temporary or otherwise as an opportunity to find ways to rebalance this workforce toward associate-level workers. Added to this, the news that the nursing regulator, perhaps under pressure to do so from the Department of Health, would include nursing associates within its registers (Nursing and Midwifery Council, 2017) appears to have consolidated the position, and status, of this new worker.

But these changes to nurse education are part of broader changes to UK higher education. The general preference for so-called market forces articulated so strongly during the Thatcher and Reagan years (these administrations – Thatcher became UK Prime Minister in 1979 and Reagan became US President in 1981 – marked the start of a shift in global politics to the "New Right" or toward neoliberal ideologies) has never really gone away. After the reorganisation toward the "internal market" of the UK NHS, successive UK governments have worked hard to reconfigure the higher-education sector as such a market. Universities now charge a fee payable by individual students and compete for their business. Instead of the nation as a whole training, and paying for, its required nursing or healthcare workforce for the benefit of the nation as a whole (i.e. as a public good), we have a new conceptualisation. This population is conceived of as a series of individuals who, in order to maximise their own personal benefit, chose freely to invest in their future on the basis that graduates *on average* earn more than non-graduates in the UK. Janet Davies, until recently general secretary of the RCN, expressed the fear that after the withdrawal of the bursary for students, nurses' relationship with the NHS will change: "carrying a heavy debt to get qualified, they will feel less obligation to work in the NHS" (Toynbee, 2107). That large numbers of nurses would move from NHS employment to work for private-sector providers seems unlikely; nevertheless the logical extension of the market approach would be that the NHS becomes simply another employer of nurses in a market place for their labour alongside various non-state providers of health services. That individual nurses would choose which employer would benefit them most would act as a force to improve conditions of work for nurses – at least according to neoliberal ideology. So power, in theory, is given to the individual consumer. But conceiving of students, or nurses, or patients for that matter, as being able – and willing – to exercise free choice does not do justice to the range of constraints facing all of them. The choice of where to study or where to work is often limited by geography (though not perhaps so much in large cities, although these can have their own transport issues), and in the case of students, by entry requirements. In a sense UK universities conspired to undermine this higher-education market by nearly all announcing that they would charge students the maximum fee permissible. The Higher Education and Research Act, which became law in April 2017, attempts to challenge this established power base and encourage entry into the sector by lowering the threshold that private providers must meet to become degree-awarding universities. The promotion of competition and choice are key concepts underpinning the Act and subsequent Bill (see https://publica tions.parliament.uk/pa/bills/cbill/2016-2017/0004/17004.pdf).

The Act also proposed the establishment of a new regulator for higher education in the form of the controversial (Adonis, 2018) Office for Students. Its task is to promote quality and greater choice for students and to encourage competition within the sector in England. But it paradoxically lacked representation of the National Union of Students, some say because the government could not risk its pretension to be acting in the interests of students being exposed as a lie (Scott, 2018) through failing to recognise student debt and senior university management pay as the top issues in the sector.

While many student nurses were highly active in protesting against the scrapping of the bursary (Gill, 2016), making it clear that fees and student debt would have prohibited them from considering entering the profession, readers will have their own views about how far student nurses and applicants for these places are becoming more demanding shoppers in the marketplace of nursing degrees.

Professional "self" regulation in the UK

In this section I want to set out how the character of professional self-regulation in the UK has been challenged and changed in recent years and what this has meant for nurse education.

Professional regulation, of course, gives professions considerable benefits. The professions are protected to such an extent that it is usually illegal for someone without the training endorsed by the relevant regulator, let's say as a nurse, to claim to be a nurse or do the work of a nurse. This has the benefit of protecting the public from bogus and possibly dangerous imposters (though it doesn't protect the public from possibly dangerous genuine nurses). In most cases this level of market closure enables professions to gain considerable status, income and power. In addition, the pact with the state includes (or has included) the ability for the professions to regulate themselves. In other words, they can set their own standards for behaviour, usually expressed in a code of practice, and discipline those within the profession whom they judge to have fallen short. More recently, and as a response to the Francis inquiry into the events in the Mid Staffordshire NHS Foundation Trust, the NMC has introduced requirements that practitioners need to demonstrate continuing competence (NMC, 2013).

Since the 1990s, however, UK governments have turned their attention to professional regulators, partly as a response to scandals where the regulator was seen as inadequate (Chief Medical Officer, 2001; Kennedy and Great Britain Department of; 2001). Repeated reviews have found the NMC and its predecessors to be inward looking, lacking adequate lay representation and dysfunctional in various ways (JM Consulting Ltd., 1998; NMC, 2011; Ford, 2012). A cycle of critical reviews followed by senior resignations has meant that between 2002 and 2012 the NMC had five chief executives. Hannah Cooke provides a compelling account of how the state has considerably strengthened its influence within professional "self" regulation in nursing (Cooke, 2012).

Other contributors to this volume have already identified how those involved in nurse education often think of the regulator's requirements as a constraint to the design of innovative curricula, despite the NMC's claim to be doing the just the opposite (Nursing and Midwifery Council, 2018: p. 3). Nurse education is extremely highly specified by the NMC. The Council regularly sets out what it considers are the adequate standards required for education and competence for registration as a nurse or midwife. The most recent set of these standards was published in 2018 (Nursing and Midwifery Council, 2018). The NMC itself is (at present) obliged to incorporate directives from the European Parliament regarding the recognition of professional qualifications within Europe. This includes specific requirements on programme length, content and ratio of theory to practice and the nature of practice learning and range of experience. The NMC's documents detail requirements for the timing of assessments and the character of the final judgement of competence to join the register. The universities that provide such courses have themselves to meet the NMC's strict requirements. Some educators feel that the considerable number of practical requirements imposed by the NMC on nurse education in the interests of patient safety and standardisation mitigate against the regulator's own expressed desire for empowered and self-critical students and graduates.

Nursing "failures" and nurse education

The second "crisis" to affect nurse education in the period covered by this chapter, in addition to the shortage of registered nurses in the workforce, is the crisis of confidence and self-confidence in nurses' established identity as the caring force in the healthcare machine. With the profession's strong identification with a compassionate orientation, the fall from grace threatened by a series of scandals that involved nurses during the 2010s was all the more shocking. Probably the first shock that nursing received during this period was the columnist Christina Patterson's BBC Radio 4 *Four Thought: Care to Be a Nurse?*[1] Christina, who had had breast cancer and then a recurrence, told in unsparing detail about her two stays in hospital. During both she was dealt with by cruel – the word she used – nurses. She ended by saying that there may be any number of structural explanations for the puzzle that people go into an apparently caring profession only to behave in a far from caring way, but she pointed to a fundamental personal responsibility. All nurses, she said, had a decision to make either to be cruel or to be kind and if they did not like the work they could leave. The broadcast went out in July 2011.

At a similar time, the events at Stafford hospital were coming to light. After considerable public pressure for an inquiry into poor care it emerged that elderly patients had been severely neglected by nursing staff over a long period of time and that excess deaths, perhaps up to 400, had occurred at the hospital between 2005 and 2008 (BBC News, 2010). Further failures appeared in the UK media (BBC Panorama, 2011) and in government-commissioned reports (Keogh, 2013). All of these showed nurses in a poor light. The public responded with outrage and incredulity at these apparently widespread acts of cruelty. The final report into the events at Stafford was published in February 2013 (Francis, 2013). The report identified the complex causes of poor medical and nursing care, detailing how the pressures on working culture from management led to atrocious failures of care delivery. The report claimed that entrants to nursing were not adequately prepared to resist the challenges of working in such NHS cultures that tolerated poor standards. The Francis proposal regarding nurse education was that: "There should be an increased focus in nurse training, education and professional development on the practical requirements of delivering compassionate care in addition to the theory" (Section 23.49: p. 1513).

The profession, clearly under government pressure even before the final report was published, redoubled its identification with caring and compassion. The Chief Nursing Officer for England published the document *Compassion in Practice* (Commissioning Board Chief Nursing Officer and DH Chief Nursing Adviser, 2012) involving the launch of the "six Cs" (caring, courage, compassion, competence, communication and commitment).The document included a call for nurse recruitment to be based on applicant "values" as well as technical skills. With these challenges to nursing's previously strongly positive public standing and the re-emergence of calls from certain quarters for nurse education to return to schools of nursing, the RCN commissioned Lord Willis to conduct an inquiry into pre-registration nursing education in the UK. He was asked specifically how nurse education should best create and maintain a workforce of "competent, compassionate nurses prepared to deliver services into the future" (Willis, 2012). Counter to the sometimes circulating misogynistic belief that too much education for nurses damages their caring instincts, the report found no evidence of this peculiar inverse relationship. On the whole, it stated, better-qualified nurses are associated with better patient outcomes.

At the same time the English Department of Health issued instructions to Health Education England (HEE) (Department of Health, 2013) to introduce measures intended to address the "failures of care" highlighted by the Francis report. This involved requiring HEE to ensure that its recruitment, selection and training should promote key values and behaviour among the NHS workforce. The section in the mandate on values and behaviours (p. 13) also included the requirement for HEE to set up and evaluate pilot schemes for prospective nursing students to work for up to a year as healthcare assistants. HEE in turn commissioned the consultancy company Work Psychology Group to look at evidence of effective ways to carry out "values based recruitment" (Health Education England, 2014). The group's review distinguishes the different concepts of values, personality, motivation and behaviour and describes the highly complex relationship between them. The reference point in the Department of Health mandate, the resulting HEE documents and the commissioned review of recruitment and values is the Francis report. It is worth noting that the Francis diagnosis of what went wrong and why problems at Stafford were not identified sooner is extremely broad, ranging from behaviour and policy from the Department of Health interpreted locally as bullying, constant NHS reorganisation, regulatory gaps, through misguided senior management actions, ineffective organisational communication systems, organisational defensiveness and secrecy to cultural tolerance of poor standards (Francis, 2013: pp. 65–66). It is hard to resist the conclusion that the political need to be seen to act in response to this very public scandal drove a costly series of initiatives focusing on recruitment where the benefit is unlikely to be strong. With the requirement for values-based recruitment a few unsuitable potential nurses may be directed away from the NHS but the rest who *are* motivated to put patient care at the centre of their attention will still be challenged by immersion in stressed and dysfunctional environments. Many commentators have argued that the problems with NHS failures do not lie primarily in the poor values of those entering the service but with how culture affects even the most highly motivated individuals (Buchanan et al., 2013; West, 2014). It is not new for universities to attempt to assess candidates' suitability for work with vulnerable patients, with everything from role play to group work to a single question at interview, but the obligation to put such assessment at centre stage is new.

Although the general movement of nurse education in the UK, USA and Australia has been toward higher levels of qualification, supported in the UK by the profession's regulator and, for the moment, by the Department of Health, challenge, as I mentioned at the outset, is never far away. The argument is not seldom voiced that a university-led education is in danger of missing the point regarding the skills and aptitudes needed by nurses to nurse. The most useful arguments made are often nuanced. For example, O'Driscoll points out some of the consequences of the "uncoupling" of education and practice following the move of nurse education into higher education (O'Driscoll, 2010). Nevertheless, the topic remains divisive. The question of the best educational preparation for nurses generally stimulates fierce and polarised debate (for just one example see Bradshaw (2018) and the resultant online responses). I have tried to set out in this chapter the context for changes to nurse education in the UK over the last 20 years. The profession's aspirations, changes in regulation, neoliberal policies affecting UK higher education, national economic performance, nursing shortages as well as contingent events such as highly publicised NHS care scandals all shift what is seen as desirable and possible in nurse education.

Note

1 The programme is currently available on the BBC website at www.bbc.co.uk/iplayer/episode/
b010mrzt/Four_Thought_Series_2_Care_to_be_a_nurse/

References

Adams R (2017 2nd Feb 2017) *Nursing degree appliactions after NHS burseries abolished.* Accessed at: www.the
guardian.com/education/2017/feb/02/nursing-degree-applications-slump-after-nhs-bursaries-abolished

Adonis A (2018 23rd January 2018) Office for students? It's the office against students and it is not going
to last. *Higher education.* Accessed at: www.theguardian.com/education/2018/jan/23/office-for-stu
dents-andrew-adonis

Allen D (2001) *The changing shape of nursing practice: the role of nurses in the hospital division of labour.*
London: Routledge.

Atkinson P, Reid M and Sheldrake P (1977) Medical mystique. *Sociology of Work and Occupations* 4 (3):
243–280.

BBC News (2009 Thursday, 12 November 2009) *Nursing to become graduate entry.* Accessed at: http://
news.bbc.co.uk/1/hi/health/8355388.stm

BBC News (2010 Monday, 8 November 2010) *Timeline: Stafford Hospital in crisis 2007-2010.* Accessed
at: http://news.bbc.co.uk/local/stoke/hi/people_and_places/newsid_8493000/8493964.stm

BBC Panorama (2011) Undercover care: the abuse exposed. Accessed at: www.bbc.co.uk/programmes/
b011pwt6

Bradshaw A (2018 June 24th 2018) To degree or not to degree: that is NOT the question for UK nursing.
Accessed at: www.timeshighereducation.com/blog/degree-or-not-degree-not-question-uk-nursing

Buchan J and Seccombe I (2006) From boom to bust? The UK nursing labour market. Review 2005/6
report for the Royal College of Nursing. Edinburgh: Queen Margaret University College.

Buchan J, Seccombe I, Gershlick B and Charlesworth A (2017) *In short supply: pay policy and nurse numbers
workforce profile and trends in the English NHS.* London: The Health Foundation.

Buchanan D, Denyer D, Jaina J, Kelliher C, Moore C, Parry E and Pilbeam C (2013) How do they
manage? A qualitative study of the realities of middle and front-line management work in health care.
Health services and delivery research. National Institute for Health Research. 1.

Chief Medical Officer (2001) *Harold Shipman's clinical practice 1974-1998: a clinical audit commissioned by the
chief medical officer.* London: Department of Health.

Commissioning Board Chief Nursing Officer and DH Chief Nursing Adviser (2012) *Compassion in practice: nursing, midwifery and care staff our vision and strategy.* London: Department of Health NHS Commissioning Board.

Committee on Nursing (1972) *Report of the committee on nursing (Chairman: Asa Briggs).* Cmnd. 5115.
London: HMSO.

Cooke H (2012) Changing discourses of blame in nursing and healthcare. In D. Holmes, T. Rudge and
A. Perron (Eds.). *(Re)Thinking Violence in Health Care Settings: A Critical Approach.* London: Routledge, pp.
47–66.

Cummings J (2016 14th October 2016) *Nursing associates – A new member of the multi-disciplinary workforce –
Jane Cummings.* Accessed at: www.england.nhs.uk/2016/10/jane-cummings-25/

Davies C (1995) *Gender and the professional predicament in nursing.* Buckingham: Open University Press.

Department of Health (2013) *Delivering high quality, effective, compassionate care: developing the right people
with the right skills and the right values.* London: Department of Health.

Department of Health (2015 7 April 2016) *NHS bursary reform: changes to healthcare education funding for
student nursing, midwifery and allied health students.* Accessed at: www.gov.uk/government/publications/
nhs-bursary-reform

Department of Health and CNO's Office (2006) *Modernising nursing careers - setting the direction.* London:
Department of Health.

Draper P (1995) The merger of United Kingdom colleges of nursing with univeristy departments of nursing: prospects, problems and promises. *Journal of Advanced Nursing* 23(3): 215–216.

Ford S (2012) Review concludes NMC is failing 'at every level'. Accessed at: www.nursingtimes.net/nursing-
practice/clinical-specialisms/management/review-concludes-nmc-is-failing-at-every-level/5046648.article

Francis R (2013) *Report of the Mid Staffordshire NHS Foundation Trust public inquiry: executive summary.*
London: House of Commons. HC 947.

Freidson E (1970) *The profession of medicine: a study of the sociology of applied knowledge.* Chicago, IL: University of Chicago Press.

Gill N (2016) Student nurses prepare to march as anti-fees campaign swells. *Guardian student.* Accessed at: www.theguardian.com/education/2016/jan/08/student-nurses-march-nhs-bursary-campaign

Global Health Workforce Alliance and World Health Organization (2013) *A universal truth: no health without a workforce.* Geneva: WHO.

Health Education England (2014) *Evaluation of Values Based Recruitment (VBR) in the NHS: literature review and evaluation criteria.* London: NHS HEE.

Health Workforce Australia (2014) *Australia's future health workforce – Nurses overview report.* Canberra: Commonwealth of Australia.

JM Consulting Ltd. (1998) The regulation of nurses, midwives and health visitors. Report on a review of the nurses, Midwives & Health Visitors Act 1997. Bristol: JM Consulting.

Melia K M (1987) *Learning and working: the occupational socialization of nurses.* London: Tavistock.

Kennedy I (2001) *The report of the public inquiry into children's heart surgery at the Bristol Royal Infirmary 1984-1995: learning from Bristol.* Command paper: CM5207. London: Department of Health, Stationery Office.

Keogh (2013) *Review into the quality of care and treatment provided by 14 hospital trusts in England: overview report.* London: NHS, p. 61.

Murray R (2017) Falling number of nurses in the NHS paints a worrying picture. Accessed at: www.kingsfund.org.uk/blog/2017/10/falling-number-nurses-nhs-paints-worrying-picture?gclid=Cj0KCQjwiJncBRC1ARIsAOvG-a5K7CIu7Zx0DyQkcPH3b_OlVDWh1kr9h0m7iafZ_cVhqVwVk4MLybMaAgwCEALw_wcB

NMC (2011 31/05/2011)NMC comment on Panorama's undercover care: the abuse exposed. Accessed at: www.nmc-uk.org/Press-and-media/Latest-news/NMC-comment-on-Panoramas-Undercover-Care-The-Abuse-Exposed/

NMC (2013) Council paper: Mid Staffordshire NHS Foundation Trust public inquiry report: Item 20 NMC/13/41 21 February 2013. Nursing and Midwifery Council.

Nursing and Midwifery Council (2017 25th January 2017) NMC agrees to regulate new nursing associate role. Accessed at: www.nmc.org.uk/news/news-and-updates/nmc-agrees-to-regulate-new-nursing-associate-role/

Nursing and Midwifery Council (2018) *Realising professionalism: standards for education and training Part 1: standards framework for nursing and midwifery education.* London: NMC.

O'Driscoll M, Allan H T and Smith P A (2010) Still looking for leadership – Who is responsible for student nurses' learning in practice? *Nurse Education Today* 30 (3): 212–217.

Royal College of Nursing (2017) *Safe and effective staffing: the real picture.* UK Policy Report. London: RCN.

Scott P (2018 9th January 2018) The universities' Faustian pact of 2010 gave us Toby Young. *Higher education.* Accessed at: www.theguardian.com/education/2018/jan/09/universities-faustian-pact-toby-young-fees-education

Toynbee P (2107 13th July 2017) Driving students away from nursing is a spectacular act of political self-harm. *First thoughts: public sector pay.* Accessed at: www.theguardian.com/commentisfree/2017/jul/13/students-nursing-political-self-harm-training-nhs

Traynor M (1999) *Managerialism and nursing: beyond profession and oppression.* London: Routledge.

Traynor M (2009) Indeterminacy and technicality revisited: how medicine and nursing have responded to the evidence based movement. *Sociology of Health & Illness* 31 (4): 494–507.

Traynor M, Nissen N, Lincoln C and Buus N (2015) Occupational closure in nursing work reconsidered: UK health care support workers and assistant practitioners: A focus group study. *Social Science & Medicine* 136: 81–88.

United Kingdom Central Council for Nursing Midwifery and Health Visiting (1986) *Project 2000: a new preparation for practice.* London: UKCC.

Walby S and J Greenwell (1994) *Medicine and nursing. professions in a changing health service.* London: Sage.

West M (2014) Michael West: collective leadership—Fundamental to creating the cultures we need in the NHS. Accessed at: http://blogs.bmj.com/bmj/2014/05/28/michael-west-collective-leadership-fundamental-to-creating-the-cultures-we-need-in-the-nhs/2015

Willis P (2012) Quality with compassion: the future of nursing education. Report of the willis commission on nursing education. London: Royal College of Nursing. 55.

Willis P (2015) *Raising the bar, shape of caring: a review of the future education and training of registered nurses and care assistants.* Leeds: Health Education England.

22

RECENT DEVELOPMENTS IN INTERPROFESSIONAL HEALTHCARE LEADERSHIP

Priya Martin and Dawn Forman

Introduction

There are repeated calls for transformation in how we deliver healthcare given the ageing population, financial pressures, increasing burden of chronic disease, maldistribution of the health workforce and siloed nature of healthcare education and practice (Frenk et al., 2010; WHO, 2010; HWA, 2013). A key to this transformation is changing the way health professionals enact leadership in healthcare settings. Nursing and other healthcare leaders play a key role in every organisation to achieve patient safety and healthy work environments (Alilyyani, Wong & Cummings, 2018). Different leadership approaches are highlighted in the recent leadership literature, including: authentic leadership (Alilyyani et al., 2018); change leadership (Scott, 2017); engaging transformational leadership (Alban-Metcalfe, 2017); reciprocal leadership (Martin & Milne, 2018); reflective leadership (Pipe, 2018); collaborative leadership (MacPhee et al., 2013); and distributed/informal leadership (Harris & Mayo, 2018). Most of these recent leadership models move away from the traditional, hierarchical styles and are based on the premise that leadership is everyone's responsibility (as opposed to being confined to those in management and leadership roles). All members of the healthcare team are called to be leaders and use evidence-based theory to inform their leadership practice (HWA, 2013; Harris & Mayo, 2018).

Leadership is the process of influencing others to understand and agree about what needs to be done and how to do it, and the process of facilitating individual and collective efforts to accomplish shared objectives (Yukl, 2012). Leaders affect people, their satisfaction, trust in management, commitment, individual and team effectiveness and the organisational culture and climate. Health LEADS Australia, a national leadership framework, has five areas of focus for leaders: *leads* self, *engages* others, *achieves* outcomes, *drives* innovation and *shapes* systems (HWA, 2013). Each focus area in turn has associated capabilities and descriptors to guide health professionals in the application of the framework (HWA, 2013). While various factors contribute to improved healthcare, leadership is said to play a central role in mobilising people towards a common goal. If this does not convincingly highlight the importance of leadership in transforming healthcare, there is research evidence to link the quality of health leadership to the quality of patient care through direct and indirect mechanisms (HWA, 2013).

Whilst leadership is discussed quite commonly, there is a need to discuss applications of the recent leadership models and strategies into practice, so that it translates to increased uptake and adherence of these approaches at the coalface. In this chapter we will investigate recent developments in leadership using two different, but commonly used, lenses:

1 Health services leadership with a focus on interprofessional education and practice:a scoping review of 114 papers on leadership in interprofessional education highlighted the move away from traditional hierarchical, individualistic leadership styles to more contemporary, reciprocal and collaborative leadership approaches (Brewer, Flavell & Smith, 2016). The strategic necessity to collaborate in looking at healthcare provision internationally, and the need for governance and leadership mechanisms to support collaboration across boundaries, are clearly recognised. Interprofessional collaborative leadership skills, development tools and models have been developed to support this change, and interprofessional curricula and competencies have been provided to healthcare professionals internationally for some time. Whilst there are parts of the world where the importance of interprofessional and collaborative ways of learning and working is still being resisted, the need for change has never been more apparent for the future of the health workforce and for the individual or community receiving healthcare delivery. Resistance to changing models of leadership is understandable, but nevertheless overcoming this resistance is vital if we are going to make the transformation which is necessary in our delivery of healthcare provision. This section will outline recent international developments in utilising leadership principles to enhance interprofessional education and collaborative practice in healthcare settings.

2 Leadership in clinical supervision: very few clinical supervision models even mention leadership, shying away from notions like responsibility, accountability and interpersonal power (Martin & Milne, 2018). A rare exception is the tandem model of clinical supervision, which explicitly positions the supervisor as leader, also embedding this perspective in the leadership literature. This model, first proposed by Milne and James in 2005, views supervisor and supervisee as two cyclists on a tandem. According to this analogy, the supervisor occupies the front seat and so takes control (steering the tandem, applying the brakes, changing the gears, etc.), assuming responsibility for ensuring that good progress is made down the developmental pathway. On the back seat of this metaphorical tandem, the supervisee is therefore equally clearly depicted as a follower. A recent study examining workplace-based supervision endorsed such leadership as crucial in driving clinical supervision outcomes (Dorsey et al., 2018). This section will explore how leadership principles can be best applied to clinical supervision partnerships to maximise outcomes for the supervisee and the organisation.

Overall, this chapter will discuss various leadership approaches from the recent literature, with a view to facilitating transformation in healthcare to meet emerging population needs. Using two lenses (health services leadership and clinical supervision), it will unpack how these leadership models and strategies can be applied in day-to-day situations at the coal face. Nurses, as part of the largest health professional workforce internationally, are ideally placed to drive this transformation in healthcare. Murray (2017) calls nurses at all levels to lead transformation in patient safety, patient-centred care, interprofessional collaborative working, quality improvement approaches and evidence-based practice. Such leadership is expected to facilitate care that is safe, effective, patient-centred, timely, efficient and equitable (Murray, 2017). To this end, time invested in furthering interprofessional education and practice and professional support mechanisms such as clinical supervision, preceptorship and mentoring is time well spent.

Part I: health services leadership with a focus on interprofessional education and practice

In 2010 the World Health Organization (WHO) produced a framework for interprofessional education and collaborative client-centred practice. In the same year Frenk et al. (2010) called for a transformation in the way health professionals were educated to achieve a more value-based, competency-acquiring, interprofessional, team-focused, leadership-skilled and globally aware professional workforce.

These initiatives promoted the development of interprofessional curriculum for many health professions across the world (Forman, Jones & Thistlethwaite, 2014; Canadian Interprofessional Conference, 2017).

Some educators have also sought to transform the way in which curriculum is designed and delivered so that health professionals are equipped with skills which not only prepare them for practice when they qualify, but enable them to adapt to and influence the changing healthcare environment of the future.

This section looks critically at the developing leadership models in a collaborative environment, and the governance mechanisms needed to support them.

Introduction

There is a plethora of examples of interprofessional curricula development (Barr & Lowe, 2013; Dunston et al., 2009, 2016) to ensure students focus on the needs of the patient or community and "learn with, from and about each other" (CAIPE, 2016).

More recently, resources to assess interprofessional competencies have been developed and research is under way to evaluate the effectiveness of these interprofessional initiatives (The iTOFT Consortium, Australia, 2015).

Whilst internationally we now have many countries seeking to ensure interprofessional competencies are included in accreditation mechanisms (The iTOFT Consortium, Australia, 2015), we still seem to be challenged in implementing interprofessional collaborative working in practice. As Dunston et al. (2017) have noted interprofessional education, as it is currently configured, has little chance of providing the kind of systemic and sustained approach to graduating a national workforce with well-developed interprofessional collaborative practice capabilities. Do we therefore need to look at the leadership aspects of interprofessional education?

Leadership models, leadership skills and leadership based on interprofessional values

Reeves, MacMillan and van Soeren (2010) looked at the social and historical aspects of interprofessional leadership; Steinert, Naismith and Mann (2012) looked at leadership skills. A series of edited books (Forman et al., 2014, Forman, Jones & Thistlethwaite, 2015, 2016) reviewed aspects of leadership development, collaborative practice and research and evaluation.

A review by Al-Sawai (2013) of the type of leadership skills needed by healthcare professionals stated that: "Collaborative healthcare leadership requires a synergistic work environment, wherein multiple parties are encouraged to work together toward the implementation of effective practices and processes. Such collaborations promote understanding of different cultures and facilitate integration and interdependency among multiple stakeholders" (p. 286).

Whilst aspects of leadership such as teamwork, motivation, emotional intelligence, mentoring, coaching, sustainability, resilience, power relationships, transformational leadership, adaptive, servant-led leadership, clinical leadership, situational leadership and distributed leadership are all documented, the collaborative leadership model for interprofessional care developed by the Canadian Interprofessional Health Leadership Collaborative (MacPhee et al., 2013) seems to be the most popular.

These collaborative leadership models are built on the foundation of shared values. Establishing common values has been seen as the route for leaders to be successful. As Gilbert et al. (2000) wrote: "True leadership describes unified action of leaders and followers (stakeholders) working together to jointly achieve mutual goals. It is collaborative" (p. 225).

Not only is this true in all industries, it is true internationally, as Crisp (2010) outlined when he pointed out: "Health leaders in poorer countries, without the resources or the baggage of rich countries, have learned to innovate, to build on the strengths of the population and their communities and develop new approaches" (p. 5).

The common values needed for leadership in interprofessional education were also articulated by Lamb et al. (2014) as being: "patient-centred service; respecting others' views, strengths and expertise; collaboratively involving patients and carers; and reflective practice" (p. 49).

Sector and international transfer of information

Interprofessional models recognise that collaborative practice must focus on patient- or community-centred care: professionals should hold shared values and have interprofessional competencies which enable them to work together. We need mechanisms to enable professionals, organisations and sectors to share information so a patient can transfer from primary to secondary care, from urban to rural, and indeed from country to country, with seamless healthcare provision.

In 2016 the WHO published a research report which drew together information across sectors and countries to review and make recommendations for their future healthcare needs and practices: "All recommendations require the upholding of rights, good governance, political commitment and intersectoral and multistakeholder cooperation" (WHO, 2016, p. 4).

In the UK Laycock, Burrows, and Dobson (2017) address the challenge of transferring information between health professionals and make several recommendations to enhance integrated care, including the development of a "skills pass", step 1 of which covers most of the aspects of leadership, safeguarding and teamwork. The report indicates that on-the-job training will be given for these competencies but what is not indicated is by whom and how these competencies will be assessed. Neither is it clear how different working environments will be taken into account and, whilst leadership is listed as a competency, it is not clear who will be leading and how this will be facilitated.

Whether the skills pass or any of the recommendations in these reports will make a difference in practice will depend on good governance and the determination of sector leadership, healthcare professional leaders and every practitioner to possess the values, skills and vision to enact collaborative practice.

Recently the governance structures for healthcare teams in Western countries have evolved from physician-led models to models where leadership can be assumed by a range of registered health professionals, including senior nurses. Within the UK leadership roles can be undertaken by any health professional but under strict governing protocols. Provided the health professional adheres to these protocols the trust or NHS will be held accountable if there is any legal challenge to the service. In Canada, leadership roles can be assumed by any health professional and legally the individual health professional is held accountable. In Australia, while the GP practice is a portal to funded primary health service, clients can also self-refer to community-based allied health teams. With the increasing development of consumer-focused care packages, community-based health teams are providing a wide range of primary health services. Australian health professionals must hold professional insurance.

The evolving models for leadership in healthcare teams vary across geographic and sectoral borders, and how these models are operationalised is not well researched. However, it is clear that various models of leadership exist and need to be carefully considered as healthcare evolves internationally. Interprofessional collaboration clearly has a role in the new healthcare models. As a consequence nurses are undertaking leadership development programmes to learn the necessary leadership skills for the variety of contexts in which they will be working (Frankel, 2008: p. 23).

The role of the client in leadership

The role of the patient, service user or client in the healthcare team continues to gather attention in health policy and practice literature. Foci include the development of shared decision-making processes between clients and their healthcare teams, the inclusion of client or families on clinical and policy development teams (Vahdat, Hamzehgardeshi, Hessam, Hamzehgardeshi, 2014; Braithwaithe, 2016) and the expansion of curriculum content to educate health professionals about client-centred collaborative care. These developments point towards recognition of the active, co-leadership role of the client and their significant others. However, while some improvements have been seen in the operationalisation of client-centred care across practice arenas, uptake has been described as patchy. Acute medical settings, emergency wards and high-dependency units delivering interventions for patients with deteriorating chronic conditions have come under particular attention for their lack of attention to the wishes and needs of patients and their families (Braithwaithe, 2016).

Even in practice settings purporting to deliver client-centred collaborative care, concerns have been raised regarding the capacity of hidden team hierarchies to exert covert pressures on clients to respond in ways that reinforce relational inequalities and stymie opportunities for shared leadership with the consumer (Vahdat et al., 2014).

The strategic necessity to collaborate in looking at healthcare provision internationally, and the need for governance and leadership mechanisms to support collaboration across boundaries, are clearly recognised. Interprofessional collaborative leadership skills development tools and models have been developed to support this change, and interprofessional curricula and competencies have been provided to healthcare professionals internationally for some time. Whilst there are parts of the world where the importance of interprofessional and collaborative ways of learning and working is still being resisted, the need for change has never been more apparent for the future of the health workforce and for the individual or community receiving healthcare delivery. Resistance to changing models of leadership is understandable, but nevertheless overcoming this resistance is vital if we are going to make the transformation which is necessary in our delivery of healthcare provision.

Part II: leadership in clinical supervision

The vital role of clinical supervision in the provision of safe and high-quality healthcare, as well as in supporting the healthcare professional, is being increasingly acknowledged (Martin, Copley & Tyack, 2014). Nurses are one of the early adopters of clinical supervision (White & Winstanley, 2014) and the nursing profession continues to add to the evidence base around clinical supervision, thereby propelling other health professionals to keep up the momentum. Clinical supervision is a process that provides time out and an opportunity for learning and development, within the context of an ongoing professional relationship usually with an experienced practitioner. The aim of this partnership is to engage in guided reflection on current practice in ways designed to develop and enhance that practice in the future (Milne, 2007; Winstanley & White, 2003). The ultimate aim of clinical supervision is to ensure that patients get the best and safest care possible. It is for this reason that many health organisations promote clinical supervision practice and training with their staff. Several organisations have clinical supervision policies, procedures and guidelines in place to encourage the uptake of clinical supervision to fulfil a clinical governance purpose.

Clinical supervision is commonly a one-to-one partnership of post-registration health professionals (and in some cases a partnership between a clinical supervisor and a pre-registration student undertaking a health professional course) but other variants of supervision do exist, such as peer group supervision. In one-to-one clinical supervision, there is a supervisor and a supervisee involved in an ongoing partnership. It is recommended that the supervisee–supervisor matching happens carefully considering the learning needs of the supervisee, supervisor–supervisee fit, learning styles, and so forth. Upon commencement of the clinical supervision partnership, a contract is developed between the two parties to guide the forthcoming sessions. These sessions are periodically evaluated and changes made to the supervision contract as required. In contrast, in peer group supervision, a group of like-minded practitioners meet regularly to receive clinical supervision. In such situations, the leadership responsibility tends to rotate with different members taking turns to lead (Martin, Milne & Reiser, 2017).

The growing practice of interprofessional supervision

At times, the best supervisor–supervisee fit is achieved with a clinical supervisor from another profession (Davys, 2017). This growing form of clinical supervision is termed interprofessional supervision and is more common in professions such as psychology and social work, and in mental health settings (Martin & Moran, 2018). Interprofessional supervision can also occur with students, where a pre-registration health professional student undertakes a clinical placement with a supervisor from another profession. An Australian study that evaluated students' perceptions of the effectiveness of an interprofessional placement for developing their practice capabilities found that these placements developed four core capabilities: person-centred care, effective communication, multidisciplinary care and professionalism (Grace & Morgan, 2015). A review of the interprofessional supervision literature (Davys & Beddoe, 2015) indicated that many post-registration health professional supervisees who received interprofessional supervision also received adjunct same-profession supervision. The review also found that, whilst some supervisees reported being satisfied with their interprofessional supervision arrangements, some expressed feelings of isolation and need for same-profession supervision (Davys & Beddoe, 2015). Whilst interprofessional supervision may not be suitable for every supervisee, it holds value for some supervisees and contexts and needs to be investigated further (Martin & Moran, 2018).

Developing leadership skills

There is much written, especially in nursing, about the role of clinical supervision in developing a health professional's leadership skills. In this context, clinical supervision sessions are used by supervisees to enhance their leadership skills in their current roles as well as to improve readiness to move up the career pathway. However, the role of leadership within clinical supervision (especially one-to-one clinical supervision) remains least explored (Martin & Milne, 2018).

With the need for transformation in the healthcare sector well highlighted, there are also calls for rethinking leadership within the clinical supervision context (Martin & Milne, 2018). Consistent with the move towards reciprocal and collaborative leadership approaches in healthcare (Brewer et al., 2016), there are calls for the supervisee and supervisor to take turns to lead in clinical supervision. Whilst there are many models of clinical supervision, many shy away from discussing leadership (Martin & Milne, 2018).

The tandem model of clinical supervision

One clinical supervision model that considers leadership is the tandem model of clinical supervision (Milne & James, 2005). This model views the supervisor and supervisee as two cyclists on a tandem. Here, the supervisor steers the tandem (exercises leadership, undertakes needs assessment, agrees on learning objectives, facilitates learning and evaluation) and the supervisee follows (uses experiencing, reflecting, conceptualising and doing). This model acknowledged that the tandem can also be cycled solo and so, by analogy, the supervisee can go on some "trips" in an empowered role. The tandem model emphasises the need for both the supervisor and supervisee to be linked together or well aligned on the journey of clinical supervision. Developing a sound supervision contract will assist in both parties finding common ground to move forward in supervision. The tandem also demonstrates the importance of the supervisory relationship between the supervisor and the supervisee (Milne & James, 2005).

To further embrace collaborative leadership, the tandem model can be extended to allow the supervisor and supervisee to switch places at times. In situations where it is appropriate for the supervisee to take the lead, the supervisee can steer the tandem. For example, when the supervisee is presenting a case for discussion or proposing a continuing professional development plan to meet learning needs, it may be appropriate for the supervisee to lead. The supervisor's role in these situations may be to provide some gentle guidance from the back wheel. A sound supervisory contract and a positive supervisory relationship are crucial factors for a supervisor–supervisee pair to reach the point where they can both take turns to lead. It must be acknowledged that not all supervisees will be ready to take turns to lead in clinical supervision. For example, new graduates, those who have moved practice settings or are new in their work roles, and those with identified performance issues may not be ready to lead until they find their feet. Supervisors need to explore this during the initial stages of the supervision arrangement and devise a plan to progressively enhance the supervisee's leadership within clinical supervision.

Rights and responsibilities in clinical supervision

Both the supervisor and the supervisee can enact leadership better within their clinical supervision if they are fully aware of their rights and responsibilities. The Victorian Alcohol and Other Drugs and Community Managed Mental Health (AOD and CMMH: Department of Health, 2013) sector clinical supervision guidelines provide a comprehensive list of rights and responsibilities of supervisors and supervisees based on the work by Carroll and Gilbert (2005). Carroll and Gilbert (2005) further discuss the rights and responsibilities of the supervisee extensively. Table 22.1 showss an adaptation of their work, as found in the AOD and CMMH clinical supervision guidelines, in conjunction with our experience.

Importance of a positive supervisory relationship

For the supervisor and supervisee to take turns leading the clinical supervision partnership, it is important to have a positive supervisory relationship. There is ample support in the literature to highlight the crucial role of a positive supervisory relationship (Martin et al., 2014), with some authors arguing that it is the most important factor that influences supervisee satisfaction and clinical supervision quality (Cheon et al., 2009). The supervisory relationship needs to have aspects of both support and challenge, embedded in an environment where communication is open and honest (Pelling, Barletta & Armstrong, 2009). For the supervisee to learn and grow, there needs to be an element of challenge that is required to propel them forward. However, it is important for this to be done in a supportive environment. Too much challenge and not enough support is likely to leave a supervisee feeling anxious, overwhelmed or threatened. On the other hand, too much support and not enough challenge may impede growth (Pelling et al., 2009). Supervisors need to ensure that a good balance is achieved between the support and challenge aspects, whilst ensuring that communication lines with the supervisee stay open. Supervisees too need to take the lead in providing honest feedback to the supervisor if a lack of support or too much challenge is perceived.

A recent review by Martin and Milne (2018) reiterates the roles of supervisees and supervisors to achieve the best possible outcomes. They encourage the supervisees to come prepared to supervision sessions, carefully think about the problems they want to discuss in supervision having critically reflected on what they already know about the situation, explore the literature for possible solutions and brainstorm with other colleagues if appropriate. This equates to taking initiative and responsibility for their own learning, thus demonstrating leadership within clinical supervision. Supervisors, in turn, are encouraged to seek continued supervision training, study guidelines and demonstrations of effective leadership and help supervisees to get better at providing feedback on supervision. Evaluation of supervision using a tool such as SAGE (supervision: adherence and guidance evaluation) is said to provide a good opportunity to review leadership roles within clinical supervision (Martin & Milne, 2018).

Conclusion

This chapter explored recent leadership approaches in the health setting, which are necessary to facilitate transformation in healthcare to meet emerging population needs. Health services leadership and clinical supervision are integral processes in the healthcare context and both can be enriched by incorporating principles of interprofessional education and practice. Nurses, at all levels, are called to display leadership in these critical aspects of healthcare to

Table 22.1 Rights and responsibilities in clinical supervision

Rights of the supervisor	Rights of the supervisee
• To be respected as a professional • To build a healthy supervisory relationship • To be informed of any constraints to a constructive supervision process • To engage actively in a two-way contracting process • To receive clear and constructive feedback about the supervision process • To break confidentiality in exceptional pre-agreed circumstances	• Be respected for being a professional • Become the professional the supervisee can be and wants to be (and not just a clone of the supervisor) • A safe, protected supervision space • Input into the supervision contract (and being aware of what is non-negotiable in the contract) • A healthy supervisory relationship/alliance • Fair and honest evaluations and reports from the supervisor • An opportunity to receive honest feedback from the supervisor on the supervisee's work and in turn share his or her views on the feedback • Work on any areas of development outlined by the supervisor • Receive clear and focused constructive feedback • Give clear and focused feedback to the supervisor • Ongoing, regular and systematic reviews of the supervisory arrangement • Awareness of the supervisee's own learning style and that of the supervisor • Mediation if the supervisory relationship breaks down (as agreed upon in the contract) • Appeal decisions made in supervision with which the supervisee has problems

Responsibilities of the supervisor	Responsibilities of the supervisee
• To be accountable to one's own profession for ensuring adequate standards • To give a clear account of one's model/philosophy and goals in the supervision process • To treat the supervisee and the supervision process with respect • To prepare adequately for supervision • To provide a safe, uninterrupted space in which supervision can take place • To provide clear and constructive feedback to the supervisee in an ongoing way	• In charge of the supervisee's own learning • Being prepared for supervision • Using supervision time effectively (including keeping the supervisor on track when required) • Presenting/discussing the supervisee's work openly and honestly • Monitoring and evaluating the supervisee's own work • Reflecting on his or her work • Delivering the best service possible to clients

(Continued)

(Cont).

- To be clear about confidentiality and any limits that apply
- To keep line management and clinical supervision matters clearly identified and separated in case of a dual role (where the clinical supervisor is also the line manager)
- To keep clients' interests at the centre of the supervision process
- To balance the *support* and *challenge* aspects of the supervision process
- To encourage the supervisee to seek professional help where needed to overcome personal obstacles that may affect the supervisee's work
- To provide clear professional boundaries around the supervisory relationship
- To maintain appropriate records
- To draw to the supervisee's attention aspects of work that may be overlooked by the supervisee
- To be aware of limitations in own knowledge and skills
- To ensure own professional development and support
- To provide the ongoing opportunity for the supervisee to reflect on and critically evaluate different aspects of his or her work
- To provide and promote opportunities for the supervisee's skill development relevant to the supervisee's work role
- To raise with the supervisee's line manager any concerns in the supervisee's performance, ethical issues or reportable issues, after discussion with the supervisee

- Creating learning partnerships with the supervisor
- Applying learning from supervision to work role
- Being aware of other stakeholders in the supervisory arrangements (clients, carers, the supervisee's profession, etc.)
- Being aware of cultural, religious, racial, age, gender and sexual orientation differences between the supervisee and others
- Creating ethical and professional work environments
- Proving a regular overview of the supervisee's work to the supervisor where appropriate

enhance patient-centred care, and the overall safety and quality of healthcare. It is in fact every health professional's responsibility to display leadership in their roles, so that the healthcare provided can effectively meet the complex healthcare needs of today's society.

References

Alban-Metcalfe J (2017) Clinical eladership: reflection saves lives. Accessed at: https://realworld-group.com/files/Real_World_Group_-_Reflection_saves_lives_-_11_Sept_17.pdf.

Alilyyani B, Wong C, & Cummings G (2018) Antecedents, mediators, and outcomes of authentic leadership in helathcare: a systematic review. *International Journal of Nursing Studies* 83: 34–64.

Al-Sawai A (2013) Leadership of healthcare professionals: where do we stand? *Oman Medical Journal* 28 (4): 285–287.

Barr H & Lowe H (2013) *Introducing interprofessional education*. CAIPE.

Braithwaithe J (2016) A sustainable healthcare system has patients at its centre. *Health Voices Journal of the Consumers Health forum of Australia* 17: 5–7.

Brewer ML, Flavell HL, & Smith M (2016) A scoping review to understand "leadership" in interprofessional education and practice. *Journal of Interprofessional Care* 30(4): 408–415.

Canadian Interprofessional Conference (2017) Twitter feed 29th August 2017.

Carroll M & Gilbert MC (2005) *On being a supervisee: creating learning partnerships*. London: Vukani.

Centre for the advancement of interprofessional education (2016) Definition Accessed at: www.caipe.org/

Cheon HS, Blumer MLC, Shih AT, Murphy MJ, & Sato M (2009) The influence of supervisor and supervisee matching, role conflict, and supervisory relationship on supervisee satisfaction. *Contemporary Family Therapy* 31: 52.

Crisp N (2010) *Turning the world upside down: a search for global health in the 21st century*. London: The Royal Society of Medicine Press.

Davys A & Beddoe L (2015) Interprofessional supervision: opportunities and challenges. In L Bostock (Ed.), *Interprofessional staff supervision in adult health and social care services* (Vol. 1, pp. 37–41). Brighton, England: Pavilion Publishing.

Davys AM (2017) Interprofessional supervision: a matter of difference. *Aotearoa New Zealand Social Work* 29(3): 79–94.

Department of Health (2013) *The Victorian alcohol and other drugs and community managed mental health*. La Trobe University. Accessed at: www.clinicalsupervisionguidelines.com.au.

Dorsey S, Kerns SEU, Lucid L, Pullmann MD, Harrison JP, Berliner L et al. (2018) Objective coding of content and techniques in workplace-based supervision of an EBT in public mental health. *Implementation Science* 13(19): 1–12.

Dunston R, Forman D, Moran M, Rogers GD, Thistlethwaite J, & Steketee C (2016) *Curriculum renewal in Interprofessional education in health: establishing leadership and capacity*. Canberra: Office for Learning and Teaching.

Dunston R, Forman D, Thistlethwaite J, Steketee C, Rogers G, & Moran M (2017) Repositioning interprofessional education from the margins to the centre of Australian health professional education – what is required? *Australian Health Review* 43: 224–229.

Dunston R, Lee A, Matthews L, Nisbet G, Pockett R, Thistlethwaite J, & White J (2009) *Interprofessional health education in Australia: the way forward*. Sydney: University of Technology Sydney and The University of Sydney.

Frenk J, Chen L, Bhutta ZA, Cohen J, Crisp N, Evans T et al. 2010. Health professionals for a new century: transforming education to strengthen health systems in an interdependent world. *The Lancet* 376(4): 1923–1958.

Forman D, Jones M, & Thistlethwaite J (2014) *Leadership development for interprofessional education and collaborative practice*. London: Palgrave MacMillan. IBSN 978-1-137-36301-5.

Forman D, Jones M, & Thistlethwaite J. (2015) *Leadership and collaboration: further developments for interprofessional education*. Basingstoke: Palgrave Macmillan.

Forman D, Jones M, & Thistlethwaite J (2016) *Leading research and evaluation in interprofessional education and collaborative practice*.Hampshire: Palgrave Macmillan.

Frankel A (2008) *What leadership styles should senior nurses develop?* This is an extended version of the article published. *Nursing Times* 104(35): 23–24.

Frenk J, Lincoln C, Zulfiqar AB, Cohen J, Crisp N, Evans T et al. (2010) Health professionals for a new century: transforming education to strengthen health systems in an interdependent world. *The Lancet* 376(9756): 1923–1958.

Gilbert JH, Camp RD, Cole CD, Bruce C, Fielding DW, & Stanton SJ (2000) Preparing students for interprofessional teamwork in healthcare. *Journal of Interprofessional Care* 14(*3*): 223–235.

Grace S & Morgan A (2015) Students' experiences of interprofessional supervision: shared characteristics of the caring professions. *Journal of Integrative Medicine and Therapy* 2(1): 1–5.

Harris J & Mayo P (2018) Taking a case study approach to assessing alternative leadership models in helathcaare. *British Journal of Nursing* 27(11): 608–613.

Health Workforce Australia (2013) health leads australia: the Australian helath leadership framework.

Lamb B, Clutton N, Carson-Stevens A, Panesar S, & Salvilla S (2014) Strength-based leadership for developing and sustaining interprofessional collaborative practice. In D Forman, M Jones, & J Thistlethwaite (Eds.), *Leadership development for interprofessional education and collaborative practice* (pp. 69–84). New York: Springer.

Laycock K, Burrows M, & Dobson B (2017) *Getting into shape delivering a workforce for integrated care.* London: The Reform Research trust.

MacPhee M, Paterson M, Tassone M, Marsh D, Berry S, Bainbridge L, & Verma S (2013) Transforming health systems through collaborative leadership: making change happen! *5th International Service Learning Symposium Paper Series.*

Martin P, Copley J, & Tyack Z (2014) Twelve tips for effective clinical supervision based on a narrative literature review and expert opinion. *Medical Teacher* 36(3): 201–207.

Martin P & Milne D (2018) Reciprocal leadership in clinical supervision come sof age. *Journal of Advanced Nursing* 74(9): 2019–2020.

Martin P, Milne D, & Reiser RP (2017) Peer supervsiion: international problems and prospects. *Journal of Advanced Nursing* 75(5): 998–999.

Martin P & Moran M (2018) Interprofessional supervsiion: one step too far? Presented at the *All Together Better Health Conference*, Auckland, New Zealand.

Milne D & James I (2005) Clinical supervision: 10 tests of the tandem model. *Clinical Psychology Forum* 151: 6–9.

Milne DL (2007) An empirical definition of clinical supervision. *British Journal of Clinical Psychology* 46: 437–447.

Murray EJ (2017) Core competencies for safe and quality nursing care. In EJ Murray (Ed.), *Nursing leadership and management for patient safety and quality care* (pp. 3–5). Philadelphia, PA: FADavis Company.

Pelling N, Barletta J, & Armstrong P (2009) *The practice of clinical supervision.* Australia: Australian Academic Press.

Pipe T (2018) Create a clearing preparing for leadership transition. *Nurse Leader* 16(5): 295–299.

Reeves S, MacMillan K, & van Soeren M (2010) Leadership of interprofessional health and social care teams: a socio-historical analysis. *Journal of Nursing Management* 18: 258–264.

Scott G (2017) Short report: reflections on leadership in transition. *Focus on Health Porfessional Education: A Multi-Disciplinary Journal* 18(3): 10–16.

Steinert Y, Naismith L, & Mann K (2012) Faculty development initiatives designed to promote leadership in medical education. A BEME systematic review: BEME Guide No. 19. *Medical Teacher* 34(6): 483–503.

The iTOFT Consortium, Australia (2015) *Work based assessment of teamwork: an interprofessional approach.* Canberra: Commonwealth of Australia, Office of Learning and Teaching.

Vahdat S, Hamzehgardeshi L, Hessam S, & Hamzehgardeshi Z (2014) Patient involvement in healthcare decision making: a review. *Iranian Red Crescent Medical Journal* 16(1): e12454.

White E & Winstanley J (2014) Clinical supervision and the helping professions: an interpretation of history. *The Clinical Supervisor* 33(1): 3–25.

Winstanley J & White E (2003) Clinical supervision: models, measures and best practice. *Nurse Researcher* 10(4): 7–38.

World Health Organisation (2010) *Framework for action on interprofessional education & collaborative practice.* Geneva: WHO.

World Health Organisation (2016) *Working for health and growth: investing in the health workforce.* Report of the High-Level Commission on Health Employment and Economic Growth. Geneva: WHO.

Yukl G (2012) *Leadership in organisations.* 8th ed. Upper Saddle River, NJ: Pearson.

23

APPROACHES FOR ADDRESSING DIVERSITY IN NURSING EDUCATION

Renee S. Kumpula

Introduction

Throughout the world, nurse educators are focused on the differences as well as the commonalities that hold all of humanity together. These differences provide opportunity to address the types of diversity within societies. To promote understanding of how to better address and provide quality healthcare, the International Council of Nurses (ICN) (2008) identified that increasing diversity in the workforce enhances the capacity of the profession and multidisciplinary teams to provide a growing continuum of human needs.

A number of healthcare leaders around the world are searching for expertise that represents the different types of diversity represented among customers, constituents, or populations (Institute of Medicine (IOM), 2011). In the United States alone, it is projected that, by 2044, more than 50% of the population will belong to non-Hispanic White groups, rendering no majority population (Colby and Ortman, 2015). With the expected increase of ethnic minority groups, the Hispanic population is projected to grow more than 50% and the African American population is projected to increase to 61.8 million from 41.2 million (Phillips and Malone, 2014). The US Census Bureau projects that one in five individuals will be foreign-born by 2060 (Colby and Ortman, 2015). Healthcare ventures, whether large medical centers, entrepreneurial neighborhood clinics or services, or remote community dispensaries, require adequate staffing and professionals who understand the nuances for patient care – and meeting real needs in real time for newer immigrant populations and the vulnerable (World Health Organisation, 2016). The Joint Commission (JC) (Wilson-Stronks et al., 2008) that accredits all healthcare organizations and patient care facilities in the United States added culturally competent care to its standards (Wilson-Stronks et al., 2008). Currently, patients in inpatient care and clients in outpatient care expect respect for their individual background, values, and belief systems along with shared concern for their priority health concerns (AHRQ, 2018; Benner et al., 2009; IHI, 2018).

Nursing is uniquely positioned to develop professionals who bring diverse and divergent points of view into the client–nurse relationship and the healthcare arena. Globally, nurses are 80% of the active workforce in healthcare and provide 90% of patient services in primary care (Enami, Thompson, & Gimbel, 2018; WHO, 2008). Of approximately 2.9 million registered nurses (RNs) in the United States, 10.7% are African American and 5.4% are Hispanic or Latino (HRSA, 2015; Salvucci and Lawless, 2016). Improved healthcare outcomes, and by extension patient safety, have been linked to the RN workforce and its educational preparation (Aiken, 2014; Hawkins et al., 2018). The Institute of Medicine (IOM) (Institute of Medicine (IOM), 2011) created an actionable plan in its *The Future of Nursing* report for improving patient care by increasing diversity in the nursing workforce. The American Association of Colleges of Nursing (AACN) (2017) delineated its statement with a mission and central tenet of promoting diversity, inclusion, and equity in academic programs, research, and nursing practice. Inherent in increasing a diverse nursing workforce is the deliberate intent to increase the number of nurses and nursing students who identify as persons of color (ICN, 2008; Institute of Medicine (IOM), 2011).

Nursing faculty and educators have recommended a number of initiatives to increase the percentage of students of diversity at all program levels (AACN, 2017; NLN 2016). Nurse leaders in higher education and practice see the importance of developing future nurses who have different cultural backgrounds and viewpoints, various life experiences, and unique perspectives for providing quality and team-based patient care (AACN, 2017; Benner, Tanner, & Chesla, 2009). Budden et al. (2016) report that approximately 20% of nurses identify as ethnic and/or racial minorities. A number of recruitment and retention initiatives are addressing the need for growing the number of diverse students in academic programs in the United States, Canada, Australia, New Zealand, and other countries (DeWitty et al., 2016a; Etowa et al., 2005; Tranter et al., 2018). Some of these include the Health Resources and Services Administration (HRSA) Kids into Health Careers initiative and Johnson & Johnson's Campaign for Nursing's Future (Gilchrist and Rector, 2007). An initiative for increasing diverse admissions includes the Urban Universities for Health (UUH) as a collaboration of the Coalition of Urban Serving Universities, the National Institute of Minority Health and Health Disparities of the National Institutes of Health (NIH), and the Association of Public and Land-grant Universities, and Association of American Medical Colleges (Relf, 2016). The partnership reports the importance of four core principles for processes in holistic admission (Relf, 2016). These admission principles include: broad-based and equitable admission selection criteria that are linked to the school of nursing and university goals; a review of evidence of each applicant's experience, academic merit, and attributes; an established process for review and consideration of potential individual contributions; and consideration of unique factors such as family background, sex, ethnicity, and race (Glazer and Bankston, 2014; Relf, 2016).

Innovation for increasing diversity in nursing involves growing the number of pipeline programs to increase access among those unrepresented in nursing programs (HRSA, 2009). Of 164 schools of nursing in the United States, one study reported 20% had established pipeline programs in place (Carthon et al., 2014). Another study identified three critical factors to predict enrollment: interest, readiness, and support (DeWitty, Tabloski, Hambrick, Shrefflet, Downing, & Huerta, 2016b).

Nursing education is not simply reliant on recruiting and admitting diverse students to reach goals for diversity but also developing an ability within all students to care for people with an array of backgrounds and belief systems different than their own (NLN, 2016). The AACN (2017) recommends that nurses espouse the value and diverse character of the entire human experience. The goal then becomes to enhance and grow both awareness and sensitivity within all professionals who will be addressing the most private and individual issues in a complex environment.

This chapter describes various pedagogical lenses for cultivating the workforce of the future. Specific considerations will be discussed in how to work with student populations, how to enhance student involvement, and how to create an equitable climate for student participation in nursing programs.

Diversity, inclusion, and equity in nursing education

The nursing student population is becoming more diverse in a number of ways. Each institution or facility has demographics that inform the types of diversity that one will encounter in the classroom. There is evidence of increasing numbers of students who qualify as a person of color, a minority, or subscribe individually to another descriptor or qualifier that may characterize them as students of diversity (AACN, 2017). Some colleges and universities allow students to define descriptors such as LGTBQ (lesbian, gay, transgender, bisexual, queer) and these become factors that affect how interaction occurs, and therefore, how the classroom is constructed and courses are designed for specific student populations. The International Council of Nurses (ICN) (2008) has recognized competencies that are essential for faculty to cultivate in student nurses and therefore require faculty development in order to facilitate successful outcomes for all students, including those of diversity.

The National League of Nursing (NLN) (2016) provided direction for nursing faculty development to co-create collaborative and positive cultures, generate partnerships in practice, promote interprofessional and culturally appropriate learning opportunities, delineate metrics for benchmarks, align with community partners, provide culturally relevant education including health disparities and care of diverse populations, initiate pathways for mentoring minority individuals, and strengthen efforts for diversity research, including variables of stereotyping and unconscious bias. With this vision, NLN (2016) posits that quality healthcare and diversity are strongly linked. This direction is consistent with findings of mentoring diverse students in clinical practice (Oikarainen et al., 2018). Critical factors identified with the clinical success of culturally and linguistically diverse students included: language proficiency of the instructor, experience working or living abroad, mentoring international students frequently, having essential knowledge of students and their cultural background, consistent and regular discussions of cultural difference with students, integrating native students with those of diversity, and receptiveness to support from colleagues (Oikarainen et al., 2018). These findings were consistent with Chang, Chen, and Hung's (2018) study of the effects of education on transcultural competence in community clinical practicum.

The new call to action for the profession is to provide meaningful content to foster culturally congruent care. Scholars may differ on whether this should be called cultural safety, cultural awareness, cultural sensitivity, cultural humility, or cultural competence, but the overarching goal is to educate nurses to provide culturally relevant and appropriate care (Arielli et al., 2012b; Burchum, 2002, Campinha-Bacote, 2010; Hussin, 2008; Olukotun, et al, 2018; Papps and Ramsden, 1996; Porta et al., 2019; Racine and Petrucka, 2011). This includes recognizing one's own values and cultural perspective, including how these beliefs intersect with healthcare provision and a public health nursing competency of being nonjudgmental. This fosters cultural sensitivity with each individual client and provision of care that aligns with the individual's cultural orientation (Porta et al., 2019). Moreover, studies suggest that diversity among health professionals is linked to improved access to care, increased choices and satisfaction, and more positive experiences in academic programs for individuals of diversity (Adams et al., 2017).

What constitutes diversity?

The AACN is the primary national body for determining best practices in undergraduate through graduate programs in the United States. In its position statement on diversity, inclusion, and equity for nursing education, *diversity* is defined as:

> a broad range of individual, population, and social characteristics, including but not limited to age; sex; race, ethnicity; sexual orientation; gender identity; family structures; geographic locations; national origin; immigrants and refugees; language, physical, functional, and learning abilities; religious beliefs; and socioeconomic status.
>
> *(American Association of Colleges of Nursing (AACN), 2017: p. 173)*

Inclusion is understood as organizational cultures and structures that support a learning environment where all diverse individuals thrive, including students, faculty, administrators, and staff (AACN, 2017). The AACN (2017) statement describes *equity* as "the ability to recognize the differences in the resources or knowledge needed to allow individuals to fully participate in society, including access to higher education, with the goal of overcoming obstacles to ensure fairness" (p. 173). This presumes fairness for all, without individuals encountering "artificial" barriers, negative stereotypes, and discrimination or prejudice (American Association of Colleges of Nursing (AACN), 2017, Metcalfe et al., 2017). Moreover, nurses should be advancing the social determinants of health, "the conditions in which people are born, grow, learn, live, work, play, worship, and age" along with considering the distribution of power, resources, and finances responsible for any inequities (American Association of Colleges of Nursing (AACN), 2017: p. 174). Similar definition statements inform international nursing in Australia, Canada, New Zealand, and the United Kingdom (ICN, 2008; WHO, 2016).

Particular student populations of diversity identify with qualifiers that may affect the learning experience. Scholars traditionally have thought of cultural and ethnic diversity in this discussion, but the literature indicates that other types of diversity demand equal attention (DeWitty et al., 2016b). Ageism affects a number of student bodies as deans and administrators see rising numbers of students with more life experience and previous degrees or past careers. Gender affects the nursing profession as more men enter the profession. Hurlbut and Revuelto (2018) posit that military veterans demonstrate more diversity than other segments of the general population, especially among younger veterans from 20 to 49 years of age, and are ripe for recruitment and success in nursing. As the male population is on the rise in programs, gender affects the classroom in nursing education (Bastable and Sopcyzk, 2014).

Faculty should consider various types of diversity, such as: how economic diversity affects student outcomes, how religious or spiritual diversity influences student ability or capacity to learn about holistic cultural care, how individual determination of sexual preference and identities affects the classroom experience, and how individual belief systems and traditions have an impact on student ability to negotiate providing the full continuum of nursing care. Students can also be educationally disadvantaged by background due to deficient schools or frequent moves and/or being the first in their family to enter higher education (Gilchrist and Rector, 2007; Zuzelo, 2005). In addition, factors such as family life and work can significantly affect student ability to succeed in programs (DeWitty et al., 2016a).

Schools of nursing are also experiencing increasing enrollment of those needing different types of accommodation, whether cognitive, physical, or behavioral (Child and Langford,

2011; Sopcyzk, 2014). Consideration of readiness of the individual includes ability in the following areas: cognitive strategies to inquire, reason, interpret, and problem solve; evidence of academic skills to employ in writing, processing information, and research; possession of academic behaviors such as self-awareness, self-control, initiative, and accountability; and contextual awareness, the ability to understand the university system, academic relationships, and coping skills (DeWitty et al., 2016b). The entirety of the diversity spectrum includes whether an individual identifies as a person of color or as a member of a majority or minority social group. Awareness of this spectrum is needed for assessment in educational design, planning nursing curricula, and successfully engaging students.

Approaches for the future

Historically, nursing education has traversed from traditional approaches to non-traditional approaches for teaching and learning in nursing education. In recent years, some have employed alternative pedagogies as a means to improve methods in nursing education as a whole. Nurse scholars have utilized critical pedagogy, feminist pedagogy, and narrative pedagogy in recent years to reform nursing education and the classroom environment (Benner et al., 2010; Diekelmann, 2005; Ironside, 2001). These efforts provide a new window of opportunity for addressing diversity in both nursing education and practice. Using alternative pedagogies is becoming more commonplace and has now been established as an approach that faculty are implementing effectively.

Alternative pedagogies

Various pedagogical perspectives and lenses provide a means to view what has been accomplished and what has yet to be addressed with more clarity. Alternative pedagogies offer both methods and strategies to improve nursing education as a whole, in addition to improving ways faculty educate students of diversity across all levels (Benner et al., 2010; Ironside, 2001). These lenses also are a means for seeing new possibilities for teaching and learning in the future.

Providing nursing education in a framework of critical pedagogy, feminist pedagogy, and narrative pedagogy allows faculty to design academic work for students to utilize their diverse life experience while completing coursework in programs of study. Alternative pedagogies also allow students to experience equity in the classroom, empowerment in their learning, and enhancement of their previous abilities while they learn to navigate resources and develop new nursing skills in the discipline.

Critical pedagogy lessons

The earliest of alternative pedagogies that moved away from traditional didactic higher education was critical pedagogy. Critical pedagogy was a means to counter the status quo at a historical juncture in time when groupthink and societal norms were allowing discrimination and oppression that were previously not tolerated (Lerner, 1997; Lewenson, 1996). Born out of Frankfurt School during two world wars, some scholars believed that political circumstances clouded the moral judgment of the majority (Brookfield and Holst, 2011; Kincheloe, 2007). There are many interpretations of critical pedagogy, but its usefulness to higher education in the West has been recognized for decades. From the German university culture, its leaders migrated to the United States as fascism overtook Europe in the 1930s (Kincheloe, 2007). Newer critical pedagogues proposed the utility of appreciating and implementing educational reform in the United States and other Western countries (Apple, 2004; Kincheloe, 2007).

In critical pedagogy, creating divergent thinking and implementing change are primary purposes. Critical pedagogues examined the power in social structures, how some were oppressed in these structures, and how cultural capital was necessary for the formation, legitimization, and perpetuating professions (Apple, 2004; Benner et al., 2010; Bourdieu & Passeron, 1990; Foucault, 1980; Freire, 1993; Kincheloe, 2007). Rather than simply establishing dialogue with students, the role of faculty grew beyond employing the Socratic method of answering questions with more questions; it became an advanced art of probing, pushing, and provoking questions and responses in order to create more tension and finding previously unconsidered solutions (Brookfield, 2014; Greene, 1998; Kincheloe, 2007; Nagda et al., 2003). Instead of a comfortable dialogue, faculty would intentionally facilitate and adjust the dialectic to continue the quest for making social change (Bruenig, 2005; Duarte, 2006). Some refer to this type of dialectic as radical; an approach that is not finished until action for change is taken (Benner et al., 2010; Brookfield and Holst, 2011; Nagda et al., 2003).

Feminist theory lessons

Feminist pedagogy is another alternative approach that gained popularity in Western cultures for finding the voice of the unheard. Situated in the feminist movement and as early as women's suffrage in the United Kingdom and United States, the pedagogy developed around the themes of disenfranchisement, being disempowered, and being marginalized in societal systems (Benner et al., 2010; Bryson, 1999; Webb, 2002). Its utility for nursing was apparent since nursing was largely a female profession that was thought to be inferior to medicine through the twentieth century. In the 1950s to 1970s, Western countries saw a shift as the nursing profession became more independent and autonomous with its own professional organizations and oversight with self-governance (Benner et al., 2010; Bradshaw & Hultquist, 2017; Loewenstein and Christian, 2017).

In feminist pedagogy, faculty found ways of understanding the nursing role and the patient "situatedness" with actual clinical experience. With feminist pedagogy, faculty could correlate the subjection of patients and nurses who both experience disempowerment in hierarchical systems such as healthcare (Bryson, 1999; Bradshaw & Hultquist, 2017). This allowed nurse researchers, in particular, to extract previously unconsidered and underrepresented perspectives of those in a lower position within a power structure, such as women, immigrant populations, and vulnerable populations within either Western countries or developing nations (Benner et al., 2010). Therefore, faculty were able to empower nursing students to see the potential, not only for becoming effective advocates in practice, but also to comprehend the value of seeking the patient narrative as central to planning effective nursing care (Ironside, 2001). This was reflected by Florence Nightingale when she established the nursing profession in Western culture (Dossey, Selanders, Beck & Atwell, 2005; Holliday and Parker, 1997). This was substantiated by nursing theorists and scholars who developed models such as Leininger's transcultural nursing theory (Leininger, 1995; Loewenstein and Christian, 2017).

Narrative pedagogy lessons

Narrative pedagogy was an approach developed specifically for nursing by a clinician and research faculty who developed the narrower pedagogy for nursing education to facilitate debriefing on clinical experiences (Diekelmann, 2001; Ironside, 2001, 2006). This pedagogy blended components of both critical and feminist schools of thought to develop a particular environment that established an equalizing environment and promoted equity and transparency. In co-creating a dialogue with students, where students' real-life experience and interpretation are welcomed, students could be guided to meaningfully debrief their learning in clinical situations within a safe and equitable learning space (Diekelmann, 2001, 2005; Ironside, 2006).

In narrative pedagogy, creating the appropriate space for students' clinical experience became paramount. Faculty would negotiate ways of working and sharing in the clinical debriefing, demonstrating openness and a welcoming demeanor for student participation. Much like Palmer's (1998) approach of positioning a subject in the center of the convening circle, teacher and students explore aspects of the subject together. All contributions were considered valid, and valued as real learning (Diekelmann, 2005; Ironside, 2006). Students were evaluated based on their participation rather than worrying about being graded on the quality of their insights, the depth of their knowledge, or the quantity of their contributions (Ironside, 2003). This paralleled the co-creating of a learning community between teacher and student and using democratic strategies in the classroom (Gillespie, 2005).

Using these approaches as lenses provides faculty more ability to co-create a learning community design with diverse learners. By using the dialectic from critical pedagogy, faculty may be better equipped to foster student ability to appraise and construct effective initiatives or arguments to advance both individual performance and teamwork in improving patient and client care. By seeking the vulnerable population's narrative from feminist pedagogy, faculty may cultivate the ability to seek the individual's story and establish the learner as central in teaching and learning. By establishing student and nurse experience as a reliable method to train and refine nursing skills, faculty may advance the capacity and feasibility of the nurse's role to be better understood, more highly valued, and more effectively integrated in interprofessional teamwork and improving patient outcomes. With this in mind, faculty can build the teacher–earner relationship with the respect and trust that are foundational for meaningful exchange in the learning space.

Creating learning environments for diversity

Nursing is both an art and a science. This is also true of creating a meaningful space for teaching and learning for those with cultural and linguistic diversity (Fuller and Mott-Smith, 2017). In educational design, it is imperative to understand and know one's audience. Effective faculty and nurse educators must know the specific audience or student population, how to include students in course design, how to create an equitable climate for maximum participation, and how to create a learning community in the classroom (Gillespie, 2005).

Engaging students

Employing students in negotiating the course environment is critical once faculty have determined some particular needs for inclusivity with an individual class or cohort. This early engagement is critical to establish an equitable exchange between teacher and student and promote opportunity for participation and subsequent learning (Gillespie, 2005; Loewenstein and Christian, 2017; Palmer, 1998 & 2017). One strategy for faculty is to start with some form of personal introductions in the learning space, including background information.

As an example, in one university, faculty had students offer their cultural background as part of the live introductions on the first day in a class with a community and population health focus. When joining the course team, a new faculty proposed the faculty team should first offer their own introductions with the same cultural information that was asked of students, which had not been done in the past. When the course team implemented this simple strategy, it established trust and enriched the dialogue for the rest of the semester; faculty had role-modeled transparency and provided information on an equal level with students.

Ensuring equity

When working with students of cultural diversity, it is imperative to attend to equity for student participation. Although faculty may call attention to students who represent different ethnic and cultural backgrounds, particular orientations, or countries of origin, this strategy may actually impede rather than facilitate the individual comfort level in participating in class. This fosters an acceptance of others and being non-judgmental as a nursing competency (Fuller and Mott-Smith, 2017; Porta et al., 2019). It is important to encourage and invite, but not insist that particular students become a representative of a group or serve as a cultural liaison (Campinha-Bacote, 2010; Warren, 2009). By role-modeling vulnerability themselves, faculty can demonstrate caring for an individual's welfare and elicit meaningful responses when respect and trust are established in the learning space. Once students of diversity understand they will not be singled out in discussion, they are more likely to freely contribute to meaningful conversations.

For example, beyond faculty elicitation, faculty can design small-group activities, including a small-group discussion and a report back to the whole class. In this way, other students have the opportunity to report the value of a diverse student's contribution. Another learning strategy is use of "1-2-4-all" and similar variations, "think-pair-share" or "write-pair-share," where learners individually respond to a faculty prompt, discuss responses with one peer, and then discuss shared responses within a small group. This can provide positive reinforcement for the individual to make future contributions in not only small-group interactions but also in larger-class discussions (Lipmanowicz & McCandless, 2013).

Creating community

There is evidence in the literature of nurse faculty co-creating a learning community in the classroom that builds upon the principles of alternative pedagogies. Creating a learning community is a group exercise and not a faculty-directed activity (Gillespie, 2005). To establish a learning community in the classroom requires specific educational design planning and constructivist strategies (Brookfield, 2014; Gillespie, 2005; Palmer, 1998 & 2017).

Several strategies can be employed to have students participate in creating the boundaries and establishing the norms for the communal learning experience (Brookfield, 2017; Gillespie, 2005; Palmer, 1998 & 2017). Although faculty may set a framework, there are some elements that can be left open-ended and structured for students to provide input. In this way, students share in joint decision making or make choices. Faculty must first determine components that must be set ahead of time for measuring student learning outcomes and what can be negotiable (Brookfield, 2017; Gillespie, 2005; Palmer, 1998 & 2017). This requires some investigation of the literature or canvassing experienced faculty who have established learning communities in collaboration with students. This often can work best in small- to moderate-sized groups where faculty can convene the entire class in a whole-group discussion (Gillespie, 2005). In auditorium environments for larger classes, the physical space can be limiting for faculty to provide students the opportunity to co-create ground rules for class discussions and share in collective decisions.

When teaching a larger class in an auditorium, faculty can leave several components of the course for students to jointly decide on some class norms and course activities. Faculty can encourage students to first individually consider and then discuss a couple of options in small groups. When bringing the session to a conclusion, students can indicate individual choice with raised hands or vote on options to secure their engagement.

While creating community, and a learning community in particular, faculty need to be cognizant that some students may not appreciate the value of group participation, collaborative decision making, and a commitment of allowing adequate time for meaningful discussion. Some students value science and the economy of time; activities to promote social community and relationships in the classroom may be perceived as busy work, a distraction, or less productive than a didactic format.

Accommodating diverse learners

Having diverse learners in academic programs requires system planning for accommodation and the delivery of student services. When acting on a mission to increase diversity in programs, educators need processes and structural supports in place (Loewenstein and Christian, 2017). Accommodation can take many forms, but support services in the college or university beyond the faculty role and the nursing program help ensure student success. DeWitty et al. (2016a) reported student retention was somewhat dependent upon unknown factors such as the workload and intensity or difficulty of the program; managing the pace and volume of the course load; and the value of prior professional experience before enrollment. Faculty of diversity were reported to contribute to student retention and progress in programs (Salvucci and Lawless, 2016). Gates (2018) identified eight factors to maintain students of diversity in programs: access to nurse faculty including faculty presence and advising, a global curriculum, diverse faculty, a bridge program, program plans for student remediation, policies supporting program completion, mentoring opportunities, and financial aid.

Facilitating student identification of learning disabilities and academic accommodation is key in guiding diverse learners (Loewenstein and Christian, 2017). Disabilities and learning deficits affect student performance and early assessment of dyslexia, testing anxiety, and other problems is key (Child and Langford, 2011). For conducting cultural assessment of individuals, the Giger–Davidhizar model provides important characteristics within six phenomena: communication, including difficulty with colloquial terms, medical jargon, and slang; time, including a predominance of past, present, or future time orientation; space, including orientation to distance in verbal or non-verbal encounters with touch and interpersonal techniques; social organization, including values and beliefs of social systems; environmental control, including having a locus of control; and biological variations, such as tolerance to lactose or other substances (Davidhazar and Shearer, 2005).

Part of the faculty role is to meet with at-risk students. However, it is proactive to educate adult learners on the importance of assessing their own preferences for learning, how they acquire new knowledge and process information, and the value of supportive services. By providing information for self-assessment and ensuring access to campus resources, faculty are better equipped to help individuals consider and self-identify areas where accommodation may be necessary (DeWitty et al., 2016b; Loewenstein and Christian, 2017).

Students benefit from support when they discover how to adapt academic goals to actual life circumstances, especially refugee students and international students. Faculty may be the first contact for introducing and conducting an appraisal of individual readiness for learning. It is critical to frame academic success as both a matter of personal accountability as well as acknowledgment of how cultural capital can affect learner outcomes (Bourdieu and Passeron, 1990; Brookfield, 2017; Brookfield & Holst, 2011; Loewenstein and Christian, 2017). This knowledge can help students to identify a need for accommodation. Each semester, faculty can explicitly describe the syllabus and provisions for accommodation as a standard practice. By normalizing the discussion of resources and the benefit of those resources for all students, some individuals may more aptly recognize a personal need for assessment and follow-up with campus services (DeWitty et al., 2016a; Loewenstein and Christian, 2017).

Multilingual considerations

Hurdles for multilingual learners can be numerous and resources for language and writing should be delineated and provided for students in all programs. The non-native language speaker includes English as Second Language (ESL), English Language Learners (ELL), Multi-Lingual Learners (MLL), English as an Additional Language (EAL), and other descriptors (Bosher, 2003; Bosher and Boyle, 2008; Tranter et al., 2018). Students who understand multiple languages sometimes require a personalized assessment of both their speaking and writing ability with recommendations for improving their skills while completing academic programs (Bosher, 2003; Davidhazar and Shearer, 2005).

Non-native learners can experience more testing anxiety than other students due to language load, which is the additional time it takes to process, comprehend, and respond in another language. Bosher (2003) showed that linguistic bias and unnecessarily complex structure, including grammatical errors and inconsistencies, can interfere with student understanding and accounted for 35% of flaws in multiple-choice tests. Linguistic modification, a form of simplification of the structure of test questions and items, can reduce any variance due to irrelevance and ensure that actual student knowledge of content will be measured. This involves reduction of the mean length of each phrase, eliminating extraneous information, and dividing compound sentences (Bosher & Boyle, 2008). This reduces the language load of test items for students. Although the language load may be a liability for diverse students, some scholars posit that multilingual learners have greater ability to manage an increased cognitive load (Bosher, 2009). Sometimes accommodation means the measures for academic performance are adjusted for students in order for them to demonstrate competency more equitably (Bosher, 2009; Fuller and Mott-Smith, 2017). For instance, some students may benefit from taking an oral exam rather than a multiple-choice exam. Sometimes more latitude can be given for written essay answers; faculty can elect to assess comprehension of course concepts rather than critiquing writing standards such as American Psychological Association (APA) (Fuller and Mott-Smith, 2017).

When educating newer immigrant populations, faculty can provide a learning environment where differences are valued and respected. An example is a university that employed a nursing theory of lived experience, The Ways of Knowing (Zander, 2005). This allowed students of any background to understand that their life experience had value in contributing to the learning of all. Culturally diverse students may tend to study and socialize primarily with other students who identify as students of color in nursing programs (Gilchrist and Rector, 2007). With the theoretical framework of Zander's

(2007) The Ways of Knowing, its application resulted in positive student learning outcomes in the program. Faculty reported that, with the new inclusive theory, students were more likely to socialize in class and organize themselves in mixed groupings without explicit faculty direction.

There is a growing recognition of emotional, behavioral, health, and illness concerns that students are managing while in academic programs. These concerns can interfere with academic success (Sopcyzk, 2014). Along with services for academic accommodation, campus services for counseling, mental health, and other health conditions are important for culturally and linguistically diverse students (Fuller and Mott-Smith, 2017; Loewenstein and Christian, 2017; Sopcyzk, 2014). Campus clinics provide assessment and health services for students with tuition. Diverse students have stress apart from academic work that affects their ability to be successful and meet the goals in the program. Universities are initiating programs to heighten awareness and improve services for students with a variety of challenges (DeWitty et al., 2016a; Sopcyzk, 2014).

Lessons for diversity in nursing education

For the current era in nursing education, there are growing practices in promoting a learning atmosphere of encouraging acceptance for all students and ensuring a just culture or cultural congruence in the classroom (Palmer, 1998 & 2017). A just culture is one that espouses fairness and equity, creates a space for free expression, and acknowledges that novices will make mistakes (Brookfield, 2014; Loewenstein and Christian, 2017). As long as discussion is respectful, students can be encouraged in the free exchange of ideas. The key for faculty is transforming early forays in academic exploration and discovery into teachable moments (Gillespie, 2005; Greene, 1998).

To explore themes of individual background and diversity requires heightened awareness along with exercising sensitivity in the learning space. Faculty can demonstrate cultural awareness by incorporating vulnerable populations and individuals of diversity in case studies, assignments, and reflective exercises (Porta et al., 2019). Olukotun et al. (2018) demonstrated the effectiveness of having students engage in reflection for them to acknowledge their own stereotypes along with becoming aware of differences, power, and those who are being marginalized (Terhune, 2006). Students learn to express their reactions toward inequity, deciding how to value and approach health disparities for diverse populations, and comparing and contrasting their own original perspectives and what to incorporate for practice (Olukotun, et al, 2018). Through strategic activities, students both developed and internalized new or adjusted values regarding diversity (Olukotun, et al, 2018). Reflection is a learned practice and there are cultural constraints on an individual's ability to reflect. Therefore, activities need to be congruent with the social context in which they were constructed (Brookfield, 2017; Palmer, 2007; Porta et al., 2019).

Employing educational design principles is imperative as diversity themes cannot be merely token elements. Rather, integrating themes of diversity into course activities requires much forethought and ongoing evaluation; it is an iterative process that requires continual realignment (Brookfield, 2014; Palmer, 2007). When applying diversity in course activities, it is likely that the initial projects may not be ready to be implemented in the classroom, much like simulation development often requires a number of modifications and revisions before being launched with students.

Lessons involving diversity include creating a respectful and inclusive learning community, engaging students in classroom activities, and encouraging acceptance and a just culture perspective when discussing ideas that are different, diverse, or divergent from the traditional, the status quo, or the assumed majority's point of view.

Challenges and barriers for faculty

While faculty may agree that addressing diversity is essential, making this actionable in the classroom environment can be another matter. Philosophically, faculty may agree that goals for increasing understandings of diversity are important and needed for the future of nursing. However, those who venture in actualizing this in teaching practice may encounter unanticipated challenges and barriers (Arielli et al., 2012a; Brookfield, 2017).

Early adopters of alternative pedagogies in nursing classrooms may be at risk in their schools of nursing or institutions. Although many uphold the goal of enrolling more students of diversity in programs, the existing structures and traditional practices may inhibit change (DeWitty et al., 2016a; Loewenstein and Christian, 2017). Having support from educational leadership is an important factor to consider when planning curricular or course changes. Faculty who secure support of stakeholders may mitigate risk (Arielli, et al. 2012a; Brookfield, 2017).

Innovative educators may be perceived to be transgressing established practices. Faculty who persevere and initiate change in the classroom traverse beyond what is known and accepted to that which is unknown and may not be accepted (Benner et al., 2010; Brookfield, 2017; Brookfield and Holst, 2011).

Unlike prescriptive and tidy traditional methods, creative and constructivist educational design can be messy. Faculty can encounter resistance when trying new strategies and methods for classroom activities (Arielli, et al, 2012b; Warren, 2009). Sometimes, even discussing a sensitive topic can create an unexpected response in the learning space (Brookfield, 2017; Brookfield and Holst, 2011). As an example, faculty can explore something like ethical quandaries and the historical lessons learned from the historical Tuskegee study. Although the purpose would be for students to understand how one's cultural or ethnic background influences perspectives and responses, discussion can quickly become emotionally charged when students misunderstand or misinterpret comments in class discussion (Brookfield and Holst, 2011). Even when faculty encounter challenges in the classroom, they promote joint discovery between student and teacher.

Regardless of the barriers, faculty can benefit from facilitating critical conversations and help students discover alternative ideas to their own perspectives (Brookfield, 2017). Through discovery of common ground and the inevitable differences among participants, rich discussion can promote growth and increased awareness for both learners and teachers.

Applications for other disciplines

The nursing profession is making strides in addressing diversity in nursing programs and increasing diversity in the nursing workforce. Current initiatives and innovative teaching and learning practices are opening pathways for interprofessional education; innovation is also producing better continuing education and professional development. Nursing's own use of narrative pedagogy and deriving profession-specific ways of debriefing students for meaningful learning provide parallel applications for other disciplines. Innovations that are under way can promote clinical reflection of students and nurses. These changes in nursing education have a positive impact on patient interactions and healthcare team behaviors.

Diversity and its complexity will continue to open new layers of understanding for nursing education and improving the human condition.

References

Adams L T, Campbell J, & Deming K (2017) Diversity: A key aspect of 21st century faculty roles as implemented in the Robert Wood Johnson Foundation Nurse Faculty Scholars Program. *Nursing Outlook* 65: 267–277.

Aiken L H (2014) Baccalaureate nurses and hospital outcomes; More evidence. *Medical Care* 52(10): 861–863.

Agency for Healthcare Research and Quality (AHRQ). (2018). *2018 Healthcare Quality and Disparities Report*. Accessed at: https://www.ahrq.gov/research/findings/nhqrdr/nhqdr18/index.html

American Association of Colleges of Nursing (AACN) (2017) AACN position statement on diversity, inclusion, and equity in academic nursing. *Journal of Professional Nursing* 33: 171–174.

Apple M W (2004) *Ideology and curriculum* (3rd ed). New York: Routledge.

Arielli D, Friedman V J, & Hirshfeld M J (2012a) Challenges on the path to cultural safety in nursing education. *International Nursing Review* 59(2): 187–193.

Arielli D, Mashiach M, Hirchfeld M J & Friedman V (2012b) Cultural safety and nursing education in divided societies. *Nursing Education Perspectives* 33(6): 364–368.

Bastable S B & Sopcyzk D L (2014) Gender, socioeconomic, and cultural attributes of the learner. In S B Bastable (Ed.), *Nurse as educator: Principles of teaching and learning for nursing practice* (4th ed., pp. 313–368). Sudbury, MA: Jones and Bartlett.

Benner P, Sutphen M, Leonard V & Day L (2010) *Educating nurses: A call for radical transformation*. San Francisco: Jossey Bass.

Benner P, Tanner C, & Chesla C (2009) *Expertise in nursing practice: Caring, clinical judgment and ethics* (2nd ed.). New York, NY: Springer.

Bosher S D (2003) Barriers to creating a more culturally diverse nursing profession: Linguistic bias in multiple-choice nursing exams. *Nursing Education Perspectives* 24(1): 25–34.

Bosher S D (2009) Removing language as a barrier to success on multiple-choice exams. In S D Bosher & M D Pharris (Eds.), *Transforming nursing education: The culturally inclusive environment* (pp. 259–284). St. Paul, MN: Springer.

Bosher S D & Boyle M (2008) The effects of linguistic modification on ESL students' comprehension of nursing course test items. *Nursing Education Perspectives* 29(3): 165–172.

Bourdieu P & Passeron J C (1990) *Reproduction in education, society, and culture* (2nd ed.). Thousand Oaks, CA: Sage.

Brookfield S D (2014) *The skillful teacher: On technique, trust, and responsiveness in the classroom*. San Francisco: Jossey-Bass.

Brookfield S D (2017) *Becoming a critically reflective teacher* (2nd ed.). San Francisco: Jossey-Bass.

Brookfield S D & Holst J D (2011) *Radicalizing learning: Adult education for a just world*. San Francisco: Jossey-Bass.

Bruenig M (2005) Turning experiential education and critical pedagogy theory into praxis. *Journal of Experiential Education* 28(2): 106–122.

Bryson V (1999) *Feminist debates: Issues of theory and practice*. New York: New York University Press.

Budden J, Moulton P, Harper K, Brunell M L & Smiley R (2016) The 2015 national nursing workforce survey. *Journal of Nursing Regulation* 7(1): S1–S90.

Burchum J L (2002) Cultural competence: An evolutionary perspective. *Nursing Forum* 37(4): 5–15.

Campinha-Bacote J (2010) A culturally conscious model of mentoring. *Nurse Educator* 35(3): 130–135.

Carthon J M B, Nguyen T H, Chittams J, Park E & Guevara J (2014) Measuring success: Results from the national survey of recruitment and retention initiatives in the nursing workforce. *Nursing Outlook* 62: 259–267.

Chang L, Chen S-C & Hung S-L (2018) Embracing diversity and transcultural society through community health practicum among college nursing students. *Nurse Education in Practice* 31: 156–160.

Child J & Langford E (2011) Exploring the learning experiences of nursing students with dyslexia. *Nursing Standard* 25(40): 39–467.

Colby S L & Ortman J M (2015) *Projections of the size and composition of the U. S. population: 2014 to 2060, current population reports*. Washington D. C.: U. S. Census Bureau, pp. 25–1163.

Davidhazar R & Shearer R (2005) When your nursing student is culturally diverse. *The Health Care Manager* 24(4): 356–363.

DeWitty V P, Huerta C G & Downing C A (2016a) New careers in nursing: Optimizing diversity and student success for the future of nursing. *Journal of Professional Nursing* 32(55): S4-S13.

DeWitty V P, Tabloski P A, Millett C M, Hambrick M E, Shrefflet M, Downing M A & Huerta C G (2016b) Diversifying the pipeline into doctoral nursing programs: Developing the doctoral advancement readiness self-assessment. *Journal of Professional Nursing* 32(55): S68-S75.

Diekelmann N L (2001) Narrative pedagogy: Heideggerian hermanuetical analyses of lived experiences of students, teachers, and clinicians. *Advanced Nursing Science* 23(3): 53–71.

Diekelmann N L (2005) Engaging the students and the teacher: Co-creating substantive reform with narrative pedagogy. *Journal of Nursing Education* 44: 249–252.

Dossey BM, Selanders L C, Beck D M, & Atwell A (2005) *Florence Nightingale today: Healing, leadership, global action.* Silver Spring, MD: American Nurses Association.

Duarte E (2006) Critical pedagogy and the praxis of worldly philosophy. *Journal of Philosophy of Education* 40(1): 105–114.

Enami A, Thompson H & Gimbel S (2018) In support of diversity in doctoral nursing education. *Journal of Advanced Nursing* 74: 758–759.

Etowa J B, Fesker S, Vukie A R, Wittstock L, & Youden S (2005) Recruitment and retention of minority students: Diversity in nursing education. *International Journal of Nursing Education Scholarship* 2(1): Article 13. doi: 10.2202/1548-923x.1111.

Foucault M (1980) *Power/Knowledge.* New York, NY: Pantheon.

Freire P (1993) *Pedagogy of the oppressed.* (M. Bergman Ramos, Trans.). New York: Continuum.

Fuller B L & Mott-Smith J A (2017) Issues influencing success: Comparing the perspectives of nurse educators and diverse nursing students. *Journal of Nursing Education* 56(7): 389–396.

Gates S A (2018) What works in promoting and maintaining diversity in nursing programs. *Nursing Forum* 53: 190–196. doi: 10.1111/nuf.12242.

Gilchrist K L & Rector C (2007) Can you keep them? Strategies to attract and retain nursing students from diverse populations: Best practices in nursing education. *Journal of Transcultural Nursing* 18: 277–285.

Gillespie M (2005) Student-teacher connection: A place of possibility. *Journal of Advanced Nursing* 52(2): 211–219.

Glazer G & Bankston K (2014) Holistic admission in the health professions: Findings from a national survey. Accessed at: http://urbanuniversitiesforhealth.org/media/documents/Holistic_Admissions_in_the_Health_Professions.pdf

Greene M (1998) *The dialectic of freedom.* New York: Columbia University.

Hawkins J E, Wiles L L, Karlowitz K, & Tufts K A (2018) Educational model to increase the number and diversity of RN to BSN graduates from a resource-limited rural community. *Nurse Educator* 43(4): 206–209.

Health Resources and Services Administration (2015) Pipeline programs to improve racial and ethnic diversity in the health professions: An inventory of federal programs, assessment of evaluation approaches, and critical review of the research literature. Washington, D.C. Accessed at: http://bhpr.hrsa.gov/healthworkforce/reports/pipelineprogdiversity.pdf

Holliday M & Parker D (1997) Florence Nightingale, feminism and nursing. *Journal of Advanced Nursing* 26(3): 483–488.

Hurlbut J M & Revuelto I (2018) Transitioning veterans into a BSN pathway: Building the program from the ground up to promote diversity and inclusion. *Medical-Surgical Nursing* 27(4): 266–269.

Hussin V (2008) Teaching the fluid process of cultural competence at the graduate level: A constructivist approach. In S D Bosher & M D Pharris (Eds.), *Transforming nursing education: The culturally inclusive environment* (pp. 363–386). St. Paul, MN: Springer.

Institute of Medicine (IOM) (2011) *The future of nursing: Leading change, advancing health.* Washington, DC: The National Academies Press. Accessed at: www.nap.edu/catalog.php?record_id=12956

International Council of Nurses (ICN) (2008) *Nursing care continuum: Framework and competencies.* Geneva, Switzerland: ICN.

Ironside P M (2001) Creating a research base for nursing education: An interpretive review of conventional, critical, feminist, postmodern, and phenomenologic pedagogies. *Advances in Nursing Science* 23: 72–87.

Ironside P M (2003) New pedagogies for teaching thinking: The lived experiences of students and teacher enacting narrative pedagogy. *Journal of Nursing Education* 42(11): 509–516.

Ironside P M (2006) Using narrative pedagogy: Learning and practising interpretive thinking. *Journal of Nursing Education* 55(4): 478–486.

Kincheloe J L (2007) *Critical Pedagogy* (3rd ed.). New York: Peter Lang.

Leininger M M (1995) *Transcultural nursing: Concepts, theories, research, and practices.* New York, NY: McGraw-Hill.

Lerner G (1997) *Why history matters.* Oxford: Oxford University Press.

Lewenson S B (1996) *Taking charge: Nursing, suffrage and feminism in America, 1873-1920.* New York: National League of Nursing Press.

Lipmanowicz H & McCandless K (2013) *The surprising powers of liberating structures; Simple rules to unleash a culture of innovation.* Seattle, WA: Liberating Structure Press.

Loewenstein A J & Christian L L (2017) Culture and diversity in the classroom. In M J Bradshaw & B L Hultquist (Eds.), *Innovative teaching strategies in nursing and related health professions* (7th ed., pp. 19–38). Burlington MA: Jones and Bartlett.

Metcalfe S E, Lasher R, Leffler L J, Langson, S, Bell R, & Hudson D (2017) Pipeline programs to increase the diversity of health professional students at Western Carolina University: Combining efforts to foster equality. *Journal of Best Practices in Health Professions Diversity* 10(2): 135–140.

Nagda B, Gurin P, & Lopez G (2003) Transformative pedagogy for democracy and social justice. *Race, Ethnicity & Education* 6(2): 165.

National League of Nursing (NLN) (2016) NLN releases a vision for achieving diversity and meaningful inclusion in nursing education. *Nursing Education Perspectives* 3: 186.

Oikarainen A, Mikkonen K, Tuomikoski A M, Elo S, Pitkanen S, Routsalainen, H & Kaarlainen M (2018) Mentors' competence in mentoring culturally and linguistically diverse nursing students during clinical placement. *Journal of Advanced Nursing* 74: 148–159. doi: 10.1111/jan.13388.

Olukotun O, Mkandawire-Vahlmu L, Kreuziger SB, Dressel A, Wesp L, Sima C, Scheer V, Weitzel R et al. (2018) Preparing culturally safe student nurses: An analysis of undergraduate cultural diversity course reflections. *Journal of Professional Nursing* 34: 245–252. doi: 10.1016/j.profnurs.2017.11.011

Palmer P (1998 & 2017) *The courage to teach: Exploring the inner landscape of a teacher's life.* San Francisco: Jossey-Bass.

Papps E & Ramsden I (1996) Cultural safety in nursing: The New Zealand experience. *International Journal for Quality in Health care* 8(5): 491–497.

Phillips J & Malone B (2014) Increasing racial/ethnic diversity in nursing to reduce health disparities and achieve health equity. *Public Health Reports* 129: 46–50.

Porta C J, Andres C C, Roth C J, Zaiser K & Kumpula R (2019) Competency 10: Demonstrates non-judgmental/unconditional acceptance of people different from self. In P A Schoon, C J Porta & M A Schaffer (Eds.), *Population-based public health clinical manual: The Henry Street model for nurses* (3rd ed., pp. 235–250). Indianapolis, In Sigma Theta Tau International.

Racine L & Petrucka P (2011) Enhancing decolonization and knowledge transfer with non-western populations; Examining congruence between primary healthcare and postcolonial feminist approaches. *Nursing Inquiry* 18(1): 12–20.

Relf M V (2016) Advancing diversity in academic nursing. *Journal of Professional Nursing* 32(55): 542–547.

Salvucci C & Lawless A (2016) Nursing faculty diversity: Barriers and perceptions on recruitment, hiring, and retention. *Journal of Cultural Diversity* 23(2): 65–75.

Sopcyzk D L (2014) Educating learners with disabilities. In S B Bastable (Ed.), *Nurse as educator: Principles of teaching and learning for nursing practice* (4th ed., pp. 369–420). Sudbury, MA: Jones and Bartlett.

Terhune C P (2006) "Can we talk?" Using critical self-reflection and dialogue to build diversity and change organizational culture in nursing schools. *Journal of Cultural Diversity* 13(3): 141–145.

Tranter S, Gaul C, McKenzie S, & Graham K (2018) Initiatives aimed at retaining ethnically diverse student nurses in undergraduate programmes: An integrative review. *Journal of Clinical Nursing* 27: 3846–3857.

Warren B J (2009) Teaching the fluid process of cultural competence at the graduate level: A constructivist approach. In S D Bosher & M D Pharris (Eds.), *Transforming nursing education: The culturally inclusive environment* (pp. 320–323). St. Paul, MN: Springer.

Webb C (2002) Feminism, nursing, and education. *Journal of Advanced Nursing* 39(2): 111–113.

Wilson-Stronks A, Lee K K, Cordero C L, Kopp A L, & Galvez E. (2008). *One size does not fit all: Meeting the health care needs of diverse populations.* Oakbrook Terrace, IL: The Joint Commission. Accessed at: https://www.jointcommission.org/assets/1/6/HLCOneSizeFinal.pdf

World Health Organisation (2016) Global strategic directions for strengthening nursing and midwifery 2016–2020. Accessed at: www.who.int/hrh/nursingmidwifery/global-strategic-midwifery2016-2020.pdf?ua=1

World Health Organization (2008) *Primary health care: Now more than ever.* Geneva: WHO. Accessed at: www.who.int/whr/2008/whr08_en.pdf

Zander P E (2005) Ways of knowing in nursing: The historical evolution of a concept. *The Journal of Theory Construction & Testing* 11(1): 7–11.

Zuzelo P R, 2005 Affirming the disadvantaged student. *Nurse Educator* 30(1): 27–31.

24

TECHNOLOGISATION OF NURSING EDUCATION

David Robertshaw

Introduction

Technology has changed the way people interact with the world. It has brought people closer together but also further apart. Technological change and advancement have been exponential since time began, gathering speed in the eighteenth-century "Age of Enlightenment" and accelerating since the middle of the twentieth century. The internet has facilitated levels of inter-connectivity hitherto unknown, yet not everyone in the world has a reliable internet connection. The advent of technology is arguably the most significant event in modern times.

Technology and the internet have made learning accessible to almost everyone and the benefit of knowledge sharing is felt globally. There are more mobile phones than people on the planet, and nurses can carry the entire contents of the world's journals, libraries, diction-aries, guidelines, policies, evidence and reports in their pocket. Instant access to information is transforming the way decisions are made and where care is delivered. Every measurement, note or image of a person can be stored digitally for the world to access and use for decision making or research purposes. The development of technology has provided the tools to ana-lyse patients (for example, electrocardiograph (ECG) machines, computed tomography (CT) scanners), to treat patients and even keep patients alive (for example, defibrillators, ventila-tors), to automate some care processes (for example, infusion pumps and monitoring sys-tems) and to help keep clearer and more succinct records of the care provided to patients and clients (for example, electronic care records).

However, technology has a darker side. Issues of privacy, hacking and downtime are constantly in the news. This has major implications for healthcare. For example, if an elec-tronic database became inaccessible, tracking a patient's history would not be possible. If an electronic drug chart was hacked, timely and correct drug administration would be inter-rupted. Patient safety is at major risk.

As an educational resource, technology allows educators to reach students in ways not before imagined or possible. For example, it is not practical to take ten students in the back of an air ambulance helicopter, but this could be simulated in a virtual environment or an immersive reality room. This method would also allow for real-time discussion and reflec-tion on the scenario to allow many students to learn. However, this technology has limita-tions. For example, virtual reality will never simulate the sensation of movement as an air ambulance hovers above a Scottish mountainside in a gale force wind.

This chapter focuses on the use of technology in nursing education. It will explore five technologies in current use, as well as consider what technologies the future may hold for nursing education. Some of these technologies require significant investment and ongoing maintenance; however, some are easy to use and are accessible for all. This is important because the resources and funding available to universities may not be available to the same extent worldwide, particularly for nurse educators working in developing countries. This chapter suggests low-fidelity or cheaper alternatives that may provide a similar experience. Simulation is not included here as it is covered in a previous chapter (Chapter 12).

Technology 1: virtual reality

Virtual reality is defined as "computer-generated simulation of a three-dimensional image or environment that can be interacted with in a seemingly real or physical way by a person using special electronic equipment, such as a helmet with a screen inside or gloves fitted with sensors" (Freina & Ott, 2015). Imagine going into the hospital for a day case procedure. When the nursing students arrive in the operating theatre, the staff provide patients with a headset that displays three-dimensional images of any environment the student chooses: a beach, a field, the stars or even the home. It would certainly make the experience of having an operation much more palatable. Virtual reality is mostly thought of in this way at the moment: a headset with a rich, interactive world that is a representation of reality. However, virtual reality is really any virtual world that a person can react with. Other examples of this include software tools like Second Life, where participants can engage in virtual worlds. Second Life hosts entire virtual worlds, and some participants have entirely separate lives in Second Life. It is possible to create simulated environments like lecture theatres and simulation facilities in which students can learn. Although virtual reality was created for leisure activities and gaming (Jeong & Lee, 2019), there are now serious applications for this technology in the world of education.

Virtual reality has several key features. For example, virtual reality deploys three-dimensional imaging, with the ability to interact with the environment. In addition, there are visual and sound inputs, and the user feels directly part of the simulation. Users can interact with the simulation fully, including the "people" and the "environment" (Mantovani et al., 2003). Virtual reality exists in three most common methods. The first method is head-based virtual reality, where a head-mounted display or goggles are worn displaying stereoscopic images, which are very close to the user's eyes. There are usually two images with lenses close to the eye, giving the illusion of three dimensions. This type is common, but there is also, secondly, a projection-based virtual reality, where projections are on a wall. This version is less immersive, but the benefit here is that the participant can move around in the space and interact with the virtual reality environment. The third most common type of virtual reality is that in a computer display: an example of this is a game environment. This type is two-dimensional, and the least immersive version of the experience (Sherman & Craig, 2003).

Virtual reality has been prohibited mainly by cost and the need for technological capability. Virtual-reality headsets cost in the region of £500 ($650) which, although not too expensive for some universities, may be prohibitive for clinical educators and those involved in everyday learning in the workplace. The other issue is that virtual-reality headsets and virtual worlds require powerful computers and individual creation of scenarios and worlds: this generally means there needs to be technical support, which is expensive, and powerful computers, which are expensive (de Faria et al., 2016). This may put this technology beyond the reach of nurse educators in lower-income countries.

Another issue with virtual reality is that the world can be so real, it confuses the student's mind. Students report simulation sickness, with nausea, vertigo and general malaise. This is due to the differences in sensory input between that which the student is seeing, and that which is received through the vestibular system (Wilson & Soranzo, 2015). Students see motion, but do not feel it. Or they feel motion, but they do not see it. Simulation sickness is commonly reported to be as high as 56% (Treleaven et al., 2015; Munafo, Diedrick & Stoffregen, 2017).

Healthcare education values personal interactions, individual connections and touch (Kelly et al., 2018). One of the main criticisms of virtual reality is that it is a representation of reality, rather than actual reality, and at the moment participants (or "players") can only have visual interaction. Increasingly the way we interact with virtual worlds is becoming more tactile, but this will take 10–20 years to become mainstream. Haptic interactivity is the next big "win" in virtual reality: developing technology that provides sensory input to the skin so that the scenario feels real. Nurses consider the human touch and personal, individual connections are important, therefore simulating these so that they are as real as possible will be a challenge. The simulation will also need to respond to the learner's interaction with it, which means the development of artificial intelligence to the point where the simulation can respond as if it were a human. Technology is approaching this point, but it is not there yet: and once this "holy grail" is achieved it will undoubtedly be expensive to use.

Although virtual reality is becoming increasingly available, in 2019 the technology is still in the early adoption phase. Students generally report positive increases in student satisfaction, self-confidence and engagement, with positive learning experiences and enhanced knowledge (Padilha et al., 2018; Verkuyl & Hughes, 2019). Despite the challenges, virtual reality is a positive development worthy of a wider rollout. The cheapest way to start with virtual reality is to use a Google Cardboard phone mount which is made out of cardboard and includes two lenses, with a mobile phone. YouTube has many virtual-reality and 360-degree videos which can be watched through this method, including of surgery.

Technology 2: augmented reality

Augmented reality has similarities with virtual reality, in that it uses computer-generated images, animations and sound, but instead of being a separate virtual world the images are overlaid with reality. Augmented reality is defined as a live direct or an indirect view of a physical, real-world environment whose elements are augmented by computer-generated sensory input, such as sound, graphics or GPS data (Grier et al., 2012). Augmented reality combines the physical world with digital media, by adding a computer-generated overlay on reality.

This combination of the real world and the virtual world allows students to explore concepts and structures in three dimensions, developing an awareness of space and place (Arvanitis et al., 2017). Augmented reality can demonstrate objects which are difficult to see in the real world (Klopfer & Squire, 2008), for example, a three-dimensional model of an aero-engine. The engine can be deconstructed, moved around and adjusted while appearing under the wing: students can interact with the engine in real time, without it ever being there. They can develop skills, knowledge and capabilities that would be hard to develop in other circumstances (Kerawalla et al., 2006; Squire & Klopfer, 2007).

Augmented reality could be used to demonstrate the three-dimensional structure of organs or other similar structures: students could dissect a body in real time, without ever harming a patient. Any structure in three dimensions can be built in augmented reality and shared with students. In this way, students are less prone to simulation sickness, as the visual model is in the real environment: sensory input from visual and vestibular systems matches.

Although augmented reality is cheap, like virtual reality some technical ability is required to start. The nursing educator would generally need to involve a technician to help design the model or implement a system using existing models. Aurasma, now known as HP Reveal, is one such tool. Aurasma requires a server to be running which hosts models, and then mobile devices use an app to "see" a printed image, on top of which appears a virtual model (Connolly & Hoskins, 2014). Other apps, for example, Layar (Liao & Humphreys, 2015) and Google Expeditions (Tudor et al., 2017), can overlay information on top of reality. One of the best tools to demonstrate augmented reality is Google Translate (Groves & Mundt, 2015), which will in real time convert one printed language to another on the screen.

Technology 3: online learning

Online learning is any form of learning conducted partly or wholly over the internet (Bates, 2015). Roffe (2004) defined distance education, of which online learning is part, as a method of teaching whereby the student and teacher are separated using technologies (Roffe, 2004). Online learning is nothing new: distance education started with correspondence, moving into radio, television and now online (Kentnor, 2015). Bates (2015) sees online learning as a continuum from blended learning involving some technology-enhanced learning or flipped classroom, through to fully online learning where there is no classroom or on-campus teaching. There is a taxonomy here from distance to co-located, and from online learning to elearning. The difference is not just in the distance: elearning (for example, mandatory learning) is often flat, boring and straightforward. Often people think online learning is elearning because that is all they have experienced. Online learning is an interactive, activity-led, social and constructivist learning experience. Although often seen as being something completely separate and different to face-to-face learning, the same principles apply and the same end goal is desired.

Online learning is also sometimes known as computer-based instruction, and it involves learning undertaken using a virtual learning environment (Vuopala, Hyvönen & Järvelä, 2016). Schools use online learning to great effect, often using virtual learning environments like Google Classroom (Iftakhar, 2016). There are free and open-source virtual learning environments like Moodle, and although this requires a server to host and run the software, once it is set up Moodle is fairly easy to run and can be used with little technical preparation or training (Rodrigues, Rocha & Abreu, 2017)

In nursing, online learning is most often used for post-registration programmes of learning, for example, top-up degrees or knowledge development courses (Hampton & Pearce, 2016). Although online learning works well in this context, the use of online learning in pre-registration programmes has been limited to a small number of niche institutions like the Open University. More popular in the United States, online learning does have great potential for pre-registration nursing and a shortened online learning pre-registration nursing programme was identified as an area of development in the NHS *Long Term Plan* (2019). Online learning should offer increased access and flexibility, allowing students to work alongside their studies. Learning can be participated in with flexibility and according to the

337

students' needs. This is at odds with the traditional model of learning, whereby many students are taught in lecture theatres or seminar rooms at prescribed times. However, given the current workforce challenges online learning may offer opportunities to include students who may not be able to attend "traditional" programmes.

Online learning offers great opportunities for people with disabilities and additional learning needs, and statistics demonstrate that the proportion of students with disabilities studying online learning programmes is higher than students on non-online learning programmes (Stone, 2017). Computers are arguably more accessible than buildings.

Some of the problems associated with online learning relate to the technology itself. Although devices are relatively cheap (online learning can be studied with a phone or tablet), online learning relies on internet connectivity which is not guaranteed for all (particularly those in developing countries or rural areas) (Liyanagunawardena & Aboshady, 2018). Technological and digital capability/literacy has historically been a challenge; however, this issue is reducing as time is advancing (Estacio, Whittle & Protheroe, 2017).

An issue that often arises is confirming the student's identity. Some degrees are fully online, and there is a moral and ethical dilemma with this: how do nurse educators know that the person who studied the programme and submitted the work was actually the person he or she said he or she was? Plagiarism of this kind is not only confined to online learning, however, as any student could submit work written by someone else and the recipient wouldn't necessarily check. There are technological tools available for nurse educators to use in examinations, where electronic proctoring involves a webcam with either automated software or a person watching who detects unusual movements (Hylton, Levy & Dringus, 2016).

Online learning is an incredibly powerful tool and looks set to be the future of education. Education is expensive because of the rooms, buildings and people it employs, whereas online learning offers an often cheaper option. Additionally, online learning is accessible by anyone with an internet connection and a device, making learning open and on demand.

Technology 4: massive open online courses

Massive open online courses (MOOCs) are a development of online learning. MOOCs are online courses which are open and accessible to anyone. MOOCs are massive, in terms of thousands of people, and often they are free. First emerging in 2008, the first MOOC was developed by George Siemens and Stephen Downes, called "Connectivism and Connective Knowledge". Connectivism, an educational theory integrating principles of chaos, network, complexity and self-organisation theories (Siemens, 2005), would go on to influence MOOC design and online learning theory for the following decade. This first course had a small number of students in the classroom with many thousands more studying at home. This model was repeated in Peter Norvig and Sebastian Thrun's course Introduction to Artificial Intelligence, attracting over 160,000 learners. A range of universities became interested in MOOCs around this time and either designed and delivered them independently or worked with commercial and public-sector organisations to do so. The range of topics and type of MOOCs began to diversify. Shortly thereafter commercial companies began to operate MOOCs, with the incorporation of Coursera, Udacity, edX and FutureLearn. These companies operate a reasonably successful commercial model of MOOCs with some including paid-for certification and micro-degrees as part of their courses. However, there has also been a high number of small independent providers, with some universities commencing delivery of MOOCs through alternative platforms and methods.

MOOCs gained popularity and were suggested as a disruptive technology that would "change the face of education" (Conole, 2013). There are signs this disruption is slowing, and education has not experienced the level of change that was expected. It is possible that MOOCs are in the "trough of disillusionment" and may return to prominence as educators and students become enlightened about the benefits of MOOCs. It is also possible that Amara's law, whereby the effect of technology is overestimated in the short run, and its effects underestimated in the long run, applies to MOOCs. Although MOOCs are in widespread use, there remains a lack of research and critical analysis of their implementation (Baturay, 2015). Over 100 million people have studied MOOCs yet there is a dearth of evaluation.

For nursing, MOOCs are an opportunity. MOOCs bring the world of universities and higher education out to everyone (Sanchez-Gordon & Lujan-Mora, 2016). Many universities are making their material free to access and study, with social elements. Examples of these include a MOOC on "Care Home Nursing: Changing Perceptions", run by the University of Dundee in Scotland with FutureLearn (Hill, 2019) and "Could You Be the Next Florence Nightingale?" by Coventry University (another UK university) with FutureLearn (FutureLearn, 2018). The University of Derby in the UK offers a range of MOOCs on its own platform, including on dementia, autism and social pedagogy. Coventry University also offers an online MSc in nursing, and has chosen to make this accessible for free via a MOOC with FutureLearn (FutureLearn, 2019a). Participants can receive an online note which, on completion of the course, permits the option of payment of a small fee for a certificate, or payment of the larger sum of £14,000 to receive a master's degree by studying the same material through FutureLearn (FutureLearn, 2019a). Although it is positive that these opportunities are open to all, this does in some way call into question the value of a degree: you can study the same material, complete the same assignments and gain the same learning for free, or you can pay £14,000 for a certificate to say you did it. Of course, without MOOCs, this kind of opportunity would not be available at all, and for nurses and students without access to funding, for example in developing countries, or those working in organisations unwilling or unable to fund further learning, MOOCs provide an opportunity for skills and knowledge development that would otherwise not exist. MOOCs are not limited to nursing; they exist in a myriad of subjects, from equine welfare and management (Coursera, 2019) to Jane Austen (FutureLearn, 2019b) to cybersecurity (FutureLearn, 2019c).

The future for MOOCs appears challenging. Many universities and commercial organisations are now questioning the value and investment of MOOCs. Funders and investors may have initially seen MOOCs as student recruitment tools: offering micro-learning opportunities, and encouraging a student to join the institution more substantively. However, in-course engagement and completion rates have been extremely low, although this is to be expected (Petronzi & Hadi, 2016). When such small numbers complete MOOCs, this leads to questions about the justifiability, profitability and purposes of MOOCs. This does de-value the corporate social responsibility aspect of MOOCs: large institutions and organisations have responsibilities to increase access and widen participation to higher education and MOOCs are a way of doing that.

Technology 5: applications (apps)

An app or application is software designed for a mobile device and increasingly the term is being used to refer to any software application. Most mobile phones and tablets have basic software installed on them, such as Google Android, and apps are the additional building blocks which extend the capability and function of the device. Apps are available for most uses, including email, calendars, texting and communication, and car insurance (where apps track how you drive (Aviva, 2018)), health insurance (where apps track what you eat and how you exercise (Pagnamenta, 2018)). There are many thousands of apps available to users, and apps are available on just about anything.

Beyond games and other utility apps, there is an opportunity for us to consider how apps might be used in nursing education. There are already many apps designed for nurses and students, and these are making information available instantly in the pocket of the user. For example, the *British National Formulary* (Royal Pharmaceutical Society of Great Britain, 2017) is moving away from printing expensive books to maintaining an app which is free to use. This allows medicines information to be available at the point of care, for free, and right up to date. Other applications are available which will index other evidence sources such as systematic reviews, randomised controlled trials and cohort studies which allow clinicians to implement evidence-based care at the bedside (BMJ, 2019). Medscape, a free application, offers articles for healthcare professionals on just about any clinical condition, disease or treatment, and the information is checked regularly for accuracy (Visser & Bouman, 2012). These apps provide instant information to be used and synthesised.

Apps also now exist to "do" something or offer a service beyond information. PainChek is an Australian-invented app which takes pictures and video of a person's face, adds information from a standardised scoring tool and will tell the user if a person is in pain or not (Atee et al., 2018). The technology is available to use for people who cannot verbalise their pain, for example, people living with dementia. This app is increasing in use and has a range of validated studies demonstrating its use (Atee et al., 2017).

Another app currently available which is transforming general practice is GP at Hand (Babylon, 2019). Owned by Babylon, this private general practice service originated in London. The service is being promoted by the NHS which will allow its patients to register with Babylon. The app asks a series of questions, and patients move through predetermined questionnaires to determine their condition and to offer health advice. The app allows patients to see a general practitioner through their smartphone, and if required they can still attend a walk-in centre after using the app. This technology looks set to revolutionise general practice, and although some practices use technology as a route of communication with their patients, deployment of an app on this scale for this purpose is new. There are many criticisms of the service. There is a view among some general practitioners that the GP at Hand service will "take away" their younger, fitter patients as they may find using the service easier (Rimmer, 2018). The issue with this is that most general practices have a balance of patients, with some patients using their services on a regular basis and others hardly ever: the two balance out (Iacobucci, 2019). Without younger or fitter people (who are more likely to be on the "hardly ever" end of the scale), the balance is unbalanced.

Although GP at Hand is an app for general practice, this has implications for nursing education. The future of healthcare is much more likely to be app- and technology-based. Nurse educators should be developing nursing students to have the skills to use technology in their daily lives. For example, consultation and record-keeping skills may require some modification to fit with an app. An immediate example of record keeping in the electronic space is practice assessment documentation. Increasingly, education providers are using apps for software like PebblePad to record their information and decisions about student attainment and achievement in practice (Haigh & Currant, 2010). This makes a lot of sense because students have historically had to carry heavy tree-based portfolios around with them hoping to gain signatures. Now, these decisions can be recorded and signed off electronically (Birks et al., 2016).

PebblePad is used for practice learning, but there are apps for use in the classroom too. Poll Everywhere is a commercial polling system for use in the classroom (Shon & Smith, 2011). Educators set activities or questions, and students can use their devices to engage with the software. Importantly, students use their own devices and answers appear immediately on the screen. This software can also be used for conferences and question-and-answer sessions.

Apps provide some great opportunities for nursing educators to bring the world's information into the pocket of users. Apps can allow for better record keeping and instant communication. Apps can help nursing students to make decisions and improve the care of patients.

Barriers and enablers to implementing technology in nursing education

Generally, the barriers to the increased technologisation of nursing education relate to a small number of issues: funding, technical capability and availability. Ironically, the greatest enabler is students who wish to use technology in their learning experiences. Students are open to the opportunities which technology presents, and generally, there is an expectation that technology will feature as part of nurse education. Nursing students have experienced technology in their prior education; schools and colleges use technology in day-to-day teaching. It is timely, therefore, for nursing educators to be using technology in the classroom and in the practice environment.

Technology is generally expensive, and this is because of the high costs of development, and the high costs of ongoing maintenance and training. All technology takes time to create, to develop and to test and this increases the cost. The higher fidelity the technology, the greater the cost. Some high-fidelity mannequins, for example, cost upwards of £50,000 and this is not unusual. The cost of developing an app that runs and is reliable is above £100,000. Participation in commercial projects, for example, virtual-reality simulations, costs in the region of £30,000–£50,000 with discounts if the partner brings new partners. This can't continue: new technologies should be open-source and released under creative commons licensing, permitting others to use, manipulate, edit and improve the technology. Some examples of these are Moodle, a free and open-source virtual learning environment that is in widespread use; OpenLabyrinth, which is a virtual patient system; and Open Journal Systems, which is a free journal-hosting, editing, and publishing platform. Wherever possible partners should co-develop products to ensure the cost is spread between partners. External funding is not always available, and therefore the greatest cost may be time (but that does cost money).

Technical capability is an ongoing issue for the adoption and implementation of technology in nursing education. The general technological and digital capability of the nursing and nursing education workforce is not as high as in other professions, which means that technology takes time to embed. However, we should balance this against the experiences and capabilities of our students who are much more likely to have technological and digital capability, not just because they are younger, but because they grew up in a world where technology was and is ubiquitous. Nurses should work with colleagues and partners in technology-enhanced learning teams, simulation teams and technician teams who may have more experience of using and implementing the technology. For universities, nurse educators could also enlist the help of colleagues from other departments and schools: interdisciplinary working is a requirement in universities, and working across disciplines to use and implement new technology is a way of doing this.

Availability of technology is a constant problem. Whether this is access to a "sim man", or server downtime, technology is not always available. Nurse educators can plan to use technologies, but they are never 100% reliable and so educators should consider secondary low-tech low-fidelity options. For example, if the app-based voting system being used doesn't work an alternative should be provided. If, when using an electronic practice assessment document for a student, the system is not accessible because of internet connection or device malfunction, an alternative should be available. Something as simple as a battery dying or the internet not being available can derail the best-laid plans of educators. These issues will become less prevalent as the use and availability of devices and the internet increase. Already, wi-fi is available in most places and it is unusual for students not to have a device of some kind. Battery life will extend as battery technology improves.

The future for technology in nursing education

The future looks exciting for technology in nursing education. The use and fidelity of technology have increased exponentially since the 1990s, and much of what we use today was not imagined ten years ago. Assuming the barriers are overcome, and technology continues to develop at pace, this section considers what the future holds for technology in nursing education.

Artificial intelligence, where computers are programmed to think, learn and change their behaviour in response to new scenarios and conditions (Russell & Norvig, 2016), will greatly affect our lives and our learning. Artificial intelligence is already being used in business and in the private sector, but its use will become more pronounced and visible in the public sector and education. For example, artificial intelligence can, today, analyse the blood results and other measurements of large patient populations and predict who is at risk of disease (Krittanawong et al., 2017). Clinicians can then provide targeted interventions. It would not be possible to see those patterns or links with the human eye. It is only by scaling up and using computers to think that patterns can be identified. Imagine if the same system could be applied to students: a university of 50,000 students or more could employ an artificial intelligence system which monitors their engagement, achievement and attainment and identifies students who need the most attention. It could also identify other factors such as the risk of mental health problems, which is a major issue of modern higher education (Auerbach et al., 2016).

Artificial intelligence could also become a virtual "person" that students could interact with: a "living", "thinking" simulation that responds to interactions. The natural leap here is in robotics: building a high-fidelity robot which emulates a person, and houses the artificial intelligence. This can now be done in virtual reality, but building a robot with artificial intelligence which looks like, thinks like and interacts like a human means there is no need for cameras strapped to a student's face giving the person simulation sickness. Students can learn in real time, in the real world, with real interactions. One of the concerns about this type of technology has been explored in films and television: if artificial intelligence like this can be created, in a body, and it thinks for itself, is it human? What happens if a student "kills" the intelligence? The scope of these questions is beyond this chapter, but it is an interesting thought experiment.

These possibilities have profound effects on nursing education. One of the major issues at the moment is placement capacity: if it were possible to build clinical environments which look like the real world (and it is), but include in them a range of virtual or artificial intelligence patients who look like, think like and are like real people, the level of separation between the simulated experience and the real experience becomes much smaller. Robotics and artificial intelligence could provide a unique solution to placement capacity availability. It is not yet possible to know how these interactions and changes will affect nursing students and how they will work in the real world, Questions such as, will nursing students feel empathy for a robot? are legitimate and requiring of research to ensure the technologisation of nurse education is a mindful and evidence-based process.

Conclusion

If well-thought-through and evidence-based, technology can be one of the greatest levers for learning. If it is not right, or it doesn't work or it is broken, technology can be one of the greatest failures for learners. It is an expectation of modern-day students that technology will feature in their learning and we, as educators, should be open and ready to use, demonstrate and implement technology. The future will hold challenges for technology in nursing education, but working with partners, with each other and with students, nurse educators can lead the way for the implementation and use of technology in learning. The ultimate goal for the use of technology should be to improve and enhance the learning of students, which in turn directly impacts the care that patients receive. Nurse education should study carefully the impact and nature of technology, and how it affects nursing students and patients alike, considering at every stage whether technology is the right pedagogy to use or not. This chapter has discussed five technologies, and considered future technologies: often no technology is needed at all. Nurse educators, who maintain professional roles as nurses, should not forget the personal interactions and relationships integral to working with and caring for patients. Technology is exciting, sexy, game changing and offers a glimpse of the future. However, nurse educators should focus on the core fundamentals of nursing: people.

References

Arvanitis T, Williams D, Knight J, Baber C, Gargalakos M, Sotiriou S, & Bogner FX (2017) Human factors and qualitative pedagogical evaluation of a mobile augmented reality system for science education used by learners with physical disabilities. *Personal and Ubiquitous Computing* 13:243–250.

Atee M, Hoti K, & Hughes JD (2018) A technical note on the PainChek™ system: a web portal and mobile medical device for assessing pain in people with dementia. *Frontiers in aging neuroscience* 10: 117.

Atee M, Hoti K, Parsons R, & Hughes JD (2017) Pain assessment in dementia: evaluation of a point-of-care technological solution. *Journal of Alzheimer's Disease* 60:137–150.

Auerbach RP, Alonso J, Axinn WG, Cuijpers P, Ebert DD, Green JG & Nock MK (2016) Mental disorders among college students in the World Health Organization world mental health surveys. *Psychological medicine* 46(14):2955–2970.

Aviva (2018) *Aviva Drive app.* Accessed at: www.aviva.co.uk/insurance/motor/aviva-drive/

Babylon (2019) *GP at Hand.* Accessed at: www.gpathand.nhs.uk/

Bates AW (2015) Teaching in a digital age. Accessed at: https://opentextbc.ca/teachinginadigitalage/

Baturay MH (2015) An Overview of the World of MOOCs. *Procedia - Social and Behavioral Sciences* 174: 427–433.

Birks M, Hartin P, Woods C, Emmanuel E, & Hitchins M (2016) Students' perceptions of the use of eportfolios in nursing and midwifery education. *Nurse Education in Practice* 18:46–51.

BMJ (2019) *Evidence on demand: health education England brings BMJ Best Practice to the bedside.* Accessed at: https://bestpractice.bmj.com/info/evidence-on-demand-health-education-england-brings-bmj-best-practice-to-the-bedside/.

Connolly E, & Hoskins J (2014) Using iPads to teach year 7 induction: with Aurasma. *School Librarian* 62 (1):6–8.

Conole G (2013). MOOCs as disruptive technologies: strategies for enhancing the learner experience and quality of MOOCs. *Revista de Educación a Distancia*, 39: 1–17.

Coursera. (2019) *Equine welfare and Management*. Accessed at: www.coursera.org/learn/equine

de Faria, JWV, Teixeira M, Júnior LDMS, Otoch JP, & Figueiredo EG (2016) Virtual and stereoscopic anatomy: when virtual reality meets medical education. *Journal Of Neurosurgery* 125(5):1105–1111.

Estacio EV, Whittle R, & Protheroe J (2017) The digital divide: examining socio-demographic factors associated with health literacy, access and use of internet to seek health information. *Journal of Health Psychology* 24(12): 1668–1675. 1359105317695429.

Freina L, & Ott M (2015) A literature review on immersive virtual reality in education: state of the art and perspectives. *eLearning & Software for Education* 1:133–141.

FutureLearn (2018) *Could you be the next Florence nightingale?* Accessed at: www.futurelearn.com/courses/nursing-and-public-health-7004-cpd-01

FutureLearn (2019a) *MSc nursing*. Accessed at: www.futurelearn.com/degrees/coventry/nursing

FutureLearn (2019b) *Jane Austen: myth, reality and global celebrity*. Accessed at: www.futurelearn.com/courses/jane-austen

FutureLearn (2019c) *Introduction to cyber security*. Accessed at: www.futurelearn.com/courses/introduction-to-cyber-security

Grier RA, Thiruvengada H, Ellis SR, Havig P, Hale KS, & Hollands JG (2012) Augmented reality – implications toward virtual reality, human perception and performance. *Proceedings of the Human Factors and Ergonomics Society Annual Meeting* 56(1):1351–1355.

Groves M & Mundt K (2015) Friend or foe? Google Translate in language for academic purposes. *English for Specific Purposes* 37:112–121.

Haigh J & Currant N (2010) *Guiding, supporting and assessing midwifery students in clinical placements*. In PebblePad Conference, Shifnal, Shropshire, UK.

Hampton D & Pearce P F (2016) Student engagement in online nursing courses. *Nurse Educator* 41 (6):294–298.

Hill G (2019) *Online course corrects care home myths*. Accessed at: www.dundee.ac.uk/news/2019/online-course-corrects-care-home-myths.php

Hylton K, Levy Y, & Dringus LP (2016) Utilizing webcam-based proctoring to deter misconduct in online exams. *Computers & Education* 92:53–63.

Iacobucci G (2019) GP at hand: patients are less sick than others but use services more, evaluation finds. *British Medical Journal* 365:l2333.

Iftakhar S (2016) Google classroom: what works and how?. *Journal of Education and Social Sciences* 3(1):12–18.

Jeong SYS, Lee KO (2019) The emergence of virtual reality simulation and its implications for the nursing profession. *Korean Journal of Women Health Nursing* 25(2):125–128.

Kelly MA, Nixon L, McClurg C, Scherpbier A, King N, & Dornan T (2018) Experience of touch in health care: a meta-ethnography across the health care professions. *Qualitative health research* 28(2):200–212.

Kentnor H (2015) Distance education and the evolution of online learning in the United States. *Curriculum and Teaching Dialogue* 17(1,2):21–34.

Kerawalla L, Luckin R, Seljeflot S, & Woolard A (2006) "Making it real": exploring the potential of augmented reality for teaching primary school science. *Virtual Reality* 10:163–174.

Klopfer E, & Squire K (2008) Environmental detectives—the development of an augmented reality platform for environmental simulations. *Educational technology research and development* 56(2):203–228.

Krittanawong C, Zhang H, Wang Z, Aydar M, & Kitai T (2017) Artificial intelligence in precision cardiovascular medicine. *Journal of the American College of Cardiology* 69(21):2657–2664.

Liao T & Humphreys L (2015) Layar-ed places: using mobile augmented reality to tactically reengage, reproduce, and reappropriate public space. *New Media & Society* 17(9):1418–1435.

Liyanagunawardena TR, & Aboshady OA (2018) Massive open online courses: a resource for health education in developing countries. *Global Health Promotion* 25(3):74–76.

Mantovani F, Castelnuovo G, Gaggioli A, & Riva G (2003) Virtual reality training for health-care professionals. *Cyber psychology and Behavior* 6:389–395.

Munafo J, Diedrick M, & Stoffregen TA (2017) The virtual reality head-mounted display Oculus Rift induces motion sickness and is sexist in its effects. *Experimental Brain Research* 235(3):889–901.

NHS. (2019) *Long Term Plan*. Available at: www.england.nhs.uk/long-term-plan/

Padilha JM, Machado PP, Ribeiro AL, Ramos J (2018) Clinical virtual simulation in nursing education. *Clinical Simulation in Nursing* 15:13–18.

Pagnamenta, R (2018) *Insurance company is using steps recorded on Fitbits and Apple Watches to reward consumers*. Accessed at: www.telegraph.co.uk/technology/2018/11/05/insurance-company-using-steps-recorded-fitbits-apple-watches/

Petronzi D & Hadi M (2016) Exploring the factors associated with MOOC engagement, retention and the wider benefits for learners. *European Journal of Open, Distance and e-Learning* 19(2):112–129.

Rimmer A (2018) Smartphone GP app service will divert funding from most needy, warns practice. *British Medical Journal (Online)* 360: k1045.

Rodrigues S, Rocha Á, & Abreu A (2017) The use of moodle in higher education evolution of teacher's practices over time. *In 2017 12th Iberian Conference on Information Systems and Technologies (CISTI)* (pp. 1–4). IEEE.

Roffe I (2004) *Innovation and e-learning: e-business for an educational enterprise.* Cardiff, UK: University of Wales Press.

Royal Pharmaceutical Society of Great Britain. (2017) *BNF Publications.* Accessed at: https://apps.apple.com/gb/app/bnf-publications/id1045514038

Russell SJ, & Norvig P (2016) *Artificial intelligence: a modern approach.* Malaysia: Pearson Education Limited.

Sanchez-Gordon S & Lujan-Mora S (2016) How could MOOCs become accessible? The case of EdX and the future of inclusive online learning. *Journal of Universal Computer Science* 22(1):55–81.

Sherman W & Craig A (2003) *Understanding virtual reality: interface, application, and design.* San Francisco: Elsevier Science.

Shon H & Smith L (2011) A review of Poll Everywhere audience response system. *Journal of Technology in Human Services* 29(3):236–245.

Siemens G (2005). Connectivism: A learning theory for the digital age. *International Journal of Instructional Technology and Distance Learning*, 2(1), 3–10.

Squire K & Klopfer E (2007) Augmented reality simulations on handheld computers. *Journal of Learning Science* 6:371–413.

Stone C (2017) *Opportunity through online learning: improving student access, participation and success in higher education.* Perth: Curtin University.

Treleaven J, Battershill J, Cole D, Fadelli C, Freestone S, Lang K, Sarig-BaHat H (2015) Simulator sickness incidence and susceptibility during neck motion-controlled virtual reality tasks. *Virtual Reality* 19 (3-4):267–275.

Tudor AD, Minocha S, Tilling S, Needham R, & Cutler M (2017) *Google expeditions and fieldwork: friends or foes?* In: ASE (The Association for Science Education, UK) Annual Conference 2017, 4–7 Jan 2017, University of Reading, UK.

Verkuyl M & Hughes M (2019) Virtual gaming simulation in nursing education: a mixed methods study. *Clinical Simulation in Nursing* 29:9–14.

Visser B J, & Bouman J (2012) There's a medical app for that. *British Medical Journal* 344:e2162.

Vuopala E, Hyvönen P, & Järvelä S (2016) Interaction forms in successful collaborative learning in virtual learning environments. *Active Learning in Higher Education* 17(1):25–38.

Wilson CJ, Soranzo A (2015) The use of virtual reality in psychology: a case study in visual perception. *Computational and Mathematical Methods in Medicine* 151702.

25

NURSING EDUCATION AND HEALTHCARE IN THE CONTEXT OF THE ECOLOGICAL APPROACH

Ruta Renigere

Introduction

The twenty-first century has revealed numerous challenges in nursing education and healthcare, including: (1) how to implement study programmes in line with the educational trends for sustainable development in nursing studies and the process of formation and development of ecological competence; (2) how to improve the nursing education process and healthcare by using the ecological approach in healthcare practice; (3) how to create and integrate theories/models of nursing education in healthcare practice to promote healing of oneself and others; and (4) how to integrate new technologies in nursing education and healthcare practice. The result of this integration should be nursing education and healthcare practice that is a complete, well-founded and unified whole.

The ecological approach in education process and healthcare must be looked at as a varied and complex system of learning, socializing and culture that includes many different subsystems. It is a way to implement sustainable development of education and sustainability/sustainable development in healthcare, promoting unity and congruence of science and healthcare. The ecological approach in education and healthcare refers to a value-oriented transformation process of students from *I-ego* to *I-eco* in their life activities and systemic thinking in social, education and healthcare environments, complementing the professional code of ethics.

The ecological approach in the process of education and healthcare should be viewed in the context of lifelong learning and further improvement of life activities. It is important to point out Klaus Mollenhauer's (1928–1998) opinion on the human ability to integrate into society, which demands the liberation of the subject. That is, to be able to make an independent and responsible decision and to be able to act freely and independently, subjects must be liberated from the conditions that limit and inhibit their activity in society (Mollenhauer, 1977).

Evaluation of many insights and research outcomes in a variety of publications has led to the definition of a hypothetical assumption that the formation and development of the ecological competence in education and healthcare can be promoted if formal, informal and non-formal education is based on the ecological approach. The ecological approach in education and healthcare is built upon three basic building blocks:

1) education for sustainable development (ESD) and sustainability/sustainable development in healthcare practice;
2) Bronfenbrenner's ecology of human development theory;
3) deep ecology and ecosophy (Naess, 2008).

In this chapter I address the ecological approach in education and healthcare practice, which is characterized by the principles developed as a result of theoretical research and the components of professional competence. From a systemic perspective, this forms ecological competence in the social and educational environment and through experience in healthcare.

Terminology in nursing and healthcare

The healthcare discipline consists of four main abstract concepts: a person, health, environment and healthcare. Nursing theories define the basic concepts in nursing, pointing out that a person is an individual or a family or a community or even the whole humanity. Nursing theories maintain that a person in healthcare is a pivotal concept and that health can be described by the state of a person's wellness that has been mutually agreed upon between the person and the nurse. It is also emphasized that environment includes the physical surrounding of a person, his or her community, or even the whole universe and everything that it comprises. Above all, healthcare is viewed not only as a nursing science or its practical application, but also as an art: the art of learning; the art of teaching or training; the art of working; the art of leading; the art of living; the art of telling; the art of choosing; it is human to make mistakes; however, it is the next highest step on the hill of humanity to recognize and learn from them.

Evaluating the concepts defined in different nursing theories and models in the context of the ecological approach, it can be concluded that such concepts as environment, a person, adaptation, beingness in human environment, human esteem, the uniqueness of a client/patient, as well as different kinds of arts in the profession of a nurse, especially the art of living, are most closely related to the ecological approach. In nursing education and healthcare, the concept of *wellness* describes the development of a balanced and harmonious personality in an ecological environment and explains a holistic healthcare model.

In Betty Neuman's systems model, a human being is looked at as an open system that cooperates with the environment to develop harmony and balance between the internal and external environment. The aim of healthcare is to preserve and maintain human systems – the stability of the endosystem in the environment accurately assessing the potential and existing stress factors in the environment. Neuman characterizes the concept of *wellness* as an antonym to the concept of illness, pointing out that it is the condition of a human body in which all system parts and subparts forming the body are in balance and harmony with the whole system. Illness, on the contrary, indicates disharmony or imbalance among parts and subparts of the client system. Wholeness is based on the interrelationships of variables which determine the amount of resistance an individual has to any stressor (Neuman, 2010).

In the context of formation of the ecological approach and research on the development of the ecological competence, it is particularly important to integrate the concept of *wellness* as a key word, which was already present in Halbert L. Dunn's (1896–1975) work on healthcare. Miller (2005) explains the essence of the concept as follows:

1) Wellness is a holistic approach to health, which includes physical, intellectual, social, cultural and spiritual aspects.
2) Intellectual wellness is each person's own responsibility; it cannot be put on somebody else's shoulders.
3) Wellness is associated with each individual's potential; it means helping someone to move towards the highest possible degree of well-being.
4) Self-knowledge and self-integration are keys to a high degree of well-being.

The dimensions characterizing wellness form a systemic and holistic view about creating a positive and supportive social, educational and healthcare environment, encompassing the physical, intellectual, spiritual and social well-being of each individual in an ecological environment. Boyden (1987) describes the concept of human wellness from a biological point of view as a condition of the soul, fit to maintain its life and reproduce. From a subjective point of view, health is viewed as a state of mind of the soul and the flesh when it is a pleasure to live.

Wellness is an active lifelong process in which a person begins to recognize her/his own choices and make decisions favouring a balanced and satisfying life, regardless of the severity of the individual's illness. Wellness is linked to a choice that relates to our lives and the priorities that determine our lifestyle. The concept of wellness focuses on commitment and the idea that the mind, body, spirit and society are interconnected and interdependent (The Center for Integrative Medicine, 2005).

Wellness from an ecological perspective is the ability of a system to maintain the interrelationship and functions in reference to the whole system. It is a state of balance between a human body and the physical, biological and social factors of the environment that ensures normal functioning of a human body. The concept of *environment* is one of the most significant concepts that demands corresponding clarity as every system is characterized by its internal and external environment.

Commitment to the ecological health theory aims to broaden the existing healthcare perspectives by incorporating broader perceptions of global ecosystems, communities and interrelationships derived from the ecological science through the theory of derivation process. When assessing the environmental definitions in the nursing theories/models, it can be concluded that the overview of these definitions reflects a consistent view of the environment as a unit or object, and rarely affects the role of biotic and abiotic interrelations or an environment within the environment. Thus, it is pointed out that the current perception of the environment in healthcare is uncertain and overwhelmed by competing short-term definitions that lack consistent epistemology of healthcare professionals; the term *ecosystem* is proposed as an alternative to the concept of the environment in the healthcare discipline (Laustsen, 2006).

Transforming ideas from the varied historic heritage of nursing theories and models and their influence on the development of nursing science and healthcare in the twenty-first century and integrating the ecological approach in education and healthcare environment, one can conclude that these ideas are becoming more topical in contemporary nursing education and healthcare. The ecological approach promotes the unity and congruence of nursing science and healthcare as the interaction between humans and the environment.

The ecology of human development in the process of education and healthcare

The ecology of human development based on the research and insights of Bronfenbrenner (Urie Bronfenbrenner, 1917–2005) and other scholars makes a significant methodological foundation for the formation of the ecological principles. Urie Bronfenbrenner (1917–2005), the author of the theory of the ecology of human development, relates his philosophy to the scientific study of the progressive mutual accommodation between an active, growing human being and the changing properties of the immediate settings in which the developing person lives. He believes that this process is affected by relations between these settings and by the larger contexts in which the settings are embedded (Bronfenbrenner, 1979).

In the context of the present research, the growing person is a student in the process of education and healthcare. During this process, a student – the growing person – acquires a more extended, differentiated and valid conception of the ecological environment and becomes motivated and able to engage in activities that in form and content sustain or restructure that environment at levels of similar or greater complexity or reveal the properties of that environment (Bronfenbrenner, 1979).

There are three main types of interaction identified between a developing, growing person and the ecological environment and setting:

1. a person keeps changing and accommodating to the environment that does not change;
2. a person changes the environment without changing himself or herself;
3. there is a mutual interaction, accommodation and development between a person and the environment.

The significant concept of *environment* receives special emphasis in the summary of the main concepts and insights of systemology. Every system is characterized by its internal and external environment. Its structure is a display of its parts forming the system. The internal environment is a whole made of its components; the external environment, in its turn, is everything that the respective system does not comprise. Every system is an externally designed internal environment separated by the system's border surface.

Transforming the definition and propositions put forward by Bronfenbrenner that there is a correlation in every place, a theoretical foundation for a dyadic correlation between the education process of students and healthcare practice can be established. When students cooperate and participate in the education process and healthcare practice, observation dyads and dyads of joint or shared activities are developed (Figure 25.1).

In the education process and healthcare practice of students, dyadic relationships provide critical context for individual development. They also provide the basic construction of a microsystem improving on a broader range of skills in interpersonal structures, triads, tetrads, and so forth. To promote psychological development, a dyad acquires different functional forms in the education process and healthcare practice of students emphasizing the potential for interaction and development.

An observation dyad in the process of a favourable interaction shapes a mutually supportive emotional attitude among students during the process of education and healthcare practice. An observation dyad plays a significant role in the process of education and healthcare practice of students as the obtained knowledge and skills do not always correspond to the real-life healthcare situations. By paying attention to and being aware of the interest shown, students can develop an attitude, motivation and appropriate behaviour, for example, by

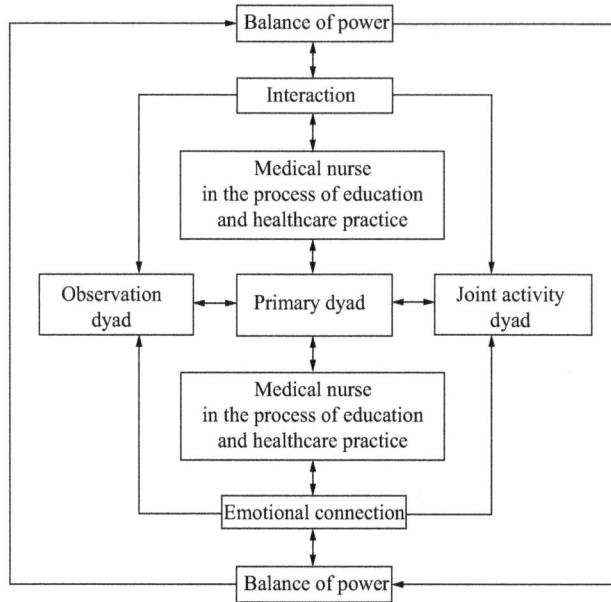

Figure 25.1 Dyadic relationships in the process of education and healthcare practice.

actively participating in the study process, joining in discussions, expressing their opinion based on their knowledge and experience and by being able to analyse and assess any problem situation critically.

A dyad of joint or shared activities is characterized by the balance of power in the subject–subject relationship – not competing but cooperating and participating. Dyads of joint or shared activities in the process of education and healthcare practice can be characterized by the application and use of the theoretical knowledge in healthcare practice. During their clinical practice, students acquire healthcare skills. Attitude, motivation and appropriate behaviour – all of these affect the dyad of joint or shared activities.

In Bronfenbrenner's bioecological theory of human development, the concept of an *endosystem* is replaced by the concept of the growing or developing person mentioned in the definitions. The concept of *a student in the process of education and healthcare practice* is applied respectively. To demonstrate the development of a student that has occurred during the process of education and healthcare practice, it is necessary to establish that a change produced in the conceptions and/or activities of a student carries over to other settings and other times. Such demonstration is referred to as developmental validity (Bronfenbrenner, 1979, Definition 9).

From a systemic point of view, an endosystem is the core of a system. The growing/ developing student in a social, educational and healthcare environment characterized by a physical, social, psychological and spiritual affiliation with this environment is like an open systemic whole in an ecological environment.

This approach corresponds to the requirements put forward by Bronfenbrenner and Morris who insist on researching simultaneously both – an individual and the environment. It is also in line with R. Lerner's view about the related systems and merging of systems (Bronfenbrenner & Morris, 2006; Lerner, 2006).

An endosystem, which the research singles out as the core of a system, merges with a *microsystem*, which is the immediate environment a student gets involved in during the process of education and healthcare practice. Bronfenbrenner emphasizes that, when analysing a microsystem, the full interpersonal system operating in the given setting must be taken into account as this system typically includes all the participants present (including the researcher) and their reciprocal relations (Bronfenbrenner, 1979). Bronfenbrenner defines four general types of interrelations between two or more settings/environments in which the developing person/student becomes an active participant during the process of education and healthcare practice. He proposes the following interconnections: (1) multisetting participation; (2) indirect linkage; (3) interesting communications; and (4) interesting knowledge.

By taking part in different education and healthcare practice environments, a student will have positive developmental effects formed as a result of different interconnections, for example, through international cooperation and student exchange programmes. Different environments/settings fit into cultural and subcultural contexts and will vary as to their ethnicity, social class, religion, age group or other background factors. Students will thus benefit from such developmental experience, but their capacity to profit will vary directly as a function of the number of transcontextual dyads, across a variety of settings, in which students in their process of education and healthcare practice have participated prior to that experience (Bronfenbrenner, 1979).

A macrosystem should be understood as a system with a wider ecological context situated furthest away from the immediate experience of students in the process of education and healthcare practice. At this level, different social factors are involved in the socialization process of a person.

Education for sustainable development and sustainability/sustainable development in healthcare

UNESCO International Commission on Education believes that future society should be a learning society and their most important conclusion is that the most significant process of sustainability/sustainable education is learning. ESD promotes the active participation of nurses in sustainable development processes in order to meet sustainability criteria in their personal lives and to jointly engage with others in sustainable development processes, both locally and globally. This makes nursing ESDan integral part of the sustainability of the healthcare process.

Sterling describes sustainable education as a change in educational culture, where sustainability theory and practice develop in a critical way. It could be transformative teaching and learning that provide an understanding of the value of knowledge, develop endurance and encompass human potential in terms of the need to achieve and strengthen social, economic and ecological well-being, recognizing that they are deeply interconnected processes (Sterling, 2001). Education is becoming one of the main mechanisms to create nurses' wellness and their quality of life. Quality of education and quality of life are the main emphases in the development of sustainable education.

Sustainability/sustainable development in nursing and healthcare must be understood in the context of globalization and global processes, which are characterized both as a process and as a state, as a system, as power and era, based on changing forms of human interaction. So far, education has been regarded as a process that allows an appropriate level of education to be achieved through the acquisition of professional knowledge and skills, while sustainability/sustainable development sets the goal of learning to be – this is the overriding task of personal development.

The concept of sustainable education and its explanation highlight several significant and topical concepts – change of attitude, environmental awareness, behaviour, responsibility and values that make the components of the principles of the ecological approach in nursing. In order to realize the tendencies of the development of sustainable education, the metacognitive understanding of what is knowledge is necessary for the learning process. Nursing education implies that learning is not only a knowledge acquisition, but also a path to individual and collective self-determination and emancipation by perceiving learning as a systemic thinking process in an education and healthcare environment based on communication, the exchange of ideas, mutual understanding, cooperation and respect. Sterling suggests that the ecological approach dimensions are closely related to the knowledge dimension and experience of the interconnected structure (Sterling, 2003).

In nursing education and healthcare, the paradigm changes from mechanical to ecological are related to three key words, relate, expand and implement, the meaning of which can be explained by three respective questions. By answering the questions: How do we perceive it? How do we imagine it? How do we do it? a vision of nursing education is shaped with a transition from the mechanical to ecological paradigm. The characteristics of the ecological paradigm are related to the development of a nurse in an ecological environment by expanding and focusing attention on inner, invisible spiritual processes through which nurses acquire, remember and use information about their internal and external setting. All learners develop and actively implement their own meaningful stimuli and a plan for lifelong and life-wide learning with the aim of developing a personality who has critical and systems thinking, independence and reflection skills, and can solve the twenty-first-century issues in social, education and healthcare environments.

An explanation of the concept of sustainable development highlights the concepts of change in attitudes, environmental awareness, behaviour, responsibility and values that are components of the principles of the ecological approach in nursing. In order to understand the complex shift in the systems of sustainability/sustainable development in nursing educa-tion and healthcare, we must begin to evaluate what needs to be changed in the process of nursing education.

Education and healthcare have been rightly considered as a continuous process of further development and improvement of nurses. This process directly influences wellness and life quality of individuals and society as a whole. The importance of sustainable education, its further development and meaningful content provide the basis for developing an ability and inner motivation for learning to learn and, by adopting systems thinking, nurses can under-stand and take part in resolving the twenty-first-century local and global healthcare issues characteristic of the multidimensional contemporary environment.

The ecological approach that is based on the ecology of education expands the view of a nurse on the ongoing processes and develops ecological consciousness. The ecological paradigm is a way of developing the potential opportunities of a nurse in a multidimensional environment on an individual and society level. The foundation of the ecological paradigm is lifelong learning and further development of a holistic healthcare model.

Comprehension models

The ecological approach involves dynamic, engaging active learning, based on the principle of acquiring wider knowledge, in order to understand the problem and situation solution in the context of a real healthcare environment. The integral part of the theory in nursing education is the healthcare practice and the context of the ecological environment.

Carper (2004) has developed four comprehension models of healthcare, which she calls fundamental patterns of knowing in nursing:

1) The first pattern of knowing is defined as empirics or the science of nursing that is based on observable and measurable information obtained by quantitative research methods. Developing Carper's patterns of knowing further, in cooperation with Chinn and Kramer; the critical questions for empiric understanding are:

    - What is it?
    - How does it work?

2) The second pattern of knowing is aesthetics or the art of nursing that includes recognizing the meaning of different health situations and reactions to them; the critical questions for aesthetic understanding are:

    - What does it mean?
    - Why is it important?

Aesthetic knowledge in nursing is related to healthcare that historically has been considered and perceived as an art and is one of the knowledge dimensions that manifests itself in a work of art. Aesthetic knowledge is characterized by subjectivity and individuality; it is unique, and its main components are intuition, interpretation, understanding and evaluation.

3) The third pattern of knowing is personal knowledge which helps nurses to get to know themselves better. The critical questions are:

    - Do I know what I am doing?
    - Am I doing what I know?

Personal knowledge, similar to aesthetic knowledge, is subjective; nurses are able to evaluate themselves critically and their attitude to others with respect and have a holistic approach to the relationship between a nurse and a patient/client. This knowledge requires self-confidence and an active empathic participation.

4) The fourth pattern of knowing is ethics or the moral component; the critical questions for this pattern of knowing are:

    - Is it right?
    - Is it responsible?

Ethical knowledge in this pattern of knowing manifests itself in following moral norms and making ethical decisions as there are many situations in healthcare practice requiring moral judgement between competing interventions. Ethical knowledge in nursing and healthcare is characterized by an ability to judge what is right and what is wrong, what are the best, most valuable and desired solutions and outcomes of healthcare (Carper, 2004; Chin & Kramer, 2004)

For nurses to really take up and develop their own personal, professional and social roles, decision making is of great importance. It is an opportunity for nurses to better understand and identify global challenges. In the twenty-first century, which is considered to be the information age, one of the prerequisites for successful learning is the critical reflection and analysis of the knowledge gained.

The principles of the ecological approach and the model of ecological competence in nursing education and healthcare

In nursing education and healthcare, the philosophical rationale behind the formation and development of the ecological approach and ecological competence is the deep ecology and ecosophy. Compared to other prominent theories, deep ecology has not crystallized into a complete system. Deep ecological thinking is a process without end. It is rather a set of prescient hints about the real connections and relations in society, culture and nature. These hints are to environmental philosophy as a tree trunk is to its roots and branches (Rothenberg, 1996). Naess believed it is important that nowadays we highly value knowledge and intellectual skills, because of the special place we human beings have among the earth's living creatures, and much more clearly than anything else, is determined by our intellectual abilities. Describing world education, it focuses on knowledge rather than recognition, on the emphasis on the abstract rather than specific themes, and the variety and scale of growth of these themes and the attention are focused primarily on an objective learning. Ecological wisdom (ecosophy) in nursing education promotes sustainable development and, as an outcome of the learning process, provides ecological knowledge and ecological skills as well as forms and develops ecological consciousness in order to emphasize morality and spirituality, which are distinctive human characteristics. The first and seventh points of Naess's and Session's eight-point platform formulate the basic philosophical principles of the ecological competence of nurses.

The first point of the platform states that the well-being and flourishing of human and non-human life on earth have value in themselves (synonyms: intrinsic value, inherent worth). These values are independent of the usefulness of the non-human world for human purposes.

The seventh point declares that the ideological change will be mainly that of appreciating quality of life (dwelling in situations of inherent value) rather than adhering to an increasingly higher standard of living. There will be a profound awareness of the difference between bigness and greatness (Næss, 2008; Sessions, 1995).

The often-cited eight-point platform developed by Naess and Sessions could make a new beginning for the ethics of a new practice in healthcare. It is an open-ended continuous attempt to apprehend the complexity and wholeness in the life of a human. Knowledge about the accurate and precise content of nature leads us to a conclusion that change is necessary in nursing education and healthcare.

Ecological consciousness and the criteria for its formation

Ecological consciousness has been developed as a tool for nurses to accumulate experience in the process of learning and cognition, to learn how to deal with problem situations, how to turn a confusing and incomprehensible situation into something that is manageable, to look for and find solutions and make mistakes. A distinguishing feature of the ecological consciousness of nurses is an ability to make a choice as all humans and their actions have significance and a purpose. The transformation from I-ego to I-eco in their life activities, in the process of their education and healthcare, is the characteristics of the endosystem environment of the ecological consciousness of nurses from a systemic point of view. It is a mistake to treat the ecological crisis only as natural hazards and pollution. The basis of ecological crisis is the present anthropocentric ecological awareness which was based on the illusion of the potential abundance of new technologies and other factors, and the development of consumer attitudes. Ecocentric ecological consciousness must replace anthropocentric ecological consciousness. Adapting the characteristics of anthropocentric and ecocentric ecological consciousness developed in line with the ideas of deep ecology and ecosophy, the ecology of education, transformative learning, ESD and the formation of ecological consciousness, the criteria and indicators of the formation and development of the ecological consciousness of nurses have been defined that help to identify the formation of the ecological consciousness of a nurse (Table 25.1).

The primary characteristics of nurses' ecological consciousness are the ability to choose because humans and their activities make sense and meaning first. The *I-ego* transformation into the *I-eco* in life, education and healthcare processes is the profile of the nurse endosystem ecological consciousness from the systemic view. The criteria for the establishment of ecological consciousness are the rationale behind the principles of the ecological approach and are consistent with the characteristics of the quality of the nursing education and healthcare.

Table 25.1 The criteria and indicators of the formation of the ecological consciousness

Criteria of the formation of ecological consciousness	Indicators of the formation of ecological consciousness
1.Self-awareness – realization of oneself as a developing/growing spiritual being in an ecosystem (not in a fixed position)	• Intrinsic motivation to learn • Systemic thinking • Critical thinking • Reflection • Awareness of the necessity for sustainable development of the environment • Independent decision making
2 Cooperation in subject–subject relationships	• Respect for human life and for living beings as a value in every cycle of life • Responsible conduct • Equal cooperation • Acceptance of pluralism • Promotion of wellness • Respect for cultural and religious diversity
3.Awareness of the highest likely potential in the development of I freedom	• Awareness of the freedom of I and we existence (including nature) • Awareness of the existence of a global environmental crisis as a result of human activities and practices and as a threat to humanity's existence • Democratic and constructive activities with an aim of protecting and sustaining the environment and solving environmental issues in everyday life activities and healthcare, primarily advocating universal values of wellness in nature and humans • An ongoing journey of self-discovery and self-knowing (through critical thinking and reflection) that leads to integration and responsible conduct in social, educational and healthcare environment

The principles of the ecological approach in nursing education and healthcare

In formulating the principles of the ecological approach, it was found that it was not possible to drastically separate the principles of the ecological approach from the principles built up for centuries in medicine and healthcare found in several documents and publications on health philosophy and medical ethics. The principles of the ecological approach in nursing education and healthcare meet the pillars of ESD and the concepts of deep ecology and ecosophy for sustainability and sustainable development in the ecosystem, characterizing ecological consciousness in nursing and the formation and development process of ecological competence (UNESCO, 2010a, 2010b, 2010c, 2010d).

The principle of developing the ability to think and the performance and experiential growth

The pillar of ESD: learning to know

By making independent decisions, nurses raise their awareness of being developing/growing spiritual beings in an ecosystem; the knowledge acquired in the process of cognition and learning gives the sense of satisfaction, stimulates the ability to think and enhances reflection and critical thinking; the knowledge-based skills/abilities further enrich the experience and performance in everyday life activities and healthcare processes.

The principle of responsibility

The pillar of ESD: learning to live together

Nurses demonstrate ongoing self-knowing, responsible and congruent, conduct and performance through functioning, and integrating into social, educational and healthcare multidimensional environment.

The principle of transformation

The pillar of ESD: learning to be

Nurses are making a conscious choice about the existence or lack of me and us according to the given situation and reaching the highest possible potential in the development of I freedom.

The principle of being aware of the cause-and-effect principle, safety advocacy, and promoting wellness

The pillar of ESD: learning to live together, learning to do

Nurses are aware of the existence of a global environmental crisis as the result of human activities and practices and as a threat to humanity's wellness in future generations, solving environmental issues, protecting and sustaining the environment in everyday life and healthcare in a democratic and constructive way, primarily advocating universal safety in different dimensions of wellness or significant fields of life, showing respect for religious and cultural diversity in multilevel communication environments, accepting pluralism and maintaining/ sustaining wellness in dyads, triads and tetrads.

The principle of the unity and wholeness of the core values in education and healthcare

Pillar of ESD: learning to transform oneself and society

By active participation in the processes of developing society wellness and maintaining sustainability of the environment, nurses adjust/attune their feelings and the core values in education and healthcare process. The defined principles of the ecological approach complement the code of ethics of nurses and integrate the criteria of ecological consciousness into a global systemic view as a development process of a spiritual harmonious being in an ecosystem. This all relates to several aspects of the process–person–context–time system, for example, a process and a person or a living being in an ecological setting (Bronfenbrenner, Morris, 2006; Tudge, Mokrova et al., 2009).

The ecological competence model

The concept of competence depends on from what aspect the competence is looked at, namely, as a result, a process and characteristics of a personal quality or the competence as an ongoing lifelong development of its components maintaining sustainability from a global point of view. From a competence point of view, analysing which key categories characterize the implementation of the competent approach in the field of education, it must be stressed that competence is a dynamic human trait that develops from a professional beginner's level and is acquired in vocational education as the highest form of competence in the direction of mastery. Incorporating the emotional, self-regulating, motivational and behavioural component into the competencies system is a methodological error because then the competent approach and professional competence are downgraded as a measurable category, singling out five components of competence:

1   readiness and motivation aspect: readiness is viewed as the ability of the entity to mobilize forces;
2   the cognitive aspect – knowledge that explains and covers competence;
3   experience and behavioural manifestation – competence in various standard and non-standard situations;
4   the attitude to the content of competence – as a matter of point and value;
5   competence in regulating the process of developing emotional willpower.

The professional competence of nurses includes several connected components that, interrelating with critical thinking, reflection and experience, highlight the essence of the nursing profession. In the context of the ecological approach, the foundation for sustainable development of nurses as a value-oriented harmonious personality in an ecological environment is characterized by 12 components of their professional competence:

1   two knowledge levels – perception and comprehension of healthcare
2   acquired theoretical knowledge manifests itself in practical skills in healthcare
3   the attitude is characterized by self-confidence and self-assessment

4 accomplishments expand the range of the given natural talents

5 willpower characterizes the level of professional development

6 the component of values is an emotional driving force and a virtue

7 motivation includes an emphasis on understanding the need for and the importance of ongoing continuous education

8 empathy is an essential professional ability

9 experience is an ongoing process of development

10 creativity in the professional activity is a spiritual process of seeking new non-standard solutions to healthcare situations

11 innovation is integration of new ideas and technologies in healthcare practice

12 cooperation in a healthcare team interacting with patients/clients, their family and relatives taking supportive and congruent action.

Critical thinking refers not only to the education process. It is a manifestation of responsible and professional conduct of a nurse in the healthcare process. Critical thinking and reflection create the interrelation of different specific components of the professional competence in the healthcare. The components of the professional competence and the criteria of the ecological consciousness determine the content of the components of the ecological competence of nurses and complement the components of the formation and development of the ecological competence.

The formation and development of ecological competence reflect an integrated collection of abilities/skills in social, educational and healthcare environments and a creative process of professional performance because of experience. The term integrated in the process of the formation and development of the ecological competence should be perceived as a necessity to be complete, well-grounded/founded, one whole consisting of many small parts making one complete whole, entire wholeness and many-sided, comprehensive and proportional (Wilber, 2008).

The components of the professional competence complement and integrate knowledge about sustainable development and sustainable processes in a social, educational and healthcare environment, the ecology of human development and deep ecology and ecosophy. This integration is characterized by five topical components: (1) a systemic view; (2) systemic thinking; (3) knowledge; (4) empathy; and (5) an ability to cooperate. Intrinsic motivation to learn is a manifestation form of the synergetic approach that reveals systemic thinking and a systemic view of a nurse in the process of self-development and self-organization in an ecological environment.

The process provides the construct for the content of the model of the ecological competence of nurses and includes the subject–subject relationship of mutual interaction and cooperation that takes place and develops over a period and provides the most important mechanism integral to personality development. The process includes the formation and development of ecological consciousness in an endosystem, enhancing the intrinsic motivation to learn and promoting systemic thinking in the social, educational and healthcare environment. By increasing the ability to learn during the developmental process, nurses also improve the skills for implementing the learning pillars of ESD – learning to be, learning to live together, learning to transform themselves and society. Ecological wisdom, which is developed in line with the principles of the ecological approach, is the characteristic parameter of emotional intelligence-empathy in social, educational and healthcare environments.

A description of the ecological competence of nurses has been developed. The ecological competence of nurses is the ability to develop their personality from I-ego to I-eco during an ongoing continuous transformation process in their lifetime, complementarily linking their personal, theoretical and practical knowledge and skills with the knowledge of ecology, developing a systemic view of the components of the professional competence on an ecosystem level from a holistic perspective and implementing the ecological approach in social, educational and healthcare environments.

Conclusion

Taking ideas from Nightingale's historic heritage and its influence on the development of nursing science and healthcare in the twenty-first century and integrating the ecological approach in education and healthcare environment, one can conclude that these ideas are still topical in contemporary nursing education and healthcare. The ecological approach promotes the unity and congruence of nursing science and healthcare as the interaction between humans and the environment, and in fact, dominates several nursing theories and models. From a historical perspective, understanding of the role of the environment has greatly influenced the development of nursing theories and models and healthcare practice. The subject–subject relationship, cooperation and interaction in the process of education and healthcare practice form positive and creative education and healthcare environments. The ecological approach in education process and healthcare should pay more attention and show more concern about the process of developing the personality of nurses, their skills of reflection and critical thinking so that they are able to implement an ecological competence model based on ecological consciousness

References

Boyden S (1987) *Western Civilization in Biological Perspective*. Oxford: Oxford University Press.

Bronfenbrenner U (1979) *The Ecology of Human Development. Experiments by Nature and Design*. Cambridge: MA Harvard University Press.

Bronfenbrenner U & Morris P A (2006) The Bioeclogical Model of Human Development. In R M Lerner & W Damon (Eds.). *Theoretical Models of Human Development, Vol. (1). The Handbook of Child Psychology* (5thEd). New York: Wiley & Sons, pp. 793–828.

Carper B A (2004) Fundamental Patterns of Knowing in Nursing. In P G Reed, N C Shearer & L HNicoll (Eds.) *Perspectives on Nursing Theory*. Philadelphia: Lippincott Williams &Wilkins, (pp. 221–228).

Chin P L & Kramer M K (2004) *Integrating Knowledge Development in Nursing (6th Ed)* St.Louis, MO: Mosby.

Laustsen G (2006) Jan-Mar Environment, Ecosystems, and Ecological 17ugust17o: A Dialoguetoward Developing Nursing Ecological Theory. *Advances in Nursing Science* 29 (1): 43–54.

Miller J W (2005) Wellness: The History and Development of a Concept. *Spektrum Freizeit*, 1: 84–102.

Mollenhauer K (1977) Interaktion und Organisation in pädagogischen Feldern. In: H Blankertz (Ed.) *(Hg.): Interaktion und Organisation in pädagogischen Feldern (= Z. f. Päd., 13. Beih.)*. Weinheim/Basel. S., pp. 39–57.

Næss A (2008) The Shallow and the Deep, Long-range Ecology Movement. A Summary Arne Naess. *Inquiry: An Interdisciplinary Journal of Philosophy* 16 (1-4): 95–100.

Neuman B (2010) *The Neuman Systems Model (3rd Ed)*. Norwalk, CT:Appleton Lange.

Lerner R M (2006) Editor's Introduction: Developmental Science, Developmental Systems and Contemporary Theories. In R M Lerner (Ed.). *Theoretical Models of Human Development. Handbook of Child Psychology*, Vol. 1 (6th Ed). Hoboken, NJ: Wiley, pp. 1–17.

Rothenberg D (1996) No World But in Things: The Poetry of Naess's Concrete Contents. *Inquiry: An Interdisciplinary Journal of Philosophy and the Social Sciences* 39 (2): 255–272.

Sessions G (1995) Ecocentrism and the Anthropocentric Detour. In G Sessions (Ed.). *Deep Ecology for the 21st Century. Readings on the Philosophy and Practice of the New Environmentalism.* Boston and London: Shambhala Publications, pp.156–183.

Sterling S (2001) *Sustainable Education. Re – visioning Learning and Change. Schumacher Briefing* (6). Bristol: Green Books.

Sterling S (2003) *Whole Systems Thinking as a Basis for Paradigm Change in Education: Explorations in the Context of Sustainability.* (PhD thesis). Centre for Research in Education andthe Environment, University of Bath. Accessed at at: www.bath.ac.uk/cree/sterling/sterlingtitle.pdf.

The Center for Integrative Medicine (2005) Accessed at: www.google.lv/search?q=integrative+medical +wellness+center&hl=lv&gbv=2&oq=integrative+medical+centre+wellness&gs_l=heirloomser p.1.0.0i22i30l3.39000.45579.0.49360.9.9.0.0.0.0.0.125.655.8j1.9.0 ... 0 ... 1ac.1.34.heirloom-serp.0.9.655GH9jrjs_9zs.

Tudge J, Mokrova I, Hatfield B & Karnik R (2009) (Eds.) Uses and Misuses of Bronfenbrenner's Bioecological Theory of Human Development. *Journal of Family Theory and Review* 1 (4): 198–210.

UNESCO. (2010a). Education. Learning to know. [Online]. Available at http://www.unesco.org/en/ education-for-sustainable-development/strategy/learning-to-know/#c16163pdf

UNESCO. (2010b). Education. Learning to do. [Online]. Available at http://www.unesco.org/en/edu cation-for-sustainable-development/strategy/learning-to-do/#c16151pdf

UNESCO (2010c). Education. Learning to be. [Online]. Available at http://www.unesco.org/en/educa tion-for-sustainable-development/strategy/learning-to-be/#c16159 pdf

UNESCO (2010d). Education. Learning to transform oneself and society. [Online]. Available at http:// www.unesco.org/en/education-for-sustainable-development/strategy/learning-to-transform/ #c16148 pdf

Wilber K (2008) *Integral Life Practice: A 21st-Century Blueprint for Physical Health, Emotional Balance, Mental Clarity, and Spiritual Awakening.* Boulder: Shambhala.

26

THINK WELL, PRACTISE WELL

Teaching nurse students to think critically

Steve Parker and Sandra Egege

Introduction

We all think. Nurse clinicians are constantly acting, and the quality of their thinking determines the quality of their actions. These actions can and do have significant consequences for the health and wellbeing of the patients and clients we care for. If we think well our actions promote positive outcomes and the lives of people using our healthcare systems are improved. If we think poorly our actions will tend to undermine those health outcomes and potentially can cause major and permanent physical, psychological and emotional injury or, in some cases, death. Given the significance of thinking in determining our actions and the serious consequences of poor thinking, it is unsurprising that there are constant global calls for critical thinking to be developed. Almost everyone agrees that critical thinking is a necessary skill in the twenty-first century.

This chapter sets out the why, what and how of teaching critical thinking skills to nursing students and nurse clinicians. We begin with the significance of critical thinking to nursing practice and include a brief discussion of some basic concepts of epistemology that are essential in understanding the broader context of critical thinking to nursing practice. This moves into a discussion of some of the cultural issues related to the teaching and learning of critical thinking, which are so relevant for a globalised and international environment.

Following this overview, we turn our attention to what is meant by critical thinking in general and then within the nursing context and discuss various approaches that have been taken to foster a critical thinking capacity and attitude. We finish by listing a variety of resources that readers can use, as well as offering practical advice on how these skills can continue to be developed.

The significance of critical thinking for nursing practice

Critical thinking is universally recognised as an essential skill for nursing practice. This can be seen when examining practice standards required by various professional nursing bodies.

For example, the Nursing and Midwifery Board of Australia (2016) practice standards for a registered nurse include "Standard 1: Thinks critically and analyses nursing practice". Baccalaureate programmes for nursing often include critical thinking skills as part of their curriculum. For example, the Bachelor of Nursing curriculum for Flinders University in South Australia has as one of its academic outcomes that students will: "use critical thinking abilities to interpret, develop, refine, enhance and validate the range of knowledge embodied in nursing practice" (Flinders University School of Nursing & Midwifery, 2012).

As Miller and Babcock (1996) argue, nurses live and practise in "a complex and changing society", "an evolving world community" and a "multicultural reality" that significantly influences the values, attitudes and practice of nurses (pp. 1–6).

Critical thinking is relevant and significant across many areas of practice. The consequences of nurse clinicians not thinking critically are serious. If nurse educators neglect the development of critical thinking in curriculum for students and clinicians, then we become potentially responsible for the ultimate consequences of students not practising the high standards of safety and professionalism required.

Another important reason for focusing on critical thinking in nursing is epistemological. Understanding why we engage in certain practices and why others are no longer considered appropriate entails understanding the process of knowledge creation that informs nursing practice. Why do we do what we do? How do we know what we know? Understanding how nursing knowledge is created and how and why what we call knowledge changes over time enables us to understand the link between that knowledge and its application in practice. This gives it a practical context. It is not enough to accept that a certain nursing intervention works for a particular patient problem most of the time. We need to have some understanding of why it works. This will enable us to think about its application and whether it might work more effectively if applied differently or even to a different but related problem.

It is important to understand that our knowledge is finite and incomplete. Even though we have gained an inordinate amount of knowledge about the human body, disease, health and healing over the last century, we know there is much more to know. We only need to reflect on the changes to nursing practice since Florence Nightingale to recognise that what we do now is better and more effective than it was. Practice has changed in line with changes to knowledge and the subsequent development of supportive technologies. Our knowledge is not complete, however, and there is still much to find out.

We also know that, as humans, we can make mistakes; we can be wrong. In nursing, this is particularly important to keep in mind, given the competing epistemological paradigms that generate knowledge. While much of nursing knowledge is derived from the empirically based scientific paradigm that informs medical knowledge (evidence-based practice), a great deal of practical nursing knowledge is derived from experience and a qualitative research framework. The nature of empirical scientific research means that its focus is on the physical domain, which remains reasonably constant across diverse contexts. The advantage of conducting research on physical objects is that they can be subjected to testing in controlled environments, variables can be isolated and data sets collected and replicated and results verified. Because of the nature of the research, the way it is conducted and the rigorous controls used to minimise human error, the claims drawn from that research are not only reliable but considered objectively true. While any findings can be questioned, the experimental process should be replicable and, if confirmed, the inferences drawn from the findings can then move into the realm of knowledge.

In addition to knowledge generated from an empirically based scientific paradigm, a great deal of nursing knowledge is derived from practice experience and qualitative research. While human bodies can be classified as physical objects open to empirical testing, they are unique in having a subjective element. As people, they can be interrogated, and the process of interrogation provides a different (often equally informative) qualitative dimension to the purely physical assessment of the medical sciences. Although qualitative research is often viewed as not providing objectively verifiable data, it contributes to an understanding of the lived experiences of patients and their health challenges. This evidence plays a crucial role in nursing practice as it informs the nurse of the effectiveness and impact of a given intervention or the care of an individual. Not all humans respond equally to similar interventions. Not all humans deal with illness in the same way.

For nursing students to apply critical thinking in practice, they need to be aware of the types of knowledge they are using that guide their practice, where it came from and how it was developed. This will allow them to recognise the strengths and the limitations of that knowledge. In this context, how the knowledge is justified – what reasons there are to accept it – will determine how reliable or strong it is. The more evidence or justification there is for a practice, the more likely it is that the practice is appropriate and effective. It is not possible to evaluate that knowledge without knowing what the justification is and how reliable the evidence is supporting it. Effective evaluation of practice requires understanding how the knowledge behind the practice became knowledge and why it still holds. This is what informs and drives practice.

Critical thinkers can apply their knowledge through their practice, critically observe the results of their actions and reflect on the effectiveness of that practice as they go. They analyse and question things. They don't always accept things at face value or because someone says this is what you should do. In the right context and done appropriately, this is a valuable trait, particularly within the area of health where individual circumstances are so important.

What is critical thinking?

Now that we have explored the significance of critical thinking for nurses, we turn to the issue of defining what critical thinking is.

When we go looking for a definition of critical thinking, we discover that there are many that have been proposed. There is a great deal of discussion, diversity of opinion and disagreement around critical thinking – its definition and the teaching of it. Like many others, Davies and Barnett (2015, p. 23) conclude that:

> theorists and educationalists who have given thought to the matter differ profoundly over fundamental aspects of critical thought or criticality. They differ over what is to count as critical thinking, over its purpose and its scope, and the way in which teaching might help to encourage it among students.

Nevertheless, universities operate on the belief that critical thinking skills can be defined, taught, acquired and applied in a range of contexts (Mulnix, 2012). The Delphi Report is the most well-known attempt to reach a consensus view of what critical thinking entails, culminating in Facione's broad definition of what falls within its boundaries (1990):

> We understand critical thinking to be purposeful, self-regulatory judgment which results in interpretation, analysis, evaluation, and inference, as well as explanation of the evidential, conceptual, methodological, criteriological, or contextual considerations upon which that judgment is based.

Following on from the Delphi Report there has been a similar attempt to develop a consensus definition of critical thinking in nursing. Scheffer and Rubenfeld (2000) carried out a five-round Delphi study across nine countries, which resulted in the following definition which, for them, includes habits of mind in addition to cognitive skills:

> Critical thinkers in nursing exhibit these habits of the mind: confidence, contextual perspective, creativity, flexibility, inquisitiveness, intellectual integrity, intuition, open-mindedness, perseverance, and reflection. Critical thinkers in nursing practice the cognitive skills of analyzing, applying standards, discriminating, information seeking, logical reasoning, predicting and transforming knowledge.

While this definition outlines the essential characteristic of critical thinkers, it is relatively abstract and does not connect these traits with the practical, real-world outcomes required by nursing practice. Consequently, we need a definition that incorporates the above but emphasises the *process* of thinking critically.

Therefore, we prefer to define critical thinking as a *process* of analysis and critique that is used to ensure that we come to the most reasonable conclusions we can about the world we live and work in, as well as the best solutions for what we want to achieve. It is a process of thinking that helps us make sure we have strong and reliable grounds for our beliefs and actions and allows us to acknowledge ambiguity or uncertainty when it exists in the real world.

Critical thinking and culture

One of the complexities of the real world in which critical thinking takes place is the diversity of cultures. Nurses often need to apply critical thinking to practice in contexts where they are challenged by multiple cultures and perspectives. There are three aspects we need to be aware of when looking at the impact that culture might have on the application of critical thinking within a health setting. The first is the cultural diversity of the patients a nurse clinician encounters; the second is the cultural diversity of the nursing staff themselves; and the third is the cultural specificity of the notion of critical thinking itself. We will look at the last aspect first as it relates directly to the teaching of critical thinking to a culturally diverse student body.

Many countries are more culturally and linguistically diverse (CALD) than they used to be, even when they are not countries with high migrant populations, because of the amount of social and political upheaval around the world. At the same time globalisation, the continuing internationalisation of universities and skills-based immigration policies have led to an increasingly diverse nursing student cohort, with large numbers of CALD students looking to gain a Western qualification in an English-speaking environment (Bednarz, Schim, & Doorenbos, 2010).

This cultural mix exposes teaching staff to an increasingly diverse student population, some of whom appear to have different academic expectations and approaches to learning. Students from Confucian-heritage cultures (CHC), for example, come from predominantly exam-based assessment pedagogies that do not appear to encourage a critical attitude. Such students desire a more structured learning environment with explicit instruction, the antithesis of what we see as a critical thinking approach (Egege & Kutieleh, 2008). Because of this, there has been a suggestion that critical thinking itself is a Western cultural concept. This is important to ascertain as the critical thinking discourse speaks of representing "universal" standards of thinking, implying a cross-cultural application (e.g., Paul and Elder,

2010). If this is not the case, then we should acknowledge its culturally specific nature when teaching critical thinking skills to a culturally diverse group. This is relevant if we want to incorporate critical thinking instruction into nursing education degrees taught in non-Western cultures by non-Western-educated staff.

How Western is the concept of critical thinking? It should be noted that the model of critical thinking used at universities has emerged from the classical Greek tradition of philosophy and its focus on argumentation, so it can be said to have Western roots. This does not mean, however, that what we view as rational or clear thinking is purely a Western concept or a prerogative of the West. All cultures have had to solve problems by finding solutions to survive. What we recognise today as science and medicine were well developed in China, India, North Africa and the Middle East centuries before Europe went through its intellectual enlightenment. Those developments necessarily built on experience and evidence of what seemed to work. So, it would be false to say that the rational thinking process and the use of justification as part of critical thinking are Western cultural innovations.

Cognition and meta-cognition are human, not cultural, capacities. The culture merely provides the opportunities to develop certain types of capacities. Having said that, the *ways* we expect students to show *evidence* of critical thinking in their *academic work* is very specific. We expect students to demonstrate their critical thinking through the "argumentative essay" using counter-argument and critique, which is part of the Socratic philosophic tradition. The expectation to "question everything", including the voice of authority, is integral to that tradition which is adversarial rather than aimed at reinforcing traditional positions (Lloyd, 1996). This process does not sit well with some cultures and political systems and needs to be explained within the context of knowledge development and models of best practice. Reflecting on and explaining the cultural and academic expressions of critical thinking that we expect and take for granted can help others to better understand and apply critical thinking in their practice as appropriate. When students from CHC backgrounds are given permission to question, critique, overtly disagree and justify their views, they perform as well as (if not better than) any other student (Biggs, 1997). This indicates that it is the method of thinking, not the capacity to think critically, that is culturally specific.

Engaging in an open process of critically examining, identifying and then explaining any cultural differences we might have empowers students from other cultures to do the same. It is important for nursing students to be aware of their own cultural beliefs and biases and how these can impact on their assessment and care of patients. The cultural diversity of nursing staff and the patient clientele does have practical implications that can lead to ill-informed actions and inappropriate interventions through misunderstandings and cultural stereotyping. In such a context, thinking critically and self-reflectively becomes essential for best practice. The patients we encounter come from a range of different cultural and religious backgrounds and this often means they may have a different approach to health and what is considered healthy practice.

We need to reflect on our own beliefs and evaluate the potential impact they may have on how we judge different cultural groups and alternative practices or different social norms. For example, cultural beliefs and practices around pregnancy, childbirth and breast-feeding can be wildly divergent. While some of these may be innocuous and have minimal impact, others may be viewed by nursing staff as potentially dangerous, detrimental to the healthy outcome of the child or "just plain wrong". We need to think carefully and critically about how we deal with cultural conflict like this, assess the benefits of intervening or not and determine to what extent our own reactions come from a narrow cultural norm or a legitimate evidence-based position. Therefore, an understanding of our own epistemological framework and what evidence grounds our practice is highly relevant.

Likewise, some cultural groups are more likely to manifest certain ailments reflective of their dietary habits and lifestyles, which can lead to stereotyping and mistaken assessment. We need to be critically aware of our epistemic beliefs and practices to see how these impact on what we consider to be good practice and whether our reactions are cultural rather than epistemologically informed. What is called "culturally congruent care" (Bednarz et al., 2010) is an attempt to conceptualise how we deal with this duality of cultural factors in an attempt to minimise their influence on nurse clinicians to enable the provision of "meaningful, beneficial and satisfying healthcare".

The role of the teacher in developing critical thinking in nurse clinicians

Once we understand the significance of teaching critical thinking to nurses, we need to ask what the role of the teacher is in supporting students to develop critical thinking skills. In our view, the best way to think about the teacher's role is as a coach. In the words of Paul and Elder (2001, p. 2), a teacher's role is to:

> design the class so that YOU model the thinking you are looking for. This requires you either to think aloud in front of the class or to present the class with thinking in written form. Once the appropriate thinking is modeled for the students, we should look for the students to engage in practice that emulates [the thinking model they have been taught].

Paul and Elder (2001) recommend that teachers should see themselves like a basketball coach by "coaching students, sitting on the sidelines, listening to peer interaction, providing feedback on the sorts of problems *in thinking* they are noticing in students". Teaching the process of thinking to students, rather than merely teaching the content of a topic, can be very challenging. This means that, as teachers, we need to think critically about our own teaching before we can be successful at teaching students how to think better; we should be able to *model* critical thinking so that students can see and hear critical thinking in action before they go ahead and practise it themselves.

How to teach critical thinking to nurse students and clinicians

Now that we have explored various aspects of critical thinking, we need to address the question of how to teach it effectively within nurse education. To do that, we will begin by discussing some of the barriers to teaching critical thinking effectively that need to be addressed or avoided and some general principles that have been found to be effective. Then we will recommend a model that we believe is practical and versatile enough to consider the cultural diversity discussed above.

There is a common assumption amongst academics that acquiring a university degree will automatically develop critical thinking skills in graduates. It is generally assumed that these skills develop either through the critical thinking demands of the course or via the process of learning the topic content itself. Research has shown that this is not the case and our assumption is false. One of the recurring problems identified in the critical thinking literature is how *unsuccessful* we have been at teaching it. Numerous studies conducted over many years indicate that university graduates are not leaving universities with well-developed critical thinking capacities, despite our efforts (Abrami et al, 2008; Willingham, 2007). A recent analysis of test results from 200 American Colleges confirmed that this was still the case (Belkin, 2017). According to Abrami et al. (2008, 2015), one of the reasons for our lack of success is the limited levels of expertise or training in what constitutes a good teaching pedagogy. As academics we are rarely taught how to incorporate critical thinking instruction into topics or what the best ways to teach it are. This has resulted in a hit-and-miss approach where some teaching of critical thinking has been very effective while others have not been effective at all (Abrami et al., 2015; Bertacchini De Oliveira et al., 2016). Given how essential critical thinking is to enabling effective nursing practice we need to find out what practices or strategies work and how we can incorporate them in our teaching without sacrificing discipline content.

Trying to ascertain what are effective teaching strategies for developing a critical thinking capacity in students, whether nursing or otherwise, is hampered by the lack of regular rigorous evaluations that have been undertaken. Even when evaluations have been conducted the evidence is often anecdotal or some form of qualitative self-assessment (Bertacchini De Oliveira et al., 2016). There have, however, been a couple of comprehensive reviews which have both managed to find rigorous studies and isolate the strategies that appear to be most effective (Abrami et al., 2015, 2008; Bertacchini De Oliveira et al., 2016; Pithers & Soden, 2000). One academic area where the teaching of critical thinking does have a distinct pedagogy and where critical thinking is the learning outcome is in non-discipline-specific stand-alone critical thinking topics. While these may be effective for developing critical thinking capacities, they are not available at all universities and may not be an option for students to take as part of their degree structure. There is also research emerging that emphasises the connection between thinking and content knowledge (Pithers & Soden, 2000). For our purposes, the more broadly applicable option for nurse educators is how to embed effective critical thinking instruction within discipline topics such as nursing topics. In that way we can ensure that more nursing students have access to explicit critical thinking instruction, can benefit from it and are able to apply it within their knowledge domain.

Things that don't work

It was clear from the reviews we accessed that there were more and *less* effective ways of teaching critical thinking, and some strategies that worked and some that did not. Pithers and Soden (2000, pp. 242–243) outlined a set of student and staff characteristics or approaches that were likely to inhibit the development of critical thinking. For *students*, being impulsive, lacking confidence, having difficulty with comprehension, being over-dependent, inflexible or dogmatic were all characteristics that impeded a critical and self-reflective approach. For *teaching staff*, believing they had nothing to learn, that they were the arbiters of critical thinking, that there was a correct approach and a right answer, that critical thinking was a means to this end, and that students "should be correct 90% of the time", were all seen as impediments to the teaching of critical thinking. Effective critical thinking requires mental flexibility and an embracing of ambiguity. These are traits that need to be encouraged in students and role-modelled by teaching staff. The world is not a static place; situations change and mistakes happen. There could be a different answer or an alternative solution.

In an attempt to see which interventions or strategies had a measurable impact on the effectiveness of teaching critical thinking, Abrami et al. (2008) identified four distinct modes of teaching intervention for critical thinking that were variously used at institutions:

1. the *generic* stand-alone critical thinking topic, already discussed above
2. the *infusion* method where critical thinking skills are *implicitly* embedded in the teaching topic content, but critical thinking is made *explicit* in the content outline
3. the *immersion* method where the teaching topic has engaging or challenging content, but critical thinking is not explicit
4. the *mixed* method where the content includes explicit critical thinking instruction and critical thinking skills are an explicit objective of teaching topic content.

Of them all, the *mixed* method was by far the most effective mode for teaching critical thinking. It produced the most statistically significant effect on critical thinking outcomes compared to the other methods. What was the *least* effective was the *immersion* method. It was also ineffective to just list critical thinking as an objective or to have it included in assignment guidelines. To be effective, critical thinking had to be *explicitly* taught within the teaching topic content. Bertacchini De Oliveira et al.'s review (2016) found that some other well-known strategies did not markedly improve critical thinking. These strategies were simulations, role-modelling, using concept maps, reflective writing or using an animated pedagogical agent. They may have an impact when used in conjunction with other strategies but the research data from their study failed to identify any significance of the strategies in isolation when compared to traditional teaching methods.

Things that do work

First, we need to be clear what it is we want students to be able to do. If all we want is for them to know the right answers and why they are right, then this will not develop their critical thinking skills. Knowledge is an essential foundation, but it is not a skill that will help students to solve practice problems or assess complex situations with multiple competing factors. Nor will setting a problem and giving students the "right" heuristic to mechanically apply. To develop their own problem-solving capacities they need to be able to think critically and thinking critically requires material that provides scope and space for students to work things through. They can benefit from having the thinking modelled and plenty of regular practice.

We know from Abrami et al.'s (2008, 2015) reviews that teaching critical thinking explicitly within the topic or subject domain is the most effective way of getting some improvement in a student's critical thinking skills. We think this is even more relevant within nursing education as it is important for students to think critically about their discipline knowledge and relate it to the context in which they will be working. While the effectiveness of that instruction will be dependent on the way critical thinking is taught, bearing in mind the attitude and expertise of the instructor, there are some effective generic strategies that can be adopted within any topic without sacrificing the knowledge we want students to master.

Drawn from the studies cited in this chapter, the following strategies have resulted in statistically significant improvements in critical thinking skills or dispositions when using validated tests:

- Problem-based learning (PBL) – this was the only strategy identified by the researchers that produced significant improvements *in isolation* (i.e., when used on its own) when compared to traditional methods such as lectures (Bertacchini De Oliveira et al., 2016).
- Authentic instruction – exposing students to authentic clinical practice examples or problems in real-life contexts produced a significant effect when compared to other methods.

- Dialogue or discussion – encouraging students to engage in discussion which is guided by the teacher who "interrogates" a point to push the discussion towards identifying assumptions, biases, contradictions or insufficient evidence, often by asking probing questions that do not threaten or make the student lose confidence. This also produced significant effects, particularly when coupled with authentic instruction.
- Using argument analysis to unpack students' thinking about points of view – this is where the teacher uses argument construction and analysis in conjunction with the Socratic method to expose and critique students' underlying assumptions and values with the aim of broadening their perspectives on issues.
- Using argument mapping – useful for identifying, analysing and mapping arguments found in texts. This has been shown to be useful as a critiquing tool to improve students' critical analysis of research findings and the quality of their own arguments.

The above strategies have been shown to produce measurable improvements in students' critical thinking skills. However, even with these strategies, there are a lot of barriers to thinking objectively that we need to make students aware of, such as perceptual limitations and personal biases. Encouraging students to engage in self-reflection and meta-cognitive thinking will help minimise the impact of these barriers. As teachers, we need to remember that critical thinking is hard work and does not come naturally. We also need to note that critical thinking is a process of making our thinking more rigorous and systematic – there is no "right" way to think but there are better ways to think and act. This requires careful and critical assessment of all relevant factors. It is the role of the lecturer to encourage this critical approach. In this context, it is better if the lecturer acts as a facilitator or coach rather than as an instructor (see section on the role of the teacher in developing critical thinking in nurse clinicians, above).

A model for teaching critical thinking

While there are many specific strategies that have been shown to be effective at teaching critical thinking, one of the issues for teachers is how to use these strategies effectively. To do that, it is useful to have a framework to guide teachers in applying these strategies. The model we recommend is one developed by Paul and Elder (2014). Paul and Elder represent their model with the diagram shown in Figure 26.1.

Critical thinkers can tease their thinking apart and examine each of the elements of thought to come to an understanding of their thinking or the thinking of others. These elements of thought also provide a framework for teasing apart the logic or structure of any topic.

While it is essential to be able to tease one's thinking apart to examine it, it is not enough just to be able to describe the structure or logic of the thinking. If thinking is to be improved, we also need to be able to evaluate the quality of thinking. So, standards of thought need to be applied to the elements of thought to evaluate the quality of the thinking.

When we consistently practise thinking critically by teasing apart our thinking and applying intellectual standards to it, we will begin to develop several intellectual traits or virtues. It almost goes without saying that a nurse with these traits is going to practise better than one without them or where they are poorly developed. This is especially obvious when we list the opposites of these traits: intellectual arrogance, intellectual cowardice, intellectual narrow-mindedness, intellectual conformity, intellectual hypocrisy, intellectual laziness, distrust of reason and evidence and intellectual unfairness. Put like this, it's obvious who we'd want caring for us in healthcare!

Critical thinkers routinely apply intellectual standards to the elements of reasoning in order to develop intellectual traits.

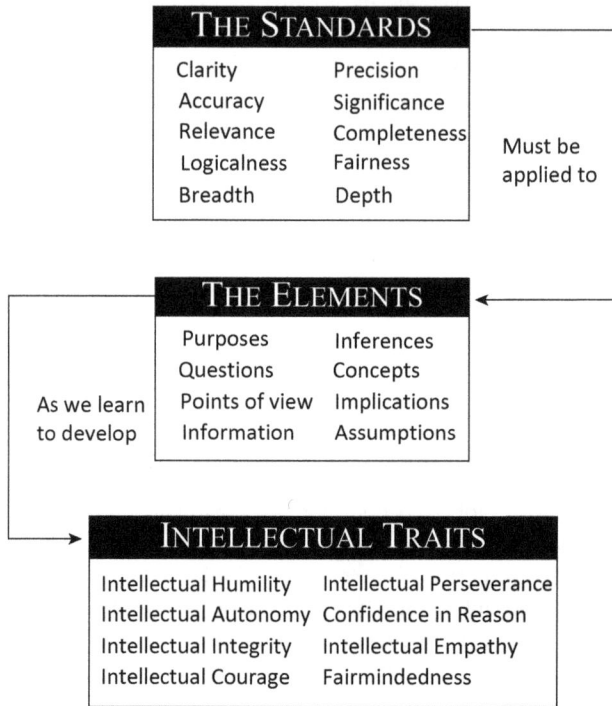

THE STANDARDS		
Clarity	Precision	
Accuracy	Significance	
Relevance	Completeness	Must be
Logicalness	Fairness	applied to
Breadth	Depth	

THE ELEMENTS		
	Purposes	Inferences
	Questions	Concepts
As we learn	Points of view	Implications
to develop	Information	Assumptions

INTELLECTUAL TRAITS	
Intellectual Humility	Intellectual Perseverance
Intellectual Autonomy	Confidence in Reason
Intellectual Integrity	Intellectual Empathy
Intellectual Courage	Fairmindedness

Figure 26.1 Paul and Elder model of critical thinking (Paul & Elder, 2014).

Teaching critical thinking using the Paul and Elder model

Applying the Paul and Elder model to teach critical thinking is all about asking the right questions. At the heart of teaching critical thinking is what is often called Socratic questioning. Socratic questioning is:

> based on the practice of disciplined, rigorously thoughtful dialogue with students. The [teacher] professes ignorance of the topic under discussion in order to elicit engaged dialogue with students. Socrates was convinced that *disciplined practice of thoughtful questioning* enables the scholar/student to examine ideas logically and to be able to determine the validity of those ideas.
>
> (*Science Education Resource Centre, 2018, emphasis supplied*)

Paul and Elder's critical thinking model is perfectly suited to the *disciplined practice of thoughtful questioning*. The elements of thought and the intellectual standards provide a rich resource for generating questions that promote a deep and meaningful dialogue with students.

Teachers who have internalised the elements of thought and the intellectual standards and routinely practise asking questions of themselves such as these will be able to conduct a dialogue with students that moves far beyond merely eliciting descriptive information from students. This dialogue with students begins the process of developing critical thinking. Ultimately, by modelling critical thinking and explicitly requiring students to think critically themselves, students will become increasingly able to think critically on their own and it will become a habit of mind.

There are many ways of using the elements of thought and intellectual standards to design or take advantage of learning moments for students. The example above illustrates the sorts of questions that can be asked of someone exploring a new skill, but the same approach can be applied to *anything*, such as reading, writing, case studies, simulations, role playing, research and problem solving, which, as discussed above, are not effective on their own. Later in this chapter, we will offer some additional ideas for embedding this approach into other learning activities.

There are many other applications of this model limited only by the imagination of the teacher or student. It can be used to guide thinking in ethics, law, clinical reasoning, research and many other areas of nursing practice.

Designing critical thinking experiences for students

We have identified several strategies that have been shown to work (see the subsection on things that do work, above). In addition, we have introduced a useful model that provides a framework for critically thinking through about nursing theory and practice. In this section, we will provide an example of how the strategies and model can be brought together to design an authentic learning experience that promotes the development of critical thinking.

When designing and implementing a learning experience, to be effective role models of critical thinking and devise authentic learning experiences, teachers need to remember the following:

- It takes *time* and *effort* to develop the intellectual traits and values described by Paul and Elder (2014).
- The acquisition of critical thinking skills is a *process*, not a mechanical application of a few tools, strategies or heuristics.
- Operating in real situations which are often indeterminate, contextual and replete with black swans (Taleb, 2010) and wicked problems ('Wicked problem,' n.d.) requires flexibility and the embracing of ambiguity.
- Thinking is fraught with preconceptions, prejudices and a tendency to egocentrism and cognitive bias, which are barriers to critical thinking.
- Examples used for learning must be authentic or closely analogous to real practice.

We urge you to be creative in how you design your classes and the learning experience you provide to students. Use a diversity of approaches and draw on the many already existing strategies and resources. Teaching critical thinking is an exciting, significant and essential activity to be engaged in. As we have stated in this chapter, it is not always easy to do or clear how best to do it. We do the best we can on the best available evidence and encourage readers to participate in the ongoing discussions and research in this field. If we, as teachers, continue to reflect on and improve our own critical thinking this will enable us to model and develop it in our students.

Thinking critically about resources and strategies

Because there are so many resources for teaching critical thinking, and they are so varied, it is useful to have a few guidelines to evaluate their suitability. Of course, when choosing strategies or resources for student learning, we recommend thinking critically about them using the framework we have suggested in this chapter. So, here are some questions to ask:

1. Does the strategy provide the opportunity for students to explicitly work through the model of critical thinking presented in this chapter (or whatever approach to critical thinking you adopt)?
2. What is the purpose of the strategy and does it align with the learning outcomes of the course or topic the student is studying?
3. Does the strategy lend itself to students overtly and explicitly teasing apart their thinking using the elements of thought and evaluating their thinking by applying the intellectual standards?
4. Does the strategy include clear instructions for using it?
5. Do the assumptions underlying the strategy align with your beliefs and values about learning?
6. Imagine you are the student. How might students experience the strategy from their perspective?
7. Does the strategy result in the outcomes you and/or the students need?

Whatever strategies for learning you decide to use, they must include students verbalising or writing out their thinking. Otherwise, it is impossible for you, as a teacher, to assess students' thinking skills or the depth and breadth of the knowledge and skills they are learning. Whatever learning strategy is engaged in, you, as a teacher, need to constantly draw attention to the activity of critical thinking and guide students through the process so they practise it repeatedly. As coaches we want students to practise critical thinking so often that it becomes a habitual part of their learning repertoire.

A final word

In this chapter, we have made suggestions about how to think about and teach critical thinking to your students and clinicians. If you adopt the suggestions we have made in this chapter, it is likely that your teaching practice will need to change. This may be just as challenging as what you will be guiding your students to do. But if we want to effectively teach critical thinking and develop nurse clinicians who can practise safely and reflectively, then we must rise to the challenges. It will require each of us to think critically about our teaching and learning approaches.

References

Abrami P C, Bernard R M, Borokhovski E, Waddington D I, Wade C A, & Persson T (2015) Strategies for teaching students to think critically: A meta-analysis. *Review of Educational Research 85*(2): 275–314.

Abrami P C, Bernard R M, Borokhovski W A, Surkes M A, Tamim R, & Zhang D (2008) Instructional interventions affecting critical thinking skills and dispositions: A stage 1 meta-analysis. *Review of Educational Research 78*(4): 1102–1134.

Bednarz H, Schim S, & Doorenbos A (2010) Cultural diversity in nursing education: Perils, pitfalls, and pearls. *Journal of Nursing Education 49*(5): 253–260.

Belkin D (2017) Exclusive test data: Many colleges fail to improve critical-thinking skills. *The Wall Street Journal*. Accessed at: www.wsj.com/articles/exclusive-test-data-many-colleges-fail-to-improve-critical-thinking-skills-1496686662

Bertacchini De Oliveira L, Johanna L, Díaz R, Da F, Carbogim C, Rogério A, & Alves De Araújo Püschel V (2016) Effectiveness of teaching strategies on the development of critical thinking in undergraduate nursing students: A meta-analysis. *Revista da Escola de Enfermagem da USP 50*(2): 350–359.

Biggs J (1997) Teaching across and within cultures: The issue of international students. In R Murray-Harvey & H C Silins (Eds.) *Learning and Teaching in Higher Education: Advancing International Perspectives* (pp. 1–22). Proceedings of the Higher Education Research and Development Society of Australasia Conference, Adelaide.

Davies M & Barnett R (2015) Introduction. In M Davies & R Barnett (Eds.) *The Palgrave Handbook of Critical Thinking in Higher Education* (pp. 1–23). New York: Palgrave Macmillan.

Egege S & Kutieleh S (2008) Dimming down difference. In L Dunn & M Wallace (Eds.) *Teaching in Transnational Higher Education: Enhancing Learning for Offshore International Students* (pp. 67–76). New York, NY: Routledge.

Facione P A (1990) Critical Thinking: A statement of expert consensus for purposes of educational assessment and instruction. Research findings and recommendations. *American Philosophical Association.* Available at 10.1016/j.tsc.2009.07.002

Flinders University School of Nursing & Midwifery (2012) *Flinders University Bachelor of Nursing curriculum 2013–2017*. Adelaide: Flinders University.

Lloyd G B (1996) *Adversaries and Authorities: Investigations into ancient Greek and Chinese Science.* Cambridge: Cambridge University Press.

Miller M A & Babcock D E (1996) *Critical Thinking Applied to Nursing.* St Louis, Missouri: Mosby.

Mulnix J W (2012) Thinking critically about critical thinking. *Educational Philosophy and Theory 44*(5): 464–479.

Nursing and Midwifery Board of Australia (2016) Registered nurse standards for practice. *Nursing and Midwifery Board of Australia.* (June), 1–8. Accessed at: www.nursingmidwiferyboard.gov.au/Codes-Guidelines-Statements/Professional-standards.aspx

Paul R & Elder L (2001) *Instructor's Manual for Critical Thinking: Tools for Taking Charge of our Learning and Your Life.* Upper Saddle River, NJ: Prentice Hall.

Paul R & Elder L (2010) Universal intellectual standards. Accessed at: www.criticalthinking.org/pages/universal-intellectual-standards/527

Paul R & Elder L (2014) *The Miniature Guide to Critical Thinking Concepts and Tools.* Accessed at: www. Foundation for Critical Thinking.org/files/Concepts_Tools.pdf

Pithers R T & Soden R (2000) Critical thinking in education: A review. *Educational Research 42*(3): 237–249.

Scheffer B K & Rubenfeld M G (2000) A consensus statement on critical thinking in nursing. *The Journal of Nursing Education 39*(8): 352–359.

Science Education Resource Centre (2018) What is socratic questioning. Accessed at: https://serc.carleton.edu/introgeo/socratic/second.html

Taleb N T (2010) *The Black Swan: The Impact of the Highly Improbable.* New York: Random House.

Wicked problem (n.d.) Accessed at: https://en.wikipedia.org/wiki/Wicked_problem

Willingham D (2007) *Critical Thinking: Why Is It So Hard to Teach?'* American Federation of Teachers, www.aft.org/sites/default/files/periodicals/Crit_Thinking.pdf

27

VOLUNTEERING AS TRANSFORMATIVE PEDAGOGY IN NURSE EDUCATION

Sue Dyson

Introduction

Where behaviourist paradigms dominate educational philosophy, the capacity for creative and innovative pedagogies for nursing is severely constrained (Ironside, 2004). Because of the need to supply nurses ready to enter the labour market, there tends to be a preoccupation with the development of technical skills, which can be easily modelled, observed and reinforced. This stands in contrast with a philosophy focused on the personal and professional development of nurses with a critical consciousness (Freire, 1970), wherein they are more prepared to question and re-invent aspects about healthcare that are in need of improvement. Behaviourism in nurse education is necessarily manifest in product-oriented curricula (Tyler, 1949), wherein success or failure is based on pre-defined measurable changes in student behaviour. Curriculum oriented more as process (Stenhouse, 1975) acknowledges principles of selecting content, developing teaching strategies and sequencing learning experiences. However, traditional process models also remain essentially behaviourist with emphasis remaining on assessing student strengths and weaknesses. Conventional behaviourist pedagogies in nurse education are perpetuated through formal regulation and control, as a means to ensure public safety and confidence in the profession. Nursing is thus defined and limited by the *regulation* of theory and practice, resulting in essentially conformist nurse education. Framing nursing curricula as a set of standards with verifiable outcome measures results in regulation acting as pseudo-pedagogy.

An alternative to conventional pedagogy is to focus on praxis in nursing, with emphasis placed on notions of a shared idea of the common good and importance of informed and committed action to the model of curriculum development. Recently, attention has been given to curriculum context, and the notion of curriculum as a social process in which personal interactions within the learning environment take on considerable significance (Howard, 2007). Conceptualising nurse education as praxis and context (Dyson, 2018) offers possibilities for further consideration of learning and teaching pedagogies, in other words more appropriate pedagogies for contemporary nursing practice. One such example is volunteering as a structured educational opportunity within the curriculum. By volunteering praxis is meant the practical application of volunteering theory, which facilitates learners' understanding of the mutual benefits of volunteering for communities and students. Conceptualising volunteering as transformative pedagogy has the potential to enable nursing students to synthesise thoughtful reflection, caring and action within a theory and research-focused curriculum. Nursing praxis (the practical application of nursing theory) is actualised through the process of student volunteering (Dyson, 2018).

This chapter is concerned with transformational critical pedagogy, which places students at the centre of learning. Nurse education is conceptualised in this chapter as a collective enterprise involving student, teacher and practitioner. Learning about nursing is considered a situated enterprise, with situation more broadly contextualised than is possible through a conventional pedagogical lens, one where nursing is necessarily contextualised as risky business. Volunteering as transformational critical pedagogy is argued as a vehicle for students to come to understand safe nursing practice (knowledge), and how to practise nursing safely (competence). The chapter begins with consideration of nursing as risky business – one which needs to be tightly controlled through regulation of the profession. I argue this has led to regulation acting as pseudo-pedagogy, which perpetuates conformist attitudes towards nurse education. In this context transformative pedagogies for nursing are stifled, in spite of the international community of nursing scholars repeatedly calling for innovative approaches to nursing pedagogy.

Nursing: a risky business

The Francis Report, published in February 2013, examined the causes of failings in care reported between 2005 and 2009 at Mid-Staffordshire NHS Foundation Trust. The public inquiry cost the UK taxpayer £13 million, sought evidence from more than 160 witnesses and resulted in 290 recommendations (Kapur, 2014). The report called for openness, transparency and candour throughout the healthcare system, improved support for compassionate caring and committed care and stronger healthcare leadership (Francis, 2013). The public have since come to understand nursing as risky business, and thus in need of tight regulation to oversee and control what nurses do. The notion of nursing as risky business underpins the Nursing and Midwifery Council's (NMC's) response to the Francis Inquiry, which was to revisit and subsequently publish new standards for pre-registration nursing education which emphasised the centrality of care and compassion in nursing (NMC, 2018).

The primacy of the concept of risk in nurse education has its origins in neo-liberal governance, where there has been a disintegration of traditional certainties, for example, professional authority (Bates & Lymbery, 2011). The decline in public trust in the nursing profession results in increased scrutiny and accountability of nurse education. Where responsibility for the production of compassionate practitioners lies with the nurse teacher the curriculum is framed within ever-tighter definitions of acceptable nursing actions in order to mitigate blame when nursing decisions lead to unwelcome consequences. The close relationship between risk and blame ensures that the search for supposedly responsible persons, in this case nurse teachers who are powerless to influence organisational factors, occurs immediately following any unwelcome event. High-profile cases and anecdotal accounts of poor care resurrect debates around the nature of nurse education. These include, but are not limited to, nursing as a vocation, whereby the moral and social meaning of nursing gives nursing vocational status

(White, 2002). A similar discourse around the modern nurse apprenticeship argues for the disparate concepts of professionalism and vocationalism to be brought together for the benefit of the nursing profession (O'Connor, 2007).

Much of what might be encountered in day-to-day nursing practice fits with Gardner's (2008) high-risk features of contemporary Western society. Unforeseen risks, lack of personal control over events or immediate threats looming larger than future threats are commonplace in nursing. However, there are also high-risk features, which occur less often but are nonetheless catastrophic; for example, the events of Mid Staffordshire NHS Foundation Trust (Francis, 2013) and Winterbourne View (CQC, 2011). In the UK, the practical element of nursing programmes occurs predominantly within NHS settings, which have become increasingly recognised as a risk, or blaming environment. In this context nurses feel they are likely to be blamed if their decisions lead to unwelcome consequences. Nurse teachers in turn feel they are likely to be blamed if the actions of nursing students lead to unwelcome consequences. Acknowledgement of the contextual factors affecting nursing work can be overlooked and their importance relegated in the aftermath of the blame game (Cleary et al., 2010). Issues of autonomy, involvement in decision making, workload issues and associated stress and burnout within the nursing profession render it difficult for nursing students to learn to practise in a safe environment. A risk-averse NHS triggers risk-averse nurse education, allowing conventional pedagogy to flourish. Conventional nursing pedagogy minimises risk, particularly around the practice component of pre-registration undergraduate programmes.

Regulation of nursing: a pseudo-pedagogy

Statutory and/or regulatory bodies exist to regulate nurse education in most countries of the Western world. In the USA, for example, the Commission on Collegiate Nursing Education (CCNE) serves this purpose by acting as the major autonomous accrediting agency for baccalaureate, graduate and residency programmes in nursing. CCNE has a remit to ensure quality and integrity of nursing programmes, and in doing so contributes to the improvement of the public's health (CCNE, 2009). In the UK, the NMC functions in a similar manner to quality assure approved programmes, and to register nurses on successful completion of approved courses. As regulator of the profession, the NMC exists to protect the public through setting education standards, shaping curriculum design and content, delineating nursing competences and approved education institutions (AEIs) to deliver pre-registration programmes. The NMC's regulatory function includes a remit to assess and quality assure practice placements for students (NMC, 2016), because 50% of pre-registration nursing courses occur in practice settings, mostly within the NHS.

Nursing programmes in the UK operate within the directives laid out in the Standards for Pre-registration Nursing Education (NMC, 2018). Failure to comply with NMC standards can ultimately lead to withdrawal of AEI status. Compliance with regulatory frameworks supports conventional pedagogy in nursing, resulting in teacher-centred curriculum design. A new ideology is necessary for a paradigm shift in nursing – moreover one with a stronger focus on student-centred nursing. Nurse education should provide active learning, critical thinking and analysis and problem-solving skills (Stanley & Dougherty, 2010), while at the same time accommodating regulatory requirements deemed necessary to protect the public, and mitigate the perception of nursing as risky business.

Pedagogy in nursing: a conventional approach

Conventional pedagogy is concerned with transmission of skills, facts and knowledge deemed a prerequisite for nursing. Pedagogy conceptualised through a conventional lens foregrounds teaching, learning and knowing about nursing as instruction. The nurse teacher acts as the instrument through which nursing knowledge is conveyed, and behaviours consistent with nursing are enforced. Conventional pedagogy in nursing facilitates regulation of nursing through the curriculum, with commodification of nurse education (Bethune & Wellard, 1997) legitimised in the production of the registered nurse. Technical rational curriculum models (Smith, 2000) facilitate this discourse, whereby the raison d'être of nurse education is to *produce* nurses who are described (in pejorative terms) as fit for purpose, fit for award and fit for practice (Benton, 2011). Curriculum conceptualised as *product* is less concerned with how to articulate a vision for nursing and nurse education than with what its objectives and content might be. On the other hand curriculum, conceptualised as *process*, takes account of the context in which learning and teaching about nursing take place. Curriculum as process allows the teacher to enter the educational setting (classroom or practice) with a considered idea of the purpose of the encounter (Dyson, 2018).

Conventional pedagogy in nursing is manifest in behaviour-driven, outcomes-focused curriculum design, which has its roots in historical notions of apprenticeship (Bradshaw, 2001), which by nature implies learning a trade from a skilled practitioner. Apprenticeship-style nurse training as an educational philosophy situates the relative status of competency over and above acquisition of theoretical knowledge. Notions of training and time served are perpetuated, with competency to practise tested through observation, complemented with practical and written examinations (Cowan et al., 2005). Competency, determined by achievement of a given set of standards, and in the UK by admission to the register (NMC, 2018), explains the commodification of nurse education. Nurses need to prove continuing fitness to practise through revalidation of competency (NMC, 2019a), paying a fee to remain on the register (NMC, 2019b).

Conventional pedagogy proliferates in nurse education because, without standards and verifiable outcome measures, the regulatory body would have difficulty in meeting its public obligation to ensure nurses provide the highest standards of care to patients and clients (NMC, 2010). Regulation serves to assure the public of the knowledge, skills and good character of all nurses admitted to the register (NMC, 2015). Pedagogy in nursing is thus characterised by the need to transmit the skills, facts and standards of moral and social conduct considered necessary for nursing. Nurse teachers, framed within conventional pedagogy, are the instrument by which nursing knowledge is conveyed and behaviours consistent with nursing are enforced. In this sense, conventional nurse education is imposed from above and outside (Dewey, 1938).

In spite of extensive calls for a new pedagogy for nursing, conventional pedagogy proliferates as nurse education continues to be tightly regulated in order to mitigate risk in nursing practice. The framework in which nurse education currently operates acts as pseudo-pedagogy, thus limiting capacity for critical pedagogies to transform nurse education.

Critical pedagogy: an opportunity for nursing

Critical pedagogy is a transformation-based approach to education, which rejects abstracted forms of commodified learning packaged as didactic instructional teaching (Cowden & Singh, 2013). Critical pedagogy draws on critical theory, which relates to an ideal standard or mode of being, grounded in justice and freedom. Critical theory raises consciousness, empowering the critical educator to challenge the taken-for-granted, while allowing structural constraints to be acknowledged (Dyson, 2018). Critical theory supports the critical educator to question the hidden assumptions and purposes of existing forms of practice.

Critical theorists, depending on disciplinary context, define critical pedagogy in different ways. Exponents of critical theory draw, for the most part, on the work of the Brazilian radical educationalist Paulo Freire. While the context in which Freire developed his ideas was radically different to the context in which nurse educators design and deliver nursing programmes – a context which differs across and within countries – nevertheless his ideas are relevant to the situation for contemporary nursing. The first of these is Freire's notion of critical consciousness, which describes individual capacity to read the world, and is deemed essential for democratic society (Freire, 1974). Critical consciousness is of immediate relevance to nurse education, where the primary purpose is to prepare nurses to work in the diverse, multicultural, complex settings which characterise nursing work. Second, Freire argued for education as a dialogic exchange between teachers and students (Freire, 1970). This is important in nursing, where student and teacher learn, question, reflect and participate in the creation of nursing knowledge.

Landers (2008) argues nurse teachers need clinical competency to support student learning, while acknowledging the teacher may only be partly familiar with many aspects of nursing. Maintaining clinical competency presents challenges for nurse teachers, who are often expert clinicians, while entering academia as novice educators. Knowledge deficit, culture and support, salary and workload all impact the ability of nurse teachers, particularly neophyte lecturers, to maintain links with clinical practice, irrespective of the desire to do so. Freire argued teachers have the central role of creating environments in which students are likely to engage in authentic learning. In other words, teachers need to identify with their students in order to bring about a mutual understanding of the goals of the education process. At the heart of Freire's pedagogy was an anti-authoritarian, dialogical and interactive approach, aimed at examining issues of relational power for students and workers (McLaren, 2009).

Critical pedagogy in nursing is important for three key reasons. First, it conceptualises pedagogy as a process of engagement between nurse teacher and nursing student. Second, engagement between nurse teacher and nursing student is based on an underlying humanistic view of the human worth and value of student and teacher (Cowden & Singh, 2013). Knowing about nursing, which comes from engagement between nurse teacher and nursing student, is understood as an exchange between people with a common purpose, rather than a financial exchange (student paying to be educated, teacher paid to educate). Third, undergraduate nursing programmes located within higher education are dependent on critical pedagogy in order to be challenging, to develop inquiring, independent minds and instil confidence in students' abilities to argue from alternative viewpoints (Hargreaves, 2008). Nurse education is a political activity which is value-laden and has multiple social meanings (Harden, 1994). As long as teachers continue to engage in conventional pedagogy to design and deliver nursing curricula students will fail to develop a critical consciousness about nursing and the context in which it occurs. A new critical pedagogy for nursing is called for (Ironside, 2004, 2006; McAllister, 2010; Dyson, 2018).

Volunteering: pedagogy and praxis

Volunteering has been defined in a number of ways around the world, including, for example, work that is carried out for the benefit of others, for society as a whole or for a specific organisation, work that is unpaid, or more specifically, work that results in the production of a public good (Dekker & Halman, 2003). In terms of support for volunteering many governments have considered policy initiatives as a means to encourage civic behaviour among young people, with student volunteering thought to be one way of doing this (Cnaan et al., 2010).

Student volunteering in the UK encompasses volunteering in local communities through programmes organised either by the student union or by institution (Student Volunteering England, 2004). In terms of international student volunteering a limited number of studies report on the extent or variability of international students volunteering in higher education, although there are international studies which report on volunteering in the population as a whole, or in the younger population (Fényes & Pusztai, 2012). Few international studies specifically examine student volunteering at subject or discipline level, for example, within nursing programmes, thus making cross-cultural comparisons within this subject area difficult. In addition, different activities and situations when aggregated into a concept of volunteering render a precise global definition problematic. Nevertheless attempts at defining volunteering around the world have recognised a number of common themes, including: it is non-obligatory; it is carried out for the benefit of others, society as a whole or a specific organisation; it is unpaid; or (less commonly) it takes place in an organised context (Dekker & Halman, 2003). The criterion of being unpaid for volunteering activities is not straightforward. Meijs et al. (2003, p. 3) accept the "availability of tangible rewards" within the remit of volunteering, while at the same time recognising the constituents of rewards for volunteering range from reimbursement of expenses to material tributes of appreciation. Quantification of acceptable remuneration for volunteering is hence difficult to determine.

In the UK, the National Union of Students (NUS) and the Association of Colleges carried out research aimed at establishing the extent of volunteering in further education in England, in order to inform strategies for expanding the number of students volunteering and volunteering opportunities. The report suggested that: (1) volunteering plays a significant role in students' lives; (2) students recognise that helping people and the community is a key aspect of volunteering, alongside gaining skills and future employability; and (3) there is a growing trend for linking volunteering to students' courses or academic qualifications (NUS, 2015). In English higher education, while there has been a long tradition of student volunteering, the situation is reported to be at a critical point, in that, without evidence of impact, continued funding and an integrated approach to its development, student volunteering will not meets its full potential (Darwen & Rannard, 1996). While there has been cross-party support to promote schemes to strengthen the role of volunteering and to promote synergies between higher education and the voluntary sector (Holdsworth & Quinn, 2010), it remains challenging to provide robust evidence on which nurse educators can incorporate volunteering opportunities into to an already pressurised undergraduate nursing curriculum (Dyson, 2018).

Many studies on the benefits of volunteering are limited in relation to the extent to which causal relationships between health, well-being and volunteering can be established. Measuring the benefits of volunteering is therefore complex, with generalisations from research on volunteering needing to be treated with caution (Mundle et al., 2012). Nevertheless, student volunteering is a form of experiential education in which learners have an opportunity to engage in activities that address human and community needs. Student volunteering has the capacity to integrate community service with academic learning, rendering it unique in relation to practice learning in undergraduate nursing programmes. When put together as a structured activity, volunteering can promote learning and development (Sheu et al., 2011).

Volunteering as pedagogy

In volunteering situations, nursing students are equal partners in the learner/teacher encounter, with learning and teaching crossing professional, disciplinary and social divides. The volunteering opportunity is independent of the requirement for achievement of nursing competencies, or for acquisition of specific nursing knowledge. Instead, knowledge about nursing is co-created during the process of volunteering without restraint of the formal curriculum. Volunteering increases students' self-confidence, and provides opportunities for greater reflection on practice through experience and action. Furthermore, the potential for development of critical perspectives and improvements in terms of meeting particular competencies is facilitated through volunteering opportunities. While student volunteering may not automatically result in learning, nor link directly to the development of caring and compassionate practice, nonetheless volunteering does provide a way for students to make sense of their experiences through opportunities intentionally designed to foster critical thinking (Dyson et al., 2017).

Exposure to volunteering empowers students to think critically and reflect on health, on education and on social problems. However, the extent to which students are able to think critically and reflect on the volunteering experience depends on the strategies used to promote critical thinking in the curriculum (Chan, 2013). Where volunteering remains an unstructured activity, or outside the curriculum, it remains difficult to evidence students' ability to adopt a critical stance towards healthcare practice. Structured volunteering, on the other hand, when followed by facilitated critical thinking and reflection on the experience, helps students to develop a more holistic view of society. Volunteering in this sense is unique in that students have the opportunity to co-create critical pedagogy, gain life experiences and have a sense of control over their learning, which is not always possible through traditional teaching (Bell et al., 2014).

Volunteering as praxis

Students benefit from volunteering while studying nursing in a number of ways. First, students are exposed to a wider variety of social groups and situations than would otherwise be the case through exposure to more conventional practice settings. Second, volunteering provides students with opportunities to break down hierarchies encountered in conventional learner/teacher relationships. Volunteering has potential to harness students' existing experience with their newly acquired knowledge and skills, framed within and scaffolded by the curriculum. Volunteering opportunities when structured within the curriculum facilitate room for creative transformative pedagogies, for example, music and percussive activities (Leonard et al., 2013), and dialogic and narrative pedagogy (Ironside & Hayden-Miles, 2012), which occur when learners and teachers come together to collectively pool insights during both the process of, and following, the volunteering experience. Integration of the theory and practice of volunteering (volunteering as praxis) facilitates students' ability to critically reflect on wider social issues and is one way in which progress towards greater compassion in nursing practice may be achieved, although research is needed to fully understand this process (Dyson, 2018).

Volunteering in the nursing curriculum

Student volunteering is not without its challenges. Nursing students, much like other students on full-time courses, often work to supplement income, and have additional caring and/or family responsibilities. For these students volunteering may be problematic.

Motivation to volunteer is linked to previous volunteering experience, ready access to information, the availability of formal volunteering programmes and support for volunteering (Jones & Hill, 2003). In the absence of access to information and support, it is unlikely students – in particular those on undergraduate nursing programmes – will engage with volunteering, and as such will miss an opportunity to appreciate how volunteering impacts learning about nursing. Structured volunteering attempts to mitigate these difficulties by supporting volunteering within the framework of the curriculum.

Access to volunteering opportunities is a further challenge when planning a nursing curriculum (McBride & Lough, 2010). While there are alternative ways through which nursing students might access volunteering, for example through student unions, university websites and through attendance at university open days, nevertheless unmotivated students are unlikely to take up volunteering, particularly when studies are seen as a priority (Dyson et al., 2017).

In addition to practical challenges for nursing students there are pedagogical challenges for nurse teachers concerning how volunteering should be positioned in the nursing curriculum, for example as a stand-alone discrete module (Bell et al., 2014) or as a continuous opportunity throughout the curriculum (Hafford-Letchfield et al., 2018). Decisions around positioning of volunteering within the curriculum lead naturally to considerations of assessment of the volunteering experience. A behaviourist teacher/content-oriented pedagogy, where the curriculum centres on a set of objectives and a range of subject matter, necessarily requires some form of assessment to verify the achievement of specified objectives. In contrast, cognitive pedagogy manifest in student/learning-oriented approaches assumes knowledge is not fixed, but is instead socially constructed and personal (Mackintosh-Franklin, 2016). Volunteering as transformative pedagogy is antithetical to assessment.

In spite of the challenges for nurse educationalists in thinking how to conceptualise volunteering in the nursing curriculum, volunteering as pedagogy is transformative, and has potential to liberate nursing students from the constraints of the formalized curriculum. Structured volunteering provides the space for students to engage with volunteering by respecting individual circumstances and life experiences, which impact student life. This is, in and of itself, a *Freirean* pedagogy reimagined within nurse education. Conscientisation in nurse education recognises nursing students not just as recipients of nurse education, but also as knowing subjects, capable of achieving a deepening awareness of both the sociocultural reality that shapes their lives and of their capacity to transform that reality (Freire, 1974).

Conclusion

All professional undergraduate nursing programmes within the UK are located within higher education, while at the same time subject to, and regulated by, statutory directives. Without verifiable outcome measures such as those set out in the Standards for Pre-registration Nursing Education (NMC, 2018), regulatory bodies perceive it difficult to address public concerns of nursing as risky business. However, in the UK at least, nursing's regulatory body does not provide specific professional guidance on the role of pedagogy or on pedagogical approaches best suited to provision of high-quality professional nurse education. This creates a challenge for nurse educators charged with designing intellectually stimulating programmes fitting for students of higher education, within the confines of conventional pedagogy, where learning is conceptualised as measurable. It is not surprising that behaviourist pedagogical approaches persist in spite of repeated calls for an alternative conceptualisation of nursing pedagogy. Where the goal of nurse education is to instruct students towards achievement of designated competencies, pedagogy becomes anti-Freirean, which is both counterintuitive and counterproductive to students' development towards emancipatory and liberatory nursing practice.

Critical pedagogy centres on hope, liberation and equality, with agency and raised consciousness taking centre stage (Luke & Gore, 1992). Volunteering is argued as one way for critical pedagogy to be made manifest in the nursing curriculum. There are other ways, for example, through critical reading, critical writing and critical reflection. Volunteering as a structured activity can incorporate all of these approaches. When followed by facilitated reflection, volunteering as a structured opportunity within the nursing curriculum has potential to counter hegemony in nurse education, perpetuated by the pseudo-pedagogy of regulation.

This chapter reiterates time is pressing. Global challenges facing nursing are rapidly impacting the nature of nursing work, and in what context nursing work occurs. Environmental change, mass migration of people, demographic change, inequalities in health, poverty, homelessness and the mental health crisis require nurse teachers to act as critical scholars, able to take critical positions and to relate their work with major social issues for the purpose of creating hope for students to transform society for the better (Giroux & Giroux, 2006). Nursing as a profession needs to resist fatalism regarding the global situation and to strive for an expanded vision for global health and global nursing through transformative nursing pedagogy.

References

Bates P & Lymbery M (2011) Managing risk in a risk averse society. In R Taylor, M Hill & F McNeil (Eds.) *Early Professional Development for Social Workers*. Birmingham: Venture Press.

Bell K, Tanner J, Rutty J, Astley-Pepper M & Hall R (2014) Successful partnerships with third sector organisations to enhance the student experience: A partnership evaluation. *Nurse Education Today* 33(3): 530–534.

Benton D (2011) Nurses fit for purpose, award and practice? *International Nursing Review* 58(3): 276.

Bethune E & Wellard S (1997) The commodification of speciality nurse education. *Contemporary Nurse* 6 (3-4): 104–109.

Bradshaw A (2001) *The Nurse Apprentice, 1860-1977*. London: Haggerston Press.

Care Quality Commission (2011) *CQC report on Winterbourne View confirms its owners failed to protect people from abuse*. Available at: www.cqc.org.uk/news/releases/cqc-report-winterbourne-view-confirms-its-owners-failed-protect-people-abuse.

Chan Z C Y (2013) A systematic review of critical thinking in nurse education. *Nurse Education Today* 33: 236–240.

Cleary M, Hunt G E & Horsfall J (2010) Identifying and addressing bullying in nursing. *Issues in Mental Health Nursing* 31(5): 331–335.

Cnaan R, Smith K A, Holmes K, Haski-Leventhal D & Handy F (2010) Motivations and benefits of student volunteering: Comparing regular, occasional, and non-volunteers in five countries. *Canadian Journal of Nonprofit and Social Economy Research* 1(1): 65–81.

Commission on Collegiate Nursing Education (2009) *Achieving Excellence in Accreditation. The First 10 years of CCNE*. Washington, DC: Commission on Collegiate Nursing Education. Available at: www.aacnnursing.org/Portals/42/CCNE/PDF/CCNE-History.pdf

Cowan D T, Norman I & Coopamah V P (2005) Competence in nursing practice: A controversial concept – a focused review of literature. *Nurse Education Today* 25: 335–362.

Cowden S & Singh G (2013) *Acts of Knowing. Critical Pedagogy in, against and Beyond the University*. London: Bloomsbury Academic.

Darwen J & Rannard A C (1996) Student volunteering in England: A critical moment. *Nurse Education Today* 16: 32–37.

Dekker P & Halman L (Eds.) (2003) *The Values of Volunteering. Cross Cultural Perspectives.* New York: Springer.

Dewey J (1938) The pattern of inquiry (from *Logic The Theory Of Inquiry* published by Henry Holt and Co.), reproduced in: L A Hickman & T M Alexander (Eds.), *The Essential Dewey (Vol 2): Ethics, Logic and Psychology* (1998) (pp. 169–179). Bloomington and Indianapolis, IN: Indiana University Press.

Dyson S E (2018) *Critical Pedagogy in Nursing: Transformational Approaches to Nurse Education in a Globalized World.* London: Palgrave Macmillan.

Dyson S E, Liu L Q, van Den Akker O & O'Driscoll M (2017) The extent, variability and attitudes towards volunteering among undergraduate nursing students: Implications for pedagogy in nurse education. *Nurse Education in Practice* 23: 15–22.

Fényes H & Pusztai G (2012) Volunteering among higher education students, focusing on the micro-level factors. *Journal of Social Work and Policy* Available at: https://dea.lib.unideb.hu/dea/bit stream/handle/2437/166283/file_up_Volunteering_FHPG_final3%20_1__corectatFH.pdf? sequence=1

Francis R (2013) *Report of the Mid Staffordshire NHS Foundation Trust Public Inquiry.* London: The Stationery Office.

Freire P (1970) *Pedagogy of the Oppressed.* New York: Seabury.

Freire P (1974) *Education for Critical Consciousness.* New York: Continuum.

Gardner D (2008) *Risk the Science and Politics of Fear.* London: Virgin Books.

Giroux H A & Giroux S S (2006) Challenging neoliberalism's new world order: The promise of critical pedagogy. *Cultural Studies, Critical Methodologies* 6(1): 21–32.

Hafford-Letchfield T, Dayananda A & Collins D (2018) Digital storytelling for interprofessional collaborative practice to develop quality and service improvements. *Social Work Education* 37(6): 804–812.

Harden J (1994) Enlightenment, empowerment and emancipation: The case for critical pedagogy in nurse education. *Nurse Education Today* 16: 32–37.

Hargreaves J (2008) Risk: The ethics of a creative curriculum. *Innovations in Education and Teaching International* 45(3): 227–234.

Holdsworth C & Quinn J (2010) Student volunteering in English higher education. *Studies in Higher Education* 35(1): 113–127.

Howard J (2007) Curriculum development. *Center for the Advancement of Teaching and Learning Elon University.* Available at: www.pdx.edu/sites/www.pdx.edu.cae/files/media_assets/Howard.pdf.

Ironside P M (2004) "Covering content" and teaching thinking: Deconstructing the additive curriculum. *Journal of Nursing Education* 43(1): 5–12.

Ironside P M (2006) Using narrative pedagogy: Learning and practising interpretive thinking. *Journal of Advanced Nursing* 55(4): 478–486.

Ironside P M & Hayden-Miles M (2012) Narrative pedagogy: Co-creating engaging learning experiences with students. In G Sherwood & S Horton-Deutsch (Eds.), *Reflective Practice: Transforming Education and Improving Outcomes* (pp. 135–148). Indianapolis: Sigma Theta Tau International.

Jones S & Hill K (2003) Understanding patterns of commitment: Motivation for community service involvement. *Journal of Higher Education* 74(5): 516–539.

Kapur N (2014) Mid Staffordshire Hospital report: What does psychology have to offer. *The Psychologist* 27: 16–20.

Landers M G (2008) The theory-practice gap in nursing: The role of the nurse teacher. *Journal of Advanced Nursing* 32(6): 1550–1556.

Leonard K, Hafford-Letchfield T & Couchman W (2013) We're all Going Bali': Utilising Gamelan as an educational resource for leadership and teamwork in post-qualifying education in health and social care. *The British Journal of Social Work* 43(1): 173–190.

Luke C & Gore J (Eds.) (1992) *Feminisms and Critical Pedagogy.* NewYork: Routledge.

Mackintosh-Franklin C (2016) Pedagogical principles underpinning undergraduate nurse education in the UK: A review. *Nurse Education Today* 40: 118–122.

McAllister M (2010) Awake and aware: Thinking constructively about the world through transformative learning. In T Warne & S McAndrew (Eds.), *Creative Approaches to Health and Social Care Education: Knowing Me, Understanding You.* Basingstoke: Palgrave Macmillan.

McBride A M & Lough B J (2010) Access to international volunteering. *Nonprofit management & leadership* 21(2): 195–208.

McLaren P (2009) Critical pedagogy: A look at the major concepts. In A Darder, M P Baltodarno & R D Torres (Eds.), *The Critical Pedagogy Reader* (2nd ed., pp. 61–83). New York: Routledge.

Meijs L C P M, Handy F, Cnaan R A, Brudney J L, Ascoli U, Ranade S, Hustinx L, Weber S & Weiss I (2003) All in eyes of the beholder? Perceptions of volunteering across eight countries. In P Dekker & L Halman (Eds.), *The Values of Volunteering. Cross Cultural Perspectives* (pp. 19–34). New York: Springer.

Mundle C, Naylor C & Buck D (2012) *Volunteering in Health and Care in England. A Summary of Key Literature*. London: The Kings Fund.

NMC (2010) *Standards for Pre-Registration Nursing Education*. London: NMC.

NMC (2015) *The Code: Professional Standards of Practice and Behaviour for Nurses and Midwives*. London: NMC. Available at www.nmc-uk.org.

NMC (2016) *Our Role in Education*. Available at https://www.nmc.org.uk/education/our-role-in-education/.

NMC (2018) *Future nurse: Standards of proficiency for registered nurses*. Available at: www.nmc.org.uk/globa lassets/sitedocuments/education-standards/future-nurse-proficiencies.pdf.

NMC (2019a) *Revalidation*. Available at: www.nmc.org.uk/globalassets/sitedocuments/revalidation/ how-to-revalidate-booklet.

NMC (2019b) Register as a nurse or midwife. Available at www.nmc.org.uk/registration/joining-the-register/register-nurse-midwife/.

NUS (2015) *Volunteering amongst further education and sixth form students* (NUS, 2015). Available at www.aoc. co.uk/sites/default/files/Volunteering%20amongst%20FE%20and%20Sixth%20Form%20students.pdf

O'Connor S J (2007) Developing professional habitus: A Bernsteinian analysis of the modern nurse apprenticeship. *Nurse Education Today* 27(7): 748–754.

Sheu L C, Zheng P, Coelho A D, Lin L D, O'Sullivan P S, O'Brien, B C, Yu A Y & Lai C J (2011) Learning through service: Student perceptions on volunteering at interprofessional Hepatitis B student-run clinics. *Journal of Cancer Education* 26: 228.

Smith M K (2000) 'Curriculum theory and practice' *the encyclopaedia of informal education*. Available at: http://infed.org/mobi/curriculum-theory-and=practice/.

Stanley M J C & Dougherty J P (2010) A paradigm shift in nursing education: A new model. *Nursing Education Perspectives* 31(6): 378–380.

Stenhouse L (1975) *An Introduction to Curriculum Research and Development*. London: Heineman.

Student Volunteering England (2004) *Student Volunteering: The National Survey*. London: Student Volunteering England.

Tyler R W (1949) *Basic Principles of Curriculum and Instruction*. Chicago: University of Chicago Press.

White K (2002) Nursing as vocation. *Nursing Ethics* 9(3): 279–290.

INDEX

For Product Safety Concerns and Information please contact our EU
representative GPSR@taylorandfrancis.com
Taylor & Francis Verlag GmbH, Kaufingerstraße 24, 80331 München, Germany